Fletcher's Introduction to Clinical Ethics

Edited by

John C. Fletcher, PhD
Edward M. Spencer, MD
Paul A. Lombardo, PhD, JD

With a Foreword by

James F. Childress, PhD

Third Edition

Hagerstown Maryland

University Publishing Group, Inc.
Hagerstown, Maryland 21740
1-800-654-8188
www.UPGBooks.com

Appendix 1 is reprinted with the permission of the JCAHO. © Joint Commission Resources: *2005 Comprehensive Accreditation Manual for Hospitals, RI
Chapter, Patient Rights and Organizational Ethics Standards.* Oakbrook Terrace, Ill.: Joint Commission on Accreditation of Healthcare Organizations,
2005, RI-1 - RI-18.

Printed in the United States of America
ISBN 1-55572-027-7

Contents

Foreword

The field of bioethics continues its creative ferment. Especially noteworthy are developments in clinical ethics, that is, ethics at the bedside. To keep pace in this rapidly changing arena, the new edition of this introductory text in clinical ethics carries forward an approach tested over time with clinicians, students in the health professions, and members of ethics committees.

The authors understand clinical ethics as a "bridge" between theoretical bioethics and the bedside. Ideas move both ways on the bridge — not merely from theorists to practitioners, but also from practitioners to theorists. In the process, both activities are enriched. While making a contribution to bioethics in general, this volume is primarily intended to provide a thoughtful, imaginative, and helpful introduction to ethics at the bedside.

Without attempting to resolve the debate about the respective roles of case-based and principle- or rule-based approaches, this text attends to both cases and general moral considerations. Examples of the latter include the enduring ethical obligations to respect privacy and confidentiality, to communicate truthfully, and to support and respect the informed consents and refusals of patients who have the capacity to make their own decisions. In addition, there is a recognition of the central place of such virtues as care, humility, courage, and practical wisdom in clinical ethics.

The six chapters in the first part of the book provide an overview of clinical ethics, relating it to professional and organizational ethics, to research and psychiatric ethics, and to the legal context in the U.S. The several ethical obligations noted above are developed in the second part of the book, while the third part focuses on ethical problems that arise in particular cases, including reproductive and life-and-death decisions. The new edition is admirably current with, and informed by, the extensive literature in clinical, ethical, and legal topics relevant to these problems.

In many ways this text serves as an important model for creative work in bioethics. First, it is interdisciplinary and interprofessional, not merely multidisciplinary and multiprofessional. Members of different disciplines and professions talked, taught, and wrote with each other to develop clear and compelling ideas about clinical ethics. This text provides the fruits of their conversations.

Second, as their conversation extended over time, so their book has now evolved to a new edition. This text displays major changes and improvements that have occurred over the more than 15 years of its development and revision.

Third, this product is the result of careful testing and assessment. Its approach and its substantive ideas were tested in the classroom as well as in practice. Some prior approaches failed, while others succeeded; some ideas flourished, while others floundered.

In short, this book reflects an ideal approach to both teaching and scholarship in bioethics. It involved a community — a small community of teachers and practitioners interested in ethics in healthcare; the members of this community worked together over time on these editions; and finally, their ideas grew out of and were tested in both the classroom and the clinical setting.

I congratulate my colleagues at the University of Virginia and elsewhere on this version, knowing they will continue to develop and test their approaches and ideas for years to come. Unfortunately, John Fletcher, the driving force behind the successive editions of this text, died over a year ago, and this edition, now entitled *Fletcher's Introduction to Clinical Ethics,* serves as a memorial to our cherished colleague and friend.

James F. Childress, PhD
The John Allen Hollingsworth Professor of Ethics
Director, Institute for Practical Ethics
and Public Life
University of Virginia
August 2005

Editor's Preface

In the spirit of the two prior editions, this third edition of *Introduction to Clinical Ethics* continues a discussion of the process and content of clinical ethics and ethics consultation — but it arrives with a mixture of sadness and hope. As colleagues and as friends, we are saddened by John Fletcher's untimely death last year. John was the book's primary editor and its unifying force. Since its first "official publication" in 1995, *Introduction to Clinical Ethics* was a project — and a discussion — that John was especially passionate about. I say "official publication," because in preceding years John used many of the chapters and cases from various contributors in a loose-leaf format; they were revised on the basis of practice in teaching clinicians and others in the health professions at the University of Virginia.

At the time of John's death, plans for the third edition were underway, but there was much that was left to be done. That the work was done, and how it was done, is testimony to John's legacy and to what "doing ethics" in a healthcare organization is all about.

Each chapter in the third edition has been either significantly revised, completely rewritten, or, in keeping pace with emerging issues, is entirely new. None of this would have been possible without a personal commitment from each contributor, and a collaborative effort. Special appreciation is due to Ed Spencer and Paul Lombardo, who both stepped forward and agreed to take on the tasks of general editors — and more. Jim Childress once again offered, graciously, to write the foreword. Leslie LeBlanc, who worked with John on the earlier two editions, assisted Ed and Paul in completing the third. We thank the Joint Commission on Accreditation of Healthcare Organizations for allowing us to include its applicable standards in appendix 1.

To each contributor we express our sincere appreciation and thanks for their willingness to be a part of, and hopefully further, the discussion.

As you may have noticed, the title of the third edition has, appropriately, been changed to *Fletcher's Introduction to Clinical Ethics*. Our thanks to the Fletcher family for agreeing to this change.

I don't know what John would have made of this, but I do hope that the discussion that is continued here — and provoked among readers — is in keeping with his spirit and his practice. And with this, I'll give John the last word — here. John wrote about three important goals of ethics consultation: this is his third goal.

> Involvement in ethics consultation necessitates reflection on one's motivation, one's personality and character, and one's strengths and weaknesses, as well as on how one knows the others involved in the case, and how motivation and intent come into play in different persons. Self-knowledge and knowledge of

others is one of the two main purposes of ethics, and the provision of guidance is the second. Neither of these goals is abstract. Respect for others presumes a capacity for and an interest in knowing them more deeply. To promote this kind of knowledge in the institution, as well as the special sources of guidance of biomedical ethics, is a goal with a practical outcome. A climate can be created in which persons become more open and capable of responding to significant ethical crises by virtue of their interest and experience in dealing with the smaller, more routine daily problems that may also be laden with ethical significance. Practice on the small problems leads to a deeper resource for responses to the large ones.*

Let the conversation continue.

Norman Quist
Publisher, University Publishing Group
August 2005

---

* J.C. Fletcher, N. Quist, and A.R. Jonsen, ed., *Ethics Consultation in Health Care* (Ann Arbor, Michigan: Health Administration Press, 1989), 183.

Part 1
Understanding the Field

1

Clinical Ethics:
History, Content, and Resources

John C. Fletcher and Edward M. Spencer

I. WHAT IS CLINICAL ETHICS?

Clinical ethics is a practical discipline that deals with real-world problems and practices in the healthcare arena. It focuses on controversies and issues surrounding the care of patients in different settings: acute care (in hospitals and clinicians' offices), long-term care, rehabilitation, home care, and hospice care.

The term "clinical" derives from the Greek word *klinikos* or "bedside," so its meaning is obvious. Not so obvious is the meaning of the word "ethics," but how this word is understood makes a real difference to the climate in which attention to moral problem solving can be effective. For some clinicians, the word ethics refers only to issues of *character*. Believing that they are already "ethical," that is, that their character traits are well formed, they misunderstand, and so often resist the work of an ethics committee. They fear that such a group will be one more source of interference with the way they practice medicine. Other clinicians link the term ethics only to specific issues in the professional relationship between themselves, patients, and other clinicians: issues such as sexual behavior, unfair fees, or self-serving referrals. The word ethics has also developed several meanings for nonclinical situations. We hear of "ethical problems" and "ethical lapses" when elected or appointed officials give special

favors or when CEOs (chief executive officers) of large corporations are caught purposefully mismanaging the resources of the corporation for personal gain.

We prefer a simple definition of ethics, which can be useful in the analysis of real-life issues. Ethics may be defined as the analysis, study, or consideration of morality; here morality refers to what is considered "good" or "right." Notice that, under this definition, the question for *morality* is, "What ought I (or we) to do in this situation? What is the right course?" while *ethics* is concerned with the question, "Why should I (or we) act in a specific manner? What justifies my action?" Morality tells what the right or good action is, while ethics considers why this action is right or good and/or why another action may be indicated. We will say more about this distinction later in this chapter.

Note that there are other ethical perspectives besides clinical ethics of importance in healthcare today. These include: professional ethics, which is concerned with the fundamental values of a profession; research ethics, which is concerned with the protection of research subjects; business ethics, which is concerned with the operation and management of healthcare-organizations (HCOs); and organizational ethics, which attempts to integrate all of the ethical perspectives in healthcare under an umbrella of "ethical climate." All are of importance in the complicated world of healthcare today. Further attention to each of these perspectives will be found in chapters 2, 3, 4, and 5. Throughout this text, we argue for an integrated approach to the ethics of healthcare; so, although we focus mainly on clinical ethics, we believe that the best strategy for considering ethical issues is to be aware of the possible impact of each of these different perspectives on the issue at hand.

This text is meant to be pragmatic and problem-centered. We believe that the best way to study clinical ethics is via attention to the most frequent and difficult ethical problems that confront clinicians, patients, and their families who are at or near the bedside — the arena of illness and healing. In these situations, decisions need to be made and actions must be taken. We call this "doing ethics," or moral problem solving.

We emphasize that it is unwise to "do ethics" by waiting for such problems to arise and addressing them only after they fester and become crises. Clinicians and institutional ethics programs need ways to address current cases and to cope with the occasional "ethics emergency." A preventive approach clearly is better than a crisis-management approach to recurrent ethical problems. "Preventive ethics" is a significant feature of clinical ethics.[1] Preventive ethics, a strong program of clinical ethics education and a supportive ethical climate within the HCO, as discussed in chapter 17, is much more feasible in HCOs that strongly support their ethics programs and reward clinicians for taking the time to develop a plan of care that includes ethical considerations.

Our readers come to the study of clinical ethics with differing motives. Some are students of medicine or nursing who are preparing to deal with ethical problems and legal concerns. Others are practicing clinicians who aim to be current on what is ethically and legally expected. Others are new or continuing members of ethics committees who seek clarity about their role and tasks.

Our experience in teaching is that, despite differing motives, our readers share five needs.

1. They need to learn to lead or participate in a process of practical moral problem solving,
2. They need to understand the major ethical obligations and responsibilities of clinicians and the accepted approaches to the most frequent ethical problems in the care of patients,
3. They need to use the resources of ethics and its concepts:

A. Major ethical principles,
B. Specific ethical considerations that carry great weight in the relations between clinicians, patients, and society, and
C. Virtues of clinicians.
4. They need to learn how to contribute to and use the resources of a program of clinical ethics in an HCO,
5. They need to learn enough about the history of clinical ethics to locate its place in the culture of HCOs and American society.

In trying to meet these needs with this textbook, we avoid giving "ready" answers for complex ethical problems. In real life, no prefabricated solutions to particular ethical problems are available. We do point out where a reasonable degree of consensus exists on a particular problem. In some problem areas, such as forgoing life-sustaining treatment for incapacitated and terminally ill patients, a consensus exists among clinicians, ethicists, and attorneys. Even so, ethical and legal challenges to this consensus, as in the *Schiavo* and *Wedland* cases (chapter 12), are ever present. There is wide variation, less consensus, or no consensus at all on other problems such as reproductive choices, physician-assisted death, or how basic healthcare ought to be equitably distributed in the U.S. However, reasoned positions have been advanced, with which students and clinicians should be familiar, and these positions are discussed in ensuing chapters.

The text appeals to ethical considerations and principles, but these are not self-explanatory and often require further analysis. Rigid formulas are no more appropriate in clinical ethics than in clinical medicine. Ethical judgments, guided by ethical principles and by practices that promote good relations between clinicians and patients, must be weighed in specific situations with particular patients. In the end, studying clinical ethics does not deliver anyone from the burdens and risks of decision making, but should enable one to help in the development of meaningful processes by which ethical decisions are made.

In the present chapter, we trace the emergence of clinical ethics and the community of persons who "do ethics" in clinical settings. We then discuss some key terms and concepts in ethics, followed by a description of the content and conceptual resources necessary for doing clinical ethics. These resources include an understanding of the basic ethical obligations of clinicians, knowledge about approaches to ethical problems that clinicians face, key ethical considerations in clinical ethics, and identification of the virtues of clinicians.

II. THE EMERGENCE OF CLINICAL ETHICS IN TEACHING, RESEARCH, AND SERVICE

In an important review of the evolution of clinical ethics,[2] Mark Siegler, Edmund D. Pellegrino, and Peter A. Singer argue that it developed in response to two perceived needs: (1) the need for bedside teaching of ethics, in the tradition of William Osler,[3] a nineteenth-century physician famous for his bedside teaching of medicine; and (2) the need for a method of ethical inquiry especially suitable to individual cases in clinical settings.[4] Implicit within both developments was the belief that ethics, properly understood, is an integral component of the practice of good clinical medicine. We would add a third perceived need: the need to create a bridge between the academic world of bioethics and medical humanities and the world of clinicians and patients.

Bioethics, as distinct from clinical ethics, began in the 1960s as an intellectual and social movement.[5] The earliest bioethicists were concerned with novel moral dilemmas and violations of the autonomy of persons — especially in settings of research and innovative therapy such as hemodialysis and transplantation for end-stage kidney disease. Coming as it did at the time of the civil rights movement, the birth of bioethics exposed great imbalances of power and authority that endangered research subjects and patients.[6]

From the origins of bioethics to the present, the concerns of individuals who work in this field have been largely with teaching, research, and social change, and this work has been done almost exclusively within higher academic centers. Within academia, bioethics became a new arena for interdisciplinary work within the larger field of ethics. Bioethics' early focus of social and institutional change was to prevent abuses and enhance the values that cluster around and guide decision making regarding human subjects of research, and, to some extent, patients. Deliberate social change in the research setting, such as prior group review of research by institutional review boards (IRBs), began in the 1960s and 1970s, well before similar changes were made in patient care settings (such as the use of ethics committees to

work on ethical issues in patient care).

These currents of change influenced clinicians and their practices, and required adaptation by clinicians and bioethicists who desired to teach, do research, and serve in clinical settings.

In particular, clinicians identified three needs of the early bioethics movement:

1. The need for a contextual approach to ethical inquiry,
2. The need to emphasize the relevance of clinical experience when doing clinical ethics, and
3. The need for an orientation toward service in clinical ethics.

The first concern was the need to develop modes of ethical inquiry that take more careful account of the variety of contexts in clinical care and the special needs of ill and suffering patients. The initial approach to bioethical inquiry used systematic reflection on moral principles and resolving ethical problems in biomedicine by weighing and balancing the claims of competing principles. The strongest advocates for a "principles approach" were Thomas L. Beauchamp and James Childress in their trendsetting work, *Principles of Biomedical Ethics* (now in its fifth edition).[7] Beauchamp and Childress advanced a simple, easily understood set of principles to be considered in ethical decision making. These principles include: (1) respect for autonomy, which obliges clinicians to respect and defend the informed choices of capable patients; (2) beneficence, which creates an obligation to benefit patients and to further their interests; (3) nonmaleficence, which asserts an obligation to prevent harm or, if risks of harm must be taken, to minimize those risks; and (4) justice, which asserts the obligation to be fair in the allocation of the benefits and burdens of society. Although valuable work was achieved by this mainstream approach, clinicians indicated the need to give more attention to the clinical context in which ethical problems are faced. Some clinicians[8] and philosophers[9] viewed this method of appealing to one or more abstract principles for justification as mechanical; as deducing ethical conclusions for concrete problematic situations from fixed moral principles or rules. Some identified a need to supply additional resources for ethical inquiry beyond highly abstract and general moral principles.

An additional resource for ethical inquiry appeared in renewed interest in *casuistry,* the time-honored art of ethical analysis by the study of cases, and the comparison of the case in question with more settled cases.[10] Clinical decision making is, after all, case-specific, so this method of analysis has much to commend it in clinical situations. Each case focuses on a specific patient who is faced with a particular illness or injury, and each case has a history that encompasses the facts that led up to the problems that need medical attention. Casuistry encourages particularistic, "bottom-up" reasoning; a principles approach supports an abstract, "top-down" decision-making process. Accordingly, casuistry is an important method of inquiry in clinical ethics. We weave cases into the discussions in this text. Several anthologies and texts have been published with rich collections of cases,[11] including two with cases in ethics consultation,[12] and one with cases for the allied health professions.[13] Like the practice of clinical medicine, casuistry builds on the accumulated experience, both individual and collective, of dealing with a variety of cases. Comparing and contrasting somewhat similar cases can help identify important ethical considerations that may not be apparent when we first focus on a particular case in isolation.

The traditional manner for considering ethical problems in clinical medicine has, until the last half of the twentieth century, been a *virtues approach,* and this approach still resonates with many. It is the basis for the traditional professional ethics of physicians and nurses. Virtue ethics focuses on the character and virtues of the clinician, and asks the question, "What kind of person should I be to do the right or good thing for my patient?" rather than focusing on a specific action and whether it is good or right. Virtue ethics in medicine has recently been criticized for supporting paternalism and denigrating autonomy (see chapter 2).

An *ethics of caring* is a prominent new mode of ethical inquiry in clinical ethics. Drawing on the writings of psychologist and educational theorist Carol Gilligan,[14] this view finds that the dominant approach of principlism tends to neglect crucial relationships and may fail to recognize the human needs and interests that also underlie the conflicts of principles. In this light, one with a "caring" perspective is concerned less with dramatic confrontations of ethical dilemmas and more with restoring and strengthening bonds between professionals, patients, and families. This perspective focuses fully on the relationships that affect an ethical problem, and, although it is of-

ten similar to a virtue approach, it emphasizes relationships rather than virtues and character traits.

Clinicians' second criticism of the bioethics movement focused on the need to deepen and enrich the study of larger issues and themes in clinical practice, and on the lack of empirical research on important ethical issues, such as decision making in critical care and at the end of life. In closing the gap between bioethics and clinical practice, clinician-ethicists — ethicists who had adapted to the clinical setting — made progress by using cases and by drawing on knowledge available only through the intimacy of the clinician-patient encounter. Five exemplary studies, among many, are informative discussions of informed consent,[15] decision making about life and death,[16] pain and suffering,[17] the use of power by clinicians,[18] and helping patients with the trauma and tasks of dying.[19] These studies draw on a variety of disciplines and experiential data obtained in clinical settings. As such, they contribute toward ethical scrutiny and inform understandings and practices in the entire clinical encounter between patients and clinicians.[20] In this way, clinical ethics strengthens the conceptual arm of the bioethics movement with experiential data and helps to motivate clinicians to reform practices.

Recently, clinical ethics has also been informed by a significant increase in empirical research on issues of concern to clinicians, patients, and our society. Here we do not give an exhaustive review, but point to the steadily growing knowledge base from empirical research on patients' capacity for healthcare decision making (chapter 9), outcomes of the informed-consent process (chapter 10), and uses of advance directives and patterns of decision making in care of critically ill and dying patients (chapter 13).

In the past decade, many more clinicians skilled in research methodology have entered the arena of clinical ethics. Their research results are published regularly in leading medical and professional journals. A noteworthy example is the Study to Understand Prognoses and Preferences for Outcomes and Risks of Treatments (SUPPORT),[21] a five-year effort that followed 9,105 adult patients in a controlled, multi-institutional assessment and trial of an intervention to improve the quality of decision making in the care of seriously ill, hospitalized adults. SUPPORT's findings were largely disappointing in terms of the ideals of shared decision making and the usefulness of advance directives, but it provides a clear baseline for new research and efforts to improve palliative care in acute-care settings.

The third criticism of the early bioethics movement was that, in addition to teaching and research, there should be clinical ethics services for clinicians and their patients. The next section is devoted to this concern.

A. The Clinical Ethics Community and Its Services

Community is meant here in a general sense — that is, a body of people sharing a common characteristic or interest who live and work in a larger society that does not fully share that characteristic or interest.[22] Members of the clinical ethics community today have a mission to teach and do research, but their most broadly shared common interest is to provide services to address ethical issues in the care of patients and in the institutions where this care is received.[23] Those who are served are those with the responsibility to make decisions whether it is the patient, clinician, or other staff member. These key decision makers need to be able to identify, analyze, and resolve ethical problems in patient care.

Well-developed clinical ethics programs typically offer five types of services:
1. Provide education in clinical ethics for clinicians, patients, surrogates, and the larger community,
2. Conduct policy studies and make recommendations for institutional and community guidelines to address various ethical issues in patient care,
3. Provide a process for case consultation at the bedside or the conference room,
4. Do targeted research on ethical problems and participate in planning for prevention of such problems, when possible,
5. Participate in ongoing evaluation.

Each service involves a complex and difficult set of tasks, which will be discussed in more detail in chapter 17. To provide any of these services requires education and training. To flourish, a clinical ethics program and its services must become more widely recognized within the HCO, the academic community, and the larger society.

Who belongs to the clinical ethics community? A sociological account of the most to the least visible would include the following.

1. The many thousands of members of ethics committees in patient care, including community members and those in regional or statewide networks to support these efforts,
2. The faculties, staffs, postgraduate fellows, and graduate students in a few centers or academic departments where study and training in clinical ethics is possible,[24]
3. The members of professional societies concerned directly with clinical ethics,
4. Educators within the nation's schools of medicine, law, and religious life that have significant interests in clinical ethics.

B. The Place of Clinical Ethics in Society

If this sketch of a clinical ethics community is reasonably accurate, what is its place and role in society? To whom is a clinical ethics program finally accountable? Whom do clinical ethicists and their colleagues serve? Differing visions of the place of clinical ethics compete in the literature: as a subspeciality of medicine,[25] as an arena for a "new breed" of healthcare consultant with an academic background,[26] or as a multidisciplinary activity that largely serves physicians.[27] None of these visions is fully satisfactory, because each locates the source of legitimation in a field or culture that is external to clinical ethics — that is, in medicine or in academics. For clinical ethics to survive and prosper, it must become a more unified multidisciplinary field and elevate its standards, especially for education and training for those who provide its services. Figure 1.1 describes the place of clinical ethics, as we see it, in society.

We use the analogy of a bridge to describe the place of clinical ethics between academic and clinical cultures, two larger and more powerful cultures. Another analogy is that of an isthmus between two large land areas (as Panama and Central America are to North and South America).

These larger cultures would benefit from increased interaction between their different practices, languages, and standards. Bioethics and medical humanities are located in academic culture. Their ways of life are guided by patterns and norms that have been forged in graduate education, by scholarly guilds, and by the political and economic arrangements of universities. The clinical world is deeply influenced by the human experience of disease and suffering, long-standing traditions of medicine and nursing, the special settings of widely varying HCOs, as well as the social and economic arrangements that structure these settings. Above these entities, however, are the larger community, region, and society that support, recognize, and legitimize each of these entities' activities. Society can govern and exercise some degree of control through law, regulation, and encouragement of the tradition of professional self-regulation.

Whom does clinical ethics serve and where is its locus of accountability? In our view, clinical ethics earns its place by serving both academic and clinical cultures, as well as the larger community, region, and society that have encouraged the development of this endeavor.

For clinical ethics to have authenticity, it must bridge the gap between the clinical world and the theoretical disciplines of bioethics and medical humanities in the academic world. Clinical ethics can contribute a body of knowledge and useful practices for clinicians and patients in different clinical settings. Clinical ethics can also contribute in several ways to bioethics and medical humanities: empirical and descriptive research on ethical problems; case narratives and stories of patients and clinicians; and translation and transmission of the ideas, concepts, and perspectives of theoretical ethics for those who interact within the clinical culture. Clinical ethics must not allow its discourse to become dominated by overly academic and theoretical concerns or to permit untrained academic professionals to attempt to provide services. By introducing the members of academic culture to the world of clinicians and patients, clinical ethics is providing a great service to the academic world.

To validate the *clinical* in clinical ethics, those who "do" clinical ethics must interact professionally and, at times, intimately with clinicians and patients in their world and know their language, practices, and beliefs. To this end, those who do clinical ethics but are not clinicians must become sufficiently educated in medicine and clinical reasoning to understand the language of diagnosis and treatment of disease, the process of medical decision making, and the social structure of a clinical culture. Because most clinical ethics programs are located in and are supported by HCOs, the danger is that the interests of the clinical or organizational culture will dominate and overwhelm clinical ethics. Wherever this danger exists, it must be overcome by the clinical ethics community's confidence and independence to challenge particular practices and characteristics of clinical culture.

The community, region, and the larger society are the ultimate sources of recognition and legitimacy for academic and clinical cultures. Likewise, the clinical ethics community needs to seek recognition for its services. It will do so not by self-proclamation, but by completing the growth process to be, by analogy, a more recognized and self-governing territory. The clinical ethics community must help its members, especially those who serve on ethics committees, to pass milestones of education and training that

Figure 1.1. The Place of Clinical Ethics in Society

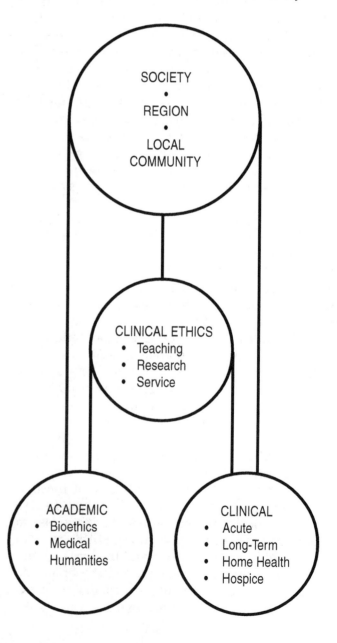

these two cultures and the larger society recognize. Chapter 17 contains practical recommendations, as well as a strategy for accreditation of education and training programs in clinical ethics.

C. Organizational Ethics

In its short lifetime, clinical ethics has mainly addressed issues in patient care and patients' rights. There is a significant need to balance attention to individual cases with ethical analysis of the organizational, management, and economic issues that affect the operation of HCOs and the healthcare system at large.[28] This need has been sharpened by standards of the Joint Commission on Accreditation of Healthcare Organizations (JCAHO) about organizational ethics — issues of institutional integrity for HCOs (see appendix 1). The JCAHO standards state that institutions that are accredited by the JCAHO must have "a functioning process to address ethical issues" that is "based on a framework that recognizes the interdependence of patient care and organizational ethical issues."[29] The JCAHO rules specifically require a process to examine ethical issues in marketing, admissions, discharge, billing, relationships with third-party payers and managed-care plans, as well as a "code of organizational ethics" that addresses each of these areas. How these and other JCAHO rules regarding patients' rights can be met by an HCO's ethics program is further described in chapter 3.

Clinical and organizational ethics can be a useful resource for clinicians, administrators, and patients involved in managed-care and other large, rapidly developing healthcare systems. Iglehart defined managed care as "a system that in varying degrees integrates the financing and delivery of medical care through contracts with selected physicians and hospitals that provide comprehensive healthcare services to enrolled members for a predetermined monthly premium."[30] He observed, "All forms of managed care represent attempts to control costs by modifying the behavior of doctors, although they do it in different ways."[31] Ethical analysis of healthcare systems draws upon some of the ethical concepts used in this text, but requires a different set of skills in describing the context of ethical problems that arise for healthcare and managed-care organizations as such. Chapter 16 examines the ethics of healthcare systems.

III. Ethics and Other Terms

How the word *ethics* is understood makes a real difference to the climate in which moral problem solving can be done effectively. Such issues and conflicts of interest are within the scope of professional ethics and the self-regulation that clinicians are supposed to exercise. Understanding ethics only within a professional framework creates questions about why "another" ethics committee is needed, when local, regional, and national medical societies already have them.

We recommend the use of the terms *clinical ethics committee* or *ethics services* to reduce misunderstanding. For such reasons, at the outset of studying clinical ethics, some important terms (such as *ethics, morality,* and *moral dilemmas*) need clarification.

A. Ethics and Morality

Although the terms *ethics* and *morality* are often used interchangeably, it is useful to distinguish between them (see the definition at the beginning of this chapter). In the ancient past, the words had similar meanings. *Ethics* stems from the Greek word *ethos,* meaning character. *Morality* is from the Latin word *mores,* meaning character, custom, or habit.[32] In the past, both terms referred to manners, character, or custom.

We now understand *morality* to mean *customary morality,* or widely shared beliefs about the moral life and norms of right and wrong conduct that prevail in a particular culture or subculture. Anthropologists have found great differences among cultures with respect to such beliefs and norms. Such moral beliefs influence how people habitually respond, without deeper reflection, to everyday moral problems.

To some it is distressing that no single unifying ethical theory or vision of the moral life prevails in this society. A pluralistic society has divergent moralities, as amply illustrated by controversy over elective abortion.[33] In the midst of heated moral controversies, a tendency can exist to impose group morality on others who differ. This urge to impose can become extreme among groups with powerful beliefs, such as when a revealed religion is seen as an absolute foundation for all of morality. Although our presentation of clinical ethics does not depend on particular religious commitments, it respects the contribution that religious traditions and thought have made to bioethics and medical humanities, and to everyday moral decisions.

At another extreme, one can subscribe to an absolute of tolerance of cultural differences and noninterference in the moral lives of others. Under this view, right and wrong are absolutely relative to culture. This type of ethical relativism empties morality of all content. Its greatest danger is to abdicate any moral standpoint in the face of great and blatant evil (for example, unspeakable crimes such as those perpetrated by the Nazis). The word *ethics* assumes some reflective and critical judgments about acts and beliefs; it means both to understand and to critique particular moralities, when necessary.

B. Moral Dilemmas

A *practical dilemma* (from the Greek *dilemmatos,* "involving two assumptions") poses a choice between two or more alternatives, all of which appear to be obligatory or desirable.[34] The decision maker is in a bind, or caught between alternatives, because circumstances prevent her or him from doing both. One kind of dilemma for busy, overcommitted people is to find that they have promised to be at two places at the same time. New information may resolve what appears at first to be a dilemma. For example, one date may have been wrongly recorded or can easily be changed. Then the dilemma dissolves. If one "horn" of a dilemma involves a matter of self-interest (a golf or tennis game) versus a moral obligation (a board meeting of a charitable organization), there is a personal dilemma but no moral dilemma, as the "right" action is known.

Beauchamp and Childress describe two forms of moral dilemmas. The difference between them is in where the sharpest point of conflict lies: within the society or within an individual. An example of the first would be that, within the larger society, some communities hold that to do act X (for example, an elective abortion) is morally right, and other communities hold that it is morally wrong; but the evidence on both sides is inconclusive and debatable. Women who look at abortion in this way and who seek moral consensus in terms of community values can be confronted by a severe dilemma posed from outside themselves. In the second form, a person can morally believe that she or he both ought and

ought not to do a specific act. In this situation, a person feels the dilemma acutely from within. Some clinicians and family members feel this kind of dilemma in cases when a dying patient has clear wishes to stop nutrition and hydration, but their own moral tradition opposes or cautions against such a choice.

1. Moral Dilemmas: Dynamics and Emotions

Moral dilemmas can also be described by tracing their personal and interpersonal dynamics. In this sense, a dilemma can occur: within a single person (intrapersonal), or between two or more persons (interpersonal).

Intrapersonal ethical dilemmas arouse powerful emotions, such as anxiety, fear of social criticism, or anger. In interpersonal conflicts, differences in the status and power of the decision makers can strongly influence the dynamics of the case. Some patients and family members feel powerless in front of clinicians and may not speak at all. They may fear alienating doctors on whom their care depends. Knowledge and skill is required to promote trust and open dialogue in such situations.[35]

One needs to heed one's feelings to engage in moral problem solving. Without a capacity to feel conflicting emotions and obligations, we may fail to recognize that moral dilemmas exist at all. Stress and exhaustion can depress emotions and desensitize clinicians to the ethical dimension of clinical care. Emotions are a key element of the moral life. The capacity to empathize with another person, or to put oneself in the other's place, is needed to be a moral person.

To allow oneself to feel conflicting emotions and conflicting obligations invites a state of moral ambiguity or uncertainty. Moral ambiguity is a "normal" stage in the process of responding to a genuine ethical problem. However, emotional responses in ethical conflicts — "shooting from the hip" or mere reaction — cut off the process of ethical deliberation (see chapter 6).

2. Problematic Responses to Moral Dilemmas

We can identify three problematic ways that clinicians respond to moral dilemmas. Each short-circuits serious ethical deliberation. These include:
1. Collapsing moral dilemmas into medical or legal questions,
2. Generalizing expertise in medicine to ethics,

3. Divorcing ethical and clinical reasoning.

As an example of collapsing moral dilemmas into medical or legal questions, George Annas identified Sherwin B. Nuland's decision to perform surgery on a 92-year-old patient who suffered intensely afterward.[36] Reflecting on his mistake in pressing his patient to concede to surgery, Nuland wrote: "Viewed by a surgeon, mine was strictly a clinical decision, and ethics should not have been a consideration."[37] Physicians habituated to such one-sided reasoning can be blind to abuse of the healer's power.[38] Another frequent response in moral dilemmas is to ask, "What does the law say?" or "Can we be sued?" Neither one of these responses is adequate to the task, although medical and legal information is certainly relevant at key points in moral problem solving.

A second problematic response is to commit the fallacy of "generalization of expertise," described long ago by Robert M. Veatch — that is, assuming that expertise about the technical facts of an area of medicine gives the physician expertise in the ethical aspects of decision making in that area.[39] This fallacy was probably at work in the early stages of the *Baby K* case,[40] discussed in chapter 13. Why did physicians of a patient carrying a fetus with anencephaly fail to develop a plan to address the ethical issues raised by the mother's strong demands for "full treatment" at birth? They fell back on their experience and expertise, and predicted that she would change her mind upon seeing the infant's head at birth. In short, they had never seen another pregnant woman make such a choice. Through this fallacious reasoning, they delayed, and then found themselves in a terrible and costly dilemma.

A third problematic response, influenced by theoretical ethics and probably transmitted in medical school courses, is to divorce ethical and clinical reasoning. The two modes of reasoning are learned at different times and remain unintegrated. In a third edition of their widely used text, Beauchamp and Childress wrote, self-critically, "We believe one of the major defects in contemporary theory in biomedical ethics is its distance from clinical practice. . . . But this defect cannot be corrected here."[41] This problem can be corrected by real collaboration between the field's theoreticians, medical and nursing school educators, and clinical ethics programs. Chapter 2 is directly relevant to the integration of clinical and ethical reasoning.

E. Learning to Frame Moral Dilemmas as Ethical Problems

How can these problematic responses be overcome? What must one know to "do" clinical ethics? What is the content of clinical ethics? A major portion of the field's content is information about types of ethical problems that are frequently faced by clinicians, patients, and patients' surrogates. Learning how to frame frequent moral dilemmas in the clinical care of patients as ethical problems, prior to moral problem solving, is the primary skill and area of knowledge involved in clinical ethics.

Working through dilemmas to identify and frame them as ethical problems is a skill that can be learned. The most frequently recurring moral dilemmas that are faced by clinicians today arise in (1) cases with circumstances that require, or seem to require, clinicians' infringements of basic obligations to patients; or (2) other particular disputes that arise in choices in diagnosis or treatment at various stages and circumstances of the life cycle.

This text presents and discusses these frequent dilemmas in the framework of ethical problems. Each ethical problem has a different history, and clinicians' approaches to these problems are constantly evolving. Because law and ethics evolve together, the development of health law is also involved in this story (see chapter 4).

IV. BASIC ETHICAL OBLIGATIONS AND ETHICAL PROBLEMS

After the clinician-patient relationship is established, we believe the following obligations are morally binding in each case:
1. Respect the patient's privacy and maintain a process that protects the patient's confidentiality,
2. Communicate honestly about all aspects of the patient's diagnosis, treatment, and prognosis,
3. Determine whether the patient is capable of sharing in decision making,
4. Conduct an ethically valid process of informed consent throughout the relationship.

An ethical problem can arise when circumstances require, or appear to require, clinicians to infringe on one or more of these basic obligations. Such circumstances occur frequently.

These obligations, the ethical problems that stem from the need to infringe on them, and exceptions to the obligations are discussed in the second part of this book, "Ethical Obligations in Each Case." Nurses and other clinicians share — with physicians — the moral responsibility to fulfill these obligations.

The third part of this book, "Ethical Problems in Particular Cases," presents a second cluster of ethical problems in the clinical setting; these problems probably occur less frequently than those presented in part 2 of the book, but they are complex and difficult to resolve when they do occur. The third part of the book discusses six substantive ethical problems that occur in individual cases.

1. When competent patients refuse medically indicated tests or treatment, for religious, cultural, or personal reasons,
2. Problems in care of suffering patients who are terminally ill, including patients' requests for assisted suicide and euthanasia, and the determination that death has occurred,
3. Decisions about forgoing life-sustaining treatment for incapacitated patients, including assessments of "medical futility."
4. Disputes about treatment of newborns, infants, and children,
5. Reproductive choices, including abortion, sterilization, prenatal diagnosis, and other uses of new reproductive technology,
6. Bedside rationing of scarce resources, such as beds in an intensive-care unit, organs, blood, and so forth.

Being familiar with these two categories of problems can enable students, clinicians, and ethics committee members to identify ethical problems in cases and engage in moral deliberation about them.

V. ETHICALLY RELEVANT CONSIDERATIONS AND VIRTUES: CARING FOR PATIENTS

"Doing" ethics requires asking questions and making judgments about what to do in particular situations and giving reasons in support of these judgments. Judgments as to the appropriate or best moral stance are typically preceded by a deliberative process. In this process, identifying the ethical problem(s) is advisable. However, to identify an ethical problem is only to begin the exploration of its significance. We then need to ask the

question, "What is ethically at stake in this case?" At this point, we recommend a review of those considerations that are most relevant to the problem(s). Ethically relevant considerations consist of the factors that help in focusing our moral judgments.

A. Eight Ethically Relevant Considerations

Below is a brief overview of eight ethical considerations that have the greatest weight and relevance in the care of patients. These considerations bridge between ethical principles, an ethics of caring and virtue, and the clinical situation. They are:

1. The balance between benefits and harms in the care of patients;
2. Disclosure, informed consent, and shared decision making;
3. The norms of family life;
4. Traditional professional responsibilities of physicians and nurses in the context of relationships with patients;
5. Professional integrity;
6. Societal norms of cost-effectiveness and allocation;
7. Cultural and religious variations; and
8. Considerations of power.

These considerations are examined in greater depth in later chapters. Other works present more broadly systematic and theoretical discussions of ethics and healthcare and the clinician-patient relationship.[42]

1. Balancing benefits and harms in the care of patients is the paramount traditional ethical consideration in the practice of clinical medicine. It carries out the claims of the ethical principles of beneficence, which aims to maximize benefits to persons, and of nonmaleficence, which aims to minimize harm or to avoid it altogether. The responsibility of all clinicians is to use their professional medical knowledge to determine what treatments maximize benefits and minimize harms to their patients. Clinicians are obligated to benefit patients or prevent harm to patients in pursuing the goals of medicine: preserving life, curing (when possible), healing, restoring or maintaining bodily functions and mental capacities, preventing disease or injury, and relieving suffering. Although patients are at the center of ethical focus in this traditional normative orientation, in contemporary medicine the interests of other parties may also be relevant to the assessment of benefits and risks (for example, the health of fetuses or live organ donors).

2. Disclosure, informed consent, and shared decision making have motivated the bioethics movement and legal thought in the past 30 years to challenge whether clinicians should have the unilateral authority to determine what medical treatment is in the best interest of patients. This threefold consideration does the work of the ethical principle of respect for autonomy. Healthcare, particularly when alternative treatments are possible, inevitably involves issues of values, which do not lie within the domain of medical knowledge. How can clinicians determine, in all cases, what is in the best interest of patients without consulting patients and adequately disclosing what they need to know to make decisions? (See chapter 10.)

The right of adult, competent patients to determine for themselves whether they will accept treatment is recognized in the legal and ethical doctrine of informed consent. To exercise voluntary consent, patients need — at least — to receive truthful disclosure from their clinicians concerning their condition, the benefits and risks of alternative treatments, and their prognosis with and without these treatments. Informed consent requires ongoing dialogue between clinicians and patients. This dialogue and its requirements is often referred to as a shared decision-making process between patients, family members or companions, and clinicians, and, in 1982, the President's Commission for the Study of Ethical Problems in Medicine and Biomedical and Behavioral Research specifically endorsed this model.[43]

3. Norms of family life are almost always at stake, since patients typically face major medical decisions as members of a family rather than as isolated individuals. Familial relationships give rise to moral responsibilities. These norms and responsibilities are nurtured by an ethics of caring. Spouses, children, and other family members provide support, help, and care for patients whose lives are disrupted by illness. Parents are intimately involved in the healthcare of their children, and family members generally have the right and the responsibility to speak for patients who are no longer capable of making decisions for themselves. Accordingly, the ethics of clinical practice must take into consideration the moral dimension of family life.

4. The relationships between clinicians and patients lie at the heart of clinical ethics, strongly informed by an ethics of caring for others. Professional healthcare providers have a fiduciary responsibility to care for sick and injured patients. The process of healing depends on the trust of patients and the trustworthiness of clinicians. Although patients are vulnerable and dependent, they are entitled to be treated with respect and as partners in the process of making healthcare decisions. In addition to being competent in the technical aspects of healthcare, clinicians are responsible for communicating with patients to enlist their participation in healthcare and for maintaining a caring presence with patients suffering from illness. To treat patients solely as diseased bodies in need of repair amounts to psychological abandonment. The ethics of clinical practice involves the way in which clinicians relate to patients in addition to the process of determining what is the right thing to do in problematic cases.

5. The professional integrity of clinicians plays an important role in determining whether treatment or care requested by patients or surrogates is ethically appropriate. The norms of professional integrity are formed and reformed, over time, and do the work of an ethics of caring for one's companions, in the moral struggles to be a good clinician. The right of patients to self-determination requires that no treatments can be imposed on competent patients without their consent. Although patients are free to refuse treatment, they are not entitled to receive whatever treatment they demand. Clinicians have no responsibility to offer or provide treatments that are medically inappropriate; for, otherwise, clinicians' integrity as professionals would be undermined.[44] Whether physicians should have the unilateral power to withhold or withdraw life-sustaining treatment on grounds of futility is a matter of current controversy. When clinicians and patients or family disagree about the appropriateness of life-sustaining treatment, ethics consultation may be indicated. In any case, clinicians are not obligated to provide treatment that they oppose for reasons of conscience.

6. Considerations of cost-effectiveness and the allocation of scarce resources are increasingly at stake in questions of the distribution of medical resources and efforts to contain the spiraling costs of healthcare. These considerations carry out the claims of the ethical principle of justice. In practice, clinicians are increasingly expected to be familiar with the costs of particular treatments and to consider these costs among the outcomes when they make decisions about treatment. Practice guidelines and managed care are two of a number of recent innovations introduced in an attempt to control costs.

Even with these efforts, the boundaries between public policy and clinical decision making are still unclear. Managed care and other cost-containment efforts are the occasion for many ethical conflicts between patients, clinicians, and third-party payers (see chapter 13). At times, clinicians cannot avoid the need to select which patients will receive scarce medical resources (see chapter 12). Equitable procedures must be applied when ethically acceptable decisions about the allocation of medical care are made. The clinician is the patient's primary advocate for access to medically indicated healthcare treatments and entitlements to coverage under private or public insurance plans.

7. Issues of cultural and/or religious variation often face clinicians who provide healthcare to patients of diverse backgrounds. Traditional cultural norms of family life may place healthcare decisions and access to information in the control of the patient's family members, rather than the patient. The concepts of patient self-determination and truthful disclosure may be foreign to the cultural practices and values of some patients. Clinicians need to apply sensitivity and tact, and perhaps religious and cultural consultation along with ethics consultation, to respond appropriately to the potentially difficult problems this may pose.

8. Considerations of power often shape or underlie ethical problems in the clinical setting and deserve special attention in furthering the principle of respect for persons and their autonomy. It is almost always the case that clinicians are in a greater position of power than patients and their family members. Sickness and disease place patients in a vulnerable and dependent position. Howard Brody examines the clinician-patient relationship from the perspective of the ways that the power of the clinician is, and should be, exercised.[45] For Brody, the *responsible use of therapeutic power* is the standard of clinical ethics. Shared decision making requires sharing power. Shared power involves recognizing the patient's moral standing and right to participate in decisions (or the proxy decision maker's right, for an incompetent patient). The major vehicle of shared power is conversation between clinician and pa-

tient. Brody writes: "The patient ideally has a right to a relationship that assures that he will be treated with respect and that medical knowledge will be used to further his own life plans and values. Both to show respect and to find out how medicine can be applied to his specific life issues, a particular sort of sustained, reasonable conversation is necessary."[46] Clinicians are obliged to examine the differentials of power among persons and groups involved in a case when ethical problems arise, to be prepared to prevent unnecessary power struggles that can end in needless lawsuits. Considerations of power are also important in the interpersonal and interprofessional relationships of physicians, nurses, students, and allied healthcare professionals.

B. The Virtues of Clinicians

The topic of clinical virtues has received less attention in the literature of bioethics than moral rules and principles.[47] *Virtues* are dispositions of character and conduct that motivate and enable clinicians to provide good care to patients. The clinical virtues function as habits that are conducive to good practice and as guides to healing and caring interactions with patients.

Faced with ethically problematic situations, clinicians can (and should) appeal to an understanding of good practice, in addition to relevant moral rules and principles. Some of the principal clinical virtues are described below, with emphasis on the virtue of caring. Clinical excellence, including the ability to respond appropriately to ethical problems in the care of patients, depends on cultivating these virtues. Clinicians who have cultivated these virtues will integrate ethics into their clinical practice and approach the care of patients in ways that minimize ethical conflicts.

1. Technical Competence

The good physician or nurse has mastered the requisite knowledge and techniques for practicing the arts of medicine or nursing. Because biomedical knowledge and techniques undergo rapid development, owing to clinical research, the good clinician must be committed to continuing education to maintain competence.

2. Objectivity and Detachment

The clinician must learn to become sufficiently distanced emotionally from the gore, pain, and invasiveness medical treatment entails to do what is needed to help the patient, while maintaining a compassionate, empathetic approach.

3. Caring

Caring is a complex perceptive and emotive disposition to relate to persons with the aim of helping them satisfy their needs. Caring individualizes and personalizes interactions with patients. It mitigates the depersonalization that is inherent in scientific medicine and institutional healthcare. Caring also counterbalances the impersonality of ethical principles and the "detachment" necessary for maintaining objectivity. By their very nature, principles consist of generalizations: they point to characteristics shared by a variety of situations. Caring gives insight into what is fitting for particular patients in particular problematic situations. Principles specify impersonal moral norms that are relevant to classes of cases. But each case has its own unique features because it involves an individual patient in a particular network of relations with others. To interact ethically with patients, clinicians must attend with care to the situations each case presents. The psychic needs of the patient as a suffering person deserve attention by clinicians, in addition to the medical needs of the patient's diseased or injured body. Caring for the patient as a person should be seen as integral to the plan of care. Caring helps the patient get better or make the best of his or her situation by relieving the distress caused by illness and its consequences — dependence, loss of control, vulnerability, and the threat of death. Lack of attention to the suffering of patients amounts to psychological abandonment.

Included within caring are the virtues of respect for patients as persons and therapeutic attentiveness. The good clinician respects patients as persons by responding to patients as individuals with life histories and inner worlds, rather than merely as bearers of disease. Therapeutic attentiveness is the disposition of the good clinician to appreciate and use the relationship with the patient as a means to promote healing and relief of suffering. This involves an empathetic presence with patients that is manifested by listening to them, acknowledging their concerns, explaining their medical situation in understandable terms, and providing reassurance.[48]

4. Clinical Benevolence

The clinician is committed to promoting the welfare of his or her patient. This is the pre-eminent traditional virtue of both medicine and nursing.

5. Subordination of Self-Interest

Clinicians may be required to subordinate their own self-interests in providing care to patients. This virtue is a necessary condition of benevolence and caring.

6. Reflective Intelligence

The good clinician is ready to anticipate problems, set reasonable goals, regard interventions as experimental, and adjust interventions in the light of experience.

7. Humility

The virtuous clinician understands the limits of medical knowledge and technique and recognizes her or his fallibility.

8. Practical Wisdom

The good clinician develops the art of clinical judgment under conditions of uncertainty and risk that characterize medicine. In the present context, the good clinician develops the ability to discern his or her appropriate role within large healthcare systems.

9. Courage

The good clinician has the mental and moral strength to venture, persevere, and withstand danger, fear, or difficulty firmly and resolutely. He or she has the courage to maintain bonds of fidelity to patients, regardless of their condition and degree of handicap. Courage is needed in taking the risks to act ethically when it may be contrary to what is legal and be the subject of legal action. Clinicians are often exposed to dangers and hazards in the care of patients, such as exposure to human immunodeficiency virus (HIV) and other infectious diseases, and the possibility of physical abuse from patients or their relatives. A final point is that courage is required to meet and cope with the costs of caring and empathy. When one is open to the often turbulent feelings and fears of others in the stress of illness, there are dangers to selfhood and even to sanity.

What is the source of authority of these ethical considerations and clinical virtues? They arise out of the practices and institutions of society in its interaction with clinical medicine. They operate as norms and standards recognized as authoritative with respect to family life, routine social interactions, religious communities, professional practices and associations, the law, and the state. The social origins of these ethical considerations and clinical virtues reflect the root meanings of ethics and morality as ethos and mores — the socially instituted norms of human conduct. The discipline of ethics, however, seeks to go beyond the "taken-for-granted" quality of everyday morality, to validate these considerations on deeper grounds of ethical principles and ethical theory. Ensuing chapters will address these issues in greater detail.

NOTES

1. For an excellent discussion of "prevention" in ethics, see L. Forrow, R.M. Arnold, and L.S. Parker, "Preventive Ethics: Expanding the Horizons of Clinical Ethics," *The Journal of Clinical Ethics* 4, no. 4 (Winter 1993): 287-94.

2. M. Siegler, E.D. Pellegrino, and P.A. Singer, "Clinical Medical Ethics," *The Journal of Clinical Ethics* 1, no. 1 (Spring 1990): 5-9.

3. M. Siegler, "A Legacy of Osler: Teaching Clinical Ethics at the Bedside," *Journal of the American Medical Association* 239 (1978): 951-6.

4. M. Siegler, "Decision Making Strategy for Clinical-Ethical Problems in Medicine," *Archives of Internal Medicine* 142 (1982): 2178-9; A.R. Jonsen, M. Siegler, and W. Winslade, *Clinical Ethics: A Practical Approach to Ethical Decisions in Clinical Medicine,* 3rd ed. (New York: McGraw-Hill, 1992).

5. R.C. Fox, "Advanced Medical Technology: Social and Ethical Implications," *Annual Review of Sociology* 2 (1976): 231-68; J.C. Fletcher, "The Bioethics Movement and Hospital Ethics Committees," *Maryland Law Review* 50 (1991): 859-88.

6. D. Rothman, *Strangers at the Bedside* (New York: Basic Books, 1991); A.R. Jonsen, ed., "The Birth of Bioethics," *Hastings Center Report* 23, no. 6 (Special supplement,1993): S1-S15.

7. T.L. Beauchamp and J.F. Childress, *Principles of Biomedical Ethics,* 4th ed. (New York: Oxford University Press, 1994), 44.

8. R. Sider and C.D. Clements, "The New Medical Ethics: A Second Opinion," *Archives of Internal Medicine* 145 (1985): 2169-73.

9. K.D. Clouser and B. Gert, "A Critique of Principlism," *Journal of Medicine and Philosophy* 15 (1990): 219-36.

10. A.R. Jonsen and S. Toulmin, *The Abuse of Casuistry* (Berkeley, Calif.: University of California Press, 1989); J.D. Arras, "Getting Down to Cases: The Revival of Casuistry in Bioethics," *Journal of Medicine and Philosophy* 16 (1991): 29-52.

11. R.M. Veatch and S.T. Fry, *Case Studies in Nursing Ethics* (Philadelphia: J.B. Lippincott, 1987); C. Levine, *Cases in Bioethics* (New York: St. Martin's Press, 1989); G. Pence, *Classic Cases in Medical Ethics,* 2nd ed. (New York: McGraw-Hill, 1993); J.C. Ahronheim, J.D. Moreno, and C. Zuckerman, *Ethics in Clinical Practice* (Boston: Little, Brown, 1994).

12. C.M. Culver, *Ethics at the Bedside* (Hanover, N.H.: University Press of New England, 1991); N. Dubler, *Ethics on Call* (New York: Harmony Books, 1992).

13. R.M. Veatch and H.E. Flack, *Case Studies in Allied Health Ethics* (Upper Saddle River, N.J.: Prentice-Hall, 1997).

14. C. Gilligan, *In a Different Voice* (Cambridge, Mass.: Harvard University Press, 1992).

15. J. Katz, *The Silent World of Doctor and Patient* (New York: Free Press, 1984).

16. B. Brody, *Life and Death Decision Making* (New York: Oxford University Press, 1988).

17. E. Cassell, *The Nature of Suffering and the Goals of Medicine* (New York: Oxford University Press, 1991).

18. H. Brody, *The Healer's Power* (New Haven, Conn.: Yale University Press, 1992).

19. T.E. Quill, *Death and Dignity: Making Choices and Taking Charge* (New York: W.W. Norton, 1993).

20. R.M. Zaner, *Ethics and the Clinical Encounter* (Englewood Cliffs, N.J.: Prentice-Hall, 1988).

21. A.F. Connors et al., "A Controlled Trial to Improve Care of Seriously Ill Hospitalized Patients," *Journal of the American Medical Association* 274, no. 20 (1995): 1591-8.

22. *Webster's Third New International Dictionary* (Chicago: Encyclopedia Britannica, 1981), 1: 460.

23. J.C. Fletcher and H. Brody, "Clinical Ethics," in *Encyclopedia of Bioethics,* 2nd ed., ed. W.T. Reich (New York: MacMillan, 1995): 399-404.

24. There are one-year, postgraduate fellowship programs in clinical ethics at the University of Chicago, Cleveland Clinic Foundation, Clinical Center of the National Institutes of Health, Harvard School of Medicine, and the University of Virginia. Some universities offer an MA degree program that focuses fully or in part on clinical

ethics: Brown University, Case Western Reserve University, Georgetown University, University of Pittsburgh, University of Minnesota, University of Tennessee, University of Virginia, Washington University, and University of Wisconsin (Milwaukee). Seven universities now offer a PhD program in biomedical ethics or bioethics, with wide variance in terms of clinical requirements: Baylor College of Medicine-Rice University, Georgetown University, Loyola University-Chicago, University of Tennessee-Knoxville, University of Texas-Houston, University of Virginia, and Washington University. See *International Directory of Bioethics Organizations* (Washington, D.C.: Kennedy Institute of Ethics, Georgetown University, 1994).

25. J. LaPuma and D. Schiedermeyer, *Ethics Consultation: A Practical Guide* (Boston: Jones and Bartlett, 1994), 58-61.

26. F.E. Baylis, ed., *The Health Care Ethics Consultant* (Totowa, N.J.: Humana Press, 1994).

27. Jonsen, Siegler, and Winslade, see note 4 above.

28. S.M. Wolf, "Health Care Reform and the Future of Physician Ethics," *Hastings Center Report* 24, no. 2 (1994): 28-41.

29. Joint Commission on Accreditation of Healthcare Organizations (JCAHO), "Patient Rights and Organizational Ethics," in *Accreditation Manual for Hospitals* (Oakbrook Terrace, Ill.: JCAHO, 1995).

30. J.K. Iglehart, "Physicians and the Growth of Managed Care," *New England Journal of Medicine* 331 (1994): 1167.

31. Ibid.

32. "Ethics and Morality," in *Encyclopedia of Ethics,* ed. L.M. Becker and C.B. Becker (New York: Garland, 1992), 329.

33. K. Luker, *Abortion and the Politics of Motherhood* (Berkeley, Calif.: University of California Press, 1984); L. Tribe, *Abortion: The Clash of Absolutes* (New York: Norton, 1991); R. Dworkin, *Life's Dominion* (New York: Alfred A. Knopf, 1993).

34. This section draws upon a discussion of dilemmas by Beauchamp and Childress. See note 7 above, pp. 11-3.

35. See R.M. Zaner, "Medicine and Dialogue," *Journal of Philosophy and Medicine* 15 (1990): 303-25. In arguing against the prevailing view of medicine as "applied biology," Zaner reconceives it essentially as "dialogue."

36. G.J. Annas, "How We Lie," *Hastings Center Report* 25 (November-December 1995): S12-S14.

37. S.B. Nuland, *How We Die* (New York: Alfred A. Knopf, 1994), 250-3, p. 253.

38. See note 18 above.

39. R.M. Veatch, "Medical Ethics: Professional or Universal," *Harvard Theological Review* 65 (1972): 531-59.

40. G.J. Annas, "Asking the Courts to Set the Standard of Emergency Care," *New England Journal of Medicine* 330 (1994): 1542-5.

41. T.L. Beauchamp and J.F. Childress, *Principles of Biomedical Ethics,* 3rd ed. (New York: Oxford University Press, 1989), 21.

42. In addition to the Beauchamp and Childress volume already cited, we recommend the following texts: B. Brody, *Life and Death Decision Making* (New York: Oxford University Press, 1988); H. Brody, *The Healer's Power* (New Haven, Conn.:, Yale University Press, 1992); E.J. Cassell, *The Nature of Suffering and the Goals of Medicine* (New York: Oxford University Press, 1991); H.T. Englehardt, Jr., *Foundations of Bioethics,* 2nd ed. (New York: Oxford University Press, 1994); H.B. Holmes and L.M. Purdy, ed., *Feminist Perspectives in Medical Ethics* (Bloomington, Ind.: Indiana University Press, 1992); E.D. Pellegrino and D.C. Thomasma, *For the Patient's Good* (New York: Oxford University Press, 1988); R.M. Veatch, *A Theory of Medical Ethics* (New York: Basic Books, 1981); R.M. Zaner, *Ethics and the Clinical Encounter* (Englewood Cliffs, N.J.: Prentice-Hall, 1988); R. Macklin, *Enemies of Patients* (New York: Oxford University Press, 1993); J.C. Ahronheim, J. Moreno, and C. Zuckerman, *Ethics in Clinical Practice* (Boston: Little, Brown, 1994).

43. President's Commission for the Study of Ethical Problems in Medicine and Biomedical and Behavioral Research, *Making Health Care Decisions,* vol. 1 (Washington, D.C.: U.S. Government Printing Office, 1982), 17-8.

44. The Virginia Health Care Decisions Act of 1992 (*Virginia Code, Annotated,* Sec. 54.1-2990 [Michie 1994]) was amended to read: "Nothing in this article shall be construed to require a physician to prescribe or render medical treatment to a patient that the physician determines to be medically or ethically inappropriate. However, in such a case, if the physician's determination is contrary to the terms of an advance directive of a qualified patient or the treatment decision of a person designated to make the decision under this article, the physician shall make a reasonable ef-

fort to transfer the patient to another physician. Nothing in this article shall be construed to condone, authorize or approve mercy killing or euthanasia, or to permit any affirmative or deliberate act or omission to end life other than to permit the natural process of dying." This provision was the first in the nation to affirm the physician's authority in the face of requests for "futile" treatment.

45. See note 18 above.

46. Ibid., 109.

47. Discussions of clinical virtues and virtue theory do, however, appear in the literature. See Beauchamp and Childress, note 7 above, pp. 366-99; W.F. May, "The Virtues in a Professional Setting," *Soundings* 68 (Fall 1984): 245-66; C.L. Bosk, *Forgive and Remember: Managing Medical Failure* (Chicago, Ill.: University of Chicago Press, 1979); J.L. Drane, *Becoming a Good Doctor: The Place of Virtue and Character in Medical Ethics* (Kansas City, Mo.: Sheed & Ward, 1988).

48. H. Zinn, "The Empathetic Physician," *Archives of Internal Medicine* 153 (1993): 306-12.

2

Professional Ethics

Edward M. Spencer

. . . If I fulfil this oath and do not violate it, may it be granted to me to enjoy life and art, being honored with fame among all men for all time to come; if I transgress it and swear falsely, may the opposite of this be true.
— The Hippocratic Oath

I will do all in my power to maintain and elevate the standard of my profession.
— The Florence Nightingale Pledge

I. INTRODUCTION

Since the late 1960s, patient care ethics in the United States has developed along two different pathways: contemporary bioethics and traditional professional ethics. Now, another pathway, healthcare organizational ethics, is under consideration, and it may supersede contemporary bioethics and traditional professional ethics. At the very least it is likely to have a significant influence on the healthcare system of the future, and so have an effect on the ethics of bedside care. In this chapter we focus on the older traditional professional ethics of medicine and nursing, but we believe it instructive, also, to consider how the development of each of these different perspectives on ethics in healthcare affects each other, and clinical care in general, and how they interact now and will interact in the future.

Contemporary bioethics began in the mid- to late-1960s with ethical questions concerning human research subjects. From the beginning, contemporary bioethics developed outside organized medicine; it involved academic philosophers, theologians, and attorneys, along with a few interested physicians and other clinicians. After addressing the ethical problems associated with research involving humans, the field of bioethics continued to develop with the organization of bioethics centers and groups, received a significant boost from several very public court cases (*Quinlan, Conroy,* and *Cruzan*),[1] and was publicly legitimized by the formation of the President's Commission for the Study of Ethical Problems in Medicine and Biomedical and Behavioral Research. The reports of the President's Commission became the foundation of the major accepted societal guidelines for decision making concerning ethical issues related to medical care, particularly those decisions that affect medical care at the end of life.

Presently, bioethicists are concerned with theoretical and practical ethical considerations of general issues and the specific problems that are associated with healthcare decisions. Largely based on concepts of "rights" or "principles," the field of bioethics directly and indirectly influences clinical ethics, which entails the practical application of bioethics theory to specific situations involving the care of patients. Contemporary bioethics has prompted the formation of institutional ethics committees, the creation of programs of ethics education and ethics consultation in healthcare settings, and many other aspects of the ethics of patient care in healthcare institutions. Most of the chapters in this text will draw upon bioethics as their theoretical base.

Organizational ethics, as applied in healthcare, is a very recent development. In the 1990s, as it became evident that the "ethical climate" of a healthcare organization often had a major effect on clinical decision making, major organizations such as the American Hospital Association (AHA) and the Joint Commission for Accreditation of Healthcare Organizations (JCAHO) began to pay much greater attention to how healthcare organizations' ethical stances affect the quality of clinical care and on the internal and external relationships of the organizations. This was (and is) a different way of looking at ethical issues in healthcare, as it introduces concepts such as systems analysis and management initiatives as a part (often a crucial part) of the analysis of ethical issues within organizations.

The more traditional clinician-based perspective is commonly called professional ethics. In the past, this conceptualization of medical ethics guided physicians, nurses, and other clinicians when they encountered situations that could be described as "ethical problems." Rather than focusing on rights or principles, or on the healthcare system and its effects, this stream of medical ethics focuses largely on maintaining the professional integrity of the individual clinician and his or her profession.

Professional organizations used traditional professional ethics in creating their professional codes. Within this tradition, codes are seen as guiding beacons for the behavior of practitioners. The codes involve advice and direction, both specific and general, concerning the proper manner of responding to a defined problem or circumstance. In addition, the codes define certain fundamental character traits of the professional practitioner.

How decisions concerning clinical care are perceived, discussed, and acted upon is directly determined by which of these differing perspectives is held to be authoritative. Contemporary bioethics emphasizes the autonomy of patients and the resulting individual rights as primary determining factors. When contemporary bioethics is used as the basis for decision making, clinical decisions require conversations and the sharing of the professional's authority. The final authority to make decisions rests with the patient, and this can lead to a clinician-patient relationship based on contractual considerations, rather than on trust.

Organizational ethics emphasizes the impact of organizational systems and the thinking that is associated with these systems on all decisions within a particular healthcare organization. The values that drive an organization are understood to be the primary determinants answers to all ethical questions, and an organization's management team has significant input to all ethically based decisions, including those that directly affect patient care.

Professional ethics concentrate on the clinician as moral agent. It asks, "What kind of a person should I be to fulfill my professional obligations?" rather than, "What should I do and how should it be done?" Contemporary bioethics perceives ethical problems as cases or situations that have discernible, consistent answers. Organizational ethics looks to an organization's values for answers. Professional ethics perceives an ethical problem as a deviation from accepted professional norms or as a lack of proper attention by a conscientious professional that has led, or may lead, to difficulty for a patient or a professional colleague.

As attention to contemporary bioethics and organizational ethics has increased, the potential for confusion has likewise increased. There is an unavoidable tension between the viewpoints of bioethics and organizational ethics and the viewpoint of professional ethics, particularly when we attempt to decide what is right in an actual situation. For example,

- Should an institutional ethics committee be concerned only with issues that involve patients' rights, or should it also be concerned with issues of professional integrity?
- Should a physician who is struggling with an ethical issue look to guidance from contemporary bioethics or to professional codes of ethics for help in understanding and addressing a problem?
- Should a hospital's values be considered in end-of-life decisions?

These and similar questions illustrate some of the sources of this tension and confusion.

Professional organizations, such as the American Medical Association (AMA), may have actually contributed to the confusion by not clearly distinguishing between professional ethics and the other two perspectives in its work. The Council on Ethical and Judicial Affairs (CEJA), AMA's group that interprets its *Code of Medical Ethics,* and issues *Current Opinions* on subjects of ethical importance, has attempted to consolidate bioethics and professional ethics by incorporating the viewpoint of contemporary bioethics into its code. In the early 1990s, CEJA added a new section to the *Code of Medical Ethics* called "Fundamental Elements of the Patient-Physician Relationship," and defined these fundamental elements in terms of the patients' rights, rather than the more traditional physicians' obligations.[2] In the 2002-2003 *Code of Medical Ethics,* "Fundamental Elements" was dropped as a part of the *Code,* but continues as part of the *Opinions.*[3] In a number of its opinions on ethical issues, CEJA has addressed bioethics issues, has used the language of bioethics, and has appealed directly to contemporary bioethics for the foundational authority for its opinions. In doing so, CEJA has gone beyond its mandated role of interpreting the *Code of Medical Ethics* and defining an ethical physician via opinions about the physician's obligations in specific circumstances.

In 1997, AMA began an Ethics Standards Group to study and promote professionalism, which, on its surface, seemed to be a response to a perceived need for some return to a traditional viewpoint. However, at the same time, the AMA initiated an Institute for Ethics that is an academic research and training center on ethics in healthcare, which has had a bioethics viewpoint in its studies and educational activities.[4]

CEJA's own confusion in distinguishing between bioethics and professional ethics is demonstrated by the turnabout in its opinions relating to the use of the organs of anencephalic infants for transplantation. This issue is an appropriate one for CEJA to consider, because as long as anencephalic infants are defined by society as "human" and "alive," the physician's traditional obligation for protection pertains. This position was the crux of the opinion issued in 1988.[5] However, the 1988 opinion was radically revised in March 1992. The following statement from the 1992 opinion demonstrates the complete reversal of the earlier position: "It is ethically permissible to consider the anencephalic as a potential organ donor, although alive still under present definitions of death."[6]

Instead of questioning society's definition concerning the humanity of the anencephalic infant, CEJA reversed a primary obligation of physicians (to protect the patient) with that single opinion. Predictably, there was significant disagreement with this action in the AMA House of Delegates and elsewhere. CEJA issued another opinion in 1996, reversing the 1992 opinion and reverting back to the 1988 position that requires determination of death prior to using the organs of anencephalic infants for transplantation.[7] This reversal demonstrates a lack of understanding within the AMA itself of the important differences between contemporary bioethics and professional medical ethics, in that a bioethics issue (defining the humanity of an anencephalic infant) was equated with interpreting the *Code of Medical Ethics* to define clearly the obligations of an ethical physician to anencephalic infants.

The AMA has paid little direct attention to organizational ethics, although it has issued several "Opinions" concerning relationships between physicians and hospitals, and the Institute of Ethics has studied and continues to study issues related to the healthcare organization and its role in decision making.

Whether there can ever be a realistic accommodation between these differing perspectives concerning the ethics of clinical care remains an open question. The attempts toward accommodation to date have fallen far short of being effective in decreasing the tension that is naturally present among these viewpoints. Contemporary bioethics — with its influence on courts and legislatures, its strong backing from most of academia, and its fundamental position emphasizing patients' rights — seems to be ascendant at present. The healthcare organization's influence on all decisions made within its walls continues to increase, and its impact on these decisions cannot be denied. So, what of a traditional view of the physician-patient relationship? Our society still shows a strong desire for a relationship between a clinician and patient based on trust rather than on negotiation grounded in "rights," or on the often more nebulous "values" of the healthcare institution. The ideal of the old-fashioned doctor still seems to strike a chord in most people, and people seldom question the desirability of healthcare professions that adhere to a fundamental internal ethos.

This chapter explores the history and fundamentals of the professional ethics viewpoint specifically for physicians and nurses. It points out the value of this viewpoint for individual patients and society and calls attention to some problematic areas. Finally, it briefly explores some possible areas of accommodation and coexistence between traditional professional ethics and contemporary bioethics and/or organizational ethics.

II. HISTORICAL BACKGROUND

A. Professional Medical Ethics

The Code of Hammurabi was the first known code of conduct for medical practitioners. Conceived by the Babylonians about 2000 BCE, it set forth in considerable detail the conduct demanded of a physician. Because it was very specific for that time and culture, it has not continued as a practical set of professional guidelines and is only of interest for historical reasons.

Portions of the body of work attributed to the Hippocratic School, such as the Hippocratic Oath, on the other hand, have continued to the present time as a basic statement of principles upon which the practice of medicine should rest. This statement of principles was likely conceived in the fifth century BCE. Unlike the Code of Hammurabi, the Hippocratic Oath set out, in brief form, a general statement of ideals that protected patients by appealing to the finer instincts of the physician, without imposing sanctions.

I swear by Apollo the Physician and Ascleplus and Hygeia and Panakeia and all the gods and goddesses, making them my witnesses, that I will fulfill according to my ability and judgment this oath and this covenant:

To hold him who has taught me this art as equal to my parents and to live my life in partnership with him, and if he is in need of money to give him a share of mine, and to regard his offspring as equal to my brothers in male lineage and to teach them this art, if they desire to learn it, without fee and covenant; to give a share of precepts and oral instructions and all the other learning to my sons and to the sons of him who has instructed me and to pupils who have signed the covenant and have taken an oath according to the medical law, but to no one else.

I will apply dietetic measures for the benefit of the sick according to my ability and judgment; I will keep them from harm and injustice.

I will neither give a deadly drug to anybody if asked for it, nor will I make a suggestion to this effect. Similarly I will not give to a woman an abortive remedy. In purity and holiness I will guard my life and my art.

I will not use the knife, not even on sufferers from stone, but will withdraw in favor of such men as are engaged in this work.

Whatever houses I may visit, I will come for the benefit of the sick, remaining free of all intentional injustice, of all mischief, and in particular of sexual relations with both female and male persons, be they free or slaves.

What I may see or hear in the course of the treatment or even outside of the treatment in regard to the life of men, which on no account one must spread abroad, I will keep to myself holding such things shameful [unspeakable] to be spoken about.

If I fulfill this oath and do not violate it, may it be granted to me to enjoy life and art, being honored with fame among all men for all time to come. If I transgress it and swear falsely, may the opposite of all this be true.[8]

Other civilizations since ancient Greece have developed written principles concerning the practice of medicine, but the Oath of Hippocrates (modified in the eleventh century to eliminate reference to pagan gods) has remained as an expression of ideal conduct for the physician. The distinguishing aspects of the Hippocratic Oath are its strong emphasis on beneficence toward the patient, on the physician's acquisition and maintenance of competence, and on certain self-serving practices to limit admission into the profession.[9]

Following Hippocrates and other early Greek philosophers, the development of the professional ethics of medicine is linked to traditional values associated with the Christian, Jewish, and Islamic religions. These ties fostered the development of compassion and other humane ideals in addition to the competence and beneficence emphasized by the Greek codes.

Al-Ruhawi, an Islamic physician, wrote what is probably the earliest systematic treatise on medical ethics in the Arabic world in the eighth century. In this treatise, al-Ruhawi tempered the ideals of the Greeks and the Islamic prophets with concrete judgments arising from bedside practices. His efforts to give realistic guidelines for action, derived from basic religious and philosophical tenets within the context of the everyday problems faced by the physician, are quite modern in their outlook.[10]

Isaac Israeli, a Jewish physician and contemporary of al-Ruhawi, also wrote extensively. His works include "The Book of Admonitions to the Physicians."[11] These admonitions, although written within the Jewish tradition, are notably secular and include issues such as thorough knowledge, attention to patients' needs, and prompt response. The admonitions relied on ancient authorities including those from the Hippocratic tradition, and emphasized the healing power of nature. Jewish religious ideals were sustained in the provocative and sobering "Daily Prayer of a Physician," attributed to Moses Maimonides, a physician and philosopher of the late twelfth century.[12] This prayer begins with references to the creation of the human body by God and its purpose as the envelope of the soul. The prayer's major theme is a request for help and support for the physician as he works to benefit mankind. It asks for inspiration leading to love of the art of medicine and God's creatures. It asks for confidence from patients so as to ensure compliance with the physician's counsel. It also asks that the physician's soul be receptive to education, be gentle and calm, and be forgiving of the arrogance of others.

In their search for professional ethics, Christian physicians attempted to reconcile the ideals of the Hippocratic tradition with their religious values. The physician was looked upon as an agent of God, with God as the ultimate healer. More practically, the physician was urged to be modest, chaste, and humble, as well as charming and affable (the latter two were hardly religious ideals). As fundamental sources of ideals, medieval physicians ignored neither the Greek philosophical legacy nor the Christian Church and its teachings, but many did attempt to apply these ideals to contemporary practice in a practical way.[13]

In this fashion, professional medical values became enmeshed with religious values. As an alternative to the priesthood, medicine was also a profession to which one could be "called," and the physician was seen as a conduit for God's power to heal the sick.

In the late eighteenth century, John Gregory, a Scottish physician and philosopher, advanced a virtue-based concept of what it means to be a physician and the character necessary to fulfill the professional obligations.[14] The next significant contribution to the development of modern professional medical ethics was made by the English physician, Thomas Percival, when he published his *Code of Medical Ethics* in 1803.[15] This was a "scheme of professional conduct relative to hospitals and other charities." Percival followed the Hippocratic tradition and included such admonitions as physicians must "keep heads clear and hands steady" by observing constant temperance. Percival's code emphasized professional etiquette.

The first items of discussion at the initial meeting of the AMA in 1847 were the establishment of a code of ethics and the creation of minimum requirements for medical education.[16] Certain state medical societies had formal written codes of conduct prior to the development of the AMA code, but these tended to be provincial. The AMA's *Principles of Medical Ethics* were based on Percival's code to a larger extent than any of the previously established state codes. To some extent, the AMA *Principles* were used to exclude those who were trained in other schools or philosophies of medical practice.[17] In general, the language and concepts of the original AMA code remained unchanged until recently. It included matters of professional etiquette as well as principles related to the care of patients.

In 1957, the AMA revised the format of the *Principles* to include 10 short sections, preceded by a preamble that "succinctly express[es] the fundamental concepts embodied in the present [1955] *Principles*." When presenting this change to the AMA House of Delegates, the AMA Judicial Council stated: "every basic principle has been preserved; on the other hand, as much as possible of the prolixity and ambiguity which in the past obstructed ready explanation, practical codification and particular selection of basic concepts has been eliminated."[18] In 1977, the Judicial Council recommended that the *Principles* be revised "to clarify and update the language, to eliminate reference to gender, and to seek a proper and reasonable balance between professional standards and contemporary legal standards in our changing society."[19]

The Judicial Council of the AMA has subsequently been renamed the Council on Ethical and Judicial Affairs. This is the body responsible for interpreting and recommending changes to the *Code of Medical Ethics,* for investigating general ethical conditions and all matters pertaining to the relations of physicians to one another or to the public, and for making recommendations to the House of Delegates (the ruling body of the AMA) or the constituent associations (those organizations that comprise the membership of the AMA, including state medical societies).

The present *Code of Medical Ethics* consists of three related parts: (1) "Principles of Medical Ethics," which is the fundamental statement of the core principles of the code; (2) "Current Opinions," which reflect the application of the principles to numerous specific ethical issues in medicine (it is here that CEJA has gone well beyond its mandate and addressed bioethics issues); and (3) "Reports" on issues of importance and interest prior to or concurrent with the issuance of an opinion.[20]

The AMA's "Principles of Medical Ethics" are as follows:

PREAMBLE:

The medical profession has long subscribed to a body of ethical statements developed primarily for the benefit of the patient. As a member of this profession, a physician must recognize responsibility not only to patients, but also to society, to other health professionals, and to self. The following Principles adopted by the American Medical Association are not laws, but standards of conduct which define the essentials of honorable behavior for the physician.

I. A physician shall be dedicated to providing competent medical care, with compassion and respect for human dignity and rights.

II. A physician shall uphold the standards of professionalism, be honest in all professional interactions, and strive to report physicians deficient in character or competence, or engaging in fraud or deception, to appropriate entities.

III. A physician shall respect the law and also recognize a responsibility to seek changes in those requirements which are contrary to the best interests of the patient.

IV. A physician shall respect the rights of patients, colleagues, and other health professionals, and shall safeguard patient confidences and privacy within the constraints of the law.

V. A physician shall continue to study, apply and advance scientific knowledge, maintain a commitment to medical education, make relevant information available to patients, colleagues, and the public, obtain consultation, and use the talents of other health professionals when indicated.

VI. A physician shall, in the provision of appropriate patient care, except in emergencies, be free to choose whom to serve, with whom to associate, and the environment in which to provide medical care.

VII. A physician shall recognize a responsibility to participate in activities contributing to the improvement of the community and the betterment of public health.

VIII. A physician shall, while caring for a patient, regard responsibility to the patient as paramount.

IX. A physician shall support access to medical care for all people.[21]

B. Professional Nursing Ethics

Contemporary bioethics has involved nurses from the beginning. The nursing profession and its major organizations have supported the clinical activities of bioethics much more than has the medical profession. The development of bioethics came at a time of significant change in attitudes toward the basic concepts of nursing professional ethics, as defined by the initial codes of the American Nurses Association (ANA). It may be that the changes in attitude toward nursing ethics meshed with perspectives in contemporary bioethics and that the timing was right for a symbiosis of the nursing profession and those involved with contemporary bioethics. Nurses may also have seen that the rights-based concepts that were being advanced by contemporary bioethics, if generally accepted, would have led to a greater sharing of clinical power by physicians and an advancement in the power allotted to nurses. Also, since nurses often work for healthcare organizations, they are therefore more aware of the influence of an organization's values on decisions that affect the ethical care of individual patients.

The origin of professional nursing ethics is usually attributed to Florence Nightingale and her concepts of responsible obedience to the physician, as developed during the Crimean War (1854-1857).[22] Nightingale is known as the founder of modern nursing because of her organizational work during the Crimean War; her subsequent activities, including founding the Nightingale Nursing School in 1860; and her concepts of preventive medicine, developed in an 1893 paper. In this famous work, she exhorted that it was important to treat the sick person rather than the disease, that prevention is much better than cure, that hospitalization does not necessarily lead to health, and that nursing must hold to its ideals as represented in the Nightingale Pledge.[23] The Nightingale Pledge is as follows:

> I solemnly pledge myself before God and in the presence of this assembly; To pass my life in purity and to practice my profession faithfully; I will abstain from whatever is deleterious and mischievous and will not take or knowingly administer any harmful drug. I will do all in my power to maintain and elevate the standard of my profession and will hold in confidence all personal matters committed to my keeping and all family affairs coming to my knowledge in the practice of my calling. With loyalty I will endeavor to aid the physician in his work, and devote myself to the welfare of those committed to my care.[24]

Nightingale's emphasis on the duty of the nurse to obey the physician has become an anachronism. However, scrutiny of her writings reveals that she did not call for blind obedience; rather, she advocated responsible obedience, with the needs of the patient being a primary consideration.

From the mid-1970s until recently, the major guiding concept in the professional ethics of nursing as articulated by the ANA has been "client advocacy." This line of thought developed at that particular time for a number of reasons: decreasing esteem for physicians; the beginnings of feminism, consumerism, and patients' rights movements; and an overall climate of increasing self-determination for patients and for healthcare professionals — including nurses, but excluding physicians. Client advocacy emphasized the autonomy and rights of the patient, as does contemporary bioethics; it is based on a freely expressed contract between the professional and the patient, which is in contrast to the earlier emphasis on care and beneficence with the physician as the final decision-making authority.[25]

As a reaction to ANA's adoption of a *Code of Ethics for Nurses* based on client advocacy in 1976, some writers focused renewed attention on caring as an important aspect of the nurse-patient encounter. Sally Gadow, a prominent proponent of this position in nursing, has written that care is the supreme covenant between the nurse and patient, and that care is the moral basis for the nurse-patient relationship.[26] Adeline Falk Rafael has attempted to combine the concepts of caring and power into a single concept that she calls "empowered caring." She sees this idea as moving beyond "power over" others to include power that enables others.[27] She believes that empowered caring should be grounded in knowledge and driven by caring. Neither Gadow nor Rafael envisioned a return to the traditional subservient position of the nurse to the physician. As attention to caring as a primary attribute of the nurse increased, the ANA revised its *Code* in 2001 to reflect this attitude. The ANA had originally adopted its code of ethics in 1950, and extensively revised it in 1976 (to client advocacy as the primary focus). The code was again extensively revised in 2001, with a middle-of-the-road approach between client advocacy and caring, and interpretive statements were added.

Provisions of *The Code of Ethics for Nurses* adopted by the ANA in 2001, are as follows:

1. The nurse, in all professional relationships, practices with compassion and respect for the inherent dignity, worth and uniqueness of every individual, unrestricted by considerations of social or economic status, personal attributes, or the nature of health problems. . . .
2. The nurse's primary commitment is to the patient, whether an individual, family, group, or community. . . .
3. The nurse promotes, advocates for, and strives to protect the health, safety, and rights of the patient. . . .
4. The nurse is responsible and accountable for individual nursing practice and determines the appropriate delegation of tasks consistent with the nurse's obligation to provide optimum patient care. . . .
5. The nurse owes the same duties to self as to others, including the responsibility to preserve integrity and safety, to maintain competence, and to continue personal and professional growth. . . .

6. The nurse participates in establishing, maintaining and improving healthcare environments and conditions of employment conducive to the provision of quality healthcare and consistent with the values of the profession through individual and collective action. . . .

7. The nurse participates in the advancement of the profession through contributions to practice, education, administration, and knowledge development. . . .

8. The nurse collaborates with other health professionals and the public in promoting community, national, and international efforts to meet health needs. . . .

9. The profession of nursing, as represented by associations and their members, is responsible for articulating nursing values, for maintaining the integrity of the profession and its practice, and for shaping social policy. . . . [The interpretive statements have not been included.][28]

III. DEFINING THE PROFESSIONAL AND THE PROFESSIONAL PRACTICE

What is a "profession"? The definitions vary widely, but most include the following elements.
1. Advanced training,
2. A well-defined and circumscribed role,
3. Continuing education,
4. Control over admission to the profession
5. Responsibility to specified individuals (patients) and to the particular group defined by the "profession,"
6. Devotion to humanistic ideals,
7. A well-defined group of necessary virtues and moral rules that define the ethical parameters of the profession.

Some definitions mention a specific or nonspecific duty to society, the secondary nature of compensation for the work of the professional, and other elements.

Robert Orr, a physician and teacher of ethics to medical students, has written: "In the classic sense being a professional implies a publicly declared vow of dedication or devotion to a way of life. It implies a special knowledge not available to the average person; it is an unequal relationship. But with that special knowledge comes a special responsibility. It is thus a fiduciary relationship in that the possessor of knowledge has a

responsibility of altruism, and the recipient of the special knowledge may thus trust the professional. In other words a professional is a trustworthy trustee."[29]

A. Physicians as Professionals

Allen Dyer, a psychiatrist and author, has stated that the medical profession is defined either by the knowledge and technical expertise of the physician or by the ethics of the professional group, specifically the fiduciary commitments of the doctor-patient relationship.[30] This distinction between knowledge and ethics is anti-Hippocratic, and would once have been unthinkable. From a traditional Hippocratic perspective, knowledge is a very personal quality that cannot be separated from the values of the knower or the user of that knowledge. However, scientific medicine has been so successful as a purveyor of technological knowledge, that it has become much easier to "uncouple" expertise and ethical responsibility. Indeed, it is easier to imagine medicine as merely the application of technology and to view medical service as a commodity, and the medical profession as a business.

It is the increasing acceptance of the separation of clinical competence from compassion and caring for the patient that has, to some extent, fostered the development of contemporary bioethics as a field that is separate from the medical profession. And it is this attitude that is feared, even looked upon with horror, by many in the profession. For most physicians, the medical profession is still defined by its internal ethics, specifically the ethic of human service. They believe that attention to appropriate professional ethical issues, by professional organizations, and attention to proper individual ethical decisions, guided by their own professional and personal conscience, are all that is needed to ensure the ethical practice of medicine. Many physicians see no need for "outsiders," such as academic ethicists or representatives of the healthcare organization, to be involved in the decision-making process in the clinical setting.

B. Professional Ethics and Medical Practice

Views regarding the practice of medicine can be classified as one of three types: (1) the scientific or technological model; (2) the participatory or community model; and (3) the classical or

Hippocratic model.[31] A brief description of each of these models follows, along with discussion of the future of physicians as professionals under each of these models.

The last 30 years have witnessed an emphasis on the *scientific model* of medical practice. This model is based on a mechanistic view of medical practice, and treats the doctor as a biotechnician. In this mode, medicine is susceptible to economic and legal control, and "informed consent," as a contract, is the major limiting factor. This model has not been satisfying for many practitioners, and it has left patients with a less-than-encouraging view of the profession and its work. Its major advantage — if it can be called that — has been to increase dramatically the use of complicated technology and the amount paid for it. Many people see this model as an aberration, and wish a return to a more humanistic approach to medical practice. This particular model contributed to the early development of contemporary bioethics, since scientific "truth" was the goal, and the character of the physician was of little importance. The traditional views of professional ethics were therefore ignored or downplayed under this model.

A second model, the *community or participatory mode of practice,* is based on the concept of equal individual worth and community-based ideals; it requires cooperation between the physician, other clinicians, and the patient and family. It is best represented by the concept of "shared decision making" as defined by the President's Commission for the Study of Ethical Problems in Medicine and Biomedical and Behavioral Research.[32] It gives equal importance to the physician and patient, and emphasizes cooperation. It exists unhappily with the more analytic mechanisms of regulation of the law, and is more comfortable in consensus-seeking endeavors. It can be seen as supportive of organizational ethics.

The *classical model* of medical practice is based on Hippocratic ideals, and begins with the ultimate worth of the doctor's activities (a calling). It depends, to some extent, on mysticism, or at least on beliefs that cannot be proved. The medical profession is seen as a closed discipline whose practitioners regard their work — the relief of human suffering — as their highest duty. The physician and patient are unequal, as are the physician and others involved in the care of the patient. This model is not comfortably responsive to outside regulation, whether it be moral, legal,

or bureaucratic. It is embodied in the quotations derived from the writings of Hippocrates: "Life is short and Art is long; the occasion fleeting; experience fallacious and judgment difficult; the physician must not only be prepared to do what is right himself, but also to make the patient, the attendants and the externals cooperate";[33] and "the physician is the servant of his Art."[34] The Hippocratic, classical ideal is broad enough to encompass ideas from research science, patient-centered but physician-directed medicine, a guild approach to practice and knowledge, and, in large measure, all of the modern approaches to healthcare. It is not broad enough to include a patient- or society-dominated approach — or even a partnership.

Although the Hippocratic ideal of medical practice has been highly criticized recently, it continues as the basic ideal of medical practice for many, both in and out of the profession. This ideal is the foundation for professional ethics in medicine, and until very recently, it has been the only authority upon which the professional codes have been built.

Historically, this ideal represents the first time that the power to heal was vested in a practitioner who was not also a shaman with the power to harm. According to the late anthropologist Margaret Mead, the Hippocratic Oath marked one of the turning points in the history of man. Mead stated: "For the first time in our tradition there was a complete separation between killing and curing. Throughout the primitive world the doctor and the sorcerer tended to be the same person. He, with power to kill had power to cure, including especially the undoing of his own killing activities. He who had power to cure would necessarily also be able to kill. With the Greeks the distinction was made clear. One profession was dedicated completely to life under all circumstances, regardless of rank, age, or intellect — the life of a slave, the life of the Emperor, the life of a child."[35]

The value of traditional medicine as a conservative cultural institution in a time of rapid fundamental changes in other major institutions is also mentioned as an important positive aspect of the traditional Hippocratic ideal.

The major criticisms of the Hippocratic ideal of medical practice are:
1. Hippocratic medicine does not fully address rights of patients and emphasizes relationships of physicians to one another.
2. The Hippocratic ideal opposes abortion and

euthanasia, and modern technology such as prenatal diagnosis, organ transplants, and heart/lung machines are difficult to fit into this schema.

3. This ideal is basically paternalistic.

These criticisms tend to be based only on the Hippocratic Oath and other writings attributed to Hippocrates, and do not consider the more common position of the modern practicing physician — that is, the Hippocratic Oath and subsequent codes should serve as professional beacons that guide the professional course. If legitimate moral ideals are confused with imperatives, they may not be recognized as goals toward which one might strive, but rather held as mandates to which one must adhere.

In specific defense of the Hippocratic ideal, as compared to the other models, the following arguments have been advanced:

1. High technology is inadequate to address the needs of many patients (the scientific model is inadequate).
2. The autonomy and rights of the patient should not always be paramount in medical decision making (professional obligations and responsibility should be considered).
3. The Oath and subsequent codes are reminders and are not meant to be a specific set of rules.
4. Paternalism and self-determination are not mutually exclusive (for example, a wise parent encourages autonomy in the child).
5. With the classical model, if there is a conflict between the best interests of the patient and those of the physician, the best interests of the patient are to have preference.

What are the attributes of the physician required by each of these models? The scientific model requires only a knowledgeable and honest scientist. The community model requires a cooperative, socially aware, and analytic clinician who attends to many aspects of living in his or her practice and is committed to the patient's rights in clinical decision making. The required attributes for the classical model seem at first to be more complex. Religious and/or mystical perspectives have in the past been associated with this mode of practice, but they have become less important in recent years. The physician may or may not be religious and still adhere to this mode of practice. Integrity and character are the major

determinants of the ideal physician in the classical model.

C. Professional Integrity

Theologian Stanley Hauerwas has said, "Integrity, not obligation, is the hallmark of the moral life."[36] Integrity is an integration of beliefs about values and purposes, by which lives are conducted. It is the psychosomatic integration of mind and body including emotions. Integrity is required of the physician who practices under any of the aforementioned models of medical practice. It is most closely associated with the classical model and is the basis for the professional ethics under this model.

The integrity of medicine as a profession and of its practitioners as professionals with professional ideals depends not only on applicable rules and principles, but also on the professional physician and his or her character. The application of professional ethics in medical care depends on this personal integrity of the individual practitioner.

D. The Concept of Medical Practice

What of the concept of "medical practice" and its effects on professional integrity and ethics? The concept has come to mean an organized activity that has, within it, certain standards of excellence that are independent of the uses to which that practice may be put by society. In other words, when one is engaged in a practice, there are internally set norms of excellence to which one must adhere. The integrity of the profession — and of the individual professional — is maintained through this concept. A professional practice is a method to maintain the tenets of the profession and the virtues of the individual professional by reminding the practitioners and the public that a practice does, in fact, exist.

Certain controversial issues have arisen in relation to the integrity of a medical practice and the ethical aspects of certain decisions and activities within this context. Two of the more important of these issues, the concept of futility and its relationship to clinical decision making and the professional's right to refuse to include certain types of patients in his or her practice, are important examples of practice-related controversies.

E. Futility

What is "futile" medical care, and how should this concept be considered in relation to the integrity of a professional and his or her practice?

The AMA defines futility in strictly physiological terms — that is, the treatment will not have the desired physiologic effect. (For example, penicillin for a viral sore throat is futile treatment; if cardiopulmonary resuscitation cannot be expected to restore cardiopulmonary function, then it is also futile treatment).

A second, more common, conceptualization of futility is that an intervention is futile if it fails to produce any benefit for the patient. (Here, consideration of quality of life, as defined by the patient and/or the patient's surrogate, come into play.)

A third definition of futility, advanced by Howard Brody, a physician-ethicist at Michigan State University School of Medicine, is that a treatment is futile if it fails to achieve any reasonable purpose of treatment, which can occur in three circumstances:

1. The probability of benefit is unacceptably low,
2. The magnitude of benefit is unacceptably small, or
3. The harm is much too great relative to any benefit.[37]

The definition that one uses is important, because, in our society, an intervention that is considered futile is often not ethically or legally required, and is, therefore, optional.

The integrity of medicine as a profession requires that members of the profession have the authority to determine what counts as truth, in the area of professional expertise. The physician has the obligation and authority to decide, within the confines of good professional practice, whether a possible treatment should be considered. If this authority is to have meaning, it must extend to decisions concerning the futility of specific interventions — particularly when considered under the strict physiologic definition of futility. Based on the same arguments, the physician as a professional has the authority to make decisions concerning futility, when defined as a lack of benefit or lack of therapeutic reasonableness, as long as the physician makes the decision after consideration of the patient's life plan. Brody argues that this is a professional decision that affects the patient's quality of life (as do essentially all professional decisions), but, when made in the context of knowledge of the patient and his or her values, is a proper decision for the physician, and it would be improper for anybody else outside a professional practice to make such a decision.[38]

In spite of these arguments, this matter is far from settled — and the debate continues. Physician and ethicist Edmund Pellegrino, discussing the concept of futility, has written: "It has been and continues to be useful, however, because it exposes the need for carefully weighing the limits of both physician and patient autonomy, the explicit meaning of participation, and the relative reliability and moral weight of objective medical and subjective value determinations. Underlying these issues are deeper philosophical questions about the nature of medical knowledge, the relationship between fact and value and the moral status of the physician's conscience in a pluralistic and democratic society like ours, which so highly prizes individual autonomy."[39]

F. Professional Refusal

Another area of controversy affecting the professional integrity of the physician and his or her practice is that of refusing to accept a particular patient into the practice. This notion is stated in the AMA *Code of Medical Ethics* as, "A physician shall, in the provision of appropriate patient care, except in emergencies, be free to choose whom to serve, with whom to associate, and the environment in which to provide medical care."[40]

Some physicians have been criticized for refusing to see patients with certain diseases, such as acquired immunodeficiency syndrome (AIDS), or for refusing to see patients based on their financial status. Are these criticisms warranted? How can behavior, which on the face of it seems "unjust," be defended as a fundamental tenet that is necessary to maintain the integrity of the profession and its members?

Although society licenses professions and allows them to operate within certain parameters, society has been loath to try to change fundamental internal professional tenets. The tendency has been to allow professions to develop their own standards for practice and to maintain these standards through self-regulation or methods prescribed by the profession.

The medical profession, through the AMA and other professional organizations, defends its stand that allows physicians to choose who shall be admitted to their practice based on the necessity to maintain the practice as an individually controlled entity, and on physicians' civil rights as individuals. Within this context, the reasons for refusing to accept certain specific patients or patients belonging to a particular group must be ethically defensible. Consider the following example. A pediatrician refuses to write a prescription for the parent of one of her 10-year-old patients on the basis that she is not as knowledgeable concerning adult patients and is therefore not as competent to treat this parent as are other, easily accessible, physicians in the immediate area. She could be prescribing less than optimum treatment when optimum treatment is available. This refusal is based on professional concepts of competence that are necessary to maintain the integrity of the profession, and, as such, is ethical.

A less clear situation occurs when a person with a particular medical-payment mechanism is refused entry into the professional practice solely on the basis of the method of payment. It has not been uncommon for some physicians to refuse to admit Medicaid and/or Medicare patients to their practices. Their reasons for this refusal include the following.

1. Treating these patients requires a significant increase in paperwork and regulatory burdens.
2. Interaction with these patients created increased external regulation.
3. Some physicians believe that Medicaid and Medicare are forms of governmental control of medical practice and that is antagonistic toward good patient care.
4. A significant decrease in income from this group of patients requires shifting costs to other patients, which many patients consider to be unfair.

When the physician continues his or her obligation to attend all people as patients in an emergency, and when adequate care is available elsewhere, this sort of refusal has been considered minimally acceptable. In defending such a refusal, physicians have correctly pointed out that they, under most conditions, are not allowed to treat Medicaid and Medicare patients for free or for a minimal, reduced fee. Bureaucratic requirements for these patients must be met or legal sanctions against the physician can be instituted.

Does a professional practice's refusal to accept certain patients contradict the professional ethical standard that patients should be treated without regard to income or ability to pay? If the refusal is based on reasons other than decreased payment for services, if there are other available avenues for the patient to receive adequate care, and if the physician would treat individual patients in this payment class under the same conditions as his or her other patients and without regard to income or payment, then many believe that this refusal is ethical and should be supported. Refusal based only on economic factors would not likely be considered ethical by any professional body.

What about refusal to treat certain patients based on their particular disease? A number of professional practices do not accept patients with AIDS. The stated reasons include the following:
1. Physicians may fear they lack expertise to treat these patients.
2. Other patients fear patients with AIDS.
3. Physicians fear possible transmission of the disease to staff and themselves.
4. Physicians fear decreased income.
5. Physicians fear negative social reactions.

There is little question that the first of these reasons, lack of expertise, is ethically sound, unless the physician is guilty of not maintaining or achieving standard competence. All of the other reasons are questionable, because the patient's well-being and needs have been made a secondary consideration to the well-being and needs of others or of the practice.

The CEJA states, "A physician may not ethically refuse to treat a patient whose condition is within the physician's realm of competence solely because the patient is (HIV) seropositive. The tradition of the AMA since 1847 is that: when an epidemic prevails, a physician must continue his labors without regard to his own health."[41]

IV. LEGAL CONSIDERATIONS

The impersonal view of physicians that can be seen in the technological model seems firmly established in most aspects of the law. In recent decisions, the courts have permitted advertising among physicians and have modified the historical professional ethics mandate to maintain absolute confidentiality. In *Tarasoff v. Regents of the University of California,* the court ruled that physicians are required to ignore patient confidentiality if significant harm to a specific person could likely be prevented.[42] There are now mandatory reporting requirements for a number of clinical situations, and mandatory review of medical records by numerous others in governmental and insurance reimbursement plans. With the passage of HIPAA (the Health Insurance Portability and Accountability Act) of 1996, and its final implementation in 2003, the government's attention to confidentiality and privacy in healthcare became more stringent. Whether any or all of these legal requirements concerning confidentiality are beneficial is still an open question.

Other individual court decisions (such as *Quinlan, Cruzan,* and *A.C.*)[43] that primarily concern decision making at the end of life seem to favor the community model of practice. These decisions have made specific reference to the advantages of hospital ethics committees and the consideration of serious end-of-life decisions by all interested parties.

Few recent court decisions favor the classical model, except to use certain professional codes as the behavioral standard to which a practitioner must adhere. Chapter 4 considers legal aspects in detail.

V. ADVICE FOR
PROFESSIONAL STUDENTS

What advice can be given to students of clinical professions, particularly medical students, concerning their duties to patients, to their profession, to society, and to themselves? Should they be concerned only with the contemporary bioethics viewpoint and its focus on patients' rights, or should they adhere to a more traditional concept of obligation to the patient, above all, as the primary determinant of ethical soundness? How much attention to the values of the organization within which one practices is indicated? These questions are not easily answered, and the answers depend upon many factors, including current law, other ethical parameters sanctioned by society, professional ethical mandates, and the conscience and character of the individual student.

Student clinicians should study and learn what these societal and professional mandates require, and the historical and other reasons for these requirements (the focus of this text). Students should observe and listen to and discuss with others, within and outside of the profession, these issues and how they do and should affect medical care. Students should consider what their chosen profession has meant historically, what they believe it means now, and how they would like to see it meet future ethical challenges. Finally, students should attempt to know themselves, be self-critical, and use their innate character as a basis for thinking about and developing their conscience and personal ethical outlook toward the profession generally, and toward their relationship to the profession and the patients it serves.

There are no magic lists of virtues, principles, case studies, organizational values statements, or codes that will guarantee success. The search for the ethics of clinical care is a continuing process that can never be totally completed, so looking for one "answer" should be discouraged. Education that is based on this textbook and similar texts and courses can be used as a beginning, but professional and personal ethical education should continue throughout one's professional career.

Albert Jonsen has written: "At a time when the genuine nobility of medicine is compromised and threatened from within and without, at a time when many of medicine's younger practitioners either have forgotten or have never learned the ethos of noblesse oblige, the challenge is the choice of an ethos — or rather the renewed commitment to an ethos."[44]

VI. FINAL CONSIDERATIONS

Beginning in the 1960s, society demanded a change from the traditional mode of medical practice, in which physicians were making newly possible life-and-death decisions for patients without inquiring about their values and desires. The pendulum swung from physician-dominated clinical decisions to patient-dominated decisions. Patient autonomy and the patient's right to make decisions became the most important aspect of the relationship, and the move from the physician as a trusted ally to the physician as a provider began. In the 1990s, further erosion of the traditional concept of the benevolent, paternalistic physician occurred when attention to the healthcare organization and its influences on decisions within its walls began.

Since the advent of contemporary bioethics, those following its lead have paid almost exclusive attention to the application of principles (particularly patient autonomy and the rights encompassed by this autonomy) as the foundation for proper ethical decision making, and have neglected the medical professional — both as an individual and as a member of a profession. Now, in addition, those with power within the healthcare organization are also exercising this power by using it to become involved in *all* decisions made within the confines of the organization.

But, there is still a reluctance to dismiss the tradition of professional ethics. Many believe this dismissal would lead to further decrease in the trusting relationship desired by many patients and their physicians. The recent perceived loss of some of the traditional virtues associated with the "old-fashioned family doctor" has caused consternation. Some also fear that, as the influence of traditional professional ethics diminishes, professional devotion to competence and compassion may also decrease.

This issue of the authority of professional ethics is not just academic; the future direction of the medical profession and the attitudes of society toward physicians and, indirectly, toward other clinicians and healthcare organizations hang in the balance. Should medicine receive its mandates on the ethics of medical care based on specific principles and procedures imposed by society, or based on the values of a healthcare organization? Or, should physicians and other clinical professionals concentrate on developing a stronger and more responsive professional ethics of their own?

A fusion of these pathways is unlikely, because their perspectives are so different. However, it may be possible to develop a positive coexistence that relegates the larger societal issues associated with medical care (such as the definition of death, the regulation of information and processes from the Human Genome Project, and issues related to financing medical care) to the bioethics community for consideration (with appropriate input from the profession but no authority for the final decision), that relegates most healthcare funding and payment issues, as well as many of the confidentiality issues, to the healthcare organization, but allows traditional professional ethics to continue to define an ethical clinician in terms of his or her professional obligations.

Edmund Pellegrino recently addressed the issue of the importance of maintaining a traditional professional ethics for medicine. In commenting on the present-day relevance of the Hippocratic Oath, he stated: "This is no mere academic skirmish. Its practical consequences affect all of society and all of us as physicians and citizens. No human being can escape the reality of being sick and being cared for. All must seriously contemplate what a divided profession without a common set of moral commitments would mean. Most important, we are obligated to ask how patients might fare in the hands of a profession with its moral fabric in tatters."[45]

NOTES

1. *In re Quinlan,* 70 N.J. 10, 355 A.2d 647 (1976); *In re Conroy,* 98 N.J. 321, 486 A.2d 1209 (1985); *Cruzan v. Harmon,* 760 S.W. 2d 408, at 411 (Mo. 1988) (*en banc*).

2. American Medical Association (AMA), Council on Ethical and Judicial Affairs (CEJA), "Fundamental Elements of the Patient-Physician Relationship," in *Code of Medical Ethics* (Chicago, Ill.: AMA, 1996), xli-xliii.

3. AMA, CEJA, "Fundamental Elements of the Patient-Physician Relationship," in *Code of Medical Ethics* (Chicago, Ill.: AMA, 2002), 281-2.

4. "Ethics Standards Group," in *Mission and Organization* (Chicago, Ill.: AMA, 2003), available at *www.ama-assn.org.*

5. AMA, CEJA, "Anencephalic Infants as Organ Donors," in *Reports* (Chicago, Ill.: AMA, December 1988).

6. AMA, CEJA, "Anencephalic Infants as Organ Donors," in *Current Opinions* (Chicago, Ill.: AMA, March 1992).

7. AMA, CEJA, "Anencephalic Neonates as Organ Donors," in *Current Opinions* (Chicago, Ill.: AMA, June 1996).

8. J. Areen et al., *Law, Science and Medicine* (Mineola, N.Y.: Foundation Press, 1984), 273.

9. Hippocrates, *The Theory and Practice of Medicine* (New York: Philosophical Library, 1964).

10. M. Levey, "Medical Ethics of Medieval Islam with Special Reference to Al-Ruhawi's Practical Ethics of the Physician," *Transactions of the American Philosophical Society* 57, part 3 (1967): 18-94.

11. I. Israeli, "The Book of Admonitions to the Physician," in C.R. Burns, *Legacies in Ethics and Medicine* (New York: Neale Watson Academic Publications, 1977).

12. M. Maimonides, "Daily Prayer of a Physician," in C.R. Burns, *Legacies in Ethics and Medicine* (New York: Neale Watson Academic Publications, 1977), 145-70.

13. Ibid., 181-203.

14. L. McCullough, *John Gregory and the In-*

vention of Professional Medical Ethics and the Profession of Medicine (Dordrecht, the Netherlands: Kluwer Academic, 1998), 1-13.

15. C. Leake, *Percival's Medical Ethics* (Baltimore, Md.: Williams & Wilkins, 1927).

16. AMA, "Principles of Medical Ethics," *http://www.ama-assn.org/ama/pub/category/4256.html.*

17. Ibid.

18. AMA, CEJA, *Code of Medical Ethics* (Chicago, Ill.: AMA, 1996), xi.

19. Ibid.

20. AMA, CEJA, *Code of Medical Ethics* (Chicago, Ill.: AMA, 2002), x-xi.

21 Ibid., xiv.

22. N.J. Bishop and S. Goldie, *A Bio-Bibliography of Florence Nightingale* (London: International Council of Nurses, 1962).

23. Ibid.

24. C.A. Quinn and M.D. Smith, *The Professional Commitment: Issues and Ethics in Nursing* (Philadelphia, Pa.: W.B. Saunders, 1987), 179.

25. G.L. Husted and J.H. Husted, *Ethical Decision Making in Nursing* (St. Louis, Mo.: Mosby-Yearbook, 1991), 27-38.

26. S. Gadow, "Covenant Without Cure: Letting Go and Holding On in Chronic Illness," in *The Ethics of Care and the Ethics of Cure: Synthesis in Chronicity,* ed. J. Watson and M. Ray (New York: National League of Nursing, 1988).

27. A.R.F. Rafael, "Power and Caring: A Dialectic in Nursing," *Advances in Nursing Science* 19, no. 1 (1996): 3-17.

28. *Code for Nurses* (Kansas City, Mo.: American Nurses Association, 2001).

29. R.D. Orr, "Personal and Professional Integrity in Clinical Medicine," *Update* 8, no. 4 (1992): 1-3.

30. A. Dyer, *Ethics and Psychiatry: Toward Professional Definition* (Washington, D.C.: American Psychiatric Institute, 1988), 4-5.

31. J.M. Jacob, *Doctors and Rules* (New York: Routledge, 1988).

32. President's Commission for the Study of Ethical Problems in Medicine and Biomedical and Behavioral Research, *Making Health Care Decisions,* vol. 1 (Washington, D.C.: U.S. Government Printing Office, 1982).

33. G.E.R. Lloyd, ed., *Hippocratic Writings,* J. Chadwick and W.N. Mann, tran. (New York: Penguin Books, 1978), 206.

34. Ibid.

35. M. Levine, *Psychiatry and Ethics* (New York: George Brazilier, 1972), 324-5.

36. S. Hauerwas, *Community and Character* (Notre Dame, Ind.: University of Notre Dame Press, 1981), 48.

37. H. Brody, *The Healer's Power* (New Haven, Conn.: Yale University Press, 1992), 174.

38. Ibid., 176.

39. E.D. Pellegrino, "Ethics," *Journal of the American Medical Association* 270, no. 2 (1993): 203.

40. See note 16 above, p. xiv.

41. Ibid., 157

42. *Tarasoff v. Regents of the University of California,* 131 Cal.Rptr. 14, 551 P.2d 334 (1976).

43. See note 1 above.

44. A. Jonsen, *The New Medicine and the Old Ethics* (Cambridge, Mass.: Harvard University Press, 1990), 78.

45. E.D. Pellegrino, "Ethics," *Journal of the American Medical Association* 275, no. 23 (June 1996): 1807-9.

3

Introduction to Organizational Ethics

Ann E. Mills and Edward M. Spencer

But isn't this a text about clinical ethics?

Isn't organizational ethics just business ethics applied to healthcare administrators?

We are ethics committee members and are interested in patient care issues — we know nothing about organizational ethics — and we don't need to.

Concerns similar to those above have been voiced by people interested in the major theme of this text who are skeptical of the relevance of organizational ethics to the major issues in patient-care ethics. This chapter is meant as an answer to these and similar skeptical statements and queries as to why a chapter on organizational ethics is included.

In attempting to address these questions, we will define organizational ethics in healthcare, define how it originated and what it means today, and explain why we believe its importance will increase, not only for the business and management aspects of healthcare organizations (HCOs) and the healthcare system as a whole, but for ethical patient-care practice as well. We believe a strong case can be made that healthcare organizational ethics will be the pre-eminent ethical perspective in HCOs, and in healthcare practice generally, in the near future.

I. THE INTRODUCTION OF ORGANIZATIONAL ETHICS

Realizing that the turmoil in the healthcare market was damaging HCO relationships, and perhaps realizing that quality of care may be more than a simple resource issue,[1] the Joint Commission on Accreditation of Healthcare Organizations (JCAHO), in 1995, expanded the "Patient Rights" section of its accreditation manual to include a mandate that requires HCOs to conduct their business and patient-care practices in an "honest, decent and proper manner."[2] The JCAHO called this mandate "organization ethics." A broader, more process-oriented definition of healthcare organizational ethics has since been advanced by the Virginia Healthcare Ethics Network: "Organization ethics consists of [a set of] processes to address ethical issues associated with the business, financial, and management areas of healthcare organizations, as well as with professional, educational, and contractual relationships affecting the operation of the healthcare organization."[3]

This definition encompasses all aspects of the operation of the HCO and includes the articulation, application, and evaluation of the organization's mission and values statements. Both approaches to organizational ethics acknowledge that the quality of care experienced by patients depends in part on the values the HCO lives by and the relationships it has with its stakeholders. Both approaches insist that HCOs pay attention to these relationships by creating a positive ethical climate throughout the HCO, and developing mechanisms to assure that the values that define the ethical climate are understood by all stakeholders.

A positive ethical climate has at least two important characteristics. First, in such organizational cultures, the mission and vision of the organization inform the expectations for professional and managerial performance and are implemented in the actual practices of the organization. Second, a positive ethical climate embodies a set of values that reflect societal norms for what the organization should value; how it should prioritize its mission, vision, and goals; and how the organization and the individuals associated with it should behave. Healthcare organizational ethics directs attention to how the mission of the organization (to provide excelllent care at reasonable cost) is carried out throughout the organization in its business, clinical, and professional practices, and how the organization works to bring its activities, at all levels of function, in line with its mission of providing excellent patient care.[4]

There is a history of close scrutiny of the ethical operations of larger nonhealthcare-related corporations. Beginning shortly after the Watergate scandal in the mid-1970s, governmental "watchdog" agencies and private groups have shown increasing interest in how corporations address ethical issues. Cases of ethically problematic activities in a number of corporations received particular attention and criticism, and, within the corporations themselves, led to the development of compliance and ethics programs as attempts to meet these criticisms. Later, as we will describe in the section "Challenges," below, these programs became virtually mandatory. But HCOs have a number of features that distinguish them from more common-garden variety organizations, and these features must be taken into account in the

design and promulgation of any "ethics" program that attempts to change or enhance an HCO's ethical climate.

II. DISTINGUISHING FEATURES OF AN HCO

HCOs exhibit certain characteristics that distinguish them from other organizations. They are unlike most other non-health-related businesses; they are not identical to healthcare professional associations; as organizations they are distinct from professionals who provide medical care in these and other settings; and they are unlike other social organizations that provide specific, beneficial services for their clients.

As businesses, HCOs are distinctive because the payer for services — be it an employer, governmental agency, or insurance company — is commonly not the "consumer" of the services provided.[5] This means that the major decisions about access to, and cost of, healthcare interventions are at least partially made by an entity that may be more interested in cost distributions than in the availability and quality of interventions for individual patients. In some instances, patients, as recipients, have little clout to affect the availability of particular healthcare professionals from whom they can seek care. Nor can they be assured that they will have access to particular treatments and interventions, even though these interventions and treatments may be of proven value. In addition, patients are often vulnerable because of their illnesses. This vulnerability and the lack of the requisite knowledge to make truly informed decisions about the quality of care available further assures that patients' decision-making authority is limited.

In addition to the division of payers and consumers, the information asymmetry between professionals and patients (and indeed, between healthcare professionals and managers of nonprofessional healthcare organizations), complicates "customer" relationships, as patients are not the fiscal agents and are almost always vulnerable. There is also a supply/demand asymmetry, since an HCO ordinarily cannot respond to all consumer demands, in particular to the demands of the uninsured, without threatening its economic survival. Moreover, some patients or patient groups cannot pay for the healthcare they need or consume, while others pay for more than they consume.

It is of equal importance that healthcare professionals, particularly doctors and nurses who are employees or who act as independent professional staff members within an HCO, have their own sets of professional ethical obligations. These independent professional standards, established by professional associations, cannot be controlled by HCOs, but are important factors in the care that HCOs provide. The tension between professional ethical mandates, particularly those that demand that the individual patient always comes first, and contractual obligations of HCOs, which often require attention to the needs of a group of "subscribers" rather than to an individual patient, is an ever-present source of conflict in today's HCO. It is obvious that HCOs cannot function without excellent professionals.

Lastly, HCOs, if they are to remain viable and fulfill their missions in today's rapidly changing healthcare arena, must plan for and respond appropriately to marketplace forces, as they maintain a coherent vision of their values and their meaning. Even religious-based HCOs and those that are community-supported must remain economically viable while they provide high-quality care, to simply survive.

In summary, HCOs serve a number of stakeholders, each with their own values, goals, and expectations. Moreover, HCOs operate within a turbulent and competitive environment that may require the making of swift and unpopular decisions. To be effective, an organizational ethics program must find ways to integrate these perspectives and the values and goals associated with them.

III. TOWARD INTEGRATION OF PATIENT-CARE ETHICS, BUSINESS ETHICS, AND PROFESSIONAL ETHICS

If an HCO is to develop a meaningful organizational ethics program with adequate mechanisms to deal with the ethical problems it will necessarily encounter, it must develop mechanisms that support the differing ethical perspectives of patient-care (clinical) ethics, business ethics, and professional ethics, and enable each perspective to enhance the overall ethics program. Organizational ethics must work to integrate these perspectives into a unified organizational ethics program, based on commonly understood organizational values that promote and sustain a positive ethical climate within each HCO.

A. Patient-Care (Clinical) Ethics

Few have suggested that a patient-care ethics committee can undertake organizational ethics development without significant modification of its mission, membership, and policies. Patient-care ethics is, after all, based on a "patients' rights" perspective, and a much broader perspective is required to respond appropriately to organizational ethics issues. Whether a patient-care ethics committee is the appropriate site for this development is still an open question, but it is one that must be addressed. Even if the patient-care ethics committee continues to operate separately from organizational ethics activities, it must be included in the development and ongoing activities of the organizational ethics program, since its accepted mission (attention to patients' rights) cannot be adequately addressed without considering organizational ethics issues, such as questions concerning adequate disclosure of the economic factors that affect the availability and cost of a particular intervention, and real or perceived conflicts of commitment and interest among healthcare professionals who work within the HCO, either as professional staff or as employees.

B. Business Ethics

Recent work in business ethics has depended heavily on a "stakeholder" concept as the basis for ethical organizational decision making. Under this model, it is the role of managers to weigh the varying obligations of an HCO to its interested and affected stakeholders, who are usually believed to include stockholders, customers, payers (if different from customers), employees, contractual partners, the local community, and the larger society. After these obligations are analyzed, a decision must be made that is based on the accepted values of the HCO.

Critics of the stakeholder concept call attention to its inability to "settle" anything, since it is only a framework for developing processes to address specific problems. However, stakeholder theory sees itself as a normative theory that specifies reciprocal accountability relationships between stakeholders and the organization in question, which provides morally relevant standards to evaluate how priorities are set and how decisions are made.[6]

There are other problems, however, with using the traditional stakeholder concept to address organizational ethics in HCOs. In many other businesses, the *role* of each stakeholder can be clearly identified. With this identification come mechanisms for each stakeholder (individual or group) to have appropriate decision-making authority in the aspects of the business that have an effect on him or her as managers, and as parts of the HCO. Under stakeholder theory, this authority is maintained by assigning rights and responsibilities, based on the particular role. This is difficult in HCOs, because of the confusion of roles of the consumer (patient), the buyer or payer (employer, government, insurance, or managed-care organization), the healthcare professional, the manager (who is sometimes a healthcare professional as well), and the HCO itself, which often functions as provider, rationer, and controller of how healthcare services are delivered. If stakeholder theory is to be effective in fostering a positive ethical climate for the HCO and in developing mechanisms to resolve differences among the various groups that comprise it, it must support organizational ethics activities that direct attention to not only the often divergent interests of these individuals and groups, but also to role confusion, to the markedly different levels of power and authority, and to the greater level of social obligation of HCOs.

C. Professional Ethics

The oldest traditional method for considering ethical issues in healthcare has been reliance on and support for the professional ethics of medicine and nursing.

Traditional professional ethics is based on the ideal that a healthcare professional should always be an advocate for the particular patient and act in that particular patient's best interest. There has always been some difficulty with this basic ideal, since few, if any, physicians and nurses have been able to act solely for the benefit of one specific patient for any significant length of time. Conflicts with another patient's needs, fiscal demands, and the personal needs of the physician or nurse have always been ethical issues for conscientious physicians and nurses. Nonetheless, the ideal of advocacy for individual patients has always been, and continues to be, a strong influence on the perceptions and reality of modern healthcare delivery.

Can this traditional professional ideal, articulated and supported in professional codes, be even the beginning of the development of a realistic

organizational ethics program in an HCO? The answer is obvious. Professional ethics focuses on obligations to specific patients, just as institutional ethics committees focus on the rights of individual patients. An institutional patient-care ethics committee may be able to change its mandate, but it is doubtful that a traditional professional ethical perspective would be able to change in such a fundamental way. Professional ethics depends on the character and virtue of the professional for its authority; patient-care ethics committees depend on the application of recognized principles that are related to individual rights for their authority. Neither, as presently constituted, can be the sole basis for organizational ethics, since the primary focus of both is the individual patient with little consideration of the effects that decisions that concern one individual may have on other individuals, or on the whole community.

In summary, patient-care and professional ethics, as currently constituted, are not sufficient as a base for organizational ethics, and business ethics, as articulated by stakeholder theory, uncovers a number of confusions that have to do with roles and responsibilities of an HCO's most important constituents — the patient and the professional. If organizational ethics is to have real meaning, as well as the ability to carry out its mandated tasks, it must be based on the consistent and accepted values of the organization that define its ethical climate, and thereby define the milieu within which decisions are made. For organizational ethics to be able to enhance and maintain an HCO's ethical climate, the HCO must institute processes to assure that the importance and requirements of an ethical climate are understood and advanced by all in the organization. This requires supporting patient, business, and professional perspectives when support enhances the organization's ethical climate. But it also requires integrating these three perspectives and mediating among them when integration or mediation is required to advance a positive ethical climate.

IV. A MODEL FOR IMPLEMENTATION

Once an organizational ethics program assumes responsibility for the positive ethical climate of an HCO, various decisions must be made: Who will be directly involved in the program? What function should they represent? Where will the organizational ethics program be located in the administrative structure? Although a program will take shape depending on the unique characteristics of the specific HCO, in our view, there are several characteristics that programs must exhibit to be effective.

Because organizational ethics represents an attempt to integrate the various perspectives of stakeholders in HCOs, a program that is most likely to be effective will be broadly representative: professional and clinical staffs, administration and finance offices, the legal office, and the board of directors. Other important functions that may be represented are human resources, quality control, risk management, and those persons responsible for budgetary issues. Clinical representation should include persons who represent physician staff and nursing staff, as well as other clinical staff, including patient representatives, chaplains, social workers, and members of the patient-care ethics committee.

Since an effective organizational ethics program must have the credibility to assess and make recommendations on controversial topics, it must report to top leadership in the HCO. We recommend that the program report directly to the board of directors (including one or more board members as a member of the program will enhance this reporting structure).

The advantages to both the HCO and the organizational ethics program itself in locating the organizational ethics program at the board level are obvious. For an organizational ethics program to succeed, its activities should be accorded prestige and authority, and prestige and authority are guaranteed for board-level activities. There should be little or no controversy regarding adequate funding for its required work, and allocation of necessary funds will be automatic with board support. When an organizational ethics program has strong support from the board, consultation with the organizational ethics program by all aspects of the HCO should rapidly become accepted and routine; acceptance and understanding of the role of the organizational ethics program should be enhanced throughout the organization; and, most importantly, there should be no undue influence by any particular department in the HCO. Locating the organizational ethics program at the board level allows it to do its work in relative harmony and understanding in all areas of the HCO, including administration, professional staff, and the legal department. Any other location for the organizational ethics program will make its task more

difficult and likely delay or impede its development.

The mandate of an organizational ethics program is to enhance and maintain a positive ethical climate, and, in so doing, to have influence on the morale, reputation, and, eventually, the competitive advantage of the healthcare organization. What kind of decision-making authority should the organizational ethics program have? Surely it is paradoxical to demand that it be granted respect, visibility, and authority, but to deny it the capacity to make decisions. Nonetheless, we believe that to maintain moral authority, an organizational ethics program should make as few decisions as possible.

Behind this paradox lies a lively debate about the proper role of ethics in institutions. On the one hand is the image of the ethics committee as a site of technical expertise, commanding a field of expert knowledge, problem-solving skills, experience, and technique, called upon to solve ethical problems as a neurologist might be called in to resolve a particular kind of medical problem. An alternative model sees the role of ethics in an institution as facilitating communication, clarifying moral positions, and arranging a safe moral space within which differences can be aired, understood, and in some (if not all) cases resolved. Both models have something to contribute to clinical ethics, and even those of us who see the task of ethics as communication and consensus building acknowledge that a considerable base of knowledge and skill is required. But the pragmatic approach to clinical ethics views expertise and experience as useful tools for achieving a procedural consensus, rather than as guarantors of the "right" answer.

To gain and retain respect in an HCO, an organizational ethics program must be perceived at all levels as representative, unbiased, independent, and with no specific agenda, beyond the articulation and maintenance of the organization's values and enhancement of the institution's positive ethical climate. Our conception of the organizational ethics program is that it facilitates and mediates change, rather than legislating it, which requires that it make few specific decisions. The decisions it may make should be procedural not policy making. Thus we suggest that the organizational ethics program have mainly an advisory function, with the actual decision-making authority maintained in the traditional areas of the HCO. Administrative and overall policy decisions should continue to be made by the governing board and administration, and medical decisions by patients, families, and healthcare professionals. Broader social and legal decisions that impact the HCO will continue to be made by the community via laws and community mores.

Finally, to be effective, the organizational ethics program must be accessible to all stakeholders in the HCO, and it must be able to balance the need for both transparency and appropriate levels of confidentiality.

V. CHALLENGES

There are a number of challenges that persons who are interested in organizational ethics must overcome for their programs to be effective. For instance, decision making in healthcare organizations is often segregated. Although some institutions recognize the importance of an integrated perspective, decision making in most large healthcare organizations is still characterized by an often bizarre administrative structure, which was developed in the late nineteenth and early twentieth centuries and which leaves administrative and budgetary matters solely in the hands of managers and gives responsibility for quality of care to physicians alone. This creates a culture of "us" and "them," in which professionals and administrators are only partially accountable for the goals of the organization. Another challenge is time. Both professionals and administrators have been overwhelmed by a barrage of new regulations, from both federal and state governments, as well as regulations forced upon them by other payers, and are unlikely to ask for or wish for new responsibilities.

Below we discuss two challenges that we see to the establishment of a fully integrated and effective organizational ethics program.

A. Healthcare Compliance Programs

Compliance activities, which we regard as one of the foremost challenges to the development of effective organizational ethics programs, are virtually mandatory under the Federal Sentencing Guidelines. (The recent U.S. Supreme Court decision in *Blakely v. Washington,* which states that a jury, not a judge, has the power to *increase* a criminal sentence based on the relevant conduct of the offender, does not diminish the importance of the Guidelines, especially as applied to organizations).[7]

In 1984 the U.S. Congress, seeking to correct what was perceived by many critics as unevenly applied justice, passed the Sentencing Reform Act of 1984 (Title II of the Comprehensive Crime Control Act of 1984). The Sentencing Reform Act established the United States Sentencing Commission, an independent agency in the judicial branch composed of seven voting and two non-voting *ex officio* members. The Commission's purpose is to establish sentencing policies and practices for the federal criminal justice system, which will assure the ends of justice by promulgating detailed guidelines that prescribe the appropriate sentences for offenders convicted of federal crimes.[8] The result of the Commission's work is the Federal Sentencing Guidelines.

In 1991, an extension of the Federal Sentencing Guidelines applied them to organizations found guilty of violating federal law.[9] The Federal Sentencing Guidelines state that an "organization" means "a person other than an individual."[10] Therefore, "persons" under this definition include corporations, partnerships, associations, joint-stock companies, unions, trusts, pension funds, unincorporated organizations, governments and their political subdivisions, and non-profit organizations.[11] Healthcare organizations, whether nonprofit or for-profit, incorporated or unincorporated, are included under this definition.

Chapter 8 of the Federal Sentencing Guidelines addresses guidelines and policy statements when the convicted defendant is an organization. According to the "Introductory Commentary" in chapter 8, even though individual agents are responsible for their own criminal conduct, organizations are additionally vicariously liable for offenses committed by their agents, and, as such, can be held culpable for an individual's actions.[12] Organizations may therefore be responsible for any financial restitution or punishment associated with an individual's criminal behavior while he or she was acting as an agent or employee of the organization. The range of fines or other punishments for the organization is based on the seriousness of the offense and the culpability of the organization.

The Guidelines, however, offer potential mitigation of organizations' culpability by tying culpability to the steps taken by the organization, prior to the offense, to prevent and detect criminal conduct, the level and extent of its involvement in or tolerance of the offense by certain personnel, and the organization's actions after an offense has been committed.[13] The Commission recognizes that an organization cannot control every action taken by every individual associated with the organization. But organizations can try to promote a climate in which it is unacceptable to break the law. Organizations can do this through effective programs to prevent and detect violations of the law.[14] Evidence that efforts in this direction have been made will reduce an organization's level of culpability, and thus possible costs to the organization.

These programs, called *corporate compliance programs,* are so important that organization attorneys who do not review compliance within their organization may be considered guilty of "recklessness."[15] If such a program is in place, then the culpability of an organization is reduced, as are the fines or punishment an organization may otherwise receive. Corporate compliance is not optional. Professionals who fail to install a comprehensive corporate compliance plan, or who neglect current regulations, are gambling with their professional and personal future, as well as with the future of their organization. But the Federal Sentencing Guidelines state that if an organization has in place a visible and effective compliance program, fines may be mitigated.[16] Since nothing can guarantee protection against individual wrongdoing in any organization, organizations, including HCOs, have a powerful motive to establish visible corporate compliance programs.

In the mid-1990s, at roughly the same time that chapter 8 was introduced into the Federal Sentencing Guidelines, the U.S. Department of Justice (DOJ) and the Centers for Medicare and Medicaid began an all-out assault on HCOs to prevent "fraud and abuse" in healthcare-related billing. The DOJ has called fraud and abuse a scourge against the integrity of our nation's healthcare system.[17] The DOJ has stated its intention to continue to be aggressive in identifying and punishing healthcare fraud — in billing, "unbundling," kickbacks, and misrepresentation — by "individual physicians as well as multi-state publicly traded companies, medical equipment dealers, ambulance companies, and laboratories as well as the hospitals, nursing homes, and home health agencies they service."[18]

This aggressive campaign has had the effect of emphasizing for HCO executives the major avenue to avoid possible punishment for wrongdoing — a corporate compliance program. Under these conditions, it is not surprising that most HCOs have corporate compliance programs.

To date, corporate compliance programs in HCOs have a focused and specific function that is related to illegal activities: to prevent these activities and to avoid DOJ attention, or, in a worst case scenario, mitigate the punishment for wrongdoing. With this preoccupation, current HCO corporate compliance programs do not have the time to or an interest in providing mechanisms that are capable of promoting and enhancing a positive ethical climate — beyond ensuring compliance with the law. A properly structured organizational ethics program may address some of the same issues as a corporate compliance program and may have a similar administrative structure, in that, to be effective, it must report to top HCO leaders; it must ensure that avenues are open for confidential communication; and it must ensure that it is visible. Because of these similarities, many persons in leadership positions see compliance programs as providing the same functions as organizational ethics programs.

But organizational ethics programs are different: they are concerned with the ethical climate of an organization, while corporate compliance is concerned with a particular function, that is, strict adherence to often poorly understood laws and regulations (particularly regulations concerning billing practices). Nothing says, however, that organizational ethics programs cannot be integrated into expanded compliance programs — and there are good reasons to take that avenue in specific situations.[19] But changing a compliance-oriented program to a more values-oriented program will produce different outcomes; in this regard, it is interesting that work that has been done to date on the outcomes produced by a values-oriented program suggests that they are more desirable from an employer perspective.[20] Some separation of strictly compliance activities may still be necessary, because of the specificity of the legal and regulatory mandates, even if the two programs are combined within one committee.

But there are other more global challenges to the problem of establishing a positive ethical climate, along with the processes that support it. One of these challenges has to do with the implications of the quality movement.

B. The Quality Movement and Reform of the Healthcare Delivery System

The *quality movement* in healthcare began two decades ago, when a group of respected and well-known physicians began attending seminars on Demings's total quality management initiatives (TQM).[21] These initiatives were first introduced in Japan, in the automobile sector. They were widely successful, and later were widely adopted by other industries in the U.S. in the 1980s. At first they were used in the manufacturing sectors, and later were incorporated in service sectors such as banking and fast food.

At first glance, these initiatives — which emphasize standards, process control, and accountability through measurement — seem ideally suited for healthcare systems that are looking for ways to manage their populations in a cost-effective context. Standards can be introduced in the processes of care and can be used to eliminate inefficiencies and waste, thereby cutting costs. Since variances in care are widely perceived to be wasteful, TQM initiatives are seen as offering a way to control costs while maintaining quality of care. They can also be used for accountability purposes.

These initiatives can be used successfully when variances in the delivery of services can be eliminated without jeopardizing quality of care. But the delivery of quality care also requires attention to a diverse population of patients. So even if two similar patients have the same diagnosis, the results of a specific clinical intervention may vary, and the patients' values and preferences may require that they receive vastly different treatments. The only way to accommodate these differences is to allow some flexibility in delivery systems, and this begins to erode the highly structured quality initiative. Without some degree of flexibility within these systems, the need for a program to oversee the enhancement and maintenance of the ethical climate of the HCO will decrease or even disappear.

This tension between the rigidity that is needed for cost control and other desirable quality factors and a more flexible system that is needed to accommodate patients' values and preferences is seen in the concept of *evidence-based medicine.* Evidence-based medicine, a variant of TQM, is the concept that a panel sponsored by the Institute of Medicine (IOM) believes to be a primary tool in reforming the healthcare system.

A report published by the IOM in 2001 called our national healthcare system "fragmented," and, as this is the case, the IOM recommended that the system as a whole should adopt one core mission, or primary purpose: "All healthcare organizations, professional groups, and private and public purchasers should adopt as their explicit purpose to continually reduce the burden of illness, injury, and disability, and to improve the health and functioning of the people of the United States."[22] The IOM report argues that if the delivery system achieves this goal, healthcare services will be timely, efficient, effective, equitable, safe, and patient-centered.[23]

Evidence-based medicine, as defined by the IOM report, has three components, as follows.

Best research evidence, which refers to clinically relevant research from the basic health and medical sciences (but especially from patient-centered clinical research); the accuracy and precision of diagnostic tests (including clinical examination); the power of prognostic markers; and the efficacy and safety of therapeutic, rehabilitative, and preventive regimens.

Clinical expertise, which refers to the ability to use clinical skills and past experience to rapidly identify each patient's unique health state and diagnosis, individual risks and benefits of potential interventions, and personal values and expectations. Clinical expertise should ensure that care is customized to individual patients.

Patient values and preferences, which refer to the unique preferences, concerns, and expectations that each patient brings to a clinical encounter, which must be integrated into clinical decisions if they are to serve the patient. Acknowledging patients' values and preferences as the third arm of evidence-based medicine should ensure that patients remain the source of control in the delivery of care.[24]

Two of these components, clinical expertise and patients' values and preferences, call for flexibility in the delivery of care, but best research evidence calls for tighter control of the processes of care so that variances can be eliminated. The resolution of this tension in actual practice will determine whether patient-care ethics and professional ethics can truly be integrated into the ethical climate of HCOs, or whether decisions will be made based on particular "protocols" that define, in a very structured manner, what intervention is indicated, and will allow for little or no variation.

VI. THE FUTURE

Despite the pervasive influence of the above-mentioned activities, we believe that organizational ethics will come into its own and have a prominent role in healthcare delivery over the next few years.

A. Society

Our society has not made up its mind as to what represents "quality" in its healthcare delivery system, but we can say with a fair amount of certainty that most people understand what "quality" is not. Our society, to date, wants its healthcare delivered in such a way that individuals' beliefs and values are respected — and has shown resentment and anger when it believes this primary goal is being ignored.

There is little doubt that costs will continue to increase, and we, as a society, will have to come to a consensus on *how* to address these cost issues, while we respect individuals' beliefs and values as related to their healthcare decisions. We doubt that our society is ready to hand over total control of the decisions concerning individual care to third parties, whether they are physicians, managers, or bureaucrats. Thus, as in the past, the healthcare delivery system will have to continue to wrestle with the paradox described above. In our view, the processes initiated by and supported by organizational ethics can help address this paradox. But there are other trends that are only just becoming noticeable that are likely to help propel effective organizational ethics programs.

B. Federal Sentencing Guidelines

As described earlier in this chapter, chapter 8 of the Federal Sentencing Guidelines was put into place after explosive scandals in the business world shook the confidence of investors in the late 1980s. In 2004, the business and investment worlds were shaken by new scandals. Consider the ramifications of Enron. But Enron satisfied the requirements of the Federal Sentencing Guidelines. It *had* a fully functioning compliance program in place, which it in fact lauded as an "ethics" program, endorsing values including respect, integrity, and excellence.[25] But its fully functioning ethics program did not create an ethical climate that prevented wrongdoing.

The Federal Sentencing Commission learned lessons from Enron's collapse, and it has proposed amendments to strengthen the Guidelines. Specifically, in the introductory commentary to chapter 8, the Guidelines point out, "The prevention and detection of criminal conduct, as facilitated by an effective compliance and ethics program, will assist an organization in encouraging *ethical* [authors' italics] conduct and in complying with all applicable laws."[26] This is the first time that the Sentencing Commission has mentioned "ethical conduct" as one of its goals.

This language is used again in the "Commentary on Application Notes," notes in which the Guidelines address each standard and the intent of each standard. Specifically, the Application of Subsection (b)(2) is addressed to an organization's leaders, and requires them to promote an organizational culture that encourages ethical conduct and a commitment to compliance with the law."[27] Thus, the Guidelines look at more than simply activities that have to do with compliance — they look at the *culture* of an organization in promoting an appropriate ethical climate.

This new emphasis will almost certainly have an effect on the healthcare industry. An HCO that has been found guilty of fraud and abuse or an HCO that elects to pay a fine rather than undergo a government audit (and most HCOs choose to pay a fine rather than face an audit; it is not an admission of intent or of guilt, but is an admission that some billing errors will almost certainly occur) must sign a "Corporate Integrity Agreement" with the U.S. Department of Health and Human Services.[28] These corporate integrity agreements are modeled on the Federal Sentencing Guidelines, and they can be expected to change as the Guidelines change.

C. Accreditation Council for Graduate Medical Education

Medical education is playing "catch up" with other accrediting bodies in the health professions, education, and business, which have focused on outcomes in education since the 1980s. The Accreditation Council for Graduate Medical Education (ACGME) has engaged in a long-term project (the Outcome Project) to emphasize outcomes assessment in residency programs and in the accreditation process.[29] To this end, ACGME has identified six core areas or "competencies" that are expected of a new practitioner. These competencies were identified within the context of how adequately physicians are prepared to practice medicine in a rapidly changing healthcare delivery system. Having identified these competencies, educators can develop tools that measure the degree to which educational activities are successful in attaining the goals and objectives of the activities.

Two of the six competencies that have been identified by ACGME for residents and other physicians are tied directly to organizational ethics. They are the competencies related to professionalism and systems-based practice.

1. Professionalism

This ACGME competency states:

Residents must demonstrate a commitment to carrying out professional responsibilities, adherence to ethical principles, and sensitivity to a diverse patient population. Residents are expected to:

- demonstrate respect, compassion, and integrity; a responsiveness to the needs of patients and society that supercedes self-interest; accountability to patients, society, and the profession; and a commitment to excellence and on-going professional development
- demonstrate a commitment to ethical principles pertaining to provision or withholding of clinical care, confidentiality of patient information, informed consent, and business practices
- demonstrate sensitivity and responsiveness to patients' culture, age, gender, and disabilities.[30]

This competency embraces both professional ethics and patient-care ethics in its three components. But the requirement that an individual demonstrate a commitment to the ethical principles (among other things) that govern business practices is a requirement that individual professionals be aware of the mission of a *healthcare organization* and its business practices, and whether or not these practices reflect the values of the HCO in its day-to-day activities.

These values will determine the ethical climate of the organization, and this is the province of organizational ethics.

2. Systems-Based Practice

This ACGME competency states:

Residents must demonstrate an awareness of and responsiveness to the larger context and system of healthcare and the ability to effectively call on system resources to provide care that is of optimal value. Residents are expected to:

- understand how their patient care and other professional practices affect other healthcare professionals, the healthcare organization, and the larger society and how these elements of the system affect their own practice
- know how types of medical practice and delivery systems differ from one another, including methods of controlling healthcare costs and allocating resources
- practice cost-effective healthcare and resource allocation that does not compromise quality of care
- advocate for quality patient care and assist patients in dealing with system complexities
- know how to partner with healthcare managers and healthcare providers to assess, coordinate, and improve healthcare and know how these activities can affect system performance.[31]

This competency is intended to ensure (among other things) that residents and other physicians understand that the goal of the delivery system is optimal, cost-effective care. But optimal care is related to professionalism, with its commitment to clinical, professional, and business ethics, so this competency is a requirement that is characterized by these principles. Again, this is the province of organizational ethics.

VII. CONCLUSION

In presenting an overview of organizational ethics in healthcare for both the present and future, we have explored a number of issues, some of which have little bearing on the ethical treatment of individual patients today or the organizations in which this treatment occurs. But, as we hope we have shown, the healthcare system is ever-changing, and most changes have been focused on a more population-based, business perspective, which has increasingly placed constraints on decisions concerning individuals' healthcare. Attending to these changes, while maintaining a consistent ethical climate, should be a large part of the focus of an organizational ethics program. Further, each citizen should understand these changes and anticipate what they mean for both patient populations and individual patients in the future. Again, organizational ethics programs can develop and support the necessary programs and materials that will assure this understanding.

The concept of organizational ethics, as seen in a consistent values-based ethical climate, is here to stay, and will become more prominent as pressures on patients, HCOs, and healthcare practitioners increase. Those involved in organizational ethics need to understand these pressures, and, at least at the local HCO level, make some sense of them, within the context of an effective, values-based ethical climate for the parent organization.

NOTES

1. In 1990, a panel of the Institute of Medicine (IOM) defined "quality" as appropriate resource usage in medical care; this definition allows distortions in quality to be classified as "mistakes" that can be attributed to waste or to under- or over-utilization of resources. See K.N. Lohr, ed., *Medicare: A Strategy for Quality Assurance* (Washington, D.C.: National Academy Press, 1990).

2. Joint Commission on Accreditation of Healthcare Organizations (JCAHO), *Patient Rights and Organizational Ethics: Standards for Organizational Ethics. Comprehensive Manual for Hospitals* (Oakbrook Terrace, Ill.: JCAHO, 1996), 95-7.

3. E.M. Spencer et al., *Organization Ethics for Healthcare Organizations* (New York, N.Y.: Oxford University Press, 2000), 212.

4. Ibid.

5. This anomaly of the healthcare system was noted in 1995 by E. Haavi Morreim, who writes: "in this sense the term purchaser is systematically ambiguous; we could be referring either to patients or to payers." See E.H. Morreim, *Balancing Act: The New Medical Ethics of Medicine's New Economics* (Washington, D.C.: Georgetown University Press, 1995), 22.

6. R.E. Freeman, *Strategic Management: A Stakeholder Approach* (Boston: Pitman Publishing, 1984); see also W. Evan and R.E. Freeman, "A Stakeholder Theory of the Modern Corporation: Kantian Capitalism," in *Ethical Theory and Business*, 3rd ed., ed. T. Beauchamp and N. Bowie (Englewood Cliffs, N.J.: Prentice-Hall, 1993), 101-5.

7. *Blakely v. Washington* (02-1632) 111 Wash. App. 851, 47 P.3d 149, reversed and remanded. For further information see *http://supct.law. cornell.edu/supct/html/02-1632.ZS.html,* accessed 19 October 2004.

8. Federal Sentencing Guidelines, *http:// www.ussc.gov/guidelin.htm,* accessed 18 October 2004.

9. See "An Overview of the United States Sentencing Commission and the Federal Sentencing Guidelines," *http://www.ussc.gov/TRAINING/ corpover04.pdf,* accessed 17 October 2004).

10. Ibid., 2.

11. Ibid.

12. Ibid.

13. Ibid.

14. Ibid., 2-3.

15. D. Dalton, M. Metzger, and J. Hill, "U.S. Sentencing Commission Guidelines: A Wake-Up Call for Corporate America," in *Ethical Issues in Business: A Philosophical Approach,* ed. T. Donaldson and P. Werhane (Upper Saddle River, N.J.: Prentice-Hall, 1994), 331-6.

16. See note 9 above, p. 2.

17. The Social Security Act section 1128C(a), as established by the Health Insurance Portability and Accountability Act of 1996 (P.L. 104-191, HIPAA or the Act), created the Health Care Fraud and Abuse Control Program, a far-reaching program to combat fraud and abuse in healthcare, including public and private health plans. In an example of just how aggressive the program has been, in its annual report for fiscal year 2002, released in September 2003, the federal government was able to reclaim more than $1.8 billion in judgments, settlements, and administrative impositions in healthcare fraud cases and proceedings. See *http://www.usdoj.gov/dag/pubdoc/hcfac report2002.htm#1,* accessed 18 October 2004.

18. Ibid.

19. A.E. Mills and E.M. Spencer, "Organization Ethics or Compliance: Which Should Articulate Values for the U.S. Healthcare System?" *HEC Forum* 13, no. 4 (December 2001): 329-43.

20. L. Klebe-Trevino et al., "Managing Ethics

and Legal Compliance: What Works and What Hurts?" *California Management Review* 41, no. 2 (1999): 131-51.

21. G. Laffel and D. Blumenthal, "The Case for Using Industrial Quality Management Science in Health Care Organizations," *Journal of the American Medical Association* 262, no. 20 (November 1989): 2869-73.

22. IOM, Crossing *the Quality Chasm: A New Health System for the 21st Century* (Washington D.C.: National Academy Press, 2001), 6.

23. These are the characteristics that the IOM committee believes the healthcare system should reflect. Ibid., "Executive Summary,": 1-22.

24. See note 22 above, p. 76.

25. G. Hassell, "The Fall of Enron: Pressure Cooker Finally Exploded," *Houston Chronicle,* 9 December 2001.

26. See "Guideline Amendments Sent to Congress," at *http://www.ussc.gov/2004guid/RFMay04.pdf,* p. 76, accessed 19 October 2004.

27. Ibid., 109.

28. U.S. Department of Health and Human Services, see Corporate Integrity Agreements, *http://www.oig.hhs.gov/fraud/cia/index.html,* accessed 19 October 2004.

29. For information on the ACGME Outcome Project, see *http://www.acgme.org/Outcome/,* accessed 19 October 2004.

30. Ibid.

31. Ibid.

4

Law and Ethics:
An Ongoing Conversation

Paul A. Lombardo

The relationship between law and ethics is a topic that inevitably engages students of ethics, regardless of the specific discipline or the profession from which they may come. Students with clinical experience almost always have some familiarity with the law because they have been exposed to compliance officers, risk managers, and attorneys at the institutions where they work. Those people provide regular instruction on the rules and official regulations that must be obeyed, and also offer instruction on methods of avoiding legal liability. Some students have even weathered the more stressful and uniformly unpleasant arena of litigation. Their interest in the overlap between law and ethics, or perhaps the seeming lack of connection between the two areas, requires exploration.

How should we talk about law and ethics? Which comes first? When features of the law seem to conflict with ethical precepts, how can we decide between them? Should we emphasize their commonality or their differences? And is there a single, best way to characterize how they relate to each other? These are the questions this chapter confronts.

I. LAWYERS AND ETHICS

Given the general regard for lawyers in American culture, it would probably surprise most people to learn that those who practice law are told regularly that they must take moral values into account in the course of offering legal advice.[1] One typical code of conduct declares that "moral and ethical considerations impinge on most legal questions and may decisively influence how the law will be applied." It is proper, according to this official interpretation of a state legal standard, to refer to such considerations when giving legal advice.[2]

But this is not the only time when experience reveals an overlap between what many might perceive as the primary role of an attorney — as client advocate — and the role of attorney as counselor who has in mind the "big picture" extending beyond the minimal technical requirements of the law. Those who have an ongoing relationship with a lawyer may articulate this complex blend of functions in the language they use to describe their lawyer. It would not be surprising to hear the job of the attorney described as a merely technical function. The lawyer as technician should "keep us up to date on the law." At other times, the focus turns to a paternal or protective function, such as "to keep us out of trouble," or, acting as a kind of professional superego, "to be our cop." The lawyer as advocate is sometimes portrayed as an aggressive combatant, a kind of buttoned-down Samurai whose task is "to fight our battles," or as a defender called "to protect us" from external dangers and those who would do us harm. But when clients reflect on the role of lawyer as counselor, it is commonplace to hear them refer to their lawyer as the person charged with "keeping us honest" — a phrase one might more readily associate with pastoral counseling than the practice of law.

Thus while it may be rare (at least at the level of popular perceptions or stereotypes) to perceive ethics as part of the world of lawyering, our common language habits provide a clue to why we sometimes put those two enterprises together. Are they really alike? In many ways they are.

II. HOW ARE LAW AND ETHICS SIMILAR?

In a line that ties law and ethics to an evolutionary trajectory, Oliver Wendell Holmes called the law "the witness and external deposit of our moral life. Its history is the history of the moral development of the race."[3] Much of the evidence for this historical tie is the language used in each discipline. Both often use a similar language — the language of rights, rules, and principles, and a habit of using this language in a systematic, disciplined analysis. At least in the Anglo-American tradition, ethics talk often sounds a great deal like legal talk. Thus, what people think they are compelled to do by "ethical" precept, whether accurately or not, enters their consciousness as something they perceive also to be demanded legally.

A second way the two areas are similar is that both attempt to regulate individual decisions and activity. They do this by means of announcing some level of consensus on norms of behavior. We are sometimes exhorted to obey the law, and ethical codes, because they represent a widely accepted pattern of socially approved conduct. To help us down that path, both law and ethics provide incentives and disincentives for behaving in certain ways and usually announce general principles to guide behavior.

A third similarity between law and ethics is that both, by their own terms, are educative, even when nonpunitive. By announcing a standard of behavior, we learn in the realms of law and ethics what actions are socially sanctioned, as well as those that are frowned upon. Even though we may face no likelihood of being arrested, convicted, or even sued for breaches of the law, we nevertheless face the realization that our behavior is ille-

gal. The declaration of illegality provides an announcement of social disapproval for our conduct, and therefore a disincentive to engage in it, regardless of the practical consequences. Likewise, if we know something has been ruled out-of-bounds ethically, the simple moral disapproval that such a ruling represents often poses a barrier to those who might otherwise happily embrace a questionable activity. This educative function is invoked by those who wish to retain seemingly antique (and unenforced) laws on the books for no other reason than the public policy statement they make against a questionable behavior. Arguments for maintaining laws against various forms of sexual activity, for example, are regularly made by those who recognize the educative force of law. The wish to preserve older versions of ethical prescriptions as a signal against the acceptance of unprincipled "modernization" represents the same concern.

Another similarity between law and ethics falls under the heading of "education," and involves methods commonly employed to teach both law and professional ethics. In both areas, norms are disseminated by promulgation and publication of codes, commentary, and opinions discussing the reasons why certain conduct is worthy of praise or blame. Where programs of legal or ethical compliance exist, announcements of enforcement actions — naming the individuals who are subject to sanctions — are published periodically. And in both areas, formal education programs make use of the case method for instruction in proper ethical practice.

The case study method has a great deal to recommend it. It is also a major point of crossover between law and ethics. Cases — descriptions of actual or hypothetical events that implicate professional value systems and require ethical analysis — may be used to explore professional standards of behavior. Case study is valuable because concrete examples of real-life situations provide the context for ethical discussion. Participants are required to identify the relevant ethical issues that are imbedded in many facts that have some or no relevance to ethical principles. The process of analysis sensitizes participants to uncover and confront issues they may not have considered previously, nor understood to be professionally relevant. Participants have the opportunity to define their own ethical limits of behavior in relationship to colleagues. This may lead to reflection on the comparative laxity or rigidity of subjective ethical standards, and an appreciation and/ or tolerance for some ethical differences. While these examples demonstrate some points of overlap between law and ethics, there are also many points of difference.

III. HOW DO LAW AND ETHICS DIFFER?

Law is accompanied by public sanction; ethics by private; those sanctions embody differing incentives and disincentives as well. Generally speaking, law represents public social regulation that can be enforced by public officials in a public forum. Thus, criminal law is upheld by government officials — police officers and prosecutors. Breaches of the criminal law can result in public sanctions, such as confinement in jail or prison, and/or monetary fines. Breaches of civil law norms may be addressed in lawsuits brought by private individuals as plaintiffs, but they are heard in a public court and the money judgments they generate carry not only the sting of financial penalty, but also the publicity of governmental enforcement. A criminal conviction or a lawsuit for damages are powerful disincentives to potential law breakers or to those who carelessly cause injuries to others.

In contrast, when we invoke principles or rules of ethics, we often have in mind aspirational norms that carry no governmental sanction. Inattention to ethical proscriptions may subject one to private penalties such as suspension or censure by professional organizations or exclusion from specific groups, careers, or opportunities. Breaching ethics may lead to social disapproval, and loss of reputation among one's peers can sometimes make private ethical sanctions more significant than the (rarely enforced) legal sanctions that are available to Boards of Medicine or similar governmental bodies.

It is also the case that codes of ethics that have been adopted by nongovernmental organizations to apply to professionals (for example, attorneys, physicians, dentists, accountants, et cetera) are often incorporated by reference within statutes and regulations that do have legal force. The failure to adhere to ethical norms as a physician could subject one both to exclusion from membership in the local medical society (private) as well as loss of the medical license granted by the state (public). Exclusion from other public groups, such as Congress, could be a consequence of ethical lapses, even though imprisonment or other pen-

alties might not follow. In such cases, the language of exculpation we often hear, "I did nothing illegal," rings particularly hollow, as the ethical violation itself carries adequate sanction to render the violator officially powerless.

Law and ethics are often seen as having a different scope. It is common to discuss law as the floor beneath one may not fall; from this perspective the scope of the law is minimalist. In contrast, the reach of ethics is seen to be more expansive, representing broad and loftier goals to which all should aspire. Despite this distinction, we regularly merge the seemingly minimal requirements of law with the desire that higher standards should be enforced. In the face of behavior that offends our moral sensitivities, we attempt to define obligations that enforce the "spirit" rather than merely the "letter" or literal commands of the law.

IV. HOW SHOULD WE CHARACTERIZE THE RELATIONSHIP?

Considering the many ways that law and ethics overlap, it is a challenge to find an appropriate way to summarize how the two fields relate to each other. We often discuss law and ethics as if one preceded the other. The quote from Oliver Wendell Holmes, Jr., above, is one example of the perspective that puts ethical reflection and experience first as a precondition for the development of law. But does law always follow ethics, or should we look first to the law before we begin to formalize our ethical standards?

Historical examples suggest that the two fields have an interactive relationship, with law often being based in ethics, while, occasionally, ethics borrows from the law. A few examples show how the exchange actually goes "both ways."

A. Law Follows Ethics, Example I: Justice, Slavery, Civil Rights

The civil rights movement of the mid-twentieth century was based in a social ethic that emphasized equality, justice, and universal personhood, and the Civil Rights Act of 1964 was widely seen as the culmination of a long period of struggle toward social and legal equality for African-Americans. Yet that struggle began as early as the seventeenth century — before the American Declaration of Independence and the Constitution were written — when some reformers began to demand the abolition of slavery. Their voices and their insistence on an ethic of racial justice were important in the debates that occurred during the Constitutional Convention (1787), but they had relatively little impact on national law until the Constitution was amended following the Civil War (1861-1865). The Thirteenth, Fourteenth, and Fifteenth Amendments to the Constitution abolished slavery, promised equal protection of the law for persons regardless of race, and guaranteed the right to vote to all, including former slaves. Those amendments provided the formal legal basis for most of the legislation passed one hundred years later as part of the civil rights movement. As this time line shows, despite ethical condemnation of slavery in some quarters from its inception during the colonial period (1619) until American Independence (1776), slavery remained in place at the Constitutional level for almost 100 years. Even after Constitutional amendment, the legal vestiges of slavery remained in place for an additional 100 years. Ethical insight preceded the law by hundreds of years.

B. Law Follows Ethics, Example II: Evolution of Tort Law

The common law developed in England as a record of widely accepted and functionally important social mores. Common law torts (legal claims for injury to people) included actions for such disruptive behavior as battery and defamation. In its worst forms, battery involved intentional violence toward a person, an activity easily seen as worthy of condemnation. Defamation has a more complex pedigree. It involved lying about a person — but not lying generally. For a lie to qualify as defamatory, it had to harm a person's reputation. Some lies were more problematic than others, and those, known as "defamation *per se*," we considered so serious and so socially destructive that they did not require proof that the victim's reputation had been harmed. That class of defamation included acts such as disseminating falsehoods about a person's performance in their trade or profession.

Consider the harm such lies could generate in an English village of the medieval period: the defamed tradesman would lose his customers, and his family could fall into poverty. His skills would be lost to the village. The law, declared in cases by common law judges, simply codified the moral sense of the community. It condemned behavior that was considered socially dangerous, and, thus,

ethically problematic. The law followed — perhaps merely echoing what most would have considered an ethical rule.

C. Law Follows Ethics, Example III: Practice Guidelines

It is standard practice for professional groups to announce guidelines that describe a consensus among practitioners concerning best clinical practices. For example, the American Academy of Pediatrics publishes practice guidelines to assist pediatricians who treat common conditions in children. While these guidelines begin as recommendations to clarify a professional consensus on the acceptable range of standard treatments, they are inevitably later introduced during lawsuits to prove that an individual doctor's practices fell below the standard of care. The legal charge of professional negligence becomes defined with reference to the ethical requirement — described as a guideline — for delivering appropriate care.

Of course, the vector of causation can run the opposite direction as well. Sometimes it seems that law forms the basis for an ethical rule.

D. Ethics Follows Law, Example I: Informed Consent

The first announcement of the principle of voluntary, informed consent as a requirement of ethical conduct of research occurred in the legal context, drafted by the judges who presided at the trials of the Nazi doctors at Nuremberg.[4] This idea finally made its way into federal law as part of the regulations that prescribe requirements for federally funded research.[5] The next notable discussion of the concept occurred in the medical malpractice context.[6] Subsequently, cases began to recognize this standard for medical care. Only later did the serious discussion of informed consent as a necessary part of ethical medical practice begin to receive sustained attention from medical professionals and early bioethicists.

E. Ethics Follows Law, Example II: Standards of Care

The "standard of care" describes commonly accepted therapeutic practices followed by reputable professionals. Traditionally, the standard of care in medicine was decided in court via testimony from a doctor living and working in the same locality. The measure of what was prudent, appropriate, and thus "ethical" practice was defined by peers in the same specialty area. But some standards have been declared first in legal decisions and are then adopted as part of the ethical standard of care for a profession. In those cases, the shadow of the law provides a starting point for ethical discussion. The Washington state case of *Helling v. Carey* is one such case.[7]

In *Helling,* the plaintiff lost her vision due to glaucoma. She claimed her ophthalmologist was at fault, since she had regular vision tests but was never tested for the disease. The doctor defended on the grounds that glaucoma in a person under age 40, like the plaintiff, was very rare, and pressure tests to detect glaucoma in this age cohort were not routinely offered by the profession.

In a controversial decision, the court announced that despite the standard professional practice, the test was cheap and painless and should be provided. Cases of this type show the court making law that sets professional standards, declaring what is in the best interest of patients, rather than leaving that prerogative to doctors alone. The "ethical" practice of medicine finds its basis in a legal opinion.

F. Ethics Follows Law, Example III: Medical Confidentiality

The ethical prescription to keep a patient's secrets is almost universally endorsed in codes of medical ethics, and even finds some roots in the Hippocratic tradition.[8] But not until the *Tarasoff* case did most codes of ethics for psychiatrists begin consistently to include an exception that allowed disclosures in violation of promises of confidentiality when a patient had threatened to harm another person.[9] The "Tarasoff warning," initially condemned by many psychiatrists as a violation of ethical practice, is now the norm for practitioners, even though they may work in a state that does not legally require such warnings.

As these examples show, it is difficult accurately to claim that ethics comes first, then the law follows; nor is it enough to declare, as Holmes did, that the law merely memorializes settled ethical norms. Particularly today, the speed of communication may enable an ethical controversy that is discussed in academic or professional journals to appear as the foundation of a noteworthy legal case. The case can borrow the conceptual framework already established in scholarly discourse and adopt it as the structure of a legal opinion. And that opinion may itself furnish language that makes its way into professional codes of practice. A good example of this back-and-forth between law and ethics occurred in the assisted suicide cases decided by the U.S. Supreme Court in 1997.[10] The Court allowed a friend-of-the-court "Philosopher's Brief" to be submitted by a group that had developed an ethical argument in favor of allowing doctors to assist the death of a patient in some circumstances.[11] The resulting opinions written by the Court partook of a conversation between law and ethics, with concepts and language flowing in both directions.

Another example can be taken from the literature of research ethics. In his landmark *New England Journal of Medicine* article on the ethics of clinical research, Henry Beecher suggested one "cure" for investigators who violated the norms of research ethics: refuse to publish their scientific results. Part of his justification for this proposed rule was mentioned in a footnote describing the then recent *Mapp v. Ohio* decision of the U.S. Supreme Court. *Mapp* established the "exclusionary rule," stating that evidence obtained in violation of the Constitution could not be admitted at trial, no matter how critical it might be to conviction of a criminal.[12] The legal principle, noted Beecher, sounded equally useful in deterring unethical behavior among researchers.

Ultimately, this metaphor of conversation may best capture the way that ideas first generated in the world of ethics are adopted into the world of legal opinions, statutes, and regulation, or where those documents of the law set a new course of ethical practice for the medical profession.

V. ETHICS IN THE PROFESSIONS: THREE MODELS

Professional groups communicate standards and expectations through codes of ethics; those codes have both symbolic import and concrete impacts. Three types of codes are presented below. If we focus on the consequences of failing to abide by their directives, we might describe them either as "low-impact" or "high-impact" codes. Their "impact" can depend on how critical it is for a professional to belong to the organizations that create and disseminate them. The section below explores the significance they may have to professionals from a practical perspective.

A. Low-Impact Codes —
Voluntary Professional Associations

Consider these two statements on duties of confidentiality, taken from ethical codes for doctors and lawyers. "A physician shall respect the rights of patients, . . . and shall safeguard patient confidences and privacy within the constraints of the law," (American Medical Association, "Principles of Medical Ethics," in *Code of Medical Ethics,* 2004).[13] "A lawyer must preserve the confidences and secrets of a client. . . . A lawyer shall not knowingly reveal a confidence or secret of a client; use a confidence or secret of his client for the advantage of himself or a third party; or allow employees, associates from disclosing or using the confidences or secrets of a client," (American Bar Association, "Disciplinary Rule 4-101" in *Model Rules of Professional Conduct,* 1980).[14]

What consequences flow if a doctor or lawyer belonging to one of these professional associations breached the ethical prescriptions laid out in these statements on confidentiality? The American Bar Association and the American Medical Association are voluntary organizations. No lawyer or doctor is required to belong to them; each organization attracts members with a variety of educational programs, public service opportunities, publications, and practice assistance. Many members join out of the desire to be involved in professional "self-governance" through the publication of professional standards, and to associate and identify themselves among like-minded colleagues with similar backgrounds. Others join to have access to group insurance programs or to get group credit rates. Both organizations provide opportunities for publicly prominent, and in some cases, highly respected activities, and both regularly promulgate ethical pronouncements that represent a consensus of their members — and by extension, their professions.

We could describe their codes of ethics as "low-impact," from the limited perspective of the member who chose to be noncompliant with a provision the codes contain. Because neither association actively prosecutes its members for violating code provisions — censuring or expelling offenders found in breach of the code — there is not an expected organizational sanction for being noncompliant. In other words, it is unlikely that a doctor or a lawyer would be expelled from a professional society for revealing professional secrets. In most cases it is equally unlikely that a

license to practice would be at risk for a violation of these rules, and it certainly would be implausible in most circumstances that a civil or criminal action would follow.

So-called "low-impact" codes serve as symbols of the ideals of a profession. They do not necessarily have a punitive function, except insofar as the reputation of a practitioner and his or her standing in the professional community (no small consideration) depends on adherence. Changes to these codes are debated in parliamentary session, reworked, and amended to meet current controversies and crises in an evolving world of practice. They serve to alert members to consensus opinions on major ethical issues and are published regularly to educate professionals to the changing professional ethos. In some instances, discussion of new code provisions may be carried out through sophisticated commentary in the form of written exchanges published in professional journals.

The critical issue here is how professional societies punish violations of their stated professional standards. As a rule, they don't. But we should not lose sight of the fact, explored below, that the same course of conduct might well violate both a professional society code and a state practice act. In the latter case, it could lead to dire consequences, even though it might trigger no reaction in the former.

In contrast, consider a second type of ethical statement, the kind contained in the statutory or regulatory directives adopted by governmental licensing boards or commissions. Adherence to these standards is often made a condition of licensure for all professionals within a state.

B. High-Impact Codes — Mandatory Licensure Standards

When an ethical standard is written into the law as a portion of the state practice act, violation of that law is often defined as a crime and can subject the violator to loss or suspension of license, in addition to other criminal penalties. In the most dramatic cases, professionals found in violation of practice act provisions can be fined or imprisoned.[15] Such activities might also generate civil liability from clients or patients who are harmed, and result in lawsuits leading to monetary judgments.

For example, a doctor who took illegal payments in exchange for disclosing patients' records would breach the ethical duty to maintain confidentiality, and could be charged with "unprofessional conduct" under state licensing laws.[16] He or she could lose their license, be fined, and be sued by patients whose confidentiality was compromised. The language spelling out the doctor's responsibility in state law to maintain confidential information might correspond perfectly with similar language in a professional association's code. Even though most state licensing boards are subject to regular criticism for lackluster enforcement of professional standards, these potential legal penalties nevertheless provide disquieting reminders for would-be lawbreakers. Parallel provisions of legal practice acts yield similar consequences for lawyers who reveal client secrets. And both boards of medicine and the official bar within each state (usually maintained under the control of the state's highest court) regularly publish lists of offenders whose licenses have been revoked following a finding of unprofessional conduct.

Law and ethics merge again when a professional is disciplined pursuant to a practice act, since many professional societies require a license to be maintained "in good standing" as a condition of membership. Those "low-impact" codes may not subject a member to private enforcement mechanisms, but may very well provide that no one can maintain membership who has been publicly punished for violating legally mandatory professional ethical standards.

C. Private Professional Standards, Enforced

Though many professional societies and associations do not engage in ethical "enforcement" activities, a few do. For example, some state-level components of the American Dental Association conduct vigorous ethical compliance programs. They police members' behavior in areas such as delivery of substandard care, false advertising, or other kinds of unethical business practices. Such organizations, either because of their structure[17] or the kind of incentives they provide for members, are often able to maintain a high rate of membership among licensed practitioners, and organizational "ethics and professionalism" are regularly cited by members as powerful motives for maintaining membership. Their ethical standards find a middle ground between the "low-impact" and "high-impact" ethical codes, and their codes of ethics sometimes adopt state law standards of

practice as the baseline of ethical behavior. Members proven to have violated the law are deemed automatically in violation of standards of ethics. Expulsion and/or suspension of members may be accompanied by loss of practice benefits, insurance, or other important prerogatives, such as access to regularly organized educational opportunities that meet state requirements for regular continuing education.

These three models show how some ethical codes are used by specific professional groups. In the world of patient-care ethics, where issues usually develop around caregiver-to-patient relationships rather than professional-to-professional roles, all manner of ethical prescriptions may play a part in addressing ethical quandaries. Simultaneously, several different legal standards could also become factors in any particular clinical case. Perhaps because of the difficulty of drawing clear lines around what counts as "law" or "ethics" and the way the two disciplines overlap in practical application, several common misperceptions linger regarding what level of attention we should pay to the different voices of law and ethics. Those who plan, administer, or participate in clinical ethics activities and who rely on a written statement of principles or rules (such as an institutional code of ethics) and provide formalized instruction in ethics should be aware of these misperceptions.

VI. COMMON MISPERCEPTIONS

Legal rules are stated with detail and specificity and penalties follow violations of the law, so law trumps ethics as a guide of conduct.

Often the law only provides the roughest outline for deciding what proper behavior is. The law can never describe all of the situations that people encounter; it is necessarily broadly written and often ambiguous. A set of maxims, principles, or statements of values are often necessary for all the other times when law provides no effective guidance. Ethical standards and rules may function to provide guidance when the law does not.

Relying on the punitive function of law alone to guide our behavior will often leave us with no guide at all. As noted above, there may be no practical consequence to violating the law, either as a professional (whose licensing board may only rarely prosecute violators of practice acts) or as a citizen whose minor misdeeds might never appear on the "radar screen" of those who enforce the law. More importantly, ethical standards can be stated in aspirational terms, to represent a group's ideals and goals, and not merely the lowest common denominator of behavior. Legal compliance protocols should not be confused with programs of clinical ethics.

The law is concrete and clear; it is possible to instruct people in the law. Ethical standards are vague, subjective, and personal; people can't be taught ethics; they must be learned at home.

As noted above, the law is contained in a variety of governmental pronouncements, from Constitutions, to statutes, to administrative regulations. Those documents are subject to interpretation through several layers of court opinions. As often as not, the law is not clear, and even when it is, it is subject to regular change without notice. On the other hand, it is possible to define objectively what is ethical, just as it is possible to teach and learn the ethos of a profession. It is possible to teach principles, rules, and procedures, and, while both law and ethics capture their standards within those forms, it may be possible to specify a set of ethically (and legally) sound procedures that is much more detailed and clear than any law you could reference. Learning to apply such procedures to the issues that arise in clinical medicine is a skill none of us learns as children.

VII. THE LAW IS THE LAW IS THE LAW. . . .

Clear distinctions must be made between conduct that violates the criminal law and conduct that creates civil liability; similarly, we should understand when the law is allowing us to do something, and when behavior is commanded or prohibited. A caregiver who discovers evidence of child abuse, for example, is commanded to report it under penalty of criminal law. In contrast, the criminal law prohibits most people who provide treatment for substance abuse from revealing the identity of their patients. Some statutes on the confidentiality of HIV testing provide criminal penalties for disclosure of patients' identity and HIV status generally, while permitting, although not compelling, disclosure to a spouse.

Additionally, some laws permit us a range of conduct or immunize us in the face of troubling choices. For example, a common feature of state laws that define the use of advanced healthcare directives is to explicitly exempt physicians from criminal prosecution, as long as they discontinue artificial life support consistent with a patient's previously stated wishes.

As a general premise, one may not violate a criminal law and behave ethically.[18] In contrast, behavior that subjects one to civil liability (in other words, behavior that could prompt a lawsuit) could very well be ethically appropriate, and in some cases even praiseworthy. But, in most cases, the course of behavior that is legally prudent (in reference to both the criminal and civil law) is also ethically sound. It is nevertheless important to know if decisions made in the name of "ethics" are really only attempts to comply with legal commands or to avoid exposure to risk. Legal compliance and risk aversion are not the same as ethical acuity.

VIII. CONCLUSION

Decide how your ethical program relates to the law that regulates your activities. In other words, define for yourself what the relationship is between the law that already exists to regulate your behavior as a professional or caregiver within a clinical facility, and what other motives you want to provide for behavioral change in that setting. You may find that training in the pertinent law and regulations is all you want or need, or you may find it desirable to look to a more expansive, more value-oriented system of incentives and disincentives that comport with your ethical commitments.

NOTES

1. One recent poll reported that 36 percent of respondents rated lawyers as having either "low" or "very low" ethical standards, contrasted to only 16 percent who thought such standards "high" or "very high." The majority, 47 percent, found lawyers merely "average" in ethical standards. Source: Gallup, Cable News Network, "U.S.A. Today Poll," 14 November 2003.

2. Virginia *Rules of Professional Conduct (2004)*, Rule 2.1: "In representing a client, a lawyer shall exercise independent professional judgment and render candid advice. In rendering ad-

vice, a lawyer may refer not only to law but to other considerations such as moral, economic, social and political factors, that may be relevant to the client's situation." *Comment, Scope of Advice,* 2a: "It is proper for a lawyer to refer to relevant moral and ethical considerations in giving advice. Although a lawyer is not a moral advisor as such, moral and ethical considerations impinge on most legal questions and may decisively influence how the law will be applied."

3. O.W. Holmes, Jr., "The Path of Law," *Harvard Law Review* 10 (1897): 457, 459.

4. It could be argued that international law, which is often bereft of effective enforcement mechanisms, shares some of the features of ethical pronouncements. Similarly, one could argue that the legal requirement of informed consent contained in the regulations for federally funded research was derived from *The Belmont Report,* itself a discussion of ethical principles; U.S. Department of Health Education, and Welfare (DHEW), *The Belmont Report: Ethical Principles and Guidelines for the Protection of Human Subjects of Research* (Washington, D.C.: DHEW, 18 April 1979), *http:/ohsr.od.nih.gov/guidelines/belmont. html.*

5. See 45 *CFR* 46.116, "General Requirements of Informed Consent."

6. See for example, *Salgo v. Leland Stanford Bd. Trustees,* 317 P.2d 170 (Cal. 1957), *Natanson v. Kline,* 187 Kan. 186 (1960), and *Cobbs v. Grant,* 502 P.2d 1 (Cal. 1972).

7. *Helling v. Carey,* 519 P.2d 981 (Wash. 1974).

8. "What I may see or hear in the course of the treatment or even outside of the treatment in regard to the life of men, which on no account one must spread abroad, I will keep to myself holding such things shameful to be spoken about." L. Edelstein, "The Hippocratic Oath: Text, Translation and Interpretation," *Bulletin of the History of Medicine* supp. 1 (1943).

9. *Tarasoff v. Regents of University of California,* 551 P.2d 334 (Cal. 1976). See chapter 7, "Privacy and Confidentiality," for details of the *Tarasoff* case.

10. See *Vacco v. Quill,* 521 U.S. 793 (1997).

11. Amicus brief, "Assisted Suicide: The Philosophers' Brief" by R. Dworkin et al., submitted in *Vacco v. Quill.*

12. H.K. Beecher, "Ethics and Clinical Research," *New England Journal of Medicine* 274 (1966): 1354-60.

13. American Medical Association (AMA), Council on Ethical and Judicial Affairs, "Principles of Medical Ethics," in *Code of Medical Ethics* (Chicago, Ill.: AMA, 2004).

14. American Bar Association (ABA), Center for Professional Responsibility, "Disciplinary Rule 4 #101," in *Model Rules of Professional Conduct* (Chicago, Ill.: ABA Publishing, 2004).

15. For example, a doctor whose reckless standards of practice led to the death of a number of patients might be prosecuted for manslaughter, in addition to facing criminal charges for "unprofessional conduct."

16. See, for example, *California Business and Professions Code* sections 725-732, for provisions related to "unprofessional conduct" involving substance abuse, sexual misconduct, et cetera.

17. For example, the American Dental Association has a "tripartite" membership structure. A dentist cannot join a local or state dental society unless he or she also joins the national organization. Similarly, membership in the national society requires membership at the state and local levels. Thus a dentist who wishes to access the benefits (both professional and social) of belonging to an organized group of dentists must join at all three levels.

18. A discussion of civil disobedience could provide examples of behavior that are both illegal and ethical, but it should suffice to say that those would be rare, and a proper understanding of their place would require a treatise in itself.

5

Research Ethics

Erika Blacksher and Jonathan D. Moreno

Medical experimentation and the standards that govern it have undergone significant transformation in the last 150 years. During the mid-nineteenth century, the physician's role as healer and provider of care increasingly became associated with experimenter and collector of data.[1] By the end of the nineteenth century, medical experimentation had redefined the practice and image of medicine and had generated considerable agreement among professionals and the public about the ethical standards that should guide it.[2] The relative safety of untried treatments and procedures, the possibility of therapeutic benefit, and the voluntary consent of patients and subjects were considered essential for the conduct of ethical research.[3]

Remarkably, these ideas remain relevant 100 years later. Sustained analysis, discussion, and debate in the latter half of the twentieth century have, however, significantly refined and transformed these ideas. This chapter reviews the major issues in research ethics at the turn of the twentieth century. It is a contentious time in medical research. Tragic deaths, unprecedented financial incentives, entrepreneurial arrangements between academia and industry, and the conduct of clinical research in developing countries are just a few of the many events and trends that have heightened public scrutiny and fueled numerous regulatory reforms to strengthen what many argue is a broken system of protections for human subjects of research.[4]

Despite the diversity of ethical issues that trouble the research enterprise, the preponderance of U.S. bioethical guidance has focused on informed-consent doctrine.[5] Obtaining the informed consent of human subjects has been and continues to pose a formidable challenge for the research community. The challenges range from the most basic requirements to provide information that is clear and candid about the purpose, nature, and risks of research, to questions about the use of vulnerable populations and standards for assessing potential subjects' capacity for decision making. As important as informed consent is, however, it is neither sufficient, nor in all cases necessary.[6] Seven criteria are now widely agreed to be necessary and sufficient for the conduct of ethical medical research. They are:

1. Societal value,
2. Scientific validity,
3. Fair selection of subjects,
4. Favorable risk-benefit ratio,
5. Independent review,
6. Informed consent,
7. Respect for subjects.[7]

Nonetheless, because informed consent has received more explication than any other criterion, its history serves as a useful lens through which to examine other major research ethics issues. The evolution of informed-consent doctrine and practice was forged in response to the misrepresentation of research as "therapy," the exploitation and abuse of marginalized groups, and the influence of conflicts of interest. Of additional interest to readers of this clinical ethics textbook is the fact that the development of informed consent in the research context was, for much of its history, affected directly by the norms of clinical practice.

In what follows, we use a U.S. history of informed consent in the research context[8] as a framework to situate and review contemporary research ethics issues, including risk-benefit ratios, conflicts of interest, and fair subject selection. These sections are followed by a discussion of the regulatory reforms for research oversight and training that have been either proposed or put in place at the federal and local levels.

I. INFORMED CONSENT

Informed consent has evolved from mere acquiescence to become informed, comprehending, and voluntary consent. During much of this history, the norms of medical practice directly influenced researcher-physicians' practices and ideas about consent. As growing numbers of medical practitioners began to search for the underlying causes of human disease and to develop new techniques for diagnosis, treatment, and prevention for future patients, they continued to rely on an ethic intended to serve the welfare of current patients.[9] Physicians' traditional duties to promote patients' welfare and "above all, do no harm" urgently needed to be replaced with moral rules to guide interactions between clinical investigators and human subjects.

Medical researchers did not, however, wait for conceptual and ethical clarity, even as medicine emerged as a science-based field in the late 1900s. Key questions, such as what constituted an experiment, whether research offered the possibility of benefit, when potentially beneficial research could be considered standard medical care, and what it meant to volunteer for research, were mired in confusion and controversy for more than a century.

The norms of medical practice filled the void, often to the detriment of human subjects. The misconstrual of medical research as medical therapy determined *who* counted as a subject of

research, and, as such, whether consent in any form was considered necessary. Research that was thought to offer potential benefits to patient-subjects was often presented to patients as "medical therapy," which relieved researcher-physicians of the duty to seek patients' consent. This practice was justified by norms that dominated clinical practice at the time, "benevolent deception" and "therapeutic privilege." These norms not only relieved physicians of disclosing information, but obligated them to *hide* potentially harmful information from patients, or even to manipulate or threaten them to undergo treatment, all of which was thought to promote patients' welfare.[10]

Physicians' authoritarianism during this time was tempered only when the risks posed by experimental treatment were significant. When procedures were dangerous, it was recommended that "uncoerced" consent be obtained.[11] There was no expectation that patients in these instances were informed, only that they "volunteered." The term volunteer not only lacked formal definition, but a patient's ability to do so was constrained by the combination of widespread physician paternalism and the patient's fear of abandonment.

Although consent practices during this time left much to be desired, nineteenth-century *ideas* about consent standards were more rigorous. These ideas can be gleaned by examining attitudes and reactions to the use of various subject populations. For example, the use of members of groups who were deemed incapable of understanding or volunteering for research, such as children living in orphanages, poor people, the cognitively impaired, and prisoners, brought swift and uniform criticism.[12] However, researchers' use of themselves in their experiments was widely accepted and believed by some to be obligatory, although for reasons that were not analyzed or articulated at the time.[13]

Interestingly, the conditions of self-experimentation approximate current criteria of informed consent. Researchers who considered self-experimentation would know better than anyone the purpose of the research and the nature and degree of risks, thus fulfilling the criterion of full information. They were best prepared to comprehend this information and theorize as to potential consequences, fulfilling the criterion of comprehension. And their self-administered inoculations and applications demonstrated voluntariness, fulfilling the third criterion. Moreover, their action furthered their interests and promoted their values as researchers and, in this way, could be understood to promote their "autonomy," or self-determination. Standards for researchers' obligations to subjects other than themselves would not strive for these same high standards until well into the twentieth century.

Several events at the turn of the century signaled a shift toward more rigorous consent standards. Instances of self-regulation, legislative efforts to regulate human research, and four landmark court decisions regarding medical care initiated a shift in attention from a researcher's duty to obtain consent to the content and quality of consent. Proposed and implemented reforms addressed issues such as disclosure requirements; written consent forms (then usually called contracts, permits, or waivers); decision-making capacity; and fairness in subject selection, albeit all in cases of research with no intended benefits. Consent standards for potentially beneficial research would continue to languish in the shadows of therapeutic privilege and benevolent deception for decades to come.

The four court decisions concerning medical care merit note because of their almost immediate impact within the medical research arena. Between 1905 and 1914, four cases introduced important new ideas about the nature and justification of consent. The 1905 *Mohr v. Williams,* 1906 *Pratt v. Davis,* 1913 *Rolater v. Strain,* and 1914 *Schloendorff v. Society of New York Hospital* cases are largely responsible for developing the basic features of informed consent to medical care in American law.[14] Together these court decisions raised expectations for disclosure by physicians, expanded patients' rights to specify consent for particular procedures, and justified informed consent on grounds of patients' autonomy.[15] Indeed, the court's language in *Schloendorff* would become the most widely quoted in the current informed-consent literature.[16] Although technically not a consent case, Justice Benjamin Cardozo's language became a beacon for patient self-determination: "Every human being of adult years and sound mind has a right to determine what shall be done with his own body; and a surgeon who performs an operation without his patient's consent commits an assault, for which he is liable in damages."[17]

Two years later, strikingly similar language was used in the context of medical research. In 1916, the chair of the Council for the Defense of Medical Research, Walter Bradford Cannon, rec-

ommended uniform guidelines for experimentation involving human subjects and published a powerfully worded editorial in the *Journal of the American Medical Association* in response to a young researcher's experimentation on six syphilitic, paretic patients. Cannon wrote, "There is no more primitive and fundamental right which any individual possesses than that of controlling the uses to which his own body is put. Mankind has struggled for centuries for the recognition of this right. Civilized society is based on the recognition of it. The lay public is perfectly clear about it."[18] The American Medical Association (AMA) apparently did not share Cannon's convictions, leaving clinical investigators to work without guidelines until 1946, when the AMA amended its code of ethics as part of its involvement in the prosecution of Nazi physicians for atrocities committed during World War II.

The 1947 judgment in *United States v. Karl Brandt et al.* addressed not only on the defendants' guilt or innocence, but also produced 10 principles to guide justifiable research involving human subjects. These 10 principles make up what posterity has come to know as *The Nuremberg Code,* the first of which is the absolute requirement to obtain the subject's voluntary consent. The *Code* defines consent as having four fundamental characteristics: voluntary, competent, informed, and comprehending.[19]

The judges at Nuremberg appeared to have drawn the principles from two sources. One was a report prepared by physiologist Andrew Ivy, who had been appointed by the AMA to testify on medical ethics at the trial; the other, a memorandum written by a court-appointed expert, neurologist Leo Rosenberg. Ivy's report also was sent to the AMA's Judicial Council, which in December 1946 approved a distilled version of Ivy's rules and published them in the *Journal of the American Medical Association.* This was the first time formal guidelines for human subject research were available to U.S. medical researchers; they required both voluntary consent and prior animal testing. Although both Ivy and Rosenberg intended the provision to apply to both healthy volunteers and patient-subjects, the *Code* seems to have been interpreted at the time as applying only to healthy volunteers, not patient-subjects.

Despite the dramatic events that led to the formulation of the *Code,* it had little impact on U.S. physicians or the public at large. The greatest impact of the *Code* was felt within the U.S.

defense establishment as it prepared for the Cold War.[20] The newly created civilian Atomic Energy Commission (AEC) and the Department of Defense (DoD) were planning for defense against atomic, biological, and chemical warfare, and viewed human subject research as essential to their plans. The national security establishment's discussion of *The Nuremberg Code* was discovered by the Advisory Committee on Human Radiation Experiments (ACHRE), established in 1994 by President Bill Clinton, who authorized a massive declassification of relevant documents.

The work of the ACHRE shows that the AEC and DoD both developed progressive rules for research involving human subjects, though neither were widely communicated or implemented. The AEC, which was created in January 1947 to oversee the nation's nuclear stockpile, had good reasons to develop mechanisms to prevent abuses in human subject research.[21] The AEC inherited many of the contracts and programs of the Manhattan Project, which included secretive and sensitive studies involving the injection of 17 hospitalized patients with plutonium. The AEC also would be the sole distributor of radioisotopes which would be used in thousands of human radiation experiments, and would prove an equally rich source of funding for other research.

AEC General Manager Carroll Wilson spelled out rules for human subject research in two separate and slightly different letters in April and November 1947. They are significant for being the first known instance in which the term "informed consent" was used, and was the first time that *sick patients* were included in the consent provisions.[22] Although the meaning of informed consent is not explained or defined, Wilson's union of the words "informed" and "consent" predates by a decade what scholars had thought to be its earliest use.[23] Despite numerous opportunities, however, Wilson's rules were not disseminated. They penetrated only one research setting. The AEC-sponsored Oak Ridge Institute for Nuclear Studies (ORINS), which opened in 1950, implemented a local process for informing patients of research risks and requiring written documentation. A 1956 document indicated that they were "fully advised" about the "character and kind of treatment and care," which would be "for the most part experiments with no definite promise of improvement in my physical condition."[24]

The DoD standards that were ultimately signed into effect in February 1953 are also no-table. They are the only instance of a U.S. federal agency (or any agency of any government) adopting *The Nuremberg Code,* and required written and witnessed subject consent, and prohibited the use of prisoners of war in research studies. The DoD provisions were influenced by the National Institutes of Health (NIH), from which it had sought input. As the emerging leader in biomedical research with plans to open a state-of-the-science research hospital, the NIH had started drafting human research rules. When the NIH Clinical Center opened in 1953, its policy required the "voluntary agreement based on informed understanding" of all research subjects, including patient-subjects, and written consent from some patient-subjects involved in especially risky research.[25] Although the AEC's policy requiring consent from patient-subjects predates this provision by six years, the NIH policy was a far clearer expression and endorsement of the requirement to obtain consent from patient-subjects.[26]

The DoD provisions were approved by a new secretary of defense, who may have been unaware of the deep opposition to regulations of *any kind* expressed by Pentagon advisory committees.[27] In addition to this attitudinal barrier, implementation was further complicated by the communication of this policy in a top secret memo to the secretaries of the armed forces, which remained classified until August 1975. Attempts to communicate down the chain of command resulted in varied levels of awareness, inconsistent interpretations, and sporadic implementation throughout the 1950s and 1960s. By 1973, however, the Army, Navy, and Air Force had promulgated regulations that required written, informed consent from both patient-subjects and healthy volunteers.[28]

Opposition to the formalization and regulation of consent standards was also expressed outside the defense establishment. Notable critic Henry K. Beecher, a Harvard physician and researcher, was a forceful and frequent critic of both research abuses *and* rule-based regulations that were externally imposed on experimenters. Beecher was unconvinced that rules could prevent research abuses, believing instead in self-regulation by the "truly *responsible* investigator."[29] Ironically, his influence ultimately helped to promote the very regulatory regime he resisted.

Beecher's identification of research abuses prompted the U.S. Public Health Service (PHS) to commission a 1961 study of ethical and administrative practices of U.S. researchers and their institutions. The study found vast inconsistencies among institutions and concluded that "internal institutional regulation of research was generally insensitive and sporadic."[30] Moreover, transcripts revealed that subjects' status as patients not only failed to protect them, it endangered them. Physicians' interviews portray attitudes and practice patterns that are disturbing not only by today's standards but, no doubt, those of Beecher in 1960. Physicians reported discomfort with following well-established practices for protecting potential subjects and expressed arrogant and manipulative attitudes toward their patients.[31]

During the same period, physicians' practices in the clinical context were coming under intense scrutiny. The 1957 *Salgo v. Leland Stanford Jr. University Board of Trustees* ruling continued to press consent standards in the direction of patients' rights. Martin Salgo, who suffered permanent paralysis after undergoing translumbar aortography, sued his physician not only for medical negligence, but for failing to disclose the risk of paralysis. The court ruled in his favor and in its opinion created "informed consent." The court ruled that Mr. Salgo had clearly consented to the procedure but without all the pertinent facts, which the court ruled precluded his ability to make "an intelligent consent."[32] Although the phrase "informed consent" had been used a decade before in Carroll Wilson's 1947 memo to a handful of AEC contract researchers and medical advisors, *Salgo* put informed consent on the map for the mainstream U.S. medical community who were working in a clinical rather than a research context.

The *Salgo* case was not a complete victory for patients' rights. The court tempered its ruling by acknowledging "physician discretion" in disclosing information.[33] The court provided no analysis or explanation of the allowable "discretion," leaving patients' self-determination at the feet of physicians' judgments. As Jay Katz has noted of the ambiguity, "the court did not appreciate the futility of its endeavors, for it gave an undefined task to a group that has had neither the experience with nor the commitment to patient self-determination."[34]

Deference to physicians' paternalism imploded in the 1960s. A series of incendiary cases cast a bright light on researchers' struggle to balance their dual responsibilities as both investigators and physicians. Congressional hearings, scholarly critiques, print and broadcast media

coverage, and the public's outrage in response to these cases all led to significant reforms by the mid-1970s. For the first time, informed consent for human subject research was put before a public body for explicit discussion, analysis, and recommendations. The resulting reports and regulations would plant informed consent firmly in the ground of patients' autonomy and expand and elaborate on its meaning and requirements.

Tragic events surrounding the use of the sedative thalidomide set this reform process in motion. Approved for use in Europe but still experimental in the U.S., thalidomide was found to be safe for pregnant women, but in some cases was devastating to their fetuses, who were born with missing or deformed limbs. Legislative hearings revealed that pharmaceutical companies commonly gave physicians free samples of untested drugs and paid them to collect patient data, a practice that led to a small number of birth defects in newborn infants. Television coverage of these cases and corresponding public outcry helped to push the passage of the 1962 Kefauver-Harris Amendments to the Food, Drug, and Cosmetic Act, which enacted unprecedented requirements of researchers. For the first time in U.S. history, researchers were required to inform subjects of a drug's experimental nature and to obtain their subjects' consent to participate in research.[35]

Just as the *Salgo* ruling retreated from patients' consent in deference to physicians' discretion, so too did this new Food and Drug Administration (FDA) policy. Physicians were not required to obtain consent when it was "not feasible" or was deemed not in the best interest of the patient.[36] The vaguely worded best-interest clause caused enough confusion to prompt the new FDA Commissioner, James Lee Goddard, to clarify the matter in 1966. A small task force of FDA officials produced a policy that drew heavily on *The Nuremberg Code* and the recently passed World Medical Association (WMA) policy regarding human experimentation, commonly known as *The Declaration of Helsinki*. The FDA policy embraced the WMA's distinction between "therapeutic" and "nontherapeutic" research and its accompanying consent standards. *The Declaration of Helsinki* embraced the absolute requirement for consent to nontherapeutic research from *The Nuremberg Code,* but qualified consent standards for research that had therapeutic potential, thus continuing to foster the "therapeutic misconception" that has surrounded medical research since its inception.[37]

It also permitted third-party consent by a legal guardian for both types of research, another noteworthy deviation from *The Nuremberg Code.*

This FDA policy, which applied only to experimental drugs, devices, and biologics, was among the factors that fueled NIH Director James Shannon's advocacy of formal controls on human subject research. Shannon's commitment to formalizing human research rules was bolstered by unprecedented public and professional scrutiny of medical research, especially a controversial study conducted on poor, elderly patients at the Jewish Chronic Disease Hospital (JCDH), funded in part by the PHS. In this case, investigator Chester M. Southam, from the Sloan-Kettering Cancer Research Institute, directed research in which 22 indigent patients were injected with live cancer cells without their oral or written consent. He also violated other well-established duties, which included failing to disclose anything about the research, proceeding without review by the hospital's research committee and over the objections of three physicians, and using a vulnerable patient population — poor, elderly, frail patients — in research obviously not intended to benefit them, but to answer a scientific question.[38]

In response, Shannon created a committee to study the issues and make recommendations. Disappointed by the first committee's warning that policy reforms would thwart research progress and interfere with the physician-patient relationship, he and U.S. Surgeon General Luther Terry took their concerns to the National Advisory Health Council (NAHC), an advisory committee to the PHS surgeon general. The NAHC affirmed their concerns and issued a statement that recommended PHS funding be given only to investigators who were willing to meet key ethical criteria, including obtaining the informed consent of subjects.

The statement failed to define informed consent, but led to the creation of landmark government regulations. In February 1966, the new surgeon general, William H. Stewart, accepted the NAHC recommendations and issued a policy that compelled PHS grantee institutions to provide prior committee review of proposed experiments, and, for the first time, recognized patient-subjects in the consent provisions. Specifically, the PHS policy required that independent review committees at grantee institutions address the

1. Rights and welfare of the individual(s) involved,

2. Appropriateness of methods to secure informed consent, and

3. Risks and potential medical benefits of the investigation.

The policy, like the statement that inspired it, failed to address the substantive content of informed consent, leaving its meaning and criteria to determination by local committees.[39]

A detailed, substantive account of informed consent was soon after provided by the NIH Clinical Center. The new policy required an oral explanation of the research suited to subject's comprehension level; detailed disclosure regarding the nature, purpose, and risks of the study and procedures to be performed; and signed consents. The policy also addressed issues such as voluntariness and compliance with FDA policy. The policy has been described as the "most careful and comprehensive statement" on informed consent up to that point in U.S. history.[40]

Continued efforts to update federal policy culminated in the 1971 *The Institutional Guide to DHEW Policy on Protection of Human Subjects,* better known as the "Yellow Book," because of its cover. The policy expanded requirements to all Department of Health, Education, and Welfare (DHEW) programs and activities, provided detailed analyses of a number of issues, and retained the procedural requirement of committee peer review. And once again, informed consent was both strengthened and weakened. The policy required that consent be obtained from both patients and healthy volunteers or authorized representatives after explaining the procedures; describing the risks, discomforts, benefits, and alternatives; offering to answer all questions or inquiries; and ensuring subjects know that they may withdraw consent and discontinue participation at any time.[41] However, the policy permitted subjects' consent to be either oral or written, obtained after research participation if a complete and prompt briefing was done, and in some cases could be considered implicit in voluntary participation if adequately advertised.

The inadequacy of the policy would soon be illustrated. Primed in part by Beecher's high-profile activism, the U.S. government, the press, and the public were all watching when the "Willowbrook" and "Tuskegee" cases caught light. Both cases are now considered paradigmatic research ethics cases. Willowbrook raised subtle and complex questions about the selection of subjects, therapeutic benefit, and informed consent, and led to detailed regulations of research with children in 1983, discussed in more detail below. Tuskegee, however, is widely agreed to represent a blatant abuse of human subjects.

The notorious 40-year Tuskegee Syphilis Study, conducted by the PHS, breached research rules that were well-established not only by 1970, but when the research began, in 1932. Poor African-American men living in and around rural Tuskegee, Alabama, were used by PHS researchers to study the natural history of syphilis. Originally designed as a six-to eight-month study, it was extended for four decades. Some 400 syphilitic men and 200 non-syphilitic men were induced to "participate" by being told they would receive free treatment for "bad blood," a term used in the community to describe many ailments, but which the researchers assumed referred to syphilis. The researchers disclosed nothing to these men, nor sought their consent. They were not told that they had syphilis or that they would not benefit from participation in the study. Their free treatment included purely diagnostic procedures such as lumbar punctures. The research apparatus was designed to impede subjects' awareness of and access to available treatments, including penicillin, which was used in the treatment of syphilis by the late 1940s.

Despite many opportunities to halt the research, the Tuskegee Syphilis Study was not stopped until a 1972 New York Times front page article drew public attention and moral outrage. The DHEW established an ad hoc panel to review the study and the department's research rules, which found them inadequate across the board. The panel ordered the research stopped and recommended the establishment of a "permanent body with the authority to regulate at least all Federally supported research involving human subjects."[42]

The panel's call for direct oversight of all federally funded research by an independent body with punitive authority was met with a compromise, delivered in the 1974 National Research Act. The Act established the National Commission for the Protection of Human Subjects of Biomedical and Behavioral Research, a four-year advisory body, in return for the DHEW's conversion of human subject policies into regulations that were applicable to the entire department.[43] The regulations required grantee institutions to form institutional review boards (IRBs) and charged them with reviewing research proposals for their safety and informed-consent provisions. Informed-consent requirements were made slightly more stringent, and all, not just risky, research was required to undergo review. Still, the regulations did not apply to all federally funded research and suffered from ambiguities and unanswered questions that would become the work of the National Commission.

The National Commission produced 17 reports and appendices, including The Belmont Report, which remains a touchstone for U.S. human subject research.[44] The Commission addressed many issues, including the first formal attempt to clearly state the ethical import of the distinction between medical research and medical practice, the role and function of IRBs, informed consent and third-party permission, and research involving vulnerable populations. The Commission's extensive and detailed recommendations largely became policy.[45]

Central among the Commission's tasks was the development of basic ethical principles that could become the basis of research oversight, especially research with vulnerable populations. The Commission created a framework of three principles, each of which was to guide and justify a key function of the IRB process. Respect for persons, beneficence, and justice — the "Belmont principles" — were proposed as ethical guides and justifications for informed-consent provisions, risk-benefit analysis, and selection of subjects.[46] The Commission's elaboration on the intent and function of respect for persons made respect for autonomy fundamental to informed consent. "[M]ore decisively than any previous publication in case law or research ethics, the Commission's volumes reflected the view that the underlying principle and justification of informed consent requirements, at least for autonomous persons, is a moral principle of respect for autonomy, and no other."[47]

The Commission's attention to informed consent produced an analysis of its content and criteria that remains the standard. The Commission identified three necessary conditions for informed consent: information, comprehension, and voluntariness. These conditions were used to analyze consent for vulnerable classes of subjects, such as children, prisoners, and institutionalized persons with cognitive impairments. A report and two appendices are devoted to informed consent and are among the most widely read sections of the Commission's many reports.

By the time the National Commission had completed its work in 1978, informed consent had currency in mainstream American society. Scholars, courts, hospital board rooms, classrooms, and state legislatures focused on patients' rights to make autonomous decisions about their healthcare. Commentary on informed consent flooded the medical literature.[48] Three 1972 court rulings left no doubt about patients' rights to make medical decisions based on their values, and on the information that reasonable persons, not medical professionals, would need to know to make such decisions. The following year, the American Hospital Association published "A Patient's Bill of Rights," which included informed-consent provisions.[49] Between 1975 and 1977, 25 states enacted informed-consent legislation.[50]

Revised AMA policy issued in 1981 cinched the place of informed consent in modern medicine. The AMA *Code of Medical Ethics* had undergone numerous revisions since its creation in 1847, including a 1980 revision that acknowledged the physician's obligation to respect patients' rights.[51] Not until the following year, however, did the AMA issue a policy explicitly addressing informed consent, using much of the language in one of three landmark 1972 court decisions. The ruling in *Canterbury v. Spence* described consent as "the informed exercise of choice" based on "enough information to enable an intelligent choice."[52]

The National Commission's pioneering work largely became policy in 1981. New regulations from the Department of Health and Human Services (DHHS) were based on the National Commission's recommendations and were influenced by a subsequent bioethics commission, the President's Commission for the Study of Ethical Problems in Medicine and Biomedical and Behavioral Research, which worked from 1980 to 1983. Established to address unresolved and new issues, the members of the President's Commission stressed the importance of the informed-consent recommendations to federal officials drafting the regulations.[53] The subsequent regulations provided in-depth guidance on informed consent, particularly on disclosure requirements. In addition to the purpose and nature of the research, its potential risks and benefits, and the alternatives, researchers were now also obligated to provide an explanation and information about the confidentiality of records, compensation for injury and medical treatment if necessary, and a contact for pertinent questions.[54] The new regulations also required researchers to disclose information discovered during the study that would influence a subject's participation. The regulations applied to both biomedical and behavioral research, but broad exceptions for research that entailed minimal risk, such as interviews, surveys, or observational research, effectively exempted much of behavioral research.[55]

For all of this progress, significant gaps remain in informed-consent provisions. Informed consent, as a concept and as a practice, has been challenged by a number of scandals and new developments in the last decade of the twentieth century. These scandals and developments reveal the difficulty of achieving informed consent, especially for the most vulnerable classes of subjects.

The provision of accurate, complete, and candid information about the purpose and risks of research to potential subjects continues to challenge the research community. Among its many activities, the ACHRE reviewed 125 research proposals. Together with an individual committee member's separate review, they found that consent forms "are flawed in morally significant respects, not merely because they are difficult to read but because they are uninformative or even misleading."[56] Specifically, consent forms often present inadequate information about risks that might be significant to patients, lack important information about alternative treatments and preliminary data gathered from earlier experiments, and use the language of "treatment" and "therapy" to describe research that *may* yield therapeutic benefit when such benefit is not its purpose.

Two tragic cases that occurred in close proximity at the turn of the twenty-first century highlight the research community's reluctance to share risk information with potential subjects. In September 1999, 18-year-old Jessie Gelsinger died four days after receiving an infusion of new genes in a viral vector, as part of an experiment intended to determine whether this "gene therapy" might lead to a cure for an inherited liver disease, ornithine transcarbamylase deficiency. Among the many infractions committed by researchers at the University of Pennsylvania was their failure to reveal in the consent form the deaths of four monkeys subjected to similar research. They also failed to notify the FDA of "adverse events" that occurred in subjects in the study of which Gelsinger was a part.[57] The fact that Gelsinger was living a relatively healthy life, controlling his disease through medication and diet, made his enrollment in the study all the more controversial. Two years later, an asthma study with healthy volunteers at Johns Hopkins University resulted in the death of 24-year-old Ellen Roche. Like the gene therapy experiment, the study was cited with numerous infractions, including the failure to disclose risk information. The consent form failed to indicate that the drug being used to create symptoms similar to an asthma attack, hexamethonium, was not an approved medication but, rather, was intended to provoke a physiologic response.[58]

Such deficient consent practices may mislead many potential subjects into research participation. But sick patients may be particularly vulnerable to being misled. Patients with poor prognoses who have exhausted their options for medical treatment may feel that they have "no choice" but to participate in research, yet fail to understand that they are *in fact* participating in research. A study of subjects conducted by the ACHRE revealed that most patient-subjects believed they would personally benefit from participation and that their physicians would not offer them opportunities that did not benefit them.[59] A 1999 report by the National Bioethics Advisory Commission (NBAC) on research involving persons with mental disorders that may affect decision-making capacity reaffirmed these findings. In addition, NBAC found that existing policy fails to adequately guide researchers and IRBs on the complex matter of determining a potential subject's capacity for making decisions. Mental disorders can compromise decision-making capacity to varying degrees, and no consensus exists as to what degree of incapacity counts as a lack thereof.[60] NBAC made a number of recommendations, including that researchers indicate to IRBs who will conduct assessments of capacity and which method they will use. NBAC also recommended the development of more specific guidance on the definition of decisional capacity and improved assessment procedures.[61]

Questions about decision-making capacity also have been raised for another group of vulnerable potential subjects: HIV vaccine research subjects in Sub-Saharan Africa. Some African scholars have argued that severe and persistent poverty confounds not only being able to achieve the basic elements of informed consent, but decision-making capacity itself. Widespread illiteracy and language barriers may complicate disclosure re-

quirements, and desperation can render the offer of free medical care and pay coercive. However, some scholars have suggested that the precondition of informed consent — competence — may itself be at risk for this class of potential subjects. The effects of persistent and severe poverty, malnutrition, and illiteracy may render potential subjects unable, or limited in their capacity, to understand the complexities of biomedical science.[62] This possibility is exacerbated by widespread cultural beliefs about illness and causation that differ drastically from those of Western medical science.[63]

This brief history of informed consent reveals the interconnectedness of ethical challenges the research community faces. Full disclosure, a requirement of informed consent, requires that researchers themselves recognize the distinction between therapy and research, and present the risks and benefits candidly and clearly to potential subjects. Investigators may find it difficult to provide full disclosure, not only because their training as physicians cultivates the therapeutic misconception, but perhaps also because of a desire for prestige and profit. The high stakes of research, in turn, may lead even well-intended investigators to use convenient or compromised individuals for research. These issues — risk-benefit ratio, conflict of interest, and fair subject selection — are discussed below and are followed by a review of recent regulatory efforts to reform the practice and theory of ethical research.

II. RISK-BENEFIT RATIO

Historically, many medical investigators have failed repeatedly to present the risks of research to potential subjects in a clear and candid way. Although some transgressions clearly are attributable to intentional deception, others may reflect the confusion that has characterized the research enterprise since its inception. Because medical research emerged within the conceptual parameters and physical settings of clinical practice, the task of distinguishing one from the other took researchers and onlookers more than a century to do. PHS regulations in the mid-1960s, which required independent review of research protocols, recognized for the first time that research was different from therapy in important ways. A decade later, the National Commission's work represents the first explicit effort to articulate the distinction between medical therapy and medical research. As the Commission recognized, medical therapy aims to optimize the patient's care and is guided by the norms of "therapeutic beneficence" and "therapeutic nonmaleficence" — to promote the patient's good, and, above all, to do no harm.[64] Medical research, by contrast, aims to generate scientific knowledge that can serve future patients, not the patients who are currently under the physician-investigators' care. The two activities are distinct and demand distinct ethical standards. As Franklin Miller and Howard Brody note, "The basic goal and nature of the activity determines the ethical standards that ought to apply."[65]

The distinction is important and controversial. It is important because it underscores the potential for the abuse of potential subjects, which the history outlined above demonstrates is a constant danger of medical research. Whereas the interests of patients and physicians converge in medical therapy, as Miller and Brody note, in medical research these interests "are likely to diverge, even when the investigator acts with complete integrity."[66]

Still, the distinction remains controversial for practical and theoretical reasons. Clinical trials often entail a mixture of therapeutic and nontherapeutic features; that clinical trials may prove to have therapeutic benefits for patient-subjects can obfuscate the fact that their overriding purpose is to generate knowledge that will serve future patients.[67] Moreover, investigators are trained as physicians, and, as such, are socialized to understand their work in terms of promoting the health of an ill individual, despite the fact that medical research aims to generate knowledge that will enhance understanding and treatment of *future populations*. It is a conceptual shift that many researcher-physicians who attempt to balance both roles may find difficult to make.

What is more, these practical and psychosocial facts have found theoretical support in the notion of "clinical equipoise."[68] Clinical equipoise describes the medical community's uncertainty about the efficacy of various treatment options for a particular condition.[69] This uncertainty, according to its proponents, ethically justifies the placement of patient-subjects in randomized control trials (RCTs), wherein, typically, neither the physician nor the patient knows whether the patient is receiving the standard treatment or the experimental drug, thus, when there is no widely agreed upon, therapeutically preferred option, an investigator-physician is justified in enrolling, with

informed consent, patient-subjects in clinical trials that are intended to establish a superior therapeutic option or to establish that one option is not inferior to another.

Research is not, first and foremost, a therapeutic enterprise, but a scientific one. To suggest otherwise diverts attention from important ethical standards that must be met to justify experimentation involving humans. Importantly, such a confusion perpetuates the therapeutic misconception, which affects not only researchers but patient-subjects. As discussed above, the work of ACHRE demonstrated that patient-subjects more often than not believe they will benefit therapeutically from participating in research. This belief, far from an irrational hope on the part of patient-subjects, no doubt stems from the context in which they have been cared for: by professionals and in settings that carry out both research and therapy. This is why Miller and Brody argue, "Research participants need to know that the overall activity is aimed not at their own ultimate benefit, but at discovering new knowledge to help future patients," and that "investigators must themselves understand clearly the ways in which clinical research differs from clinical practice and convey this forthrightly to potential research subjects."[70]

None of this is to suggest that researchers do not have obligations to human subjects. They have many, as spelled out above, and they include the duty to promote a favorable risk-benefit ratio. Three conditions must be met to accomplish this:

1. Potential risks to individual subjects are minimized,
2. Potential benefits to subjects are enhanced, and
3. Potential benefits to individual subjects and society are proportionate to or outweigh the risks.[71]

The identification and assessment of risks should include physical, psychological, social, and economic risks.[72] Psychological harms include invasion of privacy and breach of confidentiality, as well as the stress and guilt that may accompany participation in behavioral research. Research that may result in stigmatization of individuals or groups should be handled with particular care. The last requirement to weigh potential benefits against risks is particularly difficult, as no widely agreed upon framework exists for making the necessary comparisons.[73] Nonetheless, these decisions must be made and are made everyday in the public policy arena.[74]

III. CONFLICTS OF INTEREST

As much as conceptual confusion may contribute to the misrepresentation of research, other factors may also be operative. Throughout the history of medical research, investigators have been motivated by any number of interests to undertake research, including the possibility of career advancement, prestige, and financial reward. None of these interests is, in itself, blameworthy; however, when these self-regarding interests impinge or eclipse researchers' duties to clearly and candidly convey the nature, purpose, and risks of research to potential subjects, they present a conflict of interest that demands regulation.

At least three sets of government regulations address financial conflicts of interest, but none is written with the aim of protecting potential research subjects.[75] These regulations cover research funded by or submitted to the PHS (which includes the NIH), the National Science Foundation, and the FDA, which leaves unregulated a large portion of research conducted in the U.S. Moreover, the regulations that do exist offer different thresholds as to what constitutes a financial conflict of interest, and fail to specify and limit the amount of compensation that can flow from sponsor to investigator or host institution.[76] Nowhere do regulations require disclosure of financial conflicts to IRBs or prospective research subjects.

As research has increasingly taken on an entrepreneurial character during the last two decades of the twentieth century, however, there have been several calls for reform regarding the disclosure of financial conflicts. During the 1980s and 1990s, when biotechnology and pharmaceutical industries "boomed" and private funding overtook public funding, new partnerships were forged between academia and industry that presented both individual investigators and institutions, with unprecedented financial incentives to develop and oversee research. In 2000, for example, the private sector invested between $55 billion and $60 billion in research development: twice the investment of the federal government.[77]

These partnerships, and the profits made possible by them, went relatively unquestioned until the 1999 Gelsinger case and the 2001 "Hutch" case. In the case of Jesse Gelsinger, described above, plaintiffs argued that the 18 year old's consent was not informed, not only because of a failure to report adverse events, but because the university's and researchers' extensive financial interests in the research were not disclosed.[78] Plaintiffs in the "Hutch" case made a similar argument. In this case, investigators at the famous Fred Hutchison Cancer Research Center in Seattle were positioned to earn substantial profits if the research designed to cure myelogenous leukemia was successful.[79] Plaintiffs alleged that researchers intentionally concealed their financial interests from patient-subjects, thereby not providing truly informed consent.

Controversies such as these, and growing recognition that conflicts of interest are widespread, has prompted government and nongovernmental responses. The federal Office for Human Research Protections (OHRP) issued interim guidelines in August 2000 to address financial conflicts of interest, which were then superceded by commentary on them provided by DHHS's own advisory committee, called at that time the National Human Research Protections Advisory Committee (NHRPAC). The national research community has come to consider these guidelines the "prevailing wisdom on conflict-of-interest issues."[80] NHRPAC's commentary specified at length many of the general recommendations made by OHRP's guidelines. Of particular importance is NHRPAC's clarification and specification regarding what constitutes a financial conflict and disclosure to IRBs and potential subjects during the informed-consent process.[81] Whereas the OHRP's interim guidelines spoke in general terms about financial relationships, the NHRPAC commentary carefully distinguishes financial interests that could threaten the moral and legal duties of investigators from financial relationships that characterize much of the research enterprise. NHRPAC also advises that potential subjects be informed about "real" financial conflicts of interest (that is, those identified as conflicts during the disclosure process within institutional mechanisms) and institutional strategies for managing those conflicts.[82]

The NHRPAC commentary is supported by other responses to the Gelsinger and "Hutch" cases. In late 2001, the Association of American Universities issued guidelines, and two reports were produced by the Association of American Colleges. The recommendations from both organizations are largely supportive of those issued by NHRPAC.[83] Congress has taken initial steps toward legislation that would require uniform regulations between the DHHS and FDA, and specifies the information that a clinical investigator must disclose to a potential subject, including any conflicts of interest held by the investigator.

IV. FAIR SUBJECT SELECTION

Before research reaches the stage of informed consent, criteria for the fair selection and recruitment of subjects should help to prevent the exploitation of compromised and otherwise marginalized individuals and social groups. The overarching criterion of fair selection of subjects requires that the scientific goals of the study guide the selection process.[84] Factors that are unrelated to the study's purpose — a group or individual's availability, marginalization, vulnerability, or privilege — should never serve as a legitimate basis for selection and enrollment. Because the results of the study should be generalizable to the populations who will use the intervention that is being studied, it is also important that groups and individuals not be excluded from opportunities to participate in research, unless there is a good scientific reason, or the group or individual is especially susceptible to risk.[85] Fair selection also requires, to the extent possible, that subjects who bear the risks of research reap the benefits of research, and those who benefit share some of the burdens.[86] These criteria aim to ensure the fair selection of subjects, yet they can create ethical tensions.

The requirement for generalizable results led to increased calls during the 1990s for the inclusion of women, minorities, and children in research, all of whom historically have been considered or proven to be vulnerable to research abuse. The use of children in research received heightened attention in the late 1990s, because the FDA became concerned about a lack of labeling indications for pediatric drugs, due to a lack of safety research in children.[87] The use of drugs by children requires that they be included in research, yet children are among society's most vulnerable populations. Young children not only are unable to consent to research, but are susceptible to the influence of parents, guardians, and other adults who are involved in their care. Moreover, an increasing percentage of children in the U.S. live in poverty, with no or limited access to quality healthcare, a fact likely to limit children's abil-

ity to benefit from the clinical advancements that they helped to make possible.[88]

The use and abuse of children has a long history.[89] Among the more controversial cases of the twentieth century is the research that took place at the Willowbrook State School for the Retarded. In this case, New York University researcher Saul Krugman attempted to create a prophylaxis for the fecally borne mild strain of hepatitis developed by nearly all of the Willowbrook children within six to 12 months of residency. The researchers deliberately infected some of the newly admitted children and cared for them in a well-equipped, well-staffed hepatitis unit, where the children were protected from exposure to other infectious diseases prevalent at the school. The case raises subtle questions about therapeutic benefit, validity of consent, and the fair selection of subjects, and remains a paradigmatic research ethics case. Research involving children received clarification and guidance in 1983, when the federal government adopted regulations based on the work of NBAC.[90]

Research that involves populations in developing countries has also raised questions about fair subject selection. Some believe that increasing amounts of preliminary pharmaceutical research are being conducted in the developing world, perhaps as a way to circumvent the costs and scrutiny associated with research in developed countries. These concerns have led to demands that research rules be scrupulously followed regardless of the site, that informed-consent requirements be applied even in culturally distant societies, and that communities and countries in which research is done should be compensated for their contribution to science. In 2000, the WMA approved paragraph 30 of its *Declaration of Helsinki* to establish an international standard of justice in research when persons in underdeveloped countries are recruited.[91]

V. REFORM EFFORTS: INCREASED MONITORING AND TRAINING

The federal government first attempted to regulate the research industry in 1900. Senator Jacob H. Gallinger, a physician and past surgeon general of New Hampshire, introduced a proposal to regulate research in Washington, D.C. The bill (1) addressed requirements for prior disclosure of the purpose of and procedures involved in research; (2) addressed written consent; and (3) made it illegal to do research with a long list of subjects who were seen as incapable of consent, or those who were especially vulnerable to coercion.[92] The bill failed due to fierce and effective lobbying by the AMA, which two years earlier had established a task force to track such legislative efforts.

The development of oversight mechanisms was incremental throughout the twentieth century, as the history above describes. The reform-oriented culture of the 1960s helped to usher in important measures that created a fruitful series of commissions and regulations, which culminated in the "Common Rule" in 1991.[93] These rules apply to all federally sponsored research and have binding authority. These regulations were adopted by 16 federal departments and agencies and detail how human subject research should be reviewed and conducted. The "Common Rule" applies to both intramural and extramural research. Although all 16 agencies conduct research according to the listed requirements in the "Common Rule," the administrative structure of their oversight programs varies. All must make assurances that human subject protections will be provided and enforced in order to receive federal funding.

The IRB continues to serve as the key mechanism for protecting human subjects. These committees have the authority to approve, disapprove, require modifications of, suspend, and oversee all human research conducted at the institution. IRBs have numerous responsibilities, which continue to grow in number as the research enterprise takes on new forms. In addition to ensuring the value and validity of research, a favorable risk-benefit ratio, fair subject selection, and adequate informed-consent provisions, IRBs are also now sometimes tasked with reviewing financial conflicts of interest that have been identified by institutional conflict-of-interest committees.[94]

At the same time, the IRB is widely viewed as an overtaxed and ineffective mechanism for protecting human subjects. In 1998, a report by the U.S. Inspector General's office at DHHS identified the many weaknesses of the current system, including the heavy workload of some IRBs, weak informed-consent protocols, a lack of ongoing monitoring, and a lack of external review.[95] In mid-2000, the DHHS announced a set of initiatives designed to strengthen these weaknesses. These include a requirement that the informed-consent process include a third-party observer for particu-larly complex or risky research; the disclosure of financial conflicts of interest to potential subjects, as discussed above; monitoring of investigator compliance with ethical requirements; and training in bioethics. In the private sector, two organizations were created to accredit human research protection programs, with the goal of creating uniform standards that reflect the view that all persons involved in research have a moral responsibility for the well-being of human subjects, not just the IRB.

NOTES

1. S.E. Lederer, *Subjected to Science: Human Experimentation in America Before the Second World War* (Baltimore: Johns Hopkins University Press, 1995), 2-6.

2. Ibid., 1, 7, 30, 54.

3. Ibid., 1-2.

4. E.J. Emanuel, D. Wendler, and C. Grady, "What Makes Clinical Research Ethical?" *Journal of the American Medical Association* 283, no. 20 (May 2000): 2701; I.G. Cohen, "Administrative Developments: New Human Subject Research Guidelines for IRBs," *Journal of Law, Medicine & Ethics* 28, no. 3 (Fall 2000): 305.

5. Emanuel, Wendler, and Grady, see note 4 above, p. 2701.

6. Ibid., 2.

7. Ibid.

8. E. Blacksher and J.D. Moreno, "A History of Informed Consent in Clinical Research," in *The Oxford Textbook of Clinical Research Ethics,* ed. E. Emanuel and F. Miller (Oxford, U.K.: Oxford University Press, forthcoming, 2006).

9. See note 1 above, p. 50.

10. R.R. Faden and T.L. Beauchamp, *A History and Theory of Informed Consent* (New York: Oxford University Press, 1986), 60-3.

11. See note 1 above, p. 10.

12. Ibid., chapter 5.

13. Ibid., 18-19.

14. See note 10 above, p. 120.

15. J. Katz, *The Silent World of Doctor and Patient* (New York: Free Press, 1984), 51; see note 10 above, p. 121.

16. See note 10 above, p. 123.

17. Ibid., 123.

18. W.C. Cannon, "The Right and Wrong of Making Experiments on Human Beings," *Journal of the American Medical Association* 67 (November 1916): 1372-3, p. 1373.

19. See note 10 above, p. 155.

20. R.R. Faden, S.E. Lederer, and J.D. Moreno, "U.S. Medical Researchers, the Nuremberg Doctors Trial, and the Nuremberg Code: A Review of Findings of the ACHRE," *Journal of the American Medical Association* 276, no. 20 (November 1996): 1667-71; Advisory Committee on Human Radiation Experiments, *Final Report of the Presidential Advisory Committee* (New York, N.Y.: Oxford University Press, 1996).

21. J.D. Moreno and S.E. Lederer, "Revising the History of Cold War Research Ethics," *Kennedy Institute of Ethics Journal* 6, no. 3 (September 1996): 223-43, p. 229.

22. Advisory Committee on Human Radiation Experiments, *Final Report,* see note 20 above, p. 50.

23. Ibid., 50; see note 21 above, p. 229.

24. Advisory Committee on Human Radiation Experiments, *Final Report,* see note 20 above, p. 53.

25. Ibid., 64, 500.

26. Ibid., 114.

27. Ibid., 46.

28. Ibid., 781.

29. Ibid., 90.

30. See note 10 above, p. 158.

31. Advisory Committee on Human Radiation Experiments, *Final Report,* see note 20 above, p. 83.

32. Katz, see note 15 above, p. 61.

33. Ibid., 61.

34. Ibid., 62.

35. See note 10 above, p. 203.

36. Advisory Committee on Human Radiation Experiments, *Final Report,* see note 20 above, p. 98.

37. See note 10 above, p. 156.

38. J. Arras, "The Jewish Chronic Disease Hospital," in *The Oxford Textbook of Clinical Research Ethics,* see note 8 above.

39. Advisory Committee on Human Radiation Experiments, *Final Report,* see note 20 above, p. 100.

40. See note 10 above, p. 209.

41. Ibid., 212.

42. Ibid., 166.

43. Advisory Committee on Human Radiation Experiments, *Final Report,* see note 20 above, p. 72.

44. National Commission for the Protection of Human Subjects of Biomedical and Behavioral Research, Department of Health, Education, and Welfare; *The Belmont Report: Ethical Principals and Guidelines for the Protection of Human Subjects of Research* (Washington, D.C.: U.S. Government Printing Office, 1979)

45. See note 10 above, p. 217.

46. *Belmont,* see note 44 above.

47. See note 10 above, p. 216, emphasis in original.

48. Ibid., 91.

49. American Hospital Association (AHA), *A Patient's Bill of Rights* (Chicago, Ill.: AHA, 1973).

50. Ibid., 139.

51. American Medical Association (AMA), *Code of Medical Ethics* (Chicago, Ill.: AMA, 1981).

52. *Canterbury v. Spence,* 464 F.2d 772 (D.C. Cir. 1972). *http://philosophy.wisc.edu/streiffer/BioandLawF99Folder/Readings Canterbury_v_Spence.pdf.*

53. See note 10 above, p. 221.

54. Ibid., 221,

55. Ibid., 219-221.

56. Advisory Committee on Human Radiation Experiments, *Final Report,* see note 20 above, p. 456.

57. R. Weiss and D. Nelson, "Methods Faulted in Fatal Gene Therapy, *Washington Post,* 8 December 1999, A1.

58. S. Levine, "FDA Cites Flaws in Hopkins Asthma Study," *Washington Post,* 3 July 2001, B03.

59. Advisory Committee on Human Radiation Experiments, *Final Report,* see note 20 above, p. 474.

60. National Bioethics Advisory Commission, "Report and Recommendations of the National Advisory Commission: Research Involving Persons with Mental Disorders That May Affect Decision Making Capacity, An Overview of the Issues," *http://www. georgetown.edu/research/nrcbl/nbac/capacity/Overview.htm,* p. 10.

61. Ibid., 4-7; T.L. Beauchamp and J.F. Childress, *Principles of Biomedical Ethics,* 5th ed. (New York: Oxford University Press, 2001), p. 74.

62. K. Moodley, "HIV Vaccine Trial Participation in South Africa: An Ethical Assessment," *Journal of Medicine and Philosophy* 27, no. 2 (2002): 197-215; A.A. van Niekerk, "Moral and Social Complexities of AIDS in Africa," *Journal of Medicine and Philosophy* 27, no. 2 (2002): 143-62.

63. P. de Zuleta, "Randomized Placebo-Controlled Trials and HIV-Infected Pregnant Women in Developing Countries: Ethical Imperialism or

Unethical Exploitation?" *Bioethics* 15, no. 4 (2001): 289-311.

64. F.G. Miller and H. Brody, "Therapeutic Misconception in the Ethics of Clinical Trials (A Critique of Clinical Equipoise)," *Hastings Center Report* 33, no. 3 (May-June 2003): 19-28.

65. Ibid., 22.

66. Ibid., 21.

67. Ibid., 21.

68. Ibid., 23-24.

69. Ibid., 19.

70. Ibid., 25-26.

71. Emanuel, Wendler, and Grady, see note 4 above, p. 2705.

72. S. Benbow, "Note: Conflict + Interest: Financial Incentives and Informed Consent in Human Subject Research," *Notre Dame Journal of Law, Ethics and Public Policy,* 17 (2003): 181.

73. Emanuel, Wendler, and Grady, see note 4 above, p. 2706.

74. Ibid.

75. M. Barnes and P.S. Florencio, "Symposium: New Directions in Human Subject Research: Looking Beyond the Academic Medical Center: Investigator, IRB and Institutional Financial Conflicts of Interest in Human-Subjects Research: Past, Present and Future," *Seton Hall Law Review* 32 (2003): 525.

76. Ibid., 4.

77. Ibid., 1.

78. See note 72 above, p. 2.

79. Ibid.

80. See note 75 above, p. 7.

81. Ibid., 8.

82. Ibid., 11.

83. Ibid., 13.

84. Emanuel, Wendler, and Grady, see note 4 above, p. 2704.

85. Ibid.,

86. Ibid., 2705.

87. L. Glantz, "Research with Children: (Law, Medicine, and Socially Responsible Research)," *American Journal of Law and Medicine* 24, no. 2-3 (Summer-Fall 1998): 213-44, p. 215.

88. National Center for Children in Poverty, "Fact Sheet: Low Income Children in the United States (2004)," *www.nccp.org/pub_cpf04.html.*

89. See note 87 above.

90. NBAC, see note 60 above.

91. The World Medical Association, "Declaration of Helsinki," *www.wma.net/e/ethicsunit/ helsinki.htm.*

92. See note 1 above, p. 72.

93. 56 *Federal Register* 28012, 18 June 1991; also DHHS, *CFR* Title 45, Part 46, Subpart A, *http:/ /www.hhs.gov/ohrp/human subjects/guidance/ 45cfr46.htm.*

94. See note 75 above, p.9.

95. Cohen, see note 4 above, p. 2.

6

Working with Persons Who Have Psychiatric Illness

Edmund G. Howe

I. INTRODUCTION

Careproviders, ethics consultants, and members of ethics committees may face exceptional challenges when they work with persons who have psychiatric illness.[1] This is so for a number of reasons, but the most important is that these patients tend to feel emotions more intensely than others do. When any of us experience intense emotion, we are much less likely to think clearly, and so our decision-making capacity is more likely to be impaired. When ethical problems arise for patients who have psychiatric illness, it is important that careproviders, ethics consultants, and ethics committee members know the most successful ways to respond. (Hereafter, "careproviders" will include clinicians, ethics consultants, and ethics committee members.)

The first thing that can be done to help patients — or any patient — is to establish a strong, trusting relationship, even though this may require sacrificing other values usually assigned higher priority. For example, when patients have schizophrenia, they may develop paranoid feelings toward their careproviders. This should be avoided if possible, as it can harm the relationship between patients and their careproviders. To protect their relationship with patients, careproviders may be forced to give patients less than the whole truth — for example, careproviders may choose not to tell patients that their paranoid feelings are delusional. Once a strong relationship is formed, though, it may be possible to tell patients the truth, in ever-increasing amounts, over time.

Two ways that careproviders can foster strong relationships are to "validate" patients and to give them choices. Careproviders can validate patients by affirming some aspect of what patients believe, even when the beliefs might be mistaken. It seems sensible to assume that when patients have psychiatric illnesses, careproviders should be *more* paternalistic, and offer fewer choices, but, to foster strong relationships, the opposite may be true.

This chapter will describe how careproviders can best respond to patients in general, and to patients who have specific psychiatric illnesses in particular.

II. GENERAL PRINCIPLES

Careproviders should use these principles in the order in which they are presented.

A. Acknowledge Conflicting Obligations

Careproviders should scrupulously acknowledge any conflicting obligations they may have, partly because patients who have psychiatric illness may be more "on guard" against experiencing slights than most people. All potentially threatening conflicts of interest should be disclosed as early as possible,[2] even when there is a chance that a patient may respond by ending the relationship. The following example shows how important this can be.

A patient had used up an inordinate amount of blood, and had depleted the hospital's blood supply, without much improvement in his condition. Supplies were being sought from other hospitals in the city. An ethics consultant was asked to intervene. The consultant had an unusual agenda in this case: simply to deliver the "bad news." The consultant should have recognized the unusual nature of his visit, have disclosed the actual nature of the consult with the patient, and then have asked the patient if he could help. But he didn't.

The patient sensed what the consultant was "up to" and refused to interact further with him. The result may have been the same if the consultant had shared his unusual agenda initially; if he had, however, the patient and consultant could have retained the basis of a trusting relationship.

Careproviders should disclose to a patient what they will do if they believe the patient may seriously harm another, or harm himself or herself. Patients in the latter category include those who are using substances that may kill them, which, due to addiction, they can't control. Careproviders can soften the effect of such warnings by pointing out that if the patient harms another, this will also hurt the patient; similarly, it should be pointed out that if the patient kills him- or herself, it may greatly harm loved ones.

Careproviders must be honest about their own motivations; for example, if they are acting primarily to protect themselves from being sued, they should say so. Patients know that their careproviders have various reasons for trying to help them. When careproviders are candid, patients may be more willing to work with them.

B. Be Non-Judgmental, Even in Thought

If having a hidden mixed agenda is the greatest deterrent to being able to intervene effectively with patients, judging patients is a close second. This is true even when careproviders judge patients only in their own minds. It is useful for careproviders to scrutinize their own views on psychiatric illness and to try to reduce the possibility that their relationship with patients is limited by their own unrecognized bias. It is easy for careproviders to be prone to bias, because bias exists in our culture; for example, beliefs that persons with psychiatric illness are "weak" or in some other way "inferior." Even when careproviders know that they aren't judgmental, it is wise to attend to the words that they use. Therapists who use an approach called dialectical behavior therapy to help patients with borderline personality disorder (discussed in the second section of this chapter) meet on a regular basis to discern judgmental statements they may unwittingly make,[3] because patients who have borderline personality disorder are exceptionally sensitive to being judged in a negative way.

When patients speak about themselves in a negative way, careproviders should comment on it, in part because patients' negative emotions may prevent them from being more autonomous. Careproviders can ask gently about patients' feelings in an open-ended way, such as, "What did you mean when you said that?" If a patient acknowledges a negative feeling such as shame, it can then be addressed. A careprovider can point out that no one is perfect, or relate an experience in which he or she was imperfect, or point out that many liabilities are, at the same time, strengths. These interventions take only moments, but, with this kind of support, patients usually will feel better, *and their capacity for autonomy will increase.* They will also appreciate their careprovider for such comments, which strengthens the patient/careprovider relationship.

Careproviders who act as ethics consultants should explain to patients and families what "doing an ethics consultation" means. First, they should make clear that they don't know better than patients what is right or wrong. Second, they should make clear that they do have greater expertise in how persons can make better decisions — they can give advice regarding what considerations should be "on the table." This implicitly informs patients that they are regarded as equals.

C. Validate Some Aspect of Patients' Views

If careproviders have sufficient understanding of a patient, it may be more powerful than medication, as the following case illustrates.

Mr. D had long been psychotic on a psychiatric ward. One evening, after almost all of the staff had left for the day, one psychiatrist and a cleaning person remained. Mr. D and the cleaning person were of a different race than the rest of the staff. The psychiatrist said to the cleaning person, "It's sad Mr. D has been here on the ward for so long." The cleaning person said, "He's not crazy. When you-all leave, he talks to me just like you and I are now." The psychiatrist arranged to transfer Mr. D to another hospital, where the staff and patients were the same race. Mr. D did well there, and was discharged almost immediately.

Careproviders should ask patients what their main concerns are and validate some aspect of them, as there is always *some* aspect of a patient's perspective that is sound.[4] In this way, careproviders indicate that they will be an ally. When patients have at least one other person who supports their interests, they are better able to express their true desires, even when they feel substantial fear. Careproviders may be morally obliged to validate patients for a reason put forward by John Stuart Mill: that an exception to the prohibition against violating another person's autonomy is when such a violation, in the long run, will enhance that person's autonomy.[5] When careproviders can begin a relationship with a patient by validating some aspect of a patient's perspective, it may alter the patient's ultimate outcome.[6] This case is an example.

I was the ethics consultant in a case in which the patient's entire family was at loggerheads with the staff. The staff wanted to withdraw treatments that they believed weren't effective. The patient, Miss K, was bleeding from numerous sites within her body. Surgery couldn't help, and the staff believed she was dying. Her family refused to allow treatments to be stopped. "She could survive," they said. I said to them, "You're right. She could survive. This doesn't often happen, but surely it's possible."

The family's response was not what the staff had imagined. It seemed like a miracle when the leading family member said, "Maybe we should listen to what the doctors are saying." The family, after some discussion, agreed to have their loved one's treatments withdrawn.

This kind of response to validation was not coincidental — it occurs all of the time. When people feel that they are opposed, they will defend their point of view; if they feel supported, they are more free to consider other options. As it happened, after treatments were withdrawn, Miss K got well.

It may be difficult for careproviders to validate a patient because other careproviders may

perceive this as a betrayal. If possible, careproviders should advise colleagues ahead of time that they might support the patient. Even when patients criticize members of the medical team, careproviders should try to find some validity in what they say. That may be difficult, because it is normal to defend one's colleagues. But, if this happens, patients may lose trust.

D. Give Choices

To enhance patients' trust, careproviders should give them choices whenever possible,[7] but patients who have psychiatric illness may make inferior choices. The primary concern must be the patients' outcome, however, and the key to achieving the best outcome possible is, again, to establish a trusting relationship. To do this, patients must feel safe.

Giving choices to patients who have mental illness can be a challenge. For example, some patients with schizophrenia refuse to take medication, even though it is well-established that antipsychotic medication is almost always essential to their doing well; in fact, some patients who stop medication take their own lives. But, if medication is forced, patients may see it as something that others do to them, and it is more likely that they will not be compliant, increasing the risk of morbidity and suicide over time.

The optimal, counter-intuitive alternative is for careproviders and patients to agree that patients may try to stop medication, but they agree to resume medication if they and their careprovider determine, together, that this has placed them at risk. Such a plan allows patients some degree of choice and preserves the patient/careprovider relationship. This is a paradigm for all patient/careprovider relationships: that is, whenever possible, patients should be given a choice. An example follows.

The patient, an elderly man, would no longer allow visiting nurses in his home to care for him, and the nurses asked for an ethics consult. The patient's physician, an internist, had told him that he was gradually going blind. The patient asked for a referral to an ophthalmologist, but his internist felt that his expertise was adequate, and he refused to write a referral, in part because the patient was on public assistance. To protest, the patient decided to refuse further nursing care. The ethics consultant suggested that the visiting nurses should call local ophthalmologists to ask if they would agree to examine the patient. To their surprise, they found one who examined the patient — at his home — for free. The ophthalmologist confirmed the internist's diagnosis that the patient would go blind. But, after the exam, the patient again accepted the visiting nurses in his home.

Psychiatric patients are likely to lack confidence, and are not likely to be appropriately assertive, as this example shows:

An infant was born with numerous medical problems, and died shortly after he was born. His body was cremated. A month or so afterward, his mother, who had become depressed, decided that she wanted his ashes. But, at that point, the best that could be done was to give the mother an urn that contained not only the ashes of her son, but also possibly the ashes of other babies who had been cremated after her son. The mother's careproviders informed her that they would have to meet with a special board to make this request, and the mother dropped her request.

Thus, careproviders should take exceptional initiative to act as patients' advocates and give them choices. Careproviders can use advance directives to give psychiatric patients additional choices. This is particularly important when patients have severe psychiatric illnesses such as schizophrenia or manic-depressive illness. When a patient is lucid, careproviders can ask them what they would want, should they lose touch with reality, and careproviders can follow the patient's stated wishes if this happens. This gives patients more control: they can state in advance, for example, which ward they want to go to, which doctor they would like to have, and which anti-psychotic medications they would be willing to take. These discussions may be more successful if careproviders say at the outset that it might look like they are using an advance directive to gain more control; they can then explain that they can't avoid how it "looks," but that this isn't their underlying intent. In this situation — and in general — careproviders should anticipate possible ambiguity and explain it in advance, as patients may be much less likely to then misinterpret their intent.
Careproviders should observe patients' emotional reactions when they discuss advance directives, because patients who have depression may feel worse when they talk about possibly unpleasant future events. Patients may do no more than just momentarily lower their eyes. When careproviders notice reactions like this, they can ask patients about their feelings. If patients can share their feelings, they will feel better. In general, careproviders should try to observe such reactions as they treat any patient. If they detect that patients may be feeling distress, they should interrupt the discussion — regardless of its content — and ask patients what they are feeling.

Careproviders may also want to inquire when patients appear to show no feelings, as it may indicate that they are experiencing painful memories or associations. Their conversation may appear to be "real," but something else may be going on. This will help patients respond optimally to treatment.

E. See Patients as Always Responding

Patients may respond in ways that are "negative," such as becoming angry. Careproviders often conclude that this is due to the patients' underlying psychiatric problems. While this is a sensible conclusion, as the patients do have psychiatric illness, it can be a serious mistake.[8] In fact, patients may feel hurt for reasons that careproviders wouldn't usually imagine as the following case example indicates.

A patient had overwhelming fear of a medical procedure that was necessary to save his life. His doctor referred him to a therapist, hoping he could help the patient overcome this life-threatening fear. To greet his new patient, the therapist asked, "What can I do for you?" The patient became enraged because his internal reaction was, "*You* should know how you can help me; don't ask me. You are the expert, and that's why I came to see you in the first place!" The patient didn't share this reaction, however, and the consultation was not successful.

If the careprovider had been able to detect that the patient was responding negatively, he could have asked about it. If the patient was willing to say how he felt, the careprovider could have apologized for having miscommunicated and could have clarified what it was that he'd really meant. When careproviders ask patients what they are feeling, patients may also reveal feelings that weren't caused by the careproviders' inadvertent offense, as below.

A careprovider asked a patient if she would like to pray with him. The patient looked sad, and the careprovider asked why. The patient said she felt sad because she knew why he had asked her to pray with him — it was because he knew she was dying. It was a good thing he had asked, because she wasn't dying! By asking about this, her doctor was able to straighten out this misunderstanding.

Some feelings can remain hidden for decades and appear only as a fleeting memory. But, by inquiring, careproviders can unearth these too. A well-known example is offered by the artist Edvard Munch, whose sister died of tuberculosis when he was five. Many years later, Munch visited a patient with a broken leg with his father, who was a doctor. That experience triggered his memory of his sister, and he then painted her in a famous work called *The Sick Child*.[9]

F. Recognize Counter-Transference Feelings

None of these approaches will enhance careproviders' effectiveness if they have negative feelings toward their patients, but what careproviders feel may be influenced by patients' underlying disorders. Schizophrenic patients are likely to make careproviders feel uneasy.[10] This may be because, regardless of how the patients present themselves, they have a psychotic process going on "underneath the surface." For example, a patient I treated carried on a "normal conversation" for several minutes, only to then say that she was being monitored by her dental fillings. Careproviders may feel sad when they treat patients who are depressed. If patients are suicidal, careproviders may feel dread, which may cause them to become emotionally distant. This is especially unfortunate, as such distancing may increase the risk that these patients will take their own lives.

Careproviders can attempt to mitigate against possible harms by, first, identifying their negative feelings about patients, and then reducing them by sharing them with their colleagues. If they fear that their colleagues will judge them negatively because of their feelings, they should choose a colleague who won't judge them. If careproviders begin to feel overwhelmed and find that they can't lessen their feelings, they should consult a colleague in mental health.

Careproviders should remain alert to the possibility they may act out their feelings; this can be inferred from their behavior. For example, they may be acting out their feelings if they are uncharacteristically late for appointments with a patient they dread seeing.

G. Try to Involve Patients' Families

In general, careproviders should not automatically respect all the preferences of patients who have psychiatric illness, but should instead be-

come more paternalistic than usual. For instance, if a patient does not want to involve family members, a careprovider should take the initiative to explore why. If the family is reasonably emotionally healthy, the careprovider should try to persuade the patient to involve them, on the other hand, if family members are not emotionally healthy and are critical of the patient, it may adversely affect how well the patient does.[11] When this is not the case, however, families may help. For example, when schizophrenic patients begin to become psychotic, family members often notice the initial indications. The patients may, for instance, begin to change how they dress. Families who are able to notice these initial signs may be able to help the patients come in for treatment earlier. Similarly, when ethical problems arise, family members may be able to provide vital information; that is, when patients relapse, their preferences may change. Careproviders may be able to persuade patients to involve their family members even when they have severed contact; careproviders should offer to take the initiative to try to contact the family and try to involve them on the patients' behalf.

One way for careproviders to do this is to ask the family to call or come in, and offer two assurances. First, careproviders can say that if the family decides that they want to end the meeting, they can, at any time; no questions asked. Careproviders can emphasize that they feel grateful that the family is willing to try, no matter what. Second, careproviders can say that the family may end the meeting if a conflict emerges between the patient and the family. Careproviders can explain that they want to be sure that family members aren't harmed if they are willing to be involved.

Once the patient and family are together, careproviders can insist that each person will speak only for him- or herself. At any sign of discord, careproviders can ask that comments be directed only to him or her. When one person speaks, she or he can ask the others to repeat their understanding of what was said. Family discussions can be very useful in resolving ethical problems. It is crucial that all core family members be involved, and careproviders should tell family members who may oppose such meetings that they are *the present standard of ethical care*. The outcomes may be phenomenally good, as this case shows:

A woman hadn't talked to her mother in years. Her mother had had multiple psychotic episodes, hospitalizations, and suicide attempts. After a family meeting like the one described, the daughter decided that she wanted her mother to move in with her. Her mother hasn't been psychotic, hospitalized, or suicidal since.

III. SPECIFIC CONDITIONS

There are a variety of psychiatric illnesses, and there are particular kinds of psychological interventions that are most effective for each. This section will focus on five main categories of psychiatric illness.

A. Schizophrenia

Perhaps the most difficult patients to treat are patients with paranoid schizophrenia. It is often assumed that schizophrenia is a biological illness, but this isn't true. For example, when an identical twin has schizophrenia, only about half of their twins also have it, which suggests that psychosocial influences also have a strong effect.[12] Personal interactions with these patients are important:[13] recent interventions using cognitive behavioral therapies have found that personal interaction can be effective.[14]

If a patient reports having a delusion, what is most important to the diagnosis is the report of the delusion, not its content. To understand the patient and to interact meaningfully with him or her, however, it is critical for careproviders to try to understand the meaning of the content.[15] They should also try to explore its meaning with the patient.[16] Careproviders should not confront the patients' delusions directly, however. Rather, if possible, they should validate some *aspect* of the delusion that is true. If they can do this, patients will feel more supported, and their fear may decrease. When this is possible, over time, the delusion may "dissolve."

Careproviders should also try to involve the patients' families, as mentioned above.[17] One breakthrough in treatment in recent decades has been to teach families to not be overly critical or emotionally over-reactive.[18] A second breakthrough is that the patients can gain greatly from learning new social skills.[19] This is an instance in which careproviders should particularly act as patients' advocates. Difficult ethical issues may arise regarding whether patients should be involuntarily hospitalized, given medications against their will, and restrained. The key in this issue is an established relationship. Also, as mentioned

above, patients will have increased control if careproviders discuss with them in advance what they would want done if they become psychotic.[20] Careproviders can also help patients gain control by discussing non-psychiatric advance directives with them.[21] This should be done slowly, over some time, if possible. The discussion should be interrupted regularly to allow patients to describe their feelings and associations.

Although these patients may be greatly cognitively impaired in some respects, they may not be impaired in others. Legally, they may be competent in one respect, but not competent in others, as the following illustration of this complex and difficult issue shows:

The mother of a patient who had schizophrenia became incapable of making decisions. The son believed that his mother wanted to continue all treatments. The son had some delusions, but they were not related to her situation. Some members of the ethics committee thought that, because the patient's son had delusions, he was incapable of determining what his mother would want, but they decided to respect his decision on her behalf. As it turned out, the patient got better and regained her capacity to make decisions for herself. When she did, she confirmed that her son had been right about her preferences.

B. Depression

The most important issue in treating depressed patients is to opt not to treat them because "anyone in their situation would feel depressed."[22] This is especially the case when patients want to die. When patients are dying and want treatment stopped, they may be depressed. Moreover, their depression may be highly treatable.[23] This is particularly likely, for example, when patients have had a stroke. It may not be knowable whether a patient is depressed without a trial of antidepressant medication. Ritalin or an amphetamine may help at once, while another antidepressant like an SSRI (selective serotonin reuptake inhibitor) takes longer to work. It may take weeks before it is known whether the patient will enjoy a positive result.

Such patients may not respond, however, unless they have psychotherapy or can find meaning in their life.[24] Finding new meaning may take time. An example is patients with sudden acute quadriplegia. They may want to die, for example, by having their ventilator disconnected immediately after their accident. Careproviders might believe that respecting their autonomy requires immediately granting their request. Yet, ethically, there may be greater justification in trying to persuade patients to wait.[25] Careproviders should point out that research indicates that a substantial proportion of patients in the same situation find, after some time, that their new life, though wholly different, is still worth living.

Careproviders should never hesitate to ask patients if they feel suicidal.[26] Careproviders sometimes fear that if they ask this question, it is as though they have suggested it, and patients will kill themselves as a result. *This is not the case.*

When patients who are dying want to commit suicide, it can be immensely useful for them to share these feelings,[27] because, if they can, they no longer must bear the feelings alone, which is a great benefit. On the other hand, it can be a problem when patients are being cared for by a hospice team, and one member of the team believes that all such confidences must be reported immediately. If patients are suddenly placed in a hospital on suicidal watch, their trust in the staff may be destroyed, and the ability of the staff to help them may be lost.[28] As this is the case, hospice staff should discuss this possibility among themselves ahead of time. Staff who can't bear accepting this risk may benefit patients more in some other medical role.

When dying patients express an interest in suicide, it is most important for careproviders to contact relatives who have become estranged.[29] When patients are dying, if they can share themselves with relatives in ways they have never shared before, their last days may be literally the best days of their lives and their relatives' lives. Consultants should tell patients this.

Patients may say that they aren't depressed, but that they are experiencing emotional anguish, which is made even worse due to the awareness that they are dying. They may say that they have been "depressed" before, and that they believe that the two feelings aren't the same. Because they are feeling existential emotional pain — which they experience as worse than depression — they may ask their careproviders to give them relief. Careproviders can give these patients medications that place them in a permanent state of unconsciousness, a practice some refer to as "terminal sedation."[30] It is unclear that what these patients are feeling is different from depression. What is clear, regardless, is that the patients find that living on, knowing that they will die soon, is unbearable. One approach that may be useful in this situation

is to give the patients the sedation that they request, but only for a few days. After they regain consciousness, they and their careprovider can decide whether to continue the medication. Some patients, after this kind of respite, change their minds and want to remain awake during the remaining time they have to live.

There is some uncertainty about whether patients should be informed ahead of time that terminal sedation is an option, as it may prove to be an option that some find too difficult to refuse. Careproviders should be aware that depressed patients are unduly susceptible to suggestion. Thus, careproviders should always attend to the connotations as well as the literal meaning of what they say, as in the following example:

A patient had been hospitalized for almost a year, receiving ongoing platelet infusions after an allergic reaction to a drug. Her family visited her around the clock — and were happy to do so. An ethics consultant, learning of the patient's situation, took the initiative to go to see her, to insure that she knew that she "had permission" to choose to die. "Are you sure that you want to remain alive?" he asked. She requested that her platelets be stopped the very next day, and, shortly thereafter, she died.

It may be that the patient felt she lacked "permission" to die, as the consultant suspected. It may also be, however, that his asking this question suggested to her that she should choose to die. Vulnerable to suggestion, she may have complied, even though she didn't really want to.

C. Dementia

When patients have dementia, their major problems may be emotional and behavioral, rather than mostly cognitive, as might be supposed.[31] These patients may, for example, be depressed, and, like depressed patients, they may also be aggressive.[32] Their emotions and behavior can be greatly helped when careproviders discuss what is "going on with them."[33] As for schizophrenic patients, no matter how impaired these patients are, careproviders still should respond to their psychological needs.[34] The care that they receive from their caregivers — who are often family members — is also vitally important.[35] Careproviders, therefore, should address the needs of caregivers as well as the needs of patients.

For example, when patients have had a severe head injury, careproviders should try to involve their spouses. These caregivers may have to grieve the loss of their partners as they knew them. They may feel agony, trying to recreate the patients "as they were." They may be greatly helped by careproviders who encourage them to accept that the improvement they hope for may never take place. It may save their marriages.[36]

Even when patients are legally incompetent, they may retain knowledge of their preferences; thus, their preferences still should be respected,[37] as in the following example:

A girl in her late teens was mildly mentally retarded and had cancer. She had tried several kinds of chemotherapy, but without success. The patient had suffered throughout each course, vomiting and losing her hair. When she was asked if she wanted to try an additional trial of chemotherapy, she said that she didn't. She wasn't able to articulate the relative differences in her options of taking or not taking more chemotherapy, but she clearly and repeatedly said "No."

Acting on her expressed preference made sense in this context, even though the young woman didn't know the specific consequences of the various options that were available to her. Her wishes were respected.

A "sliding scale" was used in the above case to assess the young woman's competency: in a sliding scale, when there is relatively little difference in the various possible outcomes for a patient, the level of the patient's comprehension can be lower. But when the relative differences in the possible outcomes are greater, the degree of understanding required of the patient to make decisions must be greater. When the relative consequences vary little, to respect a patient's preferences will at least respect her or his dignity.

D. Substance Abuse

When patients have problems involving substance abuse, three considerations are most important. First, what they need may depend on the stage of their illness.[38] If, for example, they deny that they are ill, what they most need is an intervention that will help them to discern that they are ill. This does not mean merely telling them this directly; as with paranoid schizophrenic patients, this may only increase their defensiveness. These patients use denial as a defense. It is more effective for careproviders to ask the patient if there is a way that they can find to work together to discern whether the patient really does have a problem. This approach gives priority to the patient overcoming her or his denial by establishing a relationship, and then giving the patient a

choice.[39] It requires that a careprovider treat the patient as an equal partner in the joint endeavor to decide who is right: the patient, who believes there is no problem, or the careprovider.

Second, when patients already know they have a problem, they may need to acquire greater skills. Careproviders can help patients gain skills by acting as advocates. This can be extremely important, because disorder often creates anger in others, and other careproviders may refuse to help them. Relapse is often part of the illness, and careproviders should expect relapse to occur repeatedly. Rather than give up after relapse, a better response is to be more optimistic; careproviders can say, for example, "Good! Now you know better what won't work for you, and so you have a better chance to succeed!" The preferences that patients have while they are addicted may be very different than the preferences they would have if they weren't. For this reason, careproviders may want to be more paternalistic than usual, which may mean testifying against patients in court, especially in life-threatening emergencies.

Third, careproviders should take the initiative to be advocates when addicts experience pain. Patients should be able to obtain pain relief. This may require finding a specialist who knows how, and is willing, to provide pain relief.[40] Careproviders can insist that an expert be brought in.[41] Careproviders shouldn't "give up" on these patients; careproviders who don't want to treat them commonly rationalize that, to get well, an addicted patient must first "hit bottom." There is a grain of truth to this; to get well, patients first must recognize that they have a problem, but otherwise this idea is untrue. The more losses patients experience, the harder it may be for them to recover. Addicted patients may lose everything, including their lives. They have a disease; they may go for months without drinking, only then to go on a binge. This seems to indicate that they have control, but that isn't the case. These patients may be vulnerable to internal and external cues that trigger profound cravings. Patients may not even know what these cues are, and so may not be able to avoid them. The best bet may be to try to enhance their capacities to withstand their cravings, regardless of when the cues occur; gaining this capacity may take time.

Again, it is most important to involve patients' families. Family members may be greatly harmed by what addicted patients do. Careproviders should explain to family members why they must retain hope, but at the same time help them to get the assistance that they need. This is important because family members may provide "ungluing" cues, as illustrated below:

One patient was doing well. He was relapsing only a few times a year. When he did, he would always get into "detox" within the first week. His family, nonetheless, had lost hope, so they tried new approaches. These included contacting the women he was dating and employers at his job. These actions seemed to help bring about further relapses.

E. Borderline Personality Disorder

One characteristic generally said to distinguish patients with personality disorders from patients who have other psychiatric disorders is that patients in the first group tend not to experience painful emotions themselves. Rather, they may feel fine and think they are fine. However, they may have repeated clashes with others and blame these clashes on others. The kind of personality disorder that is most likely to cause difficulties for careproviders is borderline personality disorder.[42] These patients' emotions tend to change rapidly — they may change from being warm one minute to enraged the next. When staff feels angry at a patient, the patient often has this disorder.[43] An example occurred at a hospice. A patient became angry at a staff member and then threw a glass at her. Many of the staff, as a result of this and other angry behaviors, felt afraid to enter the patient's room.

There are several keys to working most successfully with these patients. The first is to recognize that these patients do not become angry wholly on their own. Their inappropriate, overly intense responses always occur as a result of an interpersonal interaction. It is typical in cases like this for staff to feel abused, and, in response, to set arbitrary limits.[44] This may be to retaliate. Regardless, this angers these patients even more. An ever-increasing, negative vicious cycle then ensues. The task of careproviders here is to change their own behavior. Once careproviders recognize that a patient is angry, rather than reacting angrily, they should try to discern *what they have done*. Then, if possible, they should make amends. They may, for example, have inadvertently said something judgmental. When patients show destructive behaviors such as being inappropriately angry, careproviders must first recognize that they are doing the best that they can with the skills

that they have — and then tell the patients the same thing.

Once careproviders establish a meaningful relationship with patients, it may be possible to give patients what they most need: to educate them about how their behavior affects others. As above, after careproviders try to identify with the patient and explicitly acknowledge her or his underlying pain, the patient may become willing to truly listen to what they have to say. Then careproviders can share not only how the patient negatively affects others, but how this, in turn, adversely affects the patient. It may be assumed that these patients already know this, but quite often they don't. Rather than suggest that patients should learn other behaviors, careproviders should ask them if they are interested in discussing the relative pros and cons of their behavior. This implicitly suggests that there is some valid basis for what these patients do. It also shows respect by offering patients the opportunity to make choices. Even if patients decide to continue doing what they have been doing, it doesn't mean that careproviders have "failed" — merely by considering the pros and cons of their actions, these patients have acquired a greater capacity to reflect upon their own behavior. Also, by allying themselves with patients, careproviders will establish closer relationships. Patients may need the increased support of a relationship before they can feel safe enough to be willing or able to change. An example is self-cutting.[45] This behavior makes most careproviders frightened. It can be life-threatening, but, in many instances, it isn't. Therapists who are most successful know that patients' behavior may serve an important purpose for them; for instance, it may be self-soothing. Unless and until the patients can find another behavior that works as well or better for them, they most likely won't give it up; for example:

One patient's self-cutting had always been superficial and harmless. She indicated that she had no interest in ever taking her life. She did it alone, in her room, and she hid her superficial cuts under her clothing. But it caused her mother unbearable stress. After her daughter had been alone for any length of time in her room, the mother would demand that she strip so that the mother could see if she had cut herself. They engaged in this battle incessantly. The daughter found this behavior, and this alone, self-soothing. It was the only way she knew to allay the fear she experienced when she was under increased stress.

It was unrealistic at that time to expect the daughter to suddenly be willing and able to give this self-cutting up. Because she loved her mother, and her mother loved her, the careprovider suggested that, rather than doing this alone and feeling shame, when she felt that she must cut herself, she might instead ask her mother to be with her. The mother agreed. The daughter did feel less-intense fear when her mother was with her. In a short time, her self-cutting went away.

IV. CONCLUSION

When ethics consultants or committees see patients who have psychiatric illnesses, there is a risk that they will not give the best possible care, because many of the interventions that would be optimal in other circumstances aren't optimal with these patients. As described in this chapter, the best responses to these patients may seem counter-intuitive, but have been shown to be optimal over time.

NOTES

1. R.C. Kessler et al., "Lifetime and 12-Month Prevalence of DSM-III-R Psychiatric Disorders in the United States: Results from the National Co-Morbidity Survey," *Archives of General Psychiatry* 51 (1994): 8-19.

2. K.K. Boyd, "Power Imbalances and Therapy," *Focus* 11, no. 9 (August 1996): 1-4; J.F. Childress, "Citizen and Physician — Harmonious or Conflicting Responsibilities," *Journal of Medicine and Philosophy* 2, no. 4 (December 1977): 401-9.

3. M.M. Linehan, *Cognitive-Behavioral Treatment of Borderline Personality Disorder* (New York: Guilford Press, 1993).

4. Ibid.

5. J.S. Mill, *On Liberty* (London: Penguin, 1985), 173. The key passage is this: "If either a public authority or anyone else saw a person attempting to cross a bridge which had been ascertained to be unsafe, and there was no time to warn him of his danger, they might seize him and turn him back, without any real infringement of his liberty; for liberty consists in doing what one desires, and he does not desire to fall into the river" (p. 166).

6. J.R. Peteet, "Putting Suffering into Perspective: Implications of the Patient's World View," *Journal of Psychotherapy, Practice, and Research* 10, no. 3 (Summer 2001): 187-92.

7. W.R. Miller and S. Rollnick, *Motivational Interviewing: Preparing People for Change,* 2nd ed. (New York: Guilford Press, 2002).

8. M.J. Dewan and R.W. Pies, ed., *The Difficult-to-Treat Psychiatric Patient* (Washington, D.C.: American Psychiatric Association, 2001). This book is also highly recommended; M.C. Zanarini and K.R. Silk's chapter (179-208) on treating patients with borderline personality disorder is unsurpassed in the psychiatric literature.

9. R. Heller, *Edvard Munch* (Chicago: University of Chicago Press, 1984).

10. Warren Wright, a novelist, reports seeing Van Gogh's *Olive Trees* and finding it "jarring" for a reason he didn't then know. He discerned the reason later. The painting portrays two different "times" at once. The sun is in one place, but the shadows it should cast are not in the right place. This sense of "something being wrong" may be the same sense some have with some schizophrenic patients. J. Elkins, *Pictures and Tears* (New York: Routledge, 2004), 134-5.

11. American Psychiatric Association, "Practice Guidelines for the Treatment of Patients with Schizophrenia," *American Journal of Psychiatry* 154 (April, 1997, supp.): 1-63.

12. J. Bustillo et al., "The Psychosocial Treatment of Schizophrenia: An Update," *American Journal of Psychiatry* 158 (2001): 163-75; see also note 14 of this article.

13. J.J. Huszonek, "Establishing Therapeutic Contact with Schizophrenics: A Supervisory Approach," *American Journal of Psychotherapy* 41 (1987): 185-87.

14. T. Sensky et al., "A Randomized Controlled Trial of Cognitive Behavioral Therapy for Persistent Symptoms in Schizophrenia Resistant to Medication," *Archives of General Psychiatry* 57 (2000): 165-72.

15. A. Altman and M.A. Selzer, "Delusions in the Transference. Psychotherapy with the Paranoid Patient," *Psychiatry Clinics of North America* 18 (June 1995): 407-25.

16. P. Weiden and L. Havens, "Psychotherapeutic Management Techniques in the Treatment of Outpatients with Schizophrenia," *Hospital and Community Psychiatry* 45 (1994): 549-55.

17. G.E. Hogarty et al., "Three-Year Trials of Personal Therapy Among Schizophrenic Patients Living with or Independent of Family, I: Description of Study and Effects on Relapse Rates," *American Journal of Psychiatry* 154, no. 11 (1997): 1504-13; G.E. Hogarty et al., "Three-Year Trials of Personal Therapy Among Schizophrenic Patients Living with or Independent of Family, II: Effects on Adjustment of Patients," *American Journal of*

Psychiatry 154, no. 11 (1997): 1514-24.

18. G. Thornicroft and E. Susser, "Evidence-Based Psychotherapeutic Interventions in the Community of Care of Schizophrenia," *British Journal of Psychiatry* 178 (2001): 2-4.

19. A.S. Bellack, "Skills Training for People with Severe Mental Illness," *Psychiatry Rehabilitation Journal* 27 (2004): 375-91; R.P. Liberman, C.J. Wallace, and J. Hassell, "Rehab Rounds: Predicting Readiness and Responsiveness to Skills Training: the Micro-Module Learning Test," *Psychiatric Services* 55, no. 7 (July 2004): 764-6; S.R. Marder et al., "Two Year Outcome of Social Skills Training and Group Psychotherapy for Outpatients with Schizophrenia," *American Journal of Psychiatry* 153 (1996): 1585-92.

20. P.S. Appelbaum, "Psychiatric Advance Directives and the Treatment of Committed Patients," *Psychiatric Services* 55, no. 7 (July 2004): 751-2, 63; P. Thomas and A.B. Cahill, "Compulsion and Psychiatry — The Role of Advance Statements," *British Medical Journal* 329 (July 2004): 122-3.

21. J.M. Atkinson, H.C. Garner, and W.H. Gilmour, "Models of Advance Directives in Mental Health Care: Stakeholder Views," *Social Psychiatry and Psychiatric Epidemiology* 39, no. 8 (August 2004): 673-80.

22. American Psychiatric Association, "Practice Guidelines for the Treatment of Patients with Major Depressive Disorder," *American Journal of Psychiatry* 157 (2000): 1-45.

23. E. Tiernan et al., "Relations between Desire for Early Death, Depressive Symptoms and Antidepressant Prescribing in Terminally Ill Patients with Cancer," *Journal of the Royal Society of Medicine* 95 (2002): 386-90; L. Rosenblatt and S.D. Block, "Depression, Decision making and the Cessation of Life-Sustaining Treatment," *Western Journal of Medicine* 175 (2001): 320-5; R. DeRubeis et al., "Medications Versus Cognitive Behavior Therapy for Severely Depressed Outpatients: Mega-Analysis of Four Randomized Comparisons," *American Journal of Psychiatry* 156 (July 1999): 1007-13; G. Fava et al., "Depressive Cognitive-Behavioral Management of Drug-Resistant Major Disorder," *Journal of Clinical Psychiatry* 58 (1997): 278-82.

24. M.D. Sullivan, "Hope and Helplessness at the End of Life," *American Journal of Geriatric Psychiatry* 11, no. 4 (July-August 2003): 393-405.

25. M.J. Edwards and S.W. Tolle, "Disconnecting a Ventilator at the Request of a Patient Who Knows He Will then Die: The Doctor's Anguish," *Annals of Internal Medicine* 117 (1992): 254-6.

26. J.T. Maltsberger, "Treating the Suicidal Patient: Basic Principles," *Annals of the New York Academy of Science* 932 (April 2001): 158-68; H. Hendin et al., "Desperation and Other Affective States in Suicidal Patients," *Suicide and Life Threatening Behavior* 34, no. 4 (Winter 2004): 386-94; H. Hendin et al., "Recognizing and Responding to a Suicide Crisis," *Suicide and Life-Threatening Behavior* 31, no. 2 (Summer 2001): 15-28.

27. S.I. Byock, *Dying Well: Peace and Possibilities at the End of Life* (New York: Riverhead Books, 1997); D.P. Sulmasy, "Addressing the Religious and Spiritual Needs of Dying Patients," *Western Journal of Medicine* 175 (2001): 251-4.

28. J.T. Maltsberger, "Calculated Risk Taking in the Treatment of Suicidal Patients: Ethical and Legal Problems," *Death Studies* 18, no. 5 (September 1994): 439-52.

29. K. O'Leary and S. Beach, "Marital Therapy: A Viable Treatment for Depression and Marital Discord," *American Journal of Psychiatry* 47 (1990): 183-6.

30. T. Morita, "Palliative Sedation to Relieve Psycho-Existential Suffering of Terminally Ill Cancer Patients," *Journal of Pain and Symptom Management* 28, no. 5 (November 2004): 445-50; J. Rietjens et al., "Physician Reports of Terminal Sedation without Hydration or Nutrition for Patients Nearing Death in the Netherlands," *Annals of Internal Medicine* 141, no. 3 (August 2004): 178-85; C. Gauthier, "Active Voluntary Euthanasia, Terminal Sedation, and Assisted Suicide," *The Journal of Clinical Ethics* 12, no. 1 (Spring 2001): 43-50.

31. B. Pentland et al., "Training in Brain Injury Rehabilitation," *Disability and Rehabilitation* 25, no. 10 (2003): 544-8.

32. J. Demark, "Anger and its Management for Survivors of Acquired Brain Injury," *Brain Injury* 16, no. 2 (February 2002): 91-108; G.S. Alexopoulos et al., "Treatment for Agitation in Older Persons with Dementia: Postgraduate Medicine Special Report," *Post Graduate Medicine* (April 1998) 1-85; J.L. Fuh, "A Transcultural Study of Agitation in Dementia," *Journal of Geriatric Psychiatry and Neurology* 15, no. 3 (Fall 2002): 171-4; M.S. Mega et al., "The Spectrum of Behavioral Changes in Alzheimer's Disease," *Neurology* 46, no. 1 (1996): 130-5.

33. C.R. Hirsch and V.M. Mouratoglou, "Life Review of an Older Adult with Memory Diffi-

culty," *International Journal of Geriatric Psychiatry* 14, no. 4 (April 1999): 261-5.

34. K.C. Richards and C.K. Beck, "Progressively Lowered Stress Threshold Model: Understanding Behavioral Symptoms of Dementia," *Journal of the American Geriatric Society* 52, no. 10 (October 2004): 1755-60; S.M. Folzer, "Psychotherapy with 'Mild' Brain-injured Patients," *American Journal of Orthopsychiatry* 71, no. 2 (April 2001): 145-51.

35. J.E. Gaugler et al., "The Emotional Ramifications of Unmet Need in Dementia Caregiving," *American Journal of Alzheimer's Disease and Other Dementias* 19, no. 6 (November-December 2004): 369-80; J. Hinojosa and N.R. Dooley, "Improving Quality of life for Persons with Alzheimer's Disease and Their Family Caregivers: Brief Occupational Therapy Intervention," *American Journal of Occupational Therapy* 58, no. 5 (September-October 2004): 561-9; K.T. Kirchoff, M.K. Song, and K. Kehl, "Caring for the Family of the Critically Ill Patient," *Critical Care Clinics* 20, no. 3 (July 2004): 453-66; S.J. Farber et al., "Issues in End-of-Life Care: Patient, Caregiver, and Clinical Perceptions," *Journal of Palliative Medicine* 6, no. 1 (2003): 19-31.

36. J. Gosling, "Rearranged Marriages: Marital Relationships After Brain Injury," *Brain Injury* 13, no. 10 (October 1999): 785-96.

37. D.T. Watts, C.K. Cassel, and T. Howell, "Dangerous Behavior in a Demented Patient: Preserving Autonomy in a Patient with Diminished Capacity," *Journal of the American Geriatric Society* 37, no. 7 (July 1989): 658-62; P.S. Appelbaum and T. Grisso, "Assessing Patients' Capacities to Consent to Treatment," *New England Journal of Medicine* 319 (1988): 1635-8.

38. J.O. Prochaska, C.C. DiClemente, and J.C. Norcross, "In Search of How People Change: Applications to Addictive Behaviors," *American Psychologist* 47 (1992): 1102-14.

39. N.B. Figlie, J. Dunn, and R. Laranjeira, "Motivation for Change in Alcohol Dependent Outpatients from Brazil," *Addiction Behavior* 30, no. 1 (January 2005): 159-65; M.P. Karno and R. Longabaugh, "What Do we Know? Process Analysis and the Search for a Better Understanding of Project MATCH's Anger-by-Treatment Matching Effect," *Journal of Studies of Alcohol* 65, no. 4 (July 2004): 501-12; K. Witliewitz and A.G. Marlatt, "Relapse Prevention for Alcohol and Drug Problems: That was Zen, This is Tao," *American Psychologist* 59, no. 4 (May-June 2004): 224-35;

R. Secades-Villa, J.R. Fernande-Hermida, and C. Arnaez-Montaraz, "Motivational Interviewing and Treatment Retention Among Drug User Patients: A Pilot Study," *Substance Use and Misuse* 39, no. 9 (July 2004): 1369-78; D.A. Charney et al., "Integrated Treatment of Depression and Substance Use Disorders," *Journal of Clinical Psychiatry* 62 (2001): 672; R. McGarty, "Relevance of Ericksonian Psychotherapy to the Treatment of Chemical Dependency," *Substance Abuse Treatment* 2, no. 3 (1985): 147-51.

40. M. Sullivan and B. Ferrell, "Ethical Challenges in the Management of Chronic Nonmalignant Pain: Negotiating Through the Cloud of Doubt," *Journal of Pain* 6, no. 1 (January 2005): 2-9; B. Lo, T. Quill, and J. Tulski, "Discussing Palliative Care with Patients," *Annals of Internal Medicine* 130 (1999): 744-9.

41. T.E. Dews and N. Mekhail, "Safe Use of Opioids in Chronic Noncancer Pain," *Cleveland Clinic Journal of Medicine* 71, no. 11 (November 2004): 897-904.

42. M. Swartz et al., "Estimating the Prevalence of Borderline Personality Disorder in the Community," *Journal of Personality Disorders* 4 (1990): 257-73.

43. T. Nadelson, "Borderline Rage and the Therapist's Response," *American Journal of Psychiatry* 134, no. 7 (July 1977): 748-51.

44. F. Yeomans, "When a Therapist Overindulges a Demanding Borderline Patient," *Hospital and Community Psychiatry* 44, no. 4 (April 1993): 334-6; A. Pam, "Limit Setting: Theory, Techniques and Risks," *American Journal of Psychotherapy* 48, no. 3 (Summer 1994): 432-40.

45. K. Hawton et al., "Self-Cutting: Patient Characteristics Compared with Self-Poisoners," *Suicide and Life Threatening Behavior* 34, no. 3 (Autumn 2004): 199-208; J. Paris, "Half in Love with Easeful Death: the Meaning of Chronic Suicidality in Borderline Personality Disorder," *Harvard Review of Psychiatry* 12, no. 1 (January-February 2004): 42-8; R. Pies and A. Popli, "Self-Injurious Behavior: Pathophysiology and Implications for Treatment," *Journal of Clinical Psychiatry* 56 (1995): 1-9; B.S. Brodsky, M. Cloitre, and R.A. Dulit, "Relationship of Dissociation to Self-mutilation and Childhood Abuse in Borderline Personality Disorder," *American Journal of Psychiatry* 152, no. 12 (December 1995): 1788-92.

Part 2
Ethical Obligations in Each Case

7

Privacy and Confidentiality

Evan G. DeRenzo

I. PROTECTING PRIVACY AND CONFIDENTIALITY: THE DEFAULT POSITION

The obligation to protect patients' privacy and confidentiality is one of the most cherished and ancient values in medical ethics. While other values, such as supporting patients' autonomy and truth-telling, are more modern notions in clinical medicine, appreciation of the need to protect patients' privacy and to maintain confidentiality have been woven into medical ethics for millennia. All things being equal, the ancient requirement to protect privacy and maintain confidentiality is the default position in medical ethics.

Privacy and confidentiality are not, however, synonymous. Privacy and confidentiality are complementary. They are related but different concepts.

Privacy is related to personal integrity. Privacy is a basic human right, often explained as both a positive and a negative right. As a positive right, the right to privacy means that a person has the right to control access to and/or distribution of personal information, property, and/or knowledge of personal behaviors. The concept of a "zone" of privacy, implies that an individual has the right to set a boundary that is invaded only with his or her permission. In clinical medicine, the most obvious example of the positive right to privacy is

that patients (or their surrogates), under ordinary circumstances, determine access to and/or distribution of personal health information. Another example is control over clothing and personal belongings of a hospital in-patient or resident in a long-term care facility. Another is the patient's right to protect access to and/or distribution of knowledge about intimate behaviors such as hygiene, sexual preference or dysfunctional family interactions.

A negative right to privacy protects against interference, and calls on others to leave the patient alone. In the clinical setting, privacy as a negative right is protected by providing patients and families secluded spaces to discuss medical decisions, away from the involvement of care team members. Other examples include knocking on a patient's door before entering, or keeping a patient's room door closed or bed curtain pulled at the patient's request.

Confidentiality is a bit different. It is a process of keeping secret intimate knowledge that a patient has entrusted to a clinician. Because a patient must divulge intimate personal information and behaviors to obtain optimal treatment, the clinician has an obligation to use this knowledge for the patient's medical benefit only, and to keep this information concealed from others. Confidentiality protects the patient from harms that may be caused by releasing the intimate data that has been disclosed to, or observed by, the clinician. Confidentiality is a kind of promise on the part of the clinician (or institution) that information and/or access provided by an individual to a professional (or to the institution), within the context of a trusting (fiduciary) relationship, will not be divulged without the patient's, or rightful surrogate's, permission.

Confidentiality is maintained through hospital and out-patient clinic/office policies that articulate how and under what circumstances a patient's information may be released, and to whom such release(s) may be made. Another example is a "confidentiality campaign" that produces and posts artful reminders to clinicians to discuss patients in private places, where they cannot be overheard by those who are not involved in the patient's care. A more informal example is the simple reminder of one clinician to another to close out a computer screen on which a patient's information is visible, or to place a patient's chart back in a closed cabinet so that it cannot be seen by someone standing idly at a nursing station or reception desk.

Thus, privacy and confidentiality, although distinguishable, are closely related. They are conceptually connected, and the harms that can result from breaches in privacy or confidentiality are closely linked and can be equally grave. Because we think of privacy as a basic human right, in the medical context or any other social setting, lapses in its protection should be assumed to pose risk of serious harm. In the clinical medicine setting, specifically, harms can include threats to employability, insurability, and/or housing; disruptions in, or destruction of, a patient's personal relationships; and permanent mistrust of clinicians and the medical establishment. Breaches in confidentiality can be as harmful. Therefore, the default position is that it is always the obligation of the clinician and/or institution to protect patients' privacy and maintain confidentiality. Protecting privacy and confidentiality should be incorporated into the clinician's and organization's consideration of all interactions with patients, persons, and organizations connected to patients and their social networks.

Making this position the default, however, does not mean that there are no limits on protection of privacy and confidentiality, or that upholding these values is an absolute. There are few absolutes in ethics, and that privacy and confidentiality are not absolute should come as no sur-

prise. There are legitimate limitations on protecting privacy and confidentiality. The ethical practice of medicine calls on clinicians to appreciate where such limitations exist, and to become skilled in knowing how to manage patients' information in the face of legitimate limitations. These limitations have evolved as the practice of clinical medicine has evolved, yet their existence illuminates the ethical importance of the default position.

II. EVOLUTION OF PATIENTS' PRIVACY AND CONFIDENTIALITY: HIPPOCRATES TO HIPAA

Of all the ancient medical traditions, Greek medicine is the closest to the practice of contemporary Western medicine. Revered ethical maxims to protect patients' privacy and maintain confidentiality date to the time of Hippocrates. It is believed that Hippocrates lived from 460 to 377 BCE, and that the treatises of the Hippocratic collection, the *Corpus Hippocraticum,* were written by many different writers between 480 and 380 BCE. Emphasizing skills of observation that differentiated them from the physician-priests of pre-Hippocratic times and locales, Hippocratic physicians practiced medicine in ways that would be familiar to today's clinicians. Familiar, too, are the moral norms set out in the Hippocratic Oath, said to have been created after Hippocrates's death.[1] Many of the moral requirements set out in the Oath still stand as cornerstones of contemporary medical ethics. One of the most central is the physician's obligation to keep secret knowledge secret. Whether the physician has gained intimate information from the patient directly, or through observations of the patient and the patient's personal relationships in the course of the patient's care, the obligation to keep personal patient information secret is clear and emphatic.

This obligation extends throughout the development of medicine across time, national boundaries, and cultures. In the ninth century, in what is considered the first treatise devoted exclusively to medical ethics, the Islamic physician Ishaq ibn 'Ali al-Ruhawi lists keeping secrets as a primary obligation.[2] Published in 1772 at the University of Edinburgh, Scotland, physician John Gregory's *Lectures Upon the Duties and Qualifications of a Physician* articulated the requirement to preserve confidentiality.[3] In the 1803 medical code of ethics written by the British physician Thomas

Percival, the physician was instructed to speak softly enough to a patient so the conversation could not be overheard.[4] In 1933, Dr. Song Guobin, a Western-trained Chinese physician, in a book integrating Western medical ethics with ancient Confucian teachings, argued for the obligation of confidentiality.[5] Today, all codes of ethics for physicians and other clinical personnel emphasize patients' privacy and confidentiality. It is the determination of the parameters of privacy and confidentiality that has so markedly evolved.

Protections of privacy and confidentiality were formerly most concerned with concealing information and observations about non-medical aspects of the patient. Because medical care was delivered primarily in a patient's home, a physician was witness to non-medical information about the patient and about family interactions. The physician was admonished to keep secret these observations about intimate family interactions. Protecting medical information related to the patient was not the focus.

Today, in addition to the ancient concerns for secrecy about a patient's family interactions and intimate behaviors, there is a contemporary emphasis on personal health information. Influences on modern medicine dictate the extent to which patients' information must be protected from inappropriate disclosure. In ethical terms, these various factors may all be considered under the umbrella of the ancient Hippocratic dictum to avoid harming the patient, that is, upholding the principle of nonmaleficence. In ancient times, medicine had little to offer a patient in treatment. The greatest harms a physician could cause may well have been divulging embarrassing information about a patient's family that could produce shame and/or damage the family's and the patient's reputation in the community. Today, inappropriate disclosure of information about a patient's medical condition can result in more concrete harms, such as loss of medical or life insurance, employment, or housing. Personal data that has the highest potential for immediate and material harms has redirected the focus of concern.

There are, however, other factors in modern society that have greatly influenced evolving considerations of medical privacy and confidentiality. Three of the most important are legal influences on the practice of medicine, changes in payment source, and the move from written to electronic media. Concerning the first, especially in the United States: legal concerns have become central to the practice of medicine. Whether or not this phenomenon has produced an improvement or a decline in the quality of medicine is beyond the scope of this chapter. Nevertheless, it is critical to examine how moral considerations of privacy and confidentiality have been affected by legal considerations, most notably in the area of documentation. Physicians, nurses, and other clinical providers are repeatedly reminded to document, document, document. In the event of a lawsuit, documentation is necessary for the physician's and/or institution's defense. As far as the court is concerned, if it is not documented, it didn't happen.

The explosion in the requirement to document medical care is not only the result of the rise in medical malpractice litigation, but also is the result of changes in funding. Today, at least in affluent nations, the vast majority of medical care is paid by third-party payers. Whether government or private, medical insurers are responsible for payment to physicians, other billable clinicians, and medical facilities for a vast array of medical procedures. Without adequate documentation, coverage may be questioned and/or denied. Thus, modern medicine is awash in records that detail patients' private health information, written and electronic.

As the nineteenth century was known as the Industrial Age, the twentieth century was known as the Information Age. In medicine, the amount of personally identifiable patient information produced and stored has grown to dizzying amounts. To be a patient is to have a chart — or two or three or more — somewhere. To be a sick patient is to have volumes of information in multiple charts stored in various places. Research volunteers, sick or healthy, are followed by more charts. Before the computer, these ever-growing mountains of documented personal medical information were recorded on paper. Much continues to be handwritten. The advent of the computer, however, enabled this information to be recorded electronically as well. Medical mistakes from paper systems prompted calls to move to totally electronic patient record keeping. Currently, medical delivery systems use both paper and electronic formats to manage personal patient information for diagnosis and treatment, billing and reimbursement, regulatory compliance, and legal protections.

Adherence to traditional canons of medical ethics assures that physicians' training continues to include cultivation of habits that maximize the protection of patients' privacy and confidentiality. Advances in the collection and storage of patients' information, however, has necessitated more formalized policies and regulations. Today, virtually every clinician and healthcare facility and/or organization has formal policies and procedures to protect patients' privacy and confidentiality. All major professional healthcare organizations address the need to protect privacy and confidentiality in their codes of ethics and guidance documents for the training of clinicians in their specialties and categories. The Joint Commission on Accreditation of Healthcare Organizations (JCAHO) sets standards for protecting privacy and confidentiality that institutions meet through creating practices and policies that assist staff in meeting these standards. State legislation has included requirements to protect the privacy and confidentiality of personal patient data, albeit with great variability across states. Now legislation at the U.S. federal level has been enacted specifically addressing protection of private patient information.

Regulations issued in 1996 under the federal Health Insurance Portability and Accountability Act, HIPAA, which took effect 14 April 2003, set a uniform, federal standard for consumer privacy protections across the country.[6] HIPAA, while encouraging electronic transactions, requires safeguards for the security and confidentiality of all of the health information that is covered by the legislation. The regulations cover health plans, healthcare clearinghouses, and healthcare providers that conduct certain financial and administrative transactions electronically (for example, enrollment, billing, and eligibility verification). Most health insurers, pharmacies, doctors, and other healthcare providers are included under this legislation.

Patients' protections under HIPAA limit ways that health plans, pharmacies, hospitals, and other covered healthcare entities can use patients' personal medical information. The regulations protect medical records and other individually identifiable health information, whether it is on paper, in computers, or communicated orally. These protections govern permission to transmit and/or distribute information and provide for patients' access and rights to amend and/or correct medical records. The legislation also restricts use of patients' information for marketing purposes. Pharmacies, health plans, and other covered entities may not use patients' information for marketing without patients' explicit authorization. Some HIPAA violations carry criminal penalties with steep monetary sanctions and even the threat of prison sentences. HIPAA, although represented by the U.S. government as merely setting a national "floor" of privacy standards, has brought sweeping changes to medical practice. Attaching hefty monetary sanctions and possible jail time to certain HIPAA violations has refocused clinicians and the medical care delivery system on issues of privacy and confidentiality. But even HIPAA, with its thicket of detailed constraints and prohibitions, makes explicit that there are limitations on the privacy and confidentiality of patients' information. The regulations are clear: HIPAA does not restrict the ability of physicians, nurses, or other providers to share information that is needed to treat patients. The principle of beneficence, that is, to act in the patient's best interest, supercedes the obligation to protect privacy and maintain confidentiality when the two conflict. Nonetheless, when maintaining privacy and confidentiality does not jeopardize patients' medical needs, protecting privacy and confidentiality is paramount. Thus, despite the evolution of heightened practices to protect patients' private information, fundamental moral judgments about protecting privacy and confidentiality have changed little over the ages. As the methods of keeping information secret have become more complex, paralleling the complexity of modern healthcare delivery, the basic ethical notion of the clinician's responsibility to keep patients' information private holds firm.

III. LIMITATIONS ON PROTECTING PATIENTS' PRIVACY AND CONFIDENTIALITY

The exception to the rule is that if compelling, ethically justifiable reasons exist to share a patient's private information, it is ethically permissible to do so without the patient's (or surrogate's) permission or knowledge. There have always been and will continue to be compelling, ethically justifiable reasons to share a patient's private information or to breach a patient's confidence that do not weaken the default position. Rather, this confirms that protection of patients' privacy and confidentiality, a primary value, is not absolute. Clinicians and healthcare organizations must appreciate such exceptions to the rule.

Situations in which patients' privacy must be overridden to uphold stronger beneficence claims range from the obviously ethically acceptable to the confusing and ethically controversial. These exceptions to the rule fall into two categories: breaches made on behalf of the patient's own medical needs and breaches made for the protection of others.

A. Exceptions Based on the Needs of Individual Patient's Care

It is obviously acceptable, and often ethically obligatory, to breach a patient's privacy and confidentiality when the breach is based on the patient's care needs: there is an emergency, and there are no prior instructions to the contrary. That is, when a breach of privacy or confidentiality is made for the sole purpose of meeting individual, identifiable, emergency patient's medical needs, all other things being equal, there is no debate. Direct medical benefit under such circumstances trumps considerations of privacy and confidentiality. If, for example, an unconscious patient is brought into an emergency room and the emergency room team has information that the patient was recently treated elsewhere, it is morally incumbent on (and legally permissible for) the treating team to obtain the patient's past medical records. Such information may provide vital information about the patient's present condition and assist in making treatment decisions. Although technically it is a breach of confidentiality to divulge the patient's records without the patient's permission, this case is an ethically obligatory breach. The situation is an emergency, with no indication that the patient would have placed privacy over lifesaving treatment. The ethical value of acting in the patient's best interest for needed emergency medical care takes precedence over the obligation to keep personal medical information private.

Because privacy and confidentiality are always the default, only pertinent information should be shared and only with those who need it. Those who receive the information must protect its confidential nature. Clinicians must always use judgment in deciding just how much information to provide and to whom. A famous study published over 20 years ago found that more than 75 clinicians or hospital employees had access to a patient's medical record and concluded that protection of privacy and confidentiality was a "de-

crepit concept."[7] This does not reduce its importance. Imperfections in protection practices should not excuse inappropriate disclosure of patients' private information. Once outside the realm of *bona fide* medical emergencies, the routine care of a patient involves multiple clinicians and clinical care organizations. Medical information that poses heightened risk for stigma and the potential for discrimination, such as information pertaining to mental health or homosexuality, pose added complexities for the protection of data. When information is created and recorded that is known or is anticipated to carry stigma and potential discrimination, additional procedural and legislative protections can be expected to adhere. Great care must be taken to protect this kind of information from being inappropriately released.

Increased sensitivity to protecting personal health information can be seen in innovative healthcare system practices and policies. Today, many hospitals ensure that only hospital employees with legitimate needs for information about a particular patient have access to that patient's electronic records. Concerning paper records: hospital employees are trained that they are not allowed to peruse such records unless the care of a patient creates a legitimate need to do so. Outside the hospital setting, HIPAA has mandated that patients can request that their physicians, health plans, and other covered entities take reasonable steps to ensure confidential communications, such as asking that phone calls be made to the patient at work rather than home or *vice versa*.

Yet, no matter how hard clinicians and healthcare organizations try to only communicate with each other and, for example, to set up plans for communicating only with appropriate family members, the realities of modern hospital staffing patterns will result in something or someone falling through the cracks. Take the following situation.

Some intensive care unit (ICU) attendings change as frequently as every week. Residents and students rotate on monthly or six-week schedules with additional visiting fellows and students from outside institutions observing for a few days or an occasional week or two. Nursing shifts are staggered, with different hospitals having different systems for matching nurses to patients. Thus, just the constant change in staff and numbers of staff who would need to review a patient's record makes the contemporary medical setting vulnerable to breaches of patients' privacy and confidentiality. The more persons who have access to private patient data, the higher the risk of a breach. Even when patients and surrogates are well-informed that privacy and confidentiality cannot be guaranteed, the care team must still make every reasonable effort to protect confidential information. What is "reasonable" in such a complex environment as our modern healthcare delivery system?

What if an ICU patient requests that his diagnosis of a sexually transmitted disease be kept secret from his family, and the ICU team is successful at keeping the secret even after he dies? If the patient dies in the ICU, should the ICU physician falsify the death certificate to keep the secret? What if the patient improves sufficiently to be extubated and moved to a floor bed? How much effort should the ICU team make to assure that the new care team does not divulge the information to the patient's family?

These are questions that require refined ethical judgments and to which there are no formulaic answers. The rule of thumb here is, however, that one should maintain confidentiality about sensitive personal information, even from surrogates and others who make decisions on behalf of a patient who is unable to make his or her own decisions, unless withholding the information impairs decision making for needed medical treatment. When the medical need of a patient is at stake, there will be ethically appropriate limits on privacy and confidentiality, depending on multiple factors, arranged in sliding scale order, related to urgency and potential for clinical consequences of making or not making a treatment decision. Deciding what moral weight to assign to the particulars of a patient's clinical status will take thoughtfulness, consultation with the care team, sometimes input from an ethics committee and/or other bioethics resource personnel, and clinicians' skill in ethical argumentation to assure strong justifications for a breach of privacy or confidentiality. Cases in which breaches are justified on the basis of individual, direct patients' needs are ethically acceptable under certain circumstances that are patient-specific. Such breaches are, ordinarily, less ethically controversial and produce less moral distress in clinicians than do breaches that are justified on the basis of the needs of others.

B. Exceptions Based on the Needs of Others

Often quite controversial are breaches of privacy and confidentiality made on behalf of others. Such breaches, however, have been part of medical practice since at least the Middle Ages. Although the words "endemic" and "epidemic" come down to modern medicine with their original definitions intact from the *Airs, Waters, and Places,* a work contained in the *Corpus Hippocraticum,*[8] it was the spread of leprosy in the Middle Ages that was the beginning of systematic breaches of patients' privacy and confidentiality to protect others from sick patients, as formalized components of public health practices. To protect healthy members of a community, persons with leprosy were identified, expelled, and exiled for the rest of their lives. In 583, the Council of Lyons ordered the separation of lepers from healthy persons, a policy continued and elaborated upon by later church councils.[9] An individual who was suspected of having leprosy was examined by a special commission composed primarily of clerics and physicians, and, if he or she was determined to have leprosy, was made to wear a special, identifying costume, and then banished. This marked the beginning of the public health practice of quarantine, a practice that was refined during the Black Plague of 1348 and is still practiced today.

The early public health methods to protect the healthy from persons suspected of disease by observation, monitoring, separation, and sometimes isolation have evolved, but many practices created during the Middle Ages are still part of contemporary public health. Voluntary quarantine was instituted during the 2003 outbreak of severe acute respiratory syndrome (SARS) in Toronto. A notable example is in the area of sexually transmitted diseases.

New to the sixteenth and seventeenth centuries, or at least seemingly new at the time, was the disease that became known as syphilis. Syphilis appeared in Europe in epidemic proportions at the close of the fifteenth century, spreading quickly from Italy to Germany, France, Switzerland, Holland, and Greece. Appreciation of syphilis as a sexually transmitted disease occurred quickly, and public health measures, most notably directed at prostitution, developed rapidly.[10] Systems were created to test prostitutes for the disease and to monitor those infected. These systems for public reporting and monitoring were precursors to those in place today for a wide range of sexually transmitted diseases. Because tolerance of sexual matters characterized the period from the Renaissance to the eighteenth century, there was essentially no stigma attached to the condition. Today, however, such a diagnosis carries with it stigma, posing serious risks of material and psychosocial harms to infected persons, particularly those with human immunodeficiency virus (HIV).

The harm of breaches of confidentiality about such conditions is demonstrated by the case of the otolaryngologist and plastic surgeon William Behringer.[11]

In June 1987, Behringer, a surgeon at the Princeton Medical Center, was admitted as a patient. He was diagnosed with *Pneumocystis carinii* pneumonia (PCP) and was tested for HIV. Although he had previously given consent to be tested, with no pretest counseling, he had no opportunity to fully consider the implications of his test results. Behringer tested positive for HIV, the report was entered into his medical chart, and persons inside and outside the hospital learned of his HIV status. Soon after discharge, the calls to Behringer's office started, inquiring about his HIV status. His case load dwindled, some of his office staff quit, and he lost his hospital surgical privileges. Behringer sued the hospital for breach of confidentiality of his diagnosis and test results and for violating the New Jersey antidiscrimination statute and won.

Today, most hospitals and other healthcare organizations have stringent privacy policies about HIV testing and disease status. When reporting to public agencies is required, such as for suspected child abuse or certain communicable diseases, confidentiality becomes more difficult. When information must be reported by law, patients need to be informed before such information is generated. Since the Middle Ages, society has made it morally permissible to exchange patients' privacy and confidentiality for certain public health needs. Most patients and the public accept the necessity for this trade-off. But we uphold another important principle of medical ethics, the principle of respect for human dignity, when we give patients the respect of knowing beforehand what will happen to their private, especially sensitive, personal health information. In so doing, when the situation allows, the patient is able to exercise some control over the generation and/or dissemination of the information. Thus, the controversy is not whether or not this exchange is ethically acceptable, but under what circumstances it is warranted: if it must be made, how best can it be made? Complex political circumstances of the twenty-first century, for example, create new realities of security concerns. Expectations for placing public health above individual rights of privacy and assumptions of confidentiality will not change, but become more

entrenched, and the scope of permissible breaches will expand markedly.

Since the terrorist attack on the New York World Trade Center and the Pentagon in Arlington, Virginia, on 11 September 2001, the political climate of the U.S. has changed irreversibly. Bioterrorism, a word little heard before the attacks, is used in common parlance, prompting state and national legislation to expand the ability of federal, state, and local governments to act in the case of a bioterror attack. A prime example is the Model State Emergency Health Powers Act (MSEHPA).[12] Prepared by the Center for Law and the Public's Health at Georgetown and Johns Hopkins Universities, it was produced at the request of the U.S. Centers for Disease Control and Prevention (CDC). MSEHPA is designed to serve as a model for state legislatures to expand powers to detect and contain bioterrorism or naturally occurring outbreaks of disease. Detractors see the model as allowing too much power to be turned over to state and local officials during an emergency. Provisions for required vaccination, forced medical examination, and pharmacist reporting have produced much controversy. Nonetheless, more than 30 states and Washington, D.C. have enacted legislation patterned after MSEHPA. How these new laws will be implemented and coordinated with other related legislation, such as the HIPAA privacy legislation, when conflicts arise remains to be seen.[13] There will be increased demands on physicians and other clinical careproviders to disclose private health information.

Whether the breach of confidentiality in the public health arena is for diseases present for centuries or from the threat of bioterrorism, both are infringements of the privacy of the individual for the common good. The ethical justification for infringing on individuals' privacy and confidentiality on behalf of the publics health, has been well worked out, even if the details in specific cases remain debatable. But the twentieth century has seen the emergence of a qualitatively new kind of justification for breach of patients' confidentiality, the believable threat of harm by a patient to an identifiable third party.

The *Tarasoff v. Regents of the University of California* (1974) case that established this practice was about a college student, Prosenjit Poddar, who killed his former girlfriend, Tatiana Tarasoff.[14] Before killing her, Poddar threatened to do so in a psychotherapy session with his college mental health counselor. The therapist met the *then* standard-of-practice by giving the information to his supervisor and attempting to have his patient placed in temporary psychiatric custody. When Poddar carried out his threat, the victim's family sued the therapist. The California Supreme Court, in two separate opinions, ruled that the therapist had had a duty to warn the identified third party. The court opinions made it clear that protecting privacy and confidentiality are central obligations in mental healthcare. The courts, however, decided that an exception to the rule should have been made because of the specificity of the threat made to an identifiable individual, and because the court believed that a therapist has enough control of the situation to prevent the threat from being carried out. Under these circumstances, the court reasoned, the well-established protections for communications contained within the physician-patient relationship should be overridden.

This case radically altered privacy and confidentiality considerations when the disclosure of the intent to act violently is made within a medically privileged relationship. Prior to *Tarasoff,* the ethical norm was that if a medical professional believed a patient's threat of violence was real, he or she would prevent the violence by protecting the patient from him- or herself by voluntary, or, if needed, involuntary psychiatric commitment. Commitment would avoid the violence, placing the patient who made the threat in a safe environment where the threat could be addressed therapeutically. There would be no breach to the patient's confidence, although the patient's privacy would be infringed and his or her liberty rights constrained. In short, the traditional focus on the patient, not the individual to whom the threat of violence was directed, is preserved. *Tarasoff* changed that, seemingly irreversibly. Post-*Tarasoff,* the clinician is routinely required to consider how the patient might be a threat to an identifiable third party.

Additionally, the *Tarasoff* decision has been affirmed in a variety of cases, not only threatened violence in the mental healthcare setting, but also issues of persons with HIV who knowingly have unprotected sexual relations. Court opinions have shaped the *Tarasoff* obligation to apply if the violence is foreseeable and a therapist can control the patient enough to prevent the violence. Unfortunately, situations in which the two conditions are definitively met are few. Many in the mental health field believe that predicting when a threat of violence is real or is merely a thought that has been spoken out loud is so difficult that disclosure is ill-advised. Because the predictability of when a threat will be acted out is so poor, and

because breaches of confidentiality are known to have negative outcomes on trust in the patient-therapist relationship, risks of disclosure may outweigh the risks that a threat will become reality. Nevertheless, because the courts have repeatedly upheld the validity of the *Tarasoff* decision, the inclination to breach confidentiality and inform identifiable third parties about threats of harm has increased.

Legal opinion about when to disclose confidential information has made judgments about exceptions to the rule quite difficult. Variations in state laws that have attempted to clarify the matter have done little to make the situation easier on clinicians. Some jurisdictions, such as Washington, D.C., will not allow clinicians to disclose an infant's HIV status over a mother's objection, even to a father who lives in the same home. The State of Maryland leaves it up to clinicians' judgment whether or not to give HIV status information to a known sexual partner when the patient refuses to do so. The variable legislative terrain concerning disclosure of HIV disease status to sexual partners, the difficulty in assessing when a threat poses a real danger to another, and concerns about legal liability of the ethical acceptability of disclosures justified on the basis of the *Tarasoff* decision, require refined moral judgment. The complexities inherent in making these judgments will become ever more demanding as genetic medicine moves into the clinical care setting.

Issues around clinicians' obligations concerning disclosure of genetic information are still completely unsettled. Historically, physicians who learned that a patient had a genetic disease would have been bound not to disclose such information to others. As the genetics revolution has become more visible within the everyday practice of clinical medicine, the question of what should be the extent of a clinician's obligation to family members who may be affected by genetic disease is more frequently asked. The progression of thought in this area is in rapid transition. If the genetic condition can be predicted with reasonable certitude (that is, the condition has a dominant transmission pattern versus a genetic predisposition) and there is prophylaxis and/or treatment available, the clinician should attempt to have the patient inform family members who may be affected. The degree to which the clinician is morally obliged to seek out and inform such family members, however, is still hotly debated. Legal preference seems to favor *Tarasoff* and clinicians' obligation to breach patients' confidentiality to protect identifiable third parties from potential harm.

IV. GUIDANCE

Ancient and contemporary medical ethics require that clinicians protect patients' privacy and confidentiality. This is the default position. Every reasonable effort to protect patients' privacy and confidentiality must be made. When there is even the slightest hint that this maxim ought to be overridden, seek wise counsel. Physicians and other clinicians in training should first discuss the issue with the full care team. Obtain the advice of the supervising clinician or clinicians; but the obligation is not merely to take the advice of senior clinicians. Seniority in clinical medicine is (or should be) based on experience and excellence in clinical skills, scientific knowledge, and administrative competence. With seniority and mastery of these skills and knowledge comes a strong medical hierarchy. Traditional medical hierarchies may pose hurdles to sound moral decision making. Although skill in making moral judgments is part of the exercise of clinical skills, scientific knowledge, and administrative competence, sound moral reasoning cannot occur if traditional medical hierarchies stymie vigorous moral debate. And many, if not most, decisions in medicine are not merely scientific and technical decisions, but are medico-moral decisions, decisions that include a component of moral judgment.

Consideration of breaching privacy and confidentiality is an example of such a medico-moral decision. Except under emergency conditions, there may be reasonable ethical arguments for making or not making the breach. Thus, if there is any unease about the advice obtained, even if there seems to be a consensus among the treating team, the thoughtful and morally mature clinician should seek further counsel.

If the advice, or prevailing consensus, is markedly different from one's original best judgment, continue to consult others, preferably others knowledgeable about the patient's care and who are more senior than an immediate supervisor or those on the active treating team. If consultation has been primarily within one or two disciplines, discuss the matter with professionals who might have different perspectives and provide differing

moral insights. If there is still disagreement, or one continues to feel uncomfortable about the decision that has emerged, involve the organization's ethics committee and other bioethics resource personnel.

This process of consideration and consultation, and the recommendation to flatten traditional medical power hierarchies when medico-moral decisions must be made, calls on clinicians to do more than build skills in thinking-through the ethical implications of their actions. It calls on clinicians to muster the courage to act on their moral convictions. Although they are complex and difficult, these qualities and actions are needed to assure that the care offered to patients is optimal. Protecting privacy and confidentiality is always the default position, and any deviation needs to be well-reasoned and based on a strong ethical justification.

Departing from the default position is a serious process that should only be taken after much thought and care. In addition to consultation with appropriate others, healthcare organizations — from private practice offices to major medical centers — should have policies on privacy and confidentiality in place. Training programs must emphasize assuring that these policies are well-known and followed, and contribute positively to creating an organizational culture that upholds patients' privacy and confidentiality. These policies and procedures should include mechanisms for assuring that patients are aware of the privacy and confidentiality practices of the organization — and their limits.

Much of this information will be communicated to patients through conversation with their clinicians. But communications around these issues can be started through well-designed patient information packets. Most healthcare organizations provide such information to patients when they make an office visit or are admitted to an inpatient facility. These communiqués about privacy and confidentiality should make clear that patients have the right to:

- Privacy and confidentiality in treatment, except in life-threatening situations,
- Confidentiality of health records,
- Be informed about any legal reporting requirements concerning a patient's treatment,
- Obtain a copy of one's records upon request,
- Review and correct one's medical records,
- Give and revoke authorization for release of medical records.

But remember also that clinicians should not make promises of privacy or confidentiality that they expect, *a priori,* will be virtually impossible to keep. Conversations with patients that include assurances about what will be kept confidential should include caveats about what may not be confidential.

In sum, clinicians are required to maintain privacy of personal health information obtained through observation or patients' disclosures. This is a primary obligation, with exceptions to the rule that will continue to expand as medicine and the world become ever more complex. These exceptions do not reduce the centrality of the obligation. Instead, it means that the clinician, in consultation with others, as prudent, exercises sound ethical judgment about if and how such exceptions should be made. In so doing, the clinician will meet his or her obligations to protect patients' privacy and confidentiality.

V. CASES FOR FURTHER STUDY

Case 1

A young adult patient is brought into an emergency room, having been found unconscious at home by an uncle. The uncle reports to the emergency room team that he is visiting from out of town. He hasn't seen the patient in many years and doesn't know much about the patient's present medical status. He is able to report, however, that the patient had told him in a recent phone conversation that the patient had had some heart problems and had been in the nearby university hospital for tests.

Case 2

Mrs. Jones is an obese 50-year-old female. She is seen at the nutrition clinic that is attached to her primary care physician's office. Whenever she has consultation with her nutritionist, a copy is automatically sent to her primary care physician's office to go into her chart. Additionally, Mrs. Jones is in a supervised swimming program at a rehabilitation facility near her home. Quarterly reports from the swimming program are sent, also, to her primary care physician's office, with a copy sent to Mrs. Jones' home. At home, Mr. Jones is the one who opens the mail. Every quarter, when the swim program report arrives, he opens it and uses the information to criticize his wife's appearance. Over time, Mrs. Jones has become depressed about her lack of progress losing weight. She is now seen at her community mental health center by a psychiatrist for monitoring of her anti-depressant medications and by a psychologist for long-term psychotherapy. Although the community mental health center chart information is not ordinarily transferred outside the system, Mrs. Jones has given the facility written consent for her physician's nurse practitioner to get phone updates from the psychologist to assure continuity of care and to monitor for potential polypharmatoxicity problems, given the many medications Mrs. Jones is prescribed by her other physicians. Also, the nurse practitioner needs to coordinate with the community mental health center around issues of upcoming counseling needs if Mrs. Jones moves forward with gastric bypass surgery.

Case 3

Mr. Santini is a 32-year-old man dying of AIDS. He is in the hospital's ICU with pneumonia and on a respirator. He has been intubated for almost two weeks and is not getting better. His family, most of whom only speak Italian, are at his bed daily. Many members of the family have arrived from Italy. Before Mr. Santini was intubated, he instructed his physicians (one of the ICU attendings and the residents managing his care) not to let his family know he has AIDS. The one family member who speaks good English has been asking the nurses and residents why her brother isn't getting better.

Although the care team is struggling with their own feelings about having made a promise of confidentiality to the patient that is becoming increasingly difficult to keep — and will be divulged if the patient dies by the information on the death certificate — they are managing to keep Mr. Santini's primary diagnosis a secret. They have set up a system among themselves to assure that only one resident and/or one nurse and only one attending will provide any substantive medical updates to the family. Planning for the possibility that the time will come to recommend removal of the respirator, it has been decided that the attending will be the only clinician to make the recommendation, and it will be made on the basis that the pneumonia has overcome the patient. Walking a tightrope of attempting not to give the family an outright lie and protecting Mr. Santini's confidential diagnostic information has produced much stress on the team.

Case 4

Mrs. Jackson is a patient at your hospital. She has been referred to your institution because she has a rare genetic disease that has produced thyroid cancer. Fortunately, the variety of thyroid cancer is curable if caught early. In families where the mutation, which has a dominant inheritance pattern, is found, the practice has been to test all potentially affected family members. Those found carrying the mutation have their thyroid removed. Although being without a thyroid means that the patient will be on thyroid-replacement drugs for the rest of his/her life, that is the only sequelae of the condition. If, however, one has the mutation and that is not determined until one has an advanced malignancy, prognosis is poor. Mrs. Jackson has two children, ages 24 and 12. She refuses to inform the children because she says that she does not want to worry them. She also denies that her thyroid condition was malignant.

VI. STUDY QUESTIONS

1. What is the ethical reasoning for calling protection of privacy and confidentiality the default position?

2. Do you think privacy and confidentiality are decrepit concepts? On what do you base your view?

3. What might be an example of a case in which it would be ethically acceptable to breach a patient's privacy? How might this be ethically different from breaching a patient's confidentiality?

4. Please give an example of when it would be ethically obligatory to breach a patient's confidentiality? What is your ethical justification?

5. Please give two examples in which it would be ethically permissible to breach a patient's confidentiality. What is your ethical justification for each example? What might be ethical justifications for opposing the breach?

6. In case 1, should the emergency room team attempt to get the patient's records from another hospital? If so, what is the ethical justification? If so, what is the receiving team's obligation regarding the information about the patient that it has obtained?

7. In case 2, you are Mrs. Jones's primary care-provider. She tells you about how her husband reads the swim program reports and berates her for her lack of progress. What might you do, related to privacy and confidentiality issues, and what is your ethical basis for your recommendation(s)?

8. In case 3, what might you have done differently and why?

9. In case 4, how far should Mrs. Jackson's physician push her to inform her children that they may have a genetic mutation for a treatable disease? Does the obligation extend to assuring that Mrs. Jackson has her children tested? Is there a moral difference in your thinking for the child who is past the age of legal majority and the child who is still a minor? If so, please articulate the difference(s).

ACKNOWLEDGMENTS

The author would like to thank Jack Schwartz, JD, Assistant Attorney General and Director for Health Policy Development, Office of the Maryland Attorney General, Baltimore, Maryland, for his thoughtful and detailed review and comments on an early draft of this manuscript, and to Elizabeth Griffin, Falmouth, Massachusetts, for her excellent copy editing.

NOTES

1. E.H. Ackerknecht, *A Short History of Medicine* (Baltimore, Md.: Johns Hopkins University Press, 1982).

2. A.R. Jonsen, *A Short History of Medical Ethics* (New York: Oxford University Press, 2000).

3. Ibid

4. Ibid.

5. Ibid.

6. HIPAA Final Rule, *http://www.hhs.gov/ocr/ hipaa/finalreg.html,* accessed 1 June 2005.

7. M. Siegler, "Confidentiality in Medicine: A Decrepit Concept," *New England Journal of Medicine* 301, no. 243 (1982): 1861-2.

8. See note 1 above.

9. Ibid.

10. Ibid.

11. *Estate of Behringer v. The Medical Center at Princeton* 249 N.J. Super. 597, 592 A.2d. 1251 (1991).

12. L.O. Gostin et al., "The Model State Emergency Health Powers Act: Planning for and Response to Bioterrorism and Naturally Occurring Infectious Diseases," *Journal of the American Medical Association* 288, no. 5 (2002): 622-8.

13. J. Bruce, "Bioterrorism Meets Privacy: An Analysis of the Model State Emergency Health Powers Act and the HIPAA Privacy Rule," *Annals of Health Law* 12, no. 1 (2003): 75-120.

14. *Tarasoff v. Regents of the University of California* 131 Cal.Rptr. 14, 51 P.2d 334 (Cal. 1976) (*en banc*).

8

Communication, Truth-Telling, and Disclosure

Robert J. Boyle

CASES

AB was informed by her gynecologist that she had an ovarian tumor and needed immediate surgery. Naturally, she was upset, and, as a former cancer researcher with special knowledge of the subject, she began to ask questions. The questions and answers became prolonged, and the physician became progressively annoyed with the time the consultation was taking. He abruptly ended the session.

CD is a 40-year-old patient who was admitted for severe back pain. Admitted initially to the neurology service, he saw a neurosurgical resident and attending physician in consultation, had a physical therapy evaluation, had a psychiatric evaluation for the possibility of a non-organic cause for the pain, and finally is seeing you in the pain clinic.

What is your role in communicating with this patient? How much should you tell him? Should you leave such discussions to his primary physician? What does the patient know/not know about the results of other studies and consultations?

Mr. and Mrs. E were referred for genetic counseling because Mrs. E is 41, and she has recently learned that she is pregnant. The couple wants the child, but they are concerned about the risk of Down syndrome (trisomy 21). After counseling, the couple agrees to proceed with amniocentesis. The results show 47 chromosomes with no evidence of Down syndrome. However, the child is XYY. Some research has sug-

gested that XYY individuals have an increased tendency toward violence, sexual offenses, and criminal behavior. Because the couple expressed interest only in the risk of Down syndrome, and because the research on XYY is not conclusive, the genetics team is considering whether to disclose this result.

FG is a 75-year-old widower whose wife died with cancer several years ago after a long illness. He is admitted to the hospital for evaluation of weight loss. Tests reveal a mass in his lung. You are aware of the diagnosis. As you are about to enter his room, his two sons meet you and insist that their father not be told that he has cancer, since it will upset him terribly and they are not sure what he might do.

HK is a 70-year-old widow admitted for myocardial infarction. Evaluation reveals extremely poor myocardial function and an extremely poor prognosis. She is currently quite stable, alert, and conversant. Her physician believes that it would be inappropriate to discuss her prognosis with her or to recommend a do-not-resuscitate (DNR) order, since it may upset her and "kill her." The patient is asking her bedside nurse many questions. The nurse believes the patient needs to hear the prognosis so she can begin to make some decisions and arrangements.

LM is a 55-year-old woman who has just completed her annual checkup. You inform her that a screening mammogram would be in her best interest. She replies that her health insurance would not pay for the test unless there is a mass or other objective evidence of a tumor. She requests that you submit the request for payment using the latter criteria.

NP has recently been diagnosed with multiple sclerosis. She subscribes to a managed-care plan that will not cover some of the newer expensive treatments for this disease. The physician believes this is the best option for her disease at this time, but is reluctant to discuss the financial details of why the managed-care plan has made this choice. He knows that he would have to invest a lot of time and effort in challenging the policy.

RS was admitted to the hospital with a hypertensive crisis. The physician elects to treat the patient with diazoxide. She administers the usual dose of 100 milligrams. Shortly after, RS's blood pressure falls and she does not respond to resuscitation. The patient dies. The nurse notices that the vial actually contained 1,000 milligrams of medication, a fatal dose.

I. INTRODUCTION

A patient comes to a clinician with a problem or potential problem. The evaluation, diagnosis, and resolution of this problem calls for collaboration that is characterized by mutual acceptance, trust, and respect between patient and clinician and among clinicians from a variety of professions. The goal of this interaction should be to develop a plan of care, with the patient or surrogate as full partner, for this evaluation and treatment. Development of this plan begins as soon as the patient-clinician relationship is established. It should be a systematic and continuous plan, constantly re-evaluated and adjusted in light of medical information, changes in the patient's condition, changes in the contextual framework of the situation, and so forth. None of this planning can be accomplished without effective communication among all of the parties involved.

Clinicians must recognize that they are members of a team involved in developing a plan of care for the patient: nurse, physician, chaplain, social worker, physical therapist, consultant, medical student, dialysis technician, and so forth. Communication among all of these members is critical to the process.

With regard to the specific content of communication with a patient, anxieties and conflicts often develop around several questions: What should the patient be told? What should the family be told? Who should be told first? Who should inform the patient? When? How? Where? Can the actual truth be disclosed without destroying hope?

Can lying ever be seen as ethically justifiable — especially when it is done to protect the patient from harm?

In this chapter, we will focus on a range of issues dealing with communication, realizing that good communication is necessary for all of the issues discussed in this text, from confidentiality to reproductive choices. The cases above introduce the more general issue of communication (cases AB and CD) and proceed to more specific problems with truth-telling and disclosure (cases E, LM, and NP), the conflict engendered by a disclosure that the clinician or others believe may be harmful to the patient (cases FG and HK), and the fear of retribution for disclosing mistakes (case RS). Disclosure, as it pertains specifically to the process of informed consent, is discussed in chapter 10.

II. HISTORY

Communication and disclosure are not mentioned in the Hippocratic Oath, which states that the physician's duty is to act for the benefit of the patient. Other Hippocratic writings, in fact, speak against disclosure: "Perform [these duties] calmly and adroitly, concealing most things from the patient while you are attending to him. Give necessary orders with cheerfulness and serenity, turning his attention away from what is being done to him; sometimes reprove sharply and emphatically, and sometimes comfort . . . revealing nothing of the patient's future or present condition."[1]

Early Christian moralists, prompted by puzzling scriptural episodes of lying, began to wonder whether it is ever right to lie. According to Jonsen and Toulmin, "Although the wrongness of deception was widely recognized, the practice of deception was not uniformly condemned in the early Christian community."[2]

Yet Augustine (in the fourth century) argued powerfully for an absolute prohibition of any lie. He discussed what was to become the "classic case" through the Middle Ages until the eighteenth century: An innocent person, unjustly condemned, is hidden in your house. May you lie to the police officers who come to arrest him? Augustine asserted that even good consequences could never justify a deliberate lie. Centuries later, Immanuel Kant held that a lie is wrong even when based on benevolent motives, because it degrades the person who lies and violates the universal social duty to tell the truth.

In the Middle Ages, "casuists," moralists who applied rules of right and wrong to particular cases, gradually relaxed Augustine's radical position: an immense literature developed on ambiguity, mental reservation, "white lies," and equivocation. The genuine moral insight driving this literature was that, on occasion, part of the truth may be withheld. Concealing the truth was considered permissible when a person was questioned unjustly or when revealing it could cause great harm to another person.

The physician's conversation with a patient was intended to comfort and induce the patient to take the cure. The patient's role was one of obedience to the physician, although medicine and science had little to offer the patient at that point in history.

A code of medical ethics written by the nineteenth-century English physician Thomas Percival,[3] and the first code of the American Medical Association (AMA) that was based on it, were oblivious to the issue of disclosure and informed consent. These codes focused on words or behaviors of the physician that might upset the patient and be detrimental to the patient's recovery. According to the AMA code: "The life of a sick person can be shortened not only by the acts, but also by the words or manner of a physician. It is, therefore, a sacred duty to guard himself carefully in this respect, and to avoid all things which have a tendency to discourage the patient and depress his spirits."[4]

By 1980, the AMA code, now named "Principles," had changed minimally. However, the *Current Opinions of the Judicial Council of the AMA* did address disclosure and truth-telling: "The patient's right of self-decision can be effectively exercised only if the patient possesses enough information to enable an intelligent choice. . . . Social policy does not accept the paternalistic view that the physician may remain silent because divulgence might prompt the patient to forgo needed therapy."[5]

III. SHIFTING ATTITUDES ABOUT DIAGNOSTIC DISCLOSURES

During the past 30 years, there has been a remarkable change in physicians' attitudes about whether to tell the patient bad news, specifically a diagnosis of cancer:

- In 1953, 69 percent of physicians favored not telling.[6]

- In 1961, 88 percent of physicians favored not telling.[7]
- In 1979, 90 percent of physicians favored telling.[8]

The following reasons have been offered to account for the obvious evolution: availability of more treatment options for cancer (including experimental treatments); improved rates of survival from some forms of cancer; fear of malpractice suits; involvement of other disciplines/professions in healthcare; altered societal attitudes about cancer; and increased attention to patients' rights, including the right to information.[9]

Yet troubling conflicts persist, and clinical reality is often fraught with tensions that prompt less than complete disclosure. For example, in the 1979 study that reported that 90 percent of physicians approved of telling the diagnosis of cancer, the authors also reported that there was significant ambiguity about whether the obligation of disclosure is focused on the patient or the family. Respondents identified "a relative's wishes regarding disclosure to the patient" as one of the four most frequent factors considered in deciding whether to tell the patient the truth.[10]

Another example of the disparity between what people say and what they do comes from a 1982 survey of medical and nursing staff who cared for elderly patients who died. The authors of the study reported that only 18 percent of the respondents had discussed the diagnosis with patients, and even fewer had discussed impending death. The staff had not fully appreciated the communication needs of more than half of the dying patients.[11]

The authors of a 1989 study of physicians' attitudes toward the use of deception to resolve ethical problems in clinical practice reported that the majority indicated a willingness to misrepresent a diagnostic test to secure an insurance payment, and would mislead the wife of a gonorrhea patient to ensure her treatment and preserve the marriage. One-third would offer incomplete or misleading information to a patient's family if a mistake led to a patient's death. The authors concluded that the respondents justify their decisions in terms of the consequences and place a higher value on their patients' welfare and keeping patients' confidences than truth telling for its own sake.[12]

Likewise, the author of a 1993 study of oncologists defined three styles that physicians used to inform their patients about the cancer:

- Telling patients what they want to know,
- Telling patients what they need to know, and
- Translating information into terms that patients can take.

The styles were supported by the principles of respecting the truth, respecting patients' rights, honoring doctors' duty to inform, preserving hope, and honoring the individual contract between physician and patient. There was dramatic variation among physicians as to which style they used and which principles they emphasized. There was much more openness about diagnosis and treatment and much less about prognosis. The author noted "varying degrees of openness, willingness to spend time with the patient, sensitivity to patients' subtle cues and active elicitation of patients' desire to know."[13]

In a 2001 study regarding communication of cancer prognosis, physicians reported that they would not communicate any survival estimate 23 percent of the time and would communicate an estimate different from the one they had formulated 40 percent of the time.[14] Of the latter, they would overestimate survival 70 percent of the time. Of note, older patients were more likely to receive frank prognostic information, and female physicians were less likely to favor frank disclosure. One commentator felt that the reluctance to provide specific information was due to the physicians' uncertainty about being able to accurately predict survival times.[15]

IV. COMMUNICATION

Emanuel and Dubler have described "the ideal conception of the physician-patient relationship" as choice, competence, compassion, continuity, lack of conflict of interest, and communication.[16] A long-standing relationship between a patient and a primary-care clinician of the patient's choosing has often survived because of the trust that has developed between the parties. Predecessors of today's physicians recognized the therapeutic value of communication, albeit one-sided. Much of the aid a clinician gives a patient appears to depend upon the clinician's ability to mobilize the patient's positive expectations and faith within an emotionally supportive relationship.[17] As clinicians' relationships with patients have evolved, physicians have come to recognize that this communication is a two-way street. The clinician and

the patient each come to the relationship with a common goal, but each brings different, often overlapping, agendas. Patients bring to the relationship their perceived problems, all of their life values and goals, and their family background — a history both medical and personal. Clinicians bring their training and expertise, values and goals, and so forth. How these agendas are shared is critical to the therapeutic process.

Emanuel and Dubler define good communication as follows:

Good communication means that physicians listen to and understand the patient and communicate their understanding. This entails understanding the patient's symptoms, the patient's values, the effect of the disease on the patient's life, family, job and other pursuits and any other health related concerns the patient deems important. In addition, patients should be able to tell their physicians what kind of information they want and do not want to know.

When communication is good, patients are less likely to misinterpret the information they receive, more willing to ask for clarification when information is unclear, quicker to call if symptoms fail to resolve.[18]

This communication includes not only verbal data, but also verbal style, choice of words, demeanor, attitude, body language, et cetera. As Eric Cassell, a scholar of the nature of patient-clinician communication has asserted,

The spoken language is the basic tool of doctor-patient communication, the more one knows about it, the more effective is the tool. [Clinicians need to know] how the spoken language works in medicine: how words do their work and can have meanings and impact at many different levels, affecting even the body itself; how the attentive listener can know not only what speakers mean but what kind of people they are by their word choice; how all normal speech is logical, and what that knowledge can do for the physician.[19]

In a review of the doctor-patient relationship, Jensen concludes,

Through our verbal and nonverbal communication, we affect our patients for good or bad.

The doctor-patient rapport is indeed our most universally applicable therapeutic tool; like any potent medication, it must be used judiciously, with an understanding of the variables involved and with close scrutiny to monitor possible side effects. Even a simple word of advice may have widely varying results, depending on the doctor, the patient, and the relationship between them.[20]

Unfortunately, this communication is often inadequate. Korsch and colleagues reported that while only 6.75 percent of patients questioned the technical competence of the physician, 24 percent expressed dissatisfaction with their contact with the physician. Reasons included the physician's lack of warmth and friendliness, failure to consider the patient's concerns and expectations, use of unfamiliar terms, and lack of adequate explanations concerning the diagnosis and cause of illness.[21] Although medical education curricula now usually include training in interpersonal skills and humanistic care, the relative lack of emphasis in these areas in the face of overemphasis on specialization and technical expertise will continue to produce physicians who are limited in communication skills.[22]

Physicians usually spend less than one minute out of a 20-minute visit discussing treatment and planning and ask the patient if he or she has any questions less than 50 percent of the time.[23] Other researchers have found that physicians commonly underestimate patients' desire to communicate information and their interest in receiving it. Patients routinely fail to communicate with physicians about their frustrations in not being asked and their desire for increased information.[24]

What patients want most from a doctor's appointment is, first, a chance to tell their story, and, second, information about their problem and how to solve it. Unfortunately, the traditional approach to history-taking and patient evaluation often does not allow patients the opportunity to tell their story and does not allow the clinician, truly, to understand who the patient is. The clinician begins to acquire information and quickly fits it into the traditional model. The patient, on the other hand, may present information in a free-association, random-thought manner. Information that the patient feels is important may be neglected. The data from the history and physical are then written into the traditional format that may, in the end, not reflect what really concerns the pa-

tient and what the patient understands. Donnelly recommends recording the "story" and the patient's feelings about his or her situation in the patient's words as part of the history.[25]

The "social history" also reflects very little of who patients really are; where and how they live; how they function on a daily basis; what their life goals, values, and preferences are; whom they want involved in making decisions, and so forth. What ethnic or cultural issues are important to the patient during this illness? Clinicians are legally required to inquire about advance directives, but is this inquiry *pro forma,* or in the face of a broader discussion of issues with the patient? Researchers in a recent study reported that many patients felt their physicians were not interested in dialogue about "life-or-death" choices.[26] This information is important, if one goal of clinicians is to develop a plan of care, prospectively identifying potential ethical concerns, rather than waiting for a crisis to develop. Forrow and colleagues use the term *preventive ethics.*[27]

V. BARRIERS TO COMMUNICATION

There are institutional and economic barriers to good clinical interaction between clinicians and patients. Physicians who perform high-tech procedures and surgery earn proportionately far more per minute spent with patients than do primary-care physicians. We reward action, not communication. With new attention to primary-care services, this phenomenon may be gradually improving. However, the rapid emergence of managed care — with pressure for shorter office visits, reduced physician utilization, termination of long-standing clinician-patient relationships, and frequent changes in contracts and options — may further undermine continuity and communication. In a study of patients' recognition of their physicians' participatory decision-making style, physicians with primary-care training, lower volume practices (<70 out-patients/week), and who were satisfied with their own level of professional autonomy, scored higher. Patients whose physicians had higher scores changed physicians less frequently than those whose physicians had lower scores.[28]

A study of senior citizens identified six issues that negatively affected communication: anxiety (feeling intimidated), futility (inability to make a difference in the relationship), time (doctor's always busy), reluctance to bother the doctor, language (medical jargon), and memory (forgets intent to talk about something).[29]

Several studies have documented race and ethnicity as barriers to communication. African-American patients rate visits as less participatory when there was race discordance. Race concordant visits were usually longer and rated more positively.[30] The mechanisms at work in this finding are the focus of additional study.

The effectiveness of communication and adequate disclosure are often compromised by the complexity of the modern healthcare system. The patient who has a relationship with a single clinician or small group of clinicians and is referred to a tertiary-care center or a subspecialist may be interviewed (often briefly) and examined by multiple attending physicians, residents, nurses, and students. The patient may not feel able to relate to any of these individuals in his or her brief encounters. One clinician may assume that the other has provided the patient the necessary information (as in case CD). The importance of a primary-care team that is responsible for communication and coordination cannot be overlooked.

From another point of view, the clinician has a professional responsibility to communicate information about the patient, the patient's condition, potential treatment plans, and so forth, to other members of the healthcare team. Failure to communicate with other personnel may jeopardize the welfare and safety of the patient. As stated in the American Nurses Association's (ANA) *Code for Nurses,* "The complexity of healthcare delivery systems requires a multidisciplinary approach to delivery of services that has the strong support and active participation of all health professions."[31] In an academic medical center, new work hour limitations for residents at times require multiple changes of responsible physicians over 24 hours, with the added stresses on effective communication within the team, and the patient is more often faced with unfamiliar caregivers.

Communication among careproviders is not always encouraged or fostered. In their traditional paternalistic role, physicians have not wanted input from others who are involved in the patient's care. In addition, different professions fail to or are unwilling to recognize that each profession may have a different style, technique, or focus in regard to the information they have acquired about a situation or possible solutions to a problem. The classic conflict is between the physician and the nurse; other conflicts include those between the critical care nurse and the general ward nurse, the nurse and the physical therapist, and the physician and the social worker.

Many of the "ethical dilemmas" that lead to ethics consultation in our experience are, in fact, problems resulting from lack of effective communication within the healthcare team. How should the clinician respond when he or she feels strongly that the patient is not getting the information needed to participate as fully as possible in decision making (as in case HK)? How does the bedside nurse respond to the patient's questions about test results, when the tradition on that unit places this responsibility in the hands of the attending physician? Effective planning of the patient's overall care and communication among caregivers should facilitate resolution of these issues.

VI. CULTURE AND LANGUAGE

Communication also suffers when cultural differences or language barriers exist. What may be very important in one culture may be insignificant in another — the dynamic of the family, the role of the elderly, the importance of intellectual achievement, the value of life (however impaired), the belief in an afterlife — all may place the patient and the clinician on different planes, resulting in little effective communication about a particular situation. For example, Pellegrino suggests that in many cultures the patient implicitly delegates authority for decision making to the family, thereby enabling the patient to avoid bad news.[32] In a study of ethnicity and patients' autonomy, Korean-American and Mexican-American subjects were less likely than African-American and European-American subjects to believe that the patient should be told about a terminal prognosis and more likely to believe that the patient's family, rather than the patient, should make decisions about life support.[33]

When language barriers are present or when the clinician must rely on translation, much of the feeling, spontaneity, and true meaning of the communication may be lost. This is especially true when using telecommunication translation, rather than in-person translation.

VII. TRUTH-TELLING, LYING, AND DECEPTION

Effective communication and the patient's participation in decision making about healthcare require that communication be truthful. The information that the patient processes must be honest and as complete as necessary for valid decision making. If important information has been withheld or purposely inaccurate information given, the patient's self-determination is frustrated. There is a strong negative duty not to lie that is owed to all persons. The ordinary business of life depends on the expectation of truth-telling. Our society expects clinicians to manifest the highest standards of professional integrity. If that integrity is undermined, the individual patient's and the public's trust in the clinician and in medicine in general is undermined. There is also a positive duty to tell the truth — to inform others about what one knows, believes, or thinks, if the other person has a right to that knowledge. According to Higgs,

> The temptations to lie are common. . . . Everyday, if a meticulous health professional examines his work, there are demands that the truth be bent, folded, redirected or simply screwed up and binned. Mostly, he accepts that this is part of the job, sometimes to the point that the deception is no longer seen. It is actually part of a larger and more disreputable truth, that we all have to get by, somehow, someway, until the challenge becomes clear — an angry patient, a desperate relative, a complaint, a case in law. All of a sudden, our personal and professional standards are on the line, and we have to decide: what, and how important, is telling the truth.[34]

In the opening cases, should LM's physician have falsified the insurance claim to enable a screening mammogram to be done? Should RS's nurse or physician have informed the family of a mistake in dosage or tell them that the patient died as a complication of her disease?

VIII. DISCLOSURE

During the course of the patient-clinician interaction, the clinician possesses a tremendous amount of information, derived generally from education, training, and experience, and specifically from the history and diagnostic evaluation of a specific patient. It is obviously unrealistic to expect the clinician to share all of this information with the patient, especially when most of it may not be pertinent to the patient's situation at a particular time, or may be extremely technical. The issue is how the clinician determines how much the patient needs to know. What information can the patient demand? How much information is too much? The patient — by his or her questions, responses, and actions — guides the decision about how much information is helpful. The clinician must consider the importance of the information to each patient's specific clinical situation, personal needs, future implications of the information, and so forth. Clinicians also have to recognize that many patients now approach them with high expectation for precision, speed, and unlimited treatment options. Patients come to an appointment with notebooks full of articles from the internet, requesting medications they have seen advertised in the media.

Take, for example, the case of Mr. and Mrs. E. Although the immediate concern about Down syndrome has been answered, the clinician has additional significant information about the pregnancy. Although disclosure may cause initial confusion and require further counseling and disclosure, more harm would be done if the family later heard the result or read of its implications. This harm would be further compounded by their loss of confidence in the counselor.[35] These situations are not uncommon in everyday practice involving laboratory data, genetic testing, and antenatal diagnosis.

IX. DISCLOSING UNCERTAINTY

Uncertainty in many areas of medicine is an often-overlooked problem in full disclosure. This age-old tension between medicine as art or science continues. Katz notes that a great deal of the problem is the natural human fear of uncertainty, especially when persons are facing serious illness and really want a magical cure, rather than a scientific analysis of probabilities and statistics.[36] Beresford has described three sources of uncertainty:

- Technical uncertainty arising from inadequate scientific data,
- Personal uncertainty from not really knowing the patient's wishes, and
- Conceptual uncertainty from the problem of applying abstract criteria to clinical situations.[37]

Treatment of breast cancer, surgery *versus* angioplasty *versus* medical management for coronary artery disease, routine mammography, prostate specific antigen (PSA) screening, myringotomy tubes for children's ear infections — all represent questions that would initiate a lively debate in a gathering of clinicians. However, an individual clinician usually has made a decision about which treatment or test is best. This decision may have been based consciously or unconsciously on factors including specialty (for example, surgeons operate), previous training, peer pressure, economics, or prestige. At times uncertainty may cause disagreements in the clinical team about which test or treatment is best for a patient. Discussions between clinician and patient may highlight the fact that critical pieces of information are controversial or unknown. Prognosis or potential morbidity may be documented as statistical probabilities, but how those probabilities relate to that specific patient are impossible to predict; it is impossible to know whether a 40 percent cure rate will include a particular patient.

Many clinicians are reluctant to reveal these uncertainties to patients who, clinicians feel, may not have the capacity to understand such complex matters and who may suffer further anxiety and distrust. Conveying uncertainty may undermine the patient's faith in the ability and knowledge of the clinician, which some believe is an important therapeutic feature in the patient-clinician relationship.[38] Many patients (as well as some clinicians) continue to expect the clinician to be infallible and omniscient. Clinicians themselves may cope with the uncertainty by failing to acknowledge it fully in certain circumstances.

Katz sees potential value in disclosing uncertainty:

1. It would lighten physicians' burdens by absolving them from the responsibility for implicitly having promised more than they or medicine can deliver;
2. It would give patients a greater voice in decision making;
3. It would greatly reduce the exploitation of unwarranted certainty for purposes of control rather than care; and
4. It would significantly reduce the feelings of abandonment that patients experience whenever they sense that doctors are withdrawing behind a curtain of silence or evasion.[39]

Brody suggests that both clinicians and patients have a psychological interest in maintaining a mutual charade that medicine is much more certain and powerful than we know it to be; patients think this way so that they can hope in miracles, and clinicians so that they can think of themselves as meriting the great faith and trust that patients place in them. Moreover, more severely ill patients may regress psychologically, so that the relationship is more like a child-to-parent than an adult-to-adult relationship. (Parents often do not feel that full disclosure of information to children is necessary or helpful.) As a result of these and similar forces, both clinician and patient may find strategies to dodge or evade real honesty; these strategies, over time, often become embedded in customary medical practice and the usual expectations that patients have of clinicians.[40]

X. DECEPTION

The overriding ethical assumption is that truthfulness normally best serves the patient; the empirical evidence indicates that virtually all patients want the truth, even though many may ask the clinician to choose the best approach.

Some clinicians and many family members believe that disclosure of a terminal diagnosis is detrimental and may lead to acute decompensation, depression, or suicide. In fact, the chance of this happening is very remote. In a 17-year review of deaths by suicide, researchers found that only one could be attributed to transmission of the diagnosis of cancer.[41]

According to the President's Commission for the Study of Ethical Problems in Medicine and Biomedical and Behavioral Research:

There is very little empirical evidence to indicate whether and in what ways information can be harmful.

Not only is there no evidence of significant negative psychological consequences of receiving information, but on the contrary some strong evidence indicates that disclosure is beneficial. Several studies have focused upon the effects of giving patients information about their surgery and its recovery period. Preoperative counseling appears to reduce anxiety and complications during convalescence. Fewer analgesic medicines and days in hospital are required by those who are counseled than by those who are not. Providing information has also proved useful in burn treatment, in stress experienced by blood donors, in childbirth, and in sigmoidoscopy examinations.[42]

In a study of discussion of advance directives with patients suffering from early dementia, some family members initially predicted that patients would be upset by discussing end-of-life issues. However, at the conclusion of the study, researchers found no measurable adverse effects immediately following the discussion or after five days. All patients denied feeling worried, sad, or letdown by their doctor.[43] Likewise, a British study of geriatric patients' attitudes about resuscitation reported that 67 percent welcomed inquiry about their preferences, 78 percent wanted to participate in decisions, and 43 percent wanted to be the sole decision maker.[44]

Other studies have reported that over 90 percent of patients with Alzheimer disease[45] and over 80 percent with amyotrophic lateral sclerosis (ALS, or Lou Gehrig's disease)[46] want to be told their diagnosis.

Studies with hospitalized patients confirm that they are generally open to discussions about their preferences regarding cardiopulmonary resuscitation (CPR) and end-of-life issues and are generally not upset about such discussions. In addition, there was often a mismatch between patients' wishes and physicians' interpretation of those wishes.[47] Physicians are reluctant or unable to tell patients that they may be approaching the end of their lives.[48] Inadequately informed patients tend to be overly optimistic regarding prognosis.[49] Appropriate discussion may shift the focus of the care from cure to palliation with prevention of unnecessary pain and suffering, allowing patients and families to focus on meaningful closure.[50] Buckman has identified the difficulties clinicians have with telling bad news and has described techniques for more sensitive approaches[51] (discussed in detail in chapter 12).

Maintaining hope is a common theme in interviews with oncologists.[52] However, several studies suggest that patients look for reassurance that they will not be abandoned and everything possible will be done for them, rather than hope based on deception.[53] Others suggest that physicians find it too uncomfortable to tell patients that there is little left to be done, because it may be seen as failure on the physician's part.[54] Moreover, we know that identifying the cause of the patient's illness will help mobilize family support and cohesion. Patients desire to have a "name for their disease" as a way of contending with the unknown, which is often the source of their greatest fear. In a study of children and adolescents, both the patient and parents were relieved when they were informed of the diagnosis of cancer, because they then knew what the problem was and what to expect.[55] Adequate information allows patients to make not only medical decisions, but also decisions about aspects of their life, finances, final days, and so forth.

Some utilitarians affirm that consequences should determine the evaluation of a deception; withholding the truth is permissible when doing so will prevent direct harm. Beauchamp and Childress criticize this position; they argue that it is too complicated, even impossible, in actual experience, to balance the benefit of lying against the resulting loss of trust. They add that, even "on utilitarian grounds deception may have long-term negative effects on the patient's self-image and may threaten trust in healthcare professionals."[56] Others have argued, along the same lines, that the practice of "benevolent deception" may actually promote self-deceptive rationalization of more lies than are truly justified, as the "entire history of medicine before about 1960 is the history of routine deception and withholding of information."[57] In the words of the President's Commission for the Study of Ethical Problems in Medicine and Behavioral Research: "There is much to suggest that therapeutic privilege has been vastly overused as an excuse for not informing patients of facts they are entitled to know."[58]

Physicians may grant unjustified influence to family members in decisions about disclosure to patients (see case FG). The patient has the primary moral entitlement to the knowledge of his or her condition, and should have decision-making authority over family involvement. However, there may be situations in which the patient, for a variety of reasons, has placed authority in the hands of family members. Pellegrino suggests that such delegation may be a cultural expectation of the sick person that need not be explicit. He believes it is a "harmful misrepresentation of the moral foundations of respect for autonomy" to thrust the truth on the patient in such a situation.[59] He contends that the clinician must get to know the patient well enough through discussion to discern when, and if, the patient wants to contravene the cultural mores. Freedman reaches a very similar conclusion. He suggests "offering truth" by attempting to ascertain from the patient how much he or she wants to know. For example, "Do you have any questions you want to ask? Do you want to talk? Some patients want to know all about their disease, while others do not want to know so much, and some want to leave all of the decisions in the hands of their physician and family. What would you like?"[60] The patient is offered the opportunity to learn the truth, at whatever level of detail the patient desires. This decision should be the patient's.

Deception or flawed disclosure may take many forms:

1. *Just the facts.* This is a very complete and scientific rendition of the truth, in which medical jargon obscures the patient's comprehension and prevents the clinician from feeling discomfort or guilt. "True statements" can be deceptive if they are not authentically communicative.

2. *There's always hope.* This is the "miracles sometimes happen" dodge that represents an overly optimistic falsification of the best available clinical judgment. Fallibility and probability that are inherently part of medical practice must be honestly acknowledged by the clinician in a temperate manner.

3. *You can't tell a patient everything.* Although it may be true that "the facts are literally infinite," the ethical obligation of the clinician is not to disclose "everything"; the clinician's duty is to tell the patient what is meaningful, important, and useful to the patient in his or her condition. The inevitable selectivity and interpretive ingredients in each clinician's communication should be affirmed as the personal voice of the clinician.

4. *Omission.* Remaining silent when speech would be ethically appropriate does not change the fact that omission is a form of lying.

5. *Evasion.* Although it is true that hard news is sometimes communicated more effectively in a less blunt and more indirect manner, the language of indirection can become avoidance and self-deception. The alternative to injurious bluntness is not evasive indirection, but talk that is gentle, considerate, and open.[61]

Deception in any circumstance in the clinician-patient interaction is problematic. Even when the deception is practiced jointly by the clinician and patient, there are significant risks to the overall relationship. In a large study regarding reimbursement rules, 39 percent of physicians reported either exaggerating the severity of the condition, changing the billing diagnosis, or reporting signs or symptoms the patient did not have to help secure coverage for needed care; 37 percent reported receiving requests from patients to deceive the payor; 29 percent felt it was necessary to "game the system" to provide high-quality care.[62] If the patient knows the clinician is willing to lie to the insurance company to obtain payment for a test (case LM), there is a potential to alter the trust that may be critical in future interactions. Bloche argues that physicians do have a duty to champion patients' interests, to the limit of what is possible, without making false statements or breaching contractual duties.[63] The duty includes advocacy-oriented presentation of clinical data, including emphasis on the facts that are most favorable to the patient's case, but excludes selective withholding of data that might be material. In addition, the deceptive action risks investigation by the insurer and possibly by the federal government.[64]

XI. THERAPEUTIC ERRORS

How do clinicians approach truthful disclosure when doing so may not be to their advantage, when disclosure may end their relationship with the patient, or when disclosure may expose them to liability for a therapeutic mistake? Clinicians feel major pressure to avoid malpractice litigation. Does admitting error increase or decrease this risk (as in case RS)?

Hilfiker took an early lead in defining the complexity of dealing with errors: Was there a mistake? What were the real consequences? Was the mistake avoidable? Does the profession have a place for discussing mistakes? How can a clinician vent emotional responses?[65]

In a 1989 study, Novack and colleagues reported that one-third of the physicians who responded said that they would not disclose a fatal error to the family. However, the attitude of the majority of physicians, as noted in this study and others, would be to disclose the error.[66] Interest in the problem of medical errors increased in the 1990s, with several prominent cases and a growing body of data suggesting that this was a significant problem in the healthcare system.[67] This culminated in the 1999 Institute of Medicine (IOM) report of more than one million preventable adverse events, of which 44,000 to 98,000 were fatal per year. In addition to quantifying the problem, the IOM report also recommended a series of changes in the approach to identifying and preventing errors.[68] Simultaneously, there occurred a rather dramatic change in how individual clinicians and institutions dealt with error and how patients were informed about errors. The IOM emphasized that most errors are systems-related and are usually not related to individual negligence or misconduct. The system is remarkably complex, and clinicians are human and will make mistakes.

Professional organizations, licensing agencies, healthcare organizations, and risk-management units now strongly recommend that the clinician inform the patient of medical mistakes. There is some disagreement about whether all errors should be disclosed, or just those with clinical consequences for the patient. There are numerous minor errors. For instance, a drug may have been incorrectly ordered, incorrectly dispensed by the pharmacist, or incorrectly administered by the nurse, without causing complications for the patient. Should these events be disclosed at the risk of causing anxiety and loss of trust in the healthcare system? One study reports that 98 percent of patients said that they desired disclosure of even minor errors.[69]

Clark argues that patients need information to give informed consent, especially when they rely on caregivers to provide it. He sees this as an issue of respect: patients have a right to all of the information that directly affects their person. He also stresses the ethical obligation to correct errors or to compensate patients for errors.[70] Gillon suggests that the tendency of clinicians to close rank in their own individual and group interests is not compatible with the principle of medical beneficence.[71] He and others agree that if a mistake has been made, clinicians should, "out of common decency, let alone the principle of medical beneficence, say we are sorry."[72]

In the recent past, clinicians and institutions would shape their actions, in part, due to fear of litigation. In fact most lawyers and risk managers find that a policy of dealing honestly and openly with patients does not increase liability and probably decreases it overall.[73]

Disclosure by the clinician may also be self-therapeutic for the emotional distress and guilt that most clinicians feel after an event.[74]

XII. ETHICAL GROUNDING FOR COMMUNICATION, TRUTH-TELLING, AND DISCLOSURE

The primary ethical grounding for all of these interactions with patients is based on the principle of respect for the patient's autonomy. Adequate communication and truthful information is necessary for patients' participation in decision making, as well as their self-determination in planning their lives. Without knowing their medical condition, their prognosis, what to expect from treatment, and so forth, they cannot validly proceed. In addition, this clinical relationship and communication, both verbal and nonverbal, carries tremendous power to promote good for the patient (beneficence) and avoid harm (nonmaleficence).

The duty not to lie or deceive is similarly based. Lying violates respect for persons and may cause harm. It manipulates the patient for another's purpose. It frustrates the patient's self-determination, because it leads the patient to proceed with incorrect data. Lying undermines the trust that the patient should have in the relationship with the clinician, in past and in all future relationships.

XIII. AUTHORITATIVE STATEMENTS

The 2001 revision of the AMA *Code of Medical Ethics* affirms as the second standard of honorable behavior: "A physician shall uphold the standards of professionalism, be honest in all professional interactions, and strive to report physicians deficient in character or competence, or engaging in fraud or deception, to appropriate entities."[75]

In "Fundamental Elements of the Patient-Physician Relationship," the AMA Council on Ethical and Judicial Affairs (CEJA) elaborates on the therapeutic relationship:

The patient-physician relationship is of greatest benefit to patients when they bring medical problems to the attention of their physicians in a timely fashion, provide information about their medical condition to the best of their ability, and work with their physicians in a mutually respectful alliance. Physicians can best contribute to this alliance by serving as their patients' advocate and by fostering these rights:

1. The patient has the right to receive information from physicians and to discuss the benefits, risks, and costs of appropriate treatment alternatives. Patients should receive guidance from their physicians as to the optimal course of action. Patients are also entitled to obtain copies or summaries of their medical records, to have their questions answered, to be advised of potential conflicts of interest that their physicians might have, and to receive independent professional opinions.[76]

And also:

The relationship between patient and physician is based on trust and gives rise to physicians' ethical obligations to place patients' welfare above their own self-interest and above obligations to other groups, and to advocate for their patients' welfare.[77]

The American Nurses Association *Code for Nurses with Interpretive Statements* states,

Truthtelling and the process of reaching informed choice underlie the exercise of self-determination, which is basic to respect for persons. . . . Clients have the moral right to determine what will be done with their own person; to be given accurate information, and all the information necessary for making informed judgments.[78]

The American Hospital Association *A Patient's Bill of Rights* reads,

The patient has the right to obtain from his physicians and other direct caregivers relevant, current, and understandable information concerning his diagnosis, treatment, and prognosis.

Except in emergencies, when the patient lacks decision-making capacity and the need for treatment is urgent, the patient is entitled to the opportunity to discuss and request information related to the specific procedures and/or treatments, the risks involved, the possible length of recuperation, and the medically reasonable alternatives and their accompanying risks.[79]

The American College of Physicians "Ethics Manual," 1998, states,

The physician's primary commitment must always be to the patient's welfare and best interests, whether the physician is preventing or treating illness or helping patients to cope with illness, disability and death. The physician must support the dignity of all persons and respect their uniqueness. The interests of the patient should always be promoted regardless of financial arrangements; the health care setting; and patient characteristics, such as decision-making capacity or social status. . . .

At the beginning of a patient-physician relationship, the physician must understand the patient's complaints, underlying feelings, goals, and expectations. After patient and physician agree on the problem and the goal of therapy, the physician presents one or more courses of action. If both parties agree, the patient may authorize the physician to initiate a course of action; the physician then can accept that responsibility. The relationship has mutual obligations: The physician must be professionally competent, act responsibly and treat the patient with compassion and respect, and the patient should understand and consent to the treatment and should participate responsibly in the care. . . .

Physicians and patients may have different concepts of the meaning and resolution of medical problems. The care of the patient and the satisfaction of both parties are best served if the physician and patient discuss their expectations and concerns. Although the physician must address the patient's concerns, he or she is not required to violate fundamental personal values, standards of scientific or ethical practice, or the law. When the patient's beliefs — religious, cultural or otherwise — run counter to medical recommendations, the physician is obliged to try to understand the beliefs and viewpoints of the patient. . . .

To make health care decisions and work intelligently in partnership with the physician, the patient must be well informed. Effective physician-patient communication can dispel uncertainty and fear and enhance healing and patient satisfaction. Information should be disclosed whenever it is considered material to the patient's understanding of his or her situation, possible treatment and probable outcomes. . . .

However uncomfortable to clinician or patient, information that is essential to the patient must be disclosed. How, when, and to whom information is disclosed are important concerns that must be addressed.

Information should be given in terms the patient can understand. The physician should be sensitive to the patient's responses in setting the pace of disclosure, particularly if the illness is very serious. Disclosure should never be a mechanical or perfunctory process. Upsetting news and information should be presented to the patient in a way that minimizes distress. If the patient is unable to comprehend his or her condition, it should be fully disclosed to an appropriate surrogate.

In addition, physicians should disclose to patient information about procedural or judgment errors made in the course of care if such information is material to the patient's well-being. Errors do not necessarily constitute improper, negligent or unethical behavior, but failure to disclose them may.[80]

The American Academy of Pediatrics Committee on Bioethics, 1994, states,

There is a strong presumption that all information needed to make an appropriate decision about healthcare . . . should be provided to the patient, parents or surrogates. Experience and study suggest that most patients, family members or other decision makers want to hear the reality of their situation. Open and honest communication reduces tension in the physician-patient relationship.

Information may not be withheld on the grounds that it might cause the patient or surrogate to decline a recommended treatment or choose a treatment that the physician does not want to provide. Nor may information be withheld because its disclosure might upset the patient, parents or other decision maker. Physicians may withhold information when a competent patient clearly indicates that he or she does not wish to have the information provided, and the physician has previously offered to provide such information. Some commentators believe that parents and other surrogates do not have the same prerogative to refuse information or decline participation in decision making.

Physicians may withhold information if they believe the information would pose an immediate and/or serious threat to a patient's or surrogate's health or life. These circumstances will occur rarely, if ever. A physician who withholds information assumes the burden of supporting the decision not to make customary disclosures. The physician should withhold only the specific information that might produce a threat.[81]

In a 2002 statement, the AMA CEJA states,

The duty of patient advocacy is a fundamental element of the physician-patient relationship that should not be altered by the system of healthcare delivery in which physicians practice. Physicians must continue to place the interests of their patients first.

When managed care plans place restrictions on the care that physicians in the plan may provide to their patients, the following principles should be followed:

Regardless of any allocation guidelines or gatekeeper directives, physicians must advocate for any care they believe will materially benefit their patients.

Adequate appellate mechanisms for both patients and physicians should be in place to address disputes regarding medically necessary care. In some circumstances, physicians have an obligation to initiate appeals on behalf of their patients. Cases may arise in which a health care plan has an allocation guideline that is generally fair but in particular circumstances results in unfair denials of care, i.e., denial of care that, in the physician's judgment, would materially benefit the patient . . . . In such cases the physician's duty as patient advocate requires that the physician challenge the denial and argue for the provision of treatment in the specific case. . . . Physicians should assist patients who wish to seek additional, appropriate care outside the plan when the physician believes the care is in the patient's best interest.[82]

XIV. GUIDANCE

The clinician's goal should be an honest and tactful discussion of the medical facts — sensitive to the needs, capacities, emotions, and basic beliefs and values of the particular patient — so that the patient can participate in the decision-making process. The clinician should respect the right of the patient to obtain complete current medical information concerning diagnosis, alternatives for treatment, and prognosis, in terms the patient can be reasonably expected to understand, with open discussion of the element of uncertainty involved in the patient's care.

Truthfulness should mark the communication process between clinicians and patients; clinicians should not intentionally lie, deceive, or manipulate patients through words, actions, or silence. The "therapeutic privilege" (or "benevolent deception") may be exercised validly to withhold information only with documentation and a second opinion that disclosure would, with high probability, cause substantial harm to the patient's physical or mental well-being. The therapeutic privilege is intended to prevent direct harm to the patient; however, the moral presumption is that such cases are extremely rare, and, therefore, therapeutic privilege should never be used as an excuse to limit the patient's right to be informed.

XV. CASES FOR FURTHER STUDY

Case 1: "She'll Be Happier If She Never Knows"

It was the first time the 54-year-old patient had been hospitalized. She was born in Puerto Rico and had lived in Spanish Harlem for the past 10 years. She had come to the emergency room two weeks earlier with a severe pain and a mass in her lower right abdomen. The previous December she suffered a severe attack in the same area. Her history revealed that she was past menopause. She had worked in a nursing home and so was familiar with medical procedure.

A third-year medical student obtained the pertinent material in her medical history and talked with her briefly. She told him that she was afraid that she had cancer. When the student assured her that she would have a complete work-up, she replied sadly, "If it was cancer you doctors wouldn't tell me." The student did not comment on the patient's statement, but said that the lab tests and examinations would tell them much more about the possible causes of the pain and the mass. Two days later, the patient had been examined by medical students, the resident, the chief resident, and the attending physician. The woman was diagnosed as having a degenerating fibroid, which would explain the severe pain and the mass. It was pointed out, however, that after menopause the most common cause of a painful mass was cancer. The patient went to surgery the next morning. The same day, the medical student spoke to the resident, who reported that the patient had stage IV cancer of the cervix. They had cleaned out the entire tumor they could see, but, since it had spread to the pelvic wall, the only alternative was to try chemotherapy and radiation. The five-year survival rate of stage IV cancer at the time was not more than 20 percent.

When the patient awoke from the surgery, the medical student's first reaction was to go to her and explain the findings. He felt he should speak frankly with her, attempt to share her grief, and be there to support her. However, since he had not had much experience with cancer and this was his first patient "who had been given a death notice," he decided to speak first to the chief resident about how best to approach telling this woman. The medical student explained that she had cancer, and that he felt close enough to share some of the process. The chief resident's reaction was agitated. "Never use the word 'cancer' with a patient," he said, "because then they give up hope." He suggested using other words or medical jargon.

The student was in turmoil. He felt it was important to convey to the patient what he knew himself: that, according to the best medical understanding of her condition, she had a limited time to live; that new biomedical technology and medical discoveries meant that there were possible treatments, which could be tried; that new discoveries are continually being made. But he wanted to convey to her that the chances were that she would not live out her normal life-span — in fact, she would not survive more than a few years.

The discussion got more heated. The resident angrily asked, "I'd like to know how you'll feel when the patient jumps out the window." The student's response was that he felt he had to evaluate the patient's desire to know and that this woman had given a clear message that she wished to know.

The resident told the young student a story about a distinguished internist, the senior attending physician on the service and internationally known as author of a major medical textbook, who, while on grand rounds, asked if there was anyone present who would tell the patient they had just seen that he had cancer. When one medical student raised his hand, the internist said, "You march down to the dean's office and tell him that I said you are to be kicked out of medical school." Since an authoritarian and often hostile relation between master and student still exists in the clinical teaching setting, the student took him very seriously and turned toward the door. At that point the internist said, "Now you know what it's like to be told you have cancer. Tell a patient that, and it will destroy the last years of her life."

The student left the meeting with the resident wondering what the patient should be told and who should do the telling. He had a good idea what would be said by the senior attending physician, by the resident, and by himself. How would you advise the student?

— Adapted from a case in R.M. Veatch, *Death, Dying, and the Biological Revolution* (New Haven, Conn.: Yale University Press, 1989), 166-67.

Case 2: "Can Complicity In Deception Be Sometimes Justified?"

A five-year-old girl had been a patient in a medical center for three years because of progressive renal failure secondary to glomerulonephritis. She had been on chronic renal dialysis, and the possibility of a renal transplantation was considered. The effectiveness of this procedure in her case was questionable. On the other hand, it was the feeling of the professional staff that there was a clear possibility that a transplanted kidney would not undergo the same disease process. After discussion with the parents, it was decided to proceed with plans for transplantation.

Tissue typing was performed on the patient; it was noted that she would be difficult to match. Two siblings, age two and four, were thought to be too young to serve as donors. The girl's mother turned out not to be histocompatible. The father, however, was found to be quite compatible with his daughter. He underwent an arteriogram, and it was discovered that he had anatomically favorable circulation for transplantation.

The nephrologist met alone with the father and gave him these results. He informed the father that the prognosis for his daughter was quite uncertain. After some thought, the girl's father decided that he did not wish to donate a kidney to his daughter. He admitted that he did not have the courage and that, particularly in view of the uncertain prognosis, the very slight possibility of a cadaver kidney, and the degree of suffering his daughter had already sustained, he would prefer not to donate. The father asked the physician to tell everyone else in the family that he was not histocompatible. He was afraid that if they knew the truth, they would accuse him of allowing his daughter to die. He felt that this would "wreck the family." The physician felt very uncomfortable about this request. How would you advise him to respond?

— Adapted from a case in M.D. Levine, L. Scott, and W.J. Curran, "Ethics Rounds in a Children's Medical Center: Evaluation of a Hospital-Based Program for Continuing Education in Medical Ethics," *Pediatrics* 60 (August 1977): 205.

Case 3: "Will the Truth Spoil the Vacation In Australia?"

A 69-year-old male, estranged from his children and with no other living relatives, had a routine physical examination in preparation for a brief and much-anticipated trip to Australia. The physician suspected a serious problem and ordered more extensive testing, including further blood analysis, a bone scan, and a prostate biopsy. The results were quite conclusive: the man had an inoperable, incurable carcinoma — a small prostate nodule commonly referred to as cancer of the prostate. The carcinoma was not yet advanced and was relatively slow growing. Later, after the disease had progressed, it would be possible to provide good palliative treatment. Blood tests and X-rays showed the patient's renal function to be normal.

The physician had treated this patient for many years and knew that he was fragile in several respects. The man was quite neurotic and had an established history of psychiatric disease, although he functioned well in society and was clearly capable of rational thought and decision making. He had recently suffered a severe depressive reaction, during which he had behaved irrationally and attempted suicide. This episode immediately followed the death of his wife, who had died after a difficult and protracted battle with cancer. It was clear that he had not been equipped to deal with his wife's death, and he had been hospitalized for a short period before the suicide attempt.

Just as he was getting back on his feet, the opportunity to go to Australia materialized, and it was the first excitement he had experienced in several years. The patient also had a history of suffering prolonged and serious depression whenever informed of serious health problems. He worried excessively and often could not exercise rational control over his deliberations and decisions. His physician therefore thought that disclosure of the carcinoma under his present fragile state would almost certainly cause further irrational behavior and render the patient incapable of thinking clearly about his medical situation. When the testing had been completed and the results were known, the patient returned to his physician. He asked nervously, "Am I OK?" Without waiting for a response, he asked, "I don't have cancer, do I?" How would you advise the physician to respond?

— Adapted from a case in T.L. Beauchamp and J.F. Childress, *Principles of Biomedical Ethics* (Oxford, U.K.: Oxford University Press, 1994).

XVI. STUDY QUESTIONS

1. If, during a patient interview, you as a medical student were erroneously introduced to a patient as "Dr. So-and-So," would you correct the error or let it go? What motivates your response? Would you challenge an authority figure that misled or engaged in dysfunctional communication with a patient? Why or why not? Consider case 1, "She'll Be Happier if She Never Knows." Do the data support the resident and attending physicians' arguments in this case? What would you do if you were the medical student in the case?

2. All clinicians inevitably make mistakes in their clinical practice. You will make mistakes too. These can range from simple and uneventful medication errors, to misdiagnoses, to lethal mistakes. Consider the probability of your committing a clinical error that causes a patient moderate to severe harm. Suppose that you give a patient an intrathecal injection (into the spinal cavity) of the wrong chemotherapeutic drug, which results in your patient's paraplegia. How will you

handle this in terms of your personal feelings? Will you disclose your error? Will you say you are sorry? How will you feel about yourself?

3. Consider case 2, "Can Complicity in Deception Be Sometimes Justified?" How would you handle the situation if you were the nephrologist? What procedural safeguards could be put in place to avoid this situation happening again?

4. In case 3, "Will the Truth Spoil the Vacation in Australia?" is the therapeutic privilege the best option in this case? What are the risks and benefits of such a course of action?

NOTES

1. Hippocrates, *Decorum,* trans. W. Jones (Cambridge, Mass.: Harvard University Press, 1967), 297.

2. A.R. Jonsen and S. Toulmin, *The Abuse of Casuistry: A History of Moral Reasoning* (Berkeley, Calif.: University of California Press, 1988).

3. T. Percival, *Medical Ethics or A Code of Institutes and Precepts, Adapted to the Professional Conduct of Physicians and Surgeons* (Manchester, U.K.: S. Russell, 1803).

4. American Medical Association, *Code of Medical Ethics* (adopted May 1847), chap. 1, art. 1, sec. 4 in J. Katz, *The Silent World of Doctor and Patient* (New York: Free Press, 1984), 20.

5. American Medical Association, *Current Opinions of the Judicial Council of the AMA* (Chicago, Ill.: AMA, 1981), ¶ 8.07.

6. W.T. Fitts and I.S. Ravdin, "What Philadelphia Physicians Tell Patients about Cancer," *Journal of the American Medical Association* 15 (1953): 901.

7. D. Oken, "What to Tell Cancer Patients: A Study of Medical Attitudes," *Journal of the American Medical Association* 175 (1961): 1120.

8. D.H. Novack et al., "Changes in Physicians' Attitudes Toward Telling the Cancer Patient," *Journal of the American Medical Association* 241 (1979): 897.

9. R. Veatch and E. Tai, "Talking about Death: Patterns of Lay and Professional Change," *Annals of the American Academy of Political and Social Science* 447 (1980): 29-45.

10. See note 8 above.

11. H. Graham and B. Livesley, "Dying as a Diagnosis: Difficulties of Communication and Management in Elderly Patients," *Lancet* 2 (1982): 670-72.

12. D.H. Novack et al., "Physicians' Attitudes toward Using Deception to Resolve Difficult Ethical Problems," *Journal of the American Medical Association* 261 (1989): 2980.

13. N.T. Miyaji, "The Power of Compassion: Truth-telling Among American Doctors in the Care of Dying Patients," *Social Science and Medicine* 36 (1993): 249-64.

14. E.B. Lamont and N.A. Christakis, "Prognostic Disclosure to Patients with Cancer Near the End of Life," *Annals of Internal Medicine* 134 (2001): 1096-105.

15. P.A. Ubel, "Truth in the Most Optimistic Way," *Annals of Internal Medicine* 134 (2001): 1142-3.

16. E.J. Emanuel and N.N. Dubler, "Preserving the Physician-Patient Relationship in the Era of Managed Care," *Journal of the American Medical Association* 273 (1995): 323.

17. J.D. Frank, "The Faith That Heals," *Johns Hopkins Medical Journal* 137 (1975): 127-31.

18. See note 16 above, p. 323.

19. E.J. Cassell, *Talking with Patients* (Boston, Mass.: Massachusetts Institute of Technology Press, 1985).

20. P.S. Jensen, "The Doctor-Patient Relationship: Headed for Impasse or Improvement?" *Annals of Internal Medicine* 95 (1981): 769-71.

21. B.M. Korsch, E.K. Gozzi, and V. Francis, "Gaps in Doctor-Patient Communication," *Pediatrics* 42 (1968): 855-71.

22. See note 16 above, p. 325.

23. H. Waitzkin, "Doctor-Patient Communication: Clinical Implications of Social Science Research," *Journal of the American Medical Association* 252 (1984): 2441-6; C.H. Braddock et al., "How Doctors and Patients Discuss Routine Clinical Decisions: Informed Decision Making in the Outpatient Setting," *Journal of General Internal Medicine* 12 (1997): 339-45.

24. H.L. Hirsch, "The Physician's Duty to Stop, Look, Listen and Communicate," *Medicine and Law* 5 (1986): 449-61.

25. W.J. Donnelly, "Righting the Medical Record: Transforming Chronicle into Story," *Journal of the American Medical Association* 260 (1988): 823-5.

26. R.L. Fine, "Personal Choices: Communication between Physicians and Patients When Confronting Critical Illness," *The Journal of Clinical Ethics* 2, no. 1 (Spring 1991): 57-8.

27. L. Forrow, R.M. Arnold, and L.S. Parker, "Preventive Ethics: Expanding the Horizons of Clinical Ethics," *The Journal of Clinical Ethics* 4,

no. 4 (Winter 1993): 287-94.

28. S.H. Kaplan et al., "Characteristics of Physicians with Participatory Decision-Making Styles," *Annals of Internal Medicine* 124 (1996): 497-504.

29. A. Towle et al., "Patient Perceptions that Limit a Community-Based Intervention to Promote Participation," *Patient Education and Counseling* 50 (2003): 231-3.

30. L.A. Cooper et al., "Patient-Centered Communication, Ratings of Care, and Concordance of Patient and Physician Race," *Annals of Internal Medicine* 139 (2003): 907-15; L. Cooper-Patrick et al., "Race, Gender, and Partnership in the Patient-Physician Relationship," *Journal of the American Medical Association* 282 (1999): 583-9.

31. American Nurses Association Committee on Ethics, *Code for Nurses with Interpretive Statements* (Washington, D.C.: ANA, 1983), 16, ¶ 11.3.

32. E.D. Pellegrino, "Is Truthtelling to the Patient a Cultural Artifact?" *Journal of the American Medical Association* 268 (1992): 1734-5.

33. L.J. Blackhall et al., "Ethnicity and Attitudes toward Patient Autonomy," *Journal of the American Medical Association* 274 (1995): 820-5.

34. R. Higgs, "Truthtelling, Lying and the Doctor-Patient Relationship," in *Principles of Health Care Ethics,* ed. R. Gillon (Chichester, U.K.: John Wiley & Sons, 1994), 501.

35. R.M. Veatch, *The Patient-Physician Relation: The Patient as Partner,* part 2 (Bloomington, Ind.: Indiana University Press, 1991), 123.

36. J. Katz, *The Silent World of Doctor and Patient* (New York: Free Press, 1984), 165-206.

37. E.B. Beresford, "Uncertainty and the Shaping of Medical Decisions," *Hastings Center Report* 21 (1991): 6-11.

38. M. Parascandola, J. Hawkins, and M. Danis, "Patient Autonomy and the Challenge of Clinical Uncertainty," *Kennedy Institute of Ethics Journal* 12 (2002): 245-64.

39. See note 36, page 206.

40. H. Brody, "The Physician/Patient Relationship," in *Medical Ethics,* ed. R.M. Veatch (Boston, Mass.: Jones and Bartlett, 1989), 78-9.

41. M. Elian and G. Dean, "To Tell or Not to Tell the Diagnosis of Multiple Sclerosis," *Lancet* 2 (1985): 27.

42. President's Commission for the Study of Ethical Problems in Medicine and Biomedical and Behavioral Research, *Making Health Care Decisions,* vol. 1 (Washington, D.C.: U.S. Government Printing Office, 1982), 99-100.

43. T.E. Finucane et al., "Establishing Advance Medical Directives with Demented Patients: A Pilot Study," *The Journal of Clinical Ethics* 4, no. 1 (Spring 1993): 51-4.

44. P. Bruce-Jones et al., "Resuscitating the Elderly: What Do the Patients Want?" *Journal of Medical Ethics* 22 (1996): 154-9.

45. E. Erde, E. Nadal, and T. Scholl, "On Truthtelling and the Diagnosis of Alzheimer's Disease," *Journal of Family Practice* 26 (1988): 401-4.

46. M. Silverstein et al., "ALS and Life-Sustaining Therapy: Patients' Desire for Information, Participation in Decision-Making, and Life Sustaining Therapy," *Mayo Clinic Proceedings* 66 (1991): 906-13.

47. C. Frank et al., "Determining Resuscitation Preferences of Elderly Inpatients: A Review of the Literature," *Canadian Medical Association Journal* 169 (2003): 795-9; E.J. Emanuel et al., "Talking with Terminally Ill Patients and Their Caregivers about Death, Dying, and Bereavement," *Archives of Internal Medicine* 164 (2004): 1999-2004.

48. N.A. Christakis and T.J. Iwashyna, "Attitude and Self-reported Practice Regarding Prognostication in a National Sample of Internists," *Archives of Internal Medicine* 158 (1998): 2389-95; N.A. Christakis and E. Lamont, "Extent and Determinants of Error in Doctors' Prognoses in Terminally Ill Patients," *British Medical Journal* 320 (2000): 469-73.

49. J.C. Weeks et al., "Relationship Between Cancer Patients' Predictions of Prognosis and Their Treatment Preferences," *Journal of the American Medical Association* 279 (1998): 1709-14; T.J. Smith and K. Swisher, "Telling the Truth About Terminal Cancer," *Journal of the American Medical Association* 279 (1998): 1746-8.

50. T.E. Quill, "Initiating End-of-Life Discussions With Seriously Ill Patients," *Journal of the American Medical Association* 284 (2000): 2502-7.

51. R. Buckman, *How to Break Bad News: A Guide for Health Care Professionals* (Baltimore, Md.: Johns Hopkins University Press, 1992).

52. See note 12 above; M. Delvecchio Good et al., "American Oncology and the Discourse on Hope," *Culture, Medicine and Psychiatry* 14 (1990): 59-70; G.J. Annas, "Informed Consent, Cancer, and Truth in Prognosis," *New England Journal of Medicine* 330 (1994): 223-5.

53. J. Katz, "Legal and Ethical Issues of Informed Consent in Health Care," in *Encyclopedia of Bioethics,* ed. W.T. Reich (New York: MacMillan, 1995), 1256-63.

54. B.M. Mount, "Dealing with Our Losses," *Journal of Clinical Oncology* 4 (1986): 1127-34.

55. J. Vernick and M. Karon, "Who's Afraid of Death on a Leukemia Ward?" *American Journal of Disease of Childhood* 109 (1965): 393-7; G. Koocher, "Psychosocial Issues During the Acute Treatment of Pediatric Cancer," *Cancer* 58 (1986): 468-72.

56. T.L. Beauchamp and J.F. Childress, *Principles of Biomedical Ethics,* 3rd ed. (New York: Oxford University Press, 1989), 78-9.

57. See note 40 above, pp. 78-79.

58. See note 42 above.

59. See note 32 above, p. 1734.

60. B. Freedman, "Offering Truth: One Ethical Approach to the Uninformed Cancer Patient," *Archives of Internal Medicine* 153 (1993): 572-6.

61. Adapted from R.M. Veatch, *Death, Dying and the Biologic Revolution* (New Haven, Conn.: Yale University Press, 1976), 222-9.

62. M.K. Wynia et al., "Physician Manipulation of Reimbursement Rules for Patients," *Journal of the American Medical Association* 283 (2000): 1858-65.

63. M.G. Bloche, "Fidelity and Deceit at the Bedside," *Journal of the American Medical Association* 283 (2000): 1881-4.

64. M.T. Myers, "Lying for Patients May be a Violation of Federal Law," *Archives of Internal Medicine* 160 (2000): 2223-4.

65. D. Hilfiker, "Facing Our Mistakes," *New England Journal of Medicine* 310 (1984): 118-22.

66. See note 12 above.

67. L.L. Leap, "Error in Medicine," *Journal of the American Medical Association* 272 (1994): 1851-7; S.E. Bedell et al., "Incidence and Characteristics of Preventable Iatrogenic Cardiac Arrests," *Journal of the American Medical Association* 265 (1991): 2815-20; T.A. Brennan et al., "Incidence of Adverse Events and Negligence in Hospitalized Patients: Results of the Harvard Practice Study I," *New England Journal of Medicine* 324 (1991): 370-6.

68. L.T. Kohn, J.M. Corrigan, and M.S. Donaldson, eds., *To Err is Human: Building a Safer Health Care System* (Washington, D.C.: National Academy Press, 1999).

69. A.B. Witman, D.M. Parc, and S.B. Hardin, "How Do Patients Want Physicians to Handle Mistakes? A Survey of Internal Medicine Patients in an Academic Setting," *Archives of Internal Medicine* 156 (1996): 2565-9.

70. P.A. Clark, "Medication Errors in Family Practice, in Hospitals and After Discharge from the Hospital: An Ethical Analysis," *Journal of Law, Medicine & Ethics* 32 (2004): 349-57. 71. R. Gillon, "Doctors and Patients," *British Medical Journal* 292 (1986): 466-9.

72. L.M. Peterson and T. Brennan, "Medical Ethics and Medical Injuries: Taking Our Duties Seriously," *The Journal of Clinical Ethics* 1, no. 3 (Fall 1990): 207-11; see note 47 above.

73. L. Leape, "Reporting of Adverse Events," *New England Journal of Medicine* 347 (2002): 1633-8; M. Kapp, "Medical Errorsvs. Malpractice," *DePaul Journal of Health Care Law* 1 (1997): 751-72; S.S. Kraman and G. Hamm, "Risk Management: Extreme Honesty May Be the Best Policy," *Annals of Internal Medicine* 131 (1999): 963-7; J. Vogel and R. Delgado, "To Tell the Truth: Physicians' Duty to Disclose Medical Mistakes," *UCLA Law Review* 28 (1980): 52-94; M.E. Meaney, "Error Reduction, Patient Safety and Institutional Ethics Committees," *Journal of Law, Medicine & Ethics* 32 (2004): 358-64.

74. M.C. Newman, "The Emotional Impact of Mistakes on Family Physicians," *Archives of Family Medicine* 5 (1996): 71-5; J.F. Christensen, W. Levinson, and P.M. Dunn, "The Heart of Darkness: The Impact of Perceived Mistakes on Physicians," *Journal of General Internal Medicine* 7 (1992): 424-31; F. Rosner et al., "Disclosure and Prevention of Medical Errors," *Archives of Internal Medicine* 160 (2000): 2089-92.

75. American Medical Association, Council on Ethical and Judicial Affairs, "Principles of Medical Ethics" in *Code of Medical Ethics* (Chicago, Ill.: AMA, 2002), xiv.

76. Ibid., p. 281, ¶ 10.01.

77. Ibid., p. 285, ¶ 10.015.

78. See note 31 above, p. 2, ¶ 1.1.75.

79. American Hospital Association, *A Patient's Bill of Rights* (Chicago, Ill.: AHA, 1992), 1.

80. American College of Physicians, "Ethics Manual," *Annals of Internal Medicine* 128 (1998): 576-948.

81. Committee on Bioethics, American Academy of Pediatrics, "Guidelines on Forgoing Life-Sustaining Medical Treatment," *Pediatrics* 93 (1994): 532-6.

82. See note 76 above, pp. 219-20, ¶ 8.13.

9

Determining Patients' Capacity to Share in Decision Making

Robert J. Boyle

CASES

AB, a 90-year-old woman living alone and independently, is described as very spry and mentally "with it." She presents to the emergency room with gastrointestinal bleeding. Her surgeon advises her that, without surgery for what is presumed to be colon cancer, she will bleed to death. She refuses, stating she realizes that her "time has come." The surgeon is alarmed that this very active person is refusing the proposed treatment. He is concerned that she is "too old" to decide for herself.

CD is a 15-year-old high school student with aplastic anemia that will require a bone marrow transplant. His parents have been fully informed, but they believe that their son is too young to participate in the decision on whether to proceed.

EF is a 35-year-old construction worker who has been injured on the job. He is bleeding profusely. When brought to the emergency room, he is still alert and oriented, and informs the staff that he is a Jehovah's Witness. He refuses all blood products. His surgeon informs him that he will die without a transfusion. He understands and again refuses. The surgeon begins the process to obtain a court order to transfuse because the patient's religious beliefs are not "rational."

GH is a 40-year-old man who is unemployed and very unsophisticated. He is admitted to the hospital with severe dehy-dration and impending shock following 36 hours of vomiting. Evaluation reveals a possible small bowel obstruction. After intravenous rehydration, he feels much improved and wants to leave. His family agrees with his wishes. His physician, who is concerned that the patient may still have a bowel obstruction, obtains a court order to treat on the grounds that the patient is "retarded."

JK is a 70-year-old retired attorney who has been treated for the past two years for lymphoma. He has a previous history of moderately severe depression following the death of his wife five years ago. Over the past three weeks he has become more withdrawn, has missed several medical appointments, and has missed his usual visits to his son. He is now admitted with fever and low white blood cell count, with a probable diagnosis of septicemia. The patient refuses antibiotic therapy, saying he wants to die rather than continue treatment for his primary disease.

LM is a 78-year-old woman with progressive Alzheimer's disease who is admitted with pneumonia and other medical problems. She recognizes no one and has been incontinent for more than a year. Despite aggressive therapy, the pneumonia fails to resolve, and it is probable that she will not survive to discharge. The patient's husband has begun requesting that the physicians be less aggressive in her treatment and, in fact, decrease the intensity of her treatment. Discussion with the husband reveals that he recently proposed marriage to the couple's housekeeper. The medical staff is concerned that the husband is no longer a valid surrogate.

NP is an 18-year-old high school athlete who was injured in a motorcycle accident. His left foot was crushed, and attempts to save the limb have been unsuccessful. Infection in the foot now threatens the boy's life. However, he refuses the surgery saying, "If I cannot play sports, my life is meaningless."

QR is a 75-year-old resident in a nursing home. He was brought to the emergency room after developing respiratory distress. He has a history of severe dementia and several strokes. He was intubated and placed on a ventilator. The staff has now learned that he had no advanced directive, no designated surrogate, and no known family. He has been in the nursing home for five years.

I. INTRODUCTION

As noted in chapter 8, patients' interests and well-being are best served when they understand their situation and participate in deciding on care and treatment. This is the ethical basis for informed consent (discussed in chapter 10). Participation in decision making implies an ability (capacity) to do so.

All would agree that a patient in a coma, an infant, a severely retarded adult, a severely mentally ill patient, and a heavily intoxicated adult are not capable of decision making. But less obvious situations, similar to those presented in the cases above, are encountered frequently in the clinical setting. For example:

1. Our aging society includes increasing numbers of elderly individuals — living alone, with family, or in nursing homes — with questionable decision-making abilities.
2. Following a change of approach in the care of mental illness, many individuals with mental illness, who are able to function to varying degrees, now live on the street, in group homes, or with family.
3. Advances in medical technology have resulted in frequent major life-and-death dilemmas for patients who are no longer fully conscious or able to make decisions.
4. There are increasing numbers of individuals who have no one to make decisions for them. How does one determine whether a patient is capable or incapable of medical decision making? If the patient is not capable, who then

makes the decision? How is the decision made?

II. BACKGROUND

Society has long recognized that some of its members are unable to make decisions for themselves. Under English common law, the king had the authority and obligation to protect individuals who were incapable of protecting their own interests. This duty extended to appointing guardians to take custody of children and administer any estates with which they may have been left. Traditionally, families assumed the role of protector for members who were no longer able to care for themselves or manage their affairs. However, as patients' participation in shared decision making has increased, in the face of dramatic advances in diagnostic and therapeutic medicine, determining when a patient is unable to participate in decision making and finding an appropriate surrogate has became more critical.[1]

III. COMPETENCE VERSUS CAPACITY

The terms *capacity/incapacity* and *competence/incompetence* have different meanings in the legal context than in the medical context. Unfortunately, many writers and clinicians use the terms interchangeably.

Incompetence is the legal term used when a person has been judged by a court to be unable to take care of himself or herself or to manage his or her property. Judges base such determinations on the testimony of psychologists, psychiatrists, neurologists, other clinicians, officers of the law, or social workers. A declaration of incompetence completely negates a person's legal rights. The person who is declared incompetent may not enter a contract, hold a license, or make any other legally significant decision. Traditionally, definitions of *incompetence* have also included people whose mental capabilities might not be at issue (for example, children). People who are declared incompetent by a court usually are cared for by a court-appointed guardian.

The related but distinct term *incapacity* is used in the legal context to designate those whose individual limitations — mental or physical — do not globally restrict their cognitive abilities or life activities. Capacity is usually considered a functional matter that refers to specific functional deficits. A person may be declared incapacitated for purposes of handling financial affairs (and may have a limited guardian appointed for this purpose) while retaining the legal right to make all other decisions for himself or herself.

The terms *capacity* and *incapacity* share certain similarities in the medical and legal spheres. In the medical setting, however, the terms are used to describe the functioning of sensory and mental powers to process data and draw conclusions. Incapacity can be developmental or pathological. Developmental incapacity would include the immature mental processes of infants, children, and the developmentally retarded. Pathologic incapacity might result from some temporary or permanent deficit in psychophysiologic processes, such as encephalopathy, senile dementia, acute psychosis, or depression.[2] In this and chapter 10, the term *capacity* is used not in its strict legal sense, but from the perspective of a clinician who must make a functional analysis about a patient's decision-making ability.

IV. THE CONCEPT OF CAPACITY

Capacity is essentially the ability to make a decision. It is an absolutely basic element in the process of informed consent. Clinicians are, in simple terms, asking the question, "Should we allow this person to make this decision under these circumstances?" The consent of a person who is incapable is not valid authorization for a clinician to perform medical treatment. Conversely, a clinician who withholds treatment from an incapable patient who refuses treatment may be held liable by that patient or his or her surrogate, if the clinician does not take reasonable steps to obtain some other legally valid authorization for treatment.[3]

Any determination of capacity must address the following:
- The individual abilities of the patient;
- The requirement of the task at hand; and
- The consequences likely to flow from the decision.[4]

A. Standards for Determining Capacity

There is no "classic" definition of *capacity to make medical decisions,* nor is there a universally accepted legal definition for the term. In fact, there is considerable debate about clinical definitions of *capacity,* which is beyond the scope of this chapter.[5] A variety of often-used definitions or standards have evolved.

1. Standard Based on the Possible Outcome of the Patient's Decision

A patient is judged capable based on the outcome of his or her decision. If the decision reflects values that are not widely held or rejects conventional wisdom, the patient's capacity may be called into question. This situation often arises when the patient's decision goes against the clinician's values. Patients are less likely to have their capacity questioned if they agree with the clinician. For example, the surgeon questioned the decision of EF, the Jehovah's Witness patient who would allow himself to bleed to death rather than be transfused. In the case of GH, who wished to leave the hospital after rehydration, the patient reached a decision that his clinician opposed. The clinician then questioned his capacity on the grounds that he was "retarded."

In the case of William Bartling (*Bartling v. Superior Court*), hospital attorneys and the court redefined the legal issue of competence into a medical issue; they judged that the patient's prognosis was "optimistic" and the patient's responses were "ambivalent."[6]

Bartling was a 70-year-old man with complex medical problems, including inoperable lung cancer. Following a lung biopsy, he required intubation and mechanical ventilation in the intensive care unit (ICU). Bartling found the process of mechanical ventilation to be extremely uncomfortable and repeatedly asked that it be discontinued. He frequently removed himself from the ventilator and required hand restraints. Bartling consulted his attorney about forgoing mechanical ventilation. Bartling's physicians agreed to the plan, as long as the hospital administrator agreed. The latter also agreed, but wanted the approval of the hospital's attorney. The attorney refused permission, stating that Bartling was not terminally ill, in a persistent vegetative state, or brain dead. In a hearing, Bartling stated that he "did not wish to die," but did not "want to live on the respirator." The judge upheld the hospital attorney's position and refused to order the clinicians to discontinue mechanical ventilation or to allow Bartling's hands to be untied so that he could disconnect himself. No one questioned Bartling's competence. The patient died four months later. The case was reversed on appeal two months later.

Attorney/ethicist George Annas refers to Bartling as "The Prisoner in the ICU."[7] Annas suggests that those involved may have seen themselves as responsible for the actions of a competent patient and were more concerned with their own suffering and discomfort following the patient's death than with the suffering of the competent patient.

The "outcome standard" is rejected by most. Capacity does not necessarily mean "what is rational to me, the clinician." However, the outcome in a clinical situation may impact the level of capacity required to make decisions in that situation.

2. Standard Based on the Patient's Category or Status

A patient is judged capable based on his or her category or status; that is, the patient may be said to be incapable because he or she is mentally ill or mentally retarded (even mildly), or aged, or an adolescent minor, or critically ill (the "patient is too sick to decide"). However, many of these individuals are able to participate in decision making. There is a spectrum of ability to function in any group. A standard based on category is rejected by most.

For example, AB, the 90-year-old woman described at the beginning of this chapter who is independently living and mentally spry, is capable. She is not depressed. She understands her situation and the consequences of her refusal. Her decision is understandable. It is based on logic and fact. She is 90 and ready to die. If she had refused surgery because she does not make decisions on Tuesdays in July, the assessment might be different. In the latter case, while she may understand that she will die, her decision is not based on a rational process of decision making.

CD, the 15-year-old bone marrow transplant candidate, is capable of participating with his family in deciding on this highly invasive therapy. His status as a minor should not negate this.

While ICU patients may not recall all of their experiences in the ICU, this fact should not define all ICU patients as incapable.

3. Standard Based on the Patient's Functional Ability

The functional standard is the most widely accepted standard in determining the patients' capacity; it recognizes the patient's functional ability as a decision maker. There are a variety of definitions of this standard that help to clarify specific aspects of capacity. For example, the President's Commission for the Study of Ethical Problems in Medicine and Biomedical and Be-

havioral Research suggested that capacity is determined by whether a patient can do the following:

- *Understand information relevant to the decision.* How the information is presented is critical (see chapter 10, which discusses informed consent). Does the patient understand the problem and the proposed therapy? Is the patient alert? Is his or her attention span long enough to allow adequate intake?

- *Communicate with caregivers about the decision.* Does the patient respond? Can the patient explain the decision, or is there ambiguity, indecision, or vacillation?

- *Reason about relevant alternatives, against a background of reasonably stable personal goals and values.* Is the patient affected by psychosis, dementia, extreme phobia/panic, anxiety/euphoria, depression or anger? Does the patient have a thought disorder, short-term memory problem, depression, or waxing/waning consciousness?[8]

Appelbaum and Grisso use similar terminology:

- *Ability to communicate choices.* The patient has to maintain and communicate stable choices. Thought disorders, problems with short-term memory, or ambivalence resulting in alternating choices would affect this element. It can be tested simply by asking for a response. If there is doubt, the question can be repeated a few minutes later.

- *Ability to understand relevant information.* Deficits in attention span, intelligence, and memory may interfere. Testing might include asking the patient to paraphrase the disclosure.

- *Ability to appreciate the situation and its consequences.* Pathologic distortion, denial, or delusion would alter this element. The patient should be able to define the illness, the need for treatment, and the likely outcome.

- *Ability to rationally manipulate information.* Here the coherence and logic of one's reasoning is in question, not the outcome. Rational manipulation involves the ability to reach conclusions that are logically consistent with the starting premises. Psychosis, delirium, dementia, phobia, euphoria, depression, or anger may interfere. Patients should be able to indicate the major factors in their decisions and the importance assigned to them.[9]

White defines four broad categories of criteria for capacity:

- *"Informability."* Involves the ability to (1) receive information; (2) recognize relevant information as information; and (3) remember information.
- *Cognitive and affective capability.* Includes the ability to (1) relate situations to oneself; (2) reason about alternatives; and (3) rank alternatives ("construct personalized burden to benefit ratios for each option . . . assess the probability that each will occur . . . foresee how one's life would be variously changed"[10]). "These faculties enable patients to consider the wisdom of pursuing different alternatives, and to correlate past, present and future aspects of their lives, and to organize their lives in terms of their value structures."[11]
- *Resolution and resignation.* Incorporates the ability to (1) select an option; and (2) resign oneself to the choice. The patient reaches a conclusion, sets aside his or her uncertainties, and proceeds, even in the face of doubt.
- *Recounting one's decision-making process.* The ability to explain, by recognizable reasons, how one came to a particular decision.[12]

A number of authors in psychiatry, ethics, and law have expressed concern that the currently applied standards for determining capacity may place excess emphasis on the patient's alertness and ability to reason, while the patient may in fact have significant distortion in logic, cognitive errors, or distorted perception of his or her situation.[13] For example, NP refused surgery because he felt that without sports his life was meaningless. Individuals with head trauma may have problems with executive function, but be quite alert and oriented.

Ganzini and colleagues suggest that determinations of capacity should assess decisional autonomy, similar to the criteria above, as well as executional autonomy (the ability to actually carry out a decision). For example, if one of the issues at hand is the ability to live independently, the patient has to have the ability to appreciate his or her limitations or special care needs.[14]

B. Determining Capacity

In most clinical situations, determining capacity is not a complicated process. It is a common-sense judgment. Clinicians do it every time they interact with a patient. However, in many situations, determination of capacity may be quite problematic. Many clinical disease processes are often associated with altered mental status (such as meningitis, alcohol withdrawal, head injury, and stroke). The presence of these or other conditions does not in itself justify a determination of incapacity, but it should raise the clinician's suspicions. Likewise, a serious or life-threatening illness may lead to maladaptive behavior, with resultant post-traumatic stress disorder or depressive responses.[15]

Because depriving patients of decision-making rights is a serious infringement on their autonomy, every effort should be made to help patients perform at their best. For example, clinicians should minimize, when possible, psychoactive drugs; try to evaluate and involve the patient when he or she is "up" and not exhausted or medicated; and involve family members or other clinicians who know and can communicate well with the patient and who have the patient's trust. It may require a great deal of time, skill, and attention to determine the capacity of patients with communication disorders, such as aphasia or dysarthria. Speech therapists may provide expert assistance in enabling patients' involvement.[16]

It is important to re-evaluate patients as their situations change for better or worse. Someone who is poorly responsive today due to anxiety, depression, psychosis, or medical illness may be much improved tomorrow.

Capacity should be determined, in part, by the importance of the decision at hand. Decisions about taking a laxative and about cardiac transplant are on different levels of a "sliding scale." Drane's model defines three categories of medical situations, in which, as the consequences that may result from a decision become more serious, the capacity standards for consent or refusal become more stringent:

1. For easy, effective treatments that are not dangerous and are in the patient's best interest, awareness and assent may be all that is required,
2. For less certain treatments — when the diagnosis is doubtful, the condition is chronic, or the treatment is more dangerous or less effective — the patient must be able to understand the risks and benefits of the options and make a decision,
3. For dangerous treatments and treatments that run counter to professional and public ratio-

nality, the patient is required to show the highest standards of understanding and judgment.[17]

Drane concludes that a "properly performed competency assessment should eliminate two types of error: preventing competent persons from deciding their own treatments; and failing to protect incompetent persons from the harmful effects of a bad decision."[18] May, however, criticizes the "sliding scale" approach as an outcomes standard, allowing the patient more autonomy for low-risk decisions but restricting autonomy if the decision is riskier. He states that capacity "should not focus on the patient's abilities as such, but upon the patient's eligibility to assume decision-making responsibility."[19] This would seem to be more of an all-or-none definition.

Roth and colleagues describe a hierarchy of competency tests, which include the following:

- Evidencing a choice — a very low-level test, most respectful of autonomy, looking only for consent or denial,
- Reasonable outcome of choice,
- Choice based on rational reasons,
- Ability to understand, and
- Actual understanding, the highest test.[20]

These authors conclude that, in most situations, the test that should be applied combines elements of all the tests, and that the tests should be chosen based on the risk-benefit ratio of the treatment and whether the patient consents or refuses. Therefore, with a consent to a high-benefit and low-risk treatment, a low-level test of capacity would be applied, while a refusal may require a higher standard of capacity.

When there is doubt — due to the patient's clinical situation, the significance of the decision at hand, or dispute among careproviders (clinicians, family, or potential surrogates) — psychiatric/psychologic or neurologic consultation may be extremely important and helpful. This will allow evaluation for depression or organic brain disease. But also, in most situations, it falls to professionals to make formal determinations of capacity. In most cases, a complete mental status examination should be performed. The Mini-Mental Status Examination (MMSE), the Mattis Dementia Rating Scale, the Short Portable Mental Status Questionnaire, and the Cognitive Capacity Screening Examination are the more commonly used instruments. But again, these measure traits of mental status and are not specifically measures of decision-making capacity.[21] For example, the MMSE measures orientation in time and place, immediate recall, short-term memory, calculation, language, and constructive ability. According to Finucane and colleagues, "It can be affected by anxiety, depression, intelligence, education and the patient's sociocultural background. People with high scores may actually be [incapable] while those with relatively low scores may retain the ability to make some rational decisions. It is best to regard the MMSE as a useful but limited screening test."[22]

According to one well-known authority:

There is no international clinical, legal, philosophical or ethical consensus about competence criteria . . . there is no agreement about the threshold of decision-making or functional capacity necessary to consider a person legally or morally competent. In a given case, there may be wide consensus among clinicians, legal professionals, and ethicists that a particular person is, or is not, competent. . . . However, disagreement is likely in many cases. In part, this derives from the fact that competence determinations are not essentially factual, objective, or empirical matters but rather are value-laden judgments about the relative importance of autonomy and beneficence to the person, as assessed by the clinician or others.[23]

Numerous studies have identified the problem of application of standards by clinicians in a variety of settings, with wide variations in "accuracy" or inter-observer agreement on determinations of capacity.[24]

A variety of tools to assess capacity have been developed and standardized for general clinical use.[25] Other investigators have developed techniques for patients with specific conditions. Freedman and colleagues have suggested guidelines for assessing capacity in patients with cognitive deficits due to neurologic disorders:

- Does the patient have an adequate level of attention, or is there wandering or drifting attention?
- Is the patient able to comprehend relevant instructions; retain information long enough to evaluate it in relation to relevant, recent, and remote experiences; and express his or her wishes? Assessment might include spon-

taneous speech, auditory comprehension, writing, and reading comprehension, as well as recent and remote memory. Recent memory is important to retain information long enough to take all relevant facts into consideration. Remote memory is important for integration of current issues with past knowledge.

- Does the patient have sufficiently intact judgment? Frontal lobe dysfunction may affect ability to select goals, plan to achieve the goals, monitor performance, and evaluate consequences.[26]

Janofsky and colleagues have proposed an instrument that uses a standardized essay that would be read to patients, followed by a series of questions that correlated well with formal psychiatric determination of capacity.[27] Using a similar technique (a series of vignettes read to the patient followed by a series of questions), Fitten and colleagues[28] in a nursing home population and Marson and colleagues[29] in a population with different stages of Alzheimer's disease found that standard, indirect, cognitive screening assessment by the primary physician significantly underestimated the prevalence of impaired capacity. These authors concluded that with populations at risk for altered capacity, clinicians should more systematically and directly probe the patient's decision-making capacity when significant clinical decisions approach.

C. Depression

Depression can alter a patient's capacity for decision making. In the cases of JK and NP, clinicians might ask if these patients' refusal is rationally based on their primary disease and the discomfort they are experiencing, or is the refusal entirely or in part due to depression? Isn't a patient in this situation entitled to be depressed? Howe and colleagues note that the depressed patient may have capacity for clear thought and be able to express those thoughts, but have altered decision-making abilities due to mood and affect derangement and distorted logic.[30] Depression is relatively common; in one study, 25 percent of hospitalized cancer patients met criteria for depression, while 15 percent of elderly patients living at home met the criteria.[31] Depression in the elderly may be difficult to distinguish from dementia and, in some cases, the only means of making this differentiation may be to try antide-

pressant therapy. Depressed patients may feel hopeless and refuse treatment or food and water. They selectively perceive the more depressing or negative aspects of their environment. They tend to focus on negative feedback. They have no hope and give "logical reasons" why no therapeutic intervention can succeed. Suicidal ideation is not uncommon.

In patients with terminal illness, it is very difficult to distinguish realistic from pathological hopelessness. Depression may be a "reasonable" response to serious medical illness and may produce subtle distortions of decision making. Its diagnosis is neither necessary nor sufficient for determining that a patient is not a capable decision maker.[32]

Mild to moderate depression has little predictive value in determining preferences toward life-sustaining treatment of elderly medical patients, and these patients appear to experience no increase in desire for medical therapy after recovery from depression.[33] However, with severely depressed psychiatric in-patients, recovery from depression is associated with an increased desire for lifesaving medical therapy in patients who initially believed their situation to be hopeless and underestimated the benefit of treatment.[34] Gerety and colleagues noted similar findings in depressed nursing home patients.[35] The prognosis for depression in older individuals is worse compared to adults who are under the age of 65. In addition, prognosis is worse when acute or chronic illness is also present. Lee concludes a review of the issue, stating: "For the older patient with life-threatening illness, the literature supports vigorous treatment of depression, because the likelihood of a favorable response is high, and the risk of increased mortality for medically ill depressed, older patients is substantial. Therefore, in general, life-sustaining therapy should not be withheld until efforts have been made to reverse depression. However, this recommendation is not absolute. In some cases an older patient, although depressed, may have the capacity to refuse."[36]

In a review of depression and refusal of treatment, Sullivan and Youngner note: "It is essential for psychiatrists to accept that a seriously ill person's choice to die may be rational, especially in situations where the medical prognosis is very poor."[37] When depression compromises capacity, the authors recommend treating the depression. But they also recognize that there are times when psychiatric treatment is not appropriate, when it may intensify suicidal ideas, when the depression is absolutely treatment-resistant, or when the patient refuses treatment. They conclude:

> Psychiatrists need to recognize that some treatment refusals that result in death are legitimate, even if they are accompanied by suicidal intent. Evaluating the role of depression in these refusals and determining the effect of depression on competence are difficult tasks. They are best accomplished on the basis of a clear distinction between diagnosis of depression and assessment of competence. We must not overestimate or underestimate the value of treatment of depression for patients with severe medical illness. It is often valuable to diagnose and treat depression in the seriously ill patient, but sometimes it is valuable to accept the patient's decision to die.[38]

D. Capacity in Older Children and Adolescents

While most children would not be considered legally or ethically fully capable of making healthcare decisions, the arbitrary legal assignment of decision making at age 18 does not reflect current understanding of the cognitive development of the child. There has been a significant evolution in the desire to enhance the child's autonomy and skill as a decision maker, the recognition of the need of the minor patient to know the diagnosis and proposed treatment, and an increased role in decision making for the child-patient.[39] In the cases at the beginning of this chapter, should patient CD be included in the decision-making process about a bone marrow transplant completely, in part, or not at all?

Children begin life able to understand little about their illness; proceed to feel they caused the illness; then externalize causes, and by age 12, manifest formal logical thinking. Their cognitive development evolves from the concrete to the ability to think abstractly, reason deductively, consider multiple factors, and understand future consequences. Many factors may influence these abilities: intelligence, experience, maturity, emotional stability, or family situation. For example, the child with a chronic disease has dealt with the problems associated with the disease; has seen other patients with the disease improve or die; and, therefore, may be much better equipped to take part in decision making than a child of the

same age just hearing of his or her diagnosis. Likewise, the child whose parents have encouraged participation in other decisions relating to family or personal matters may be better prepared to make decisions. On the other hand, even the older adolescent may have trouble anticipating the future, which may cause difficulty when that adolescent attempts to weigh the effect of decisions on his or her future.

Researchers have found that children as young as age seven have developed many of the capacities needed to make good decisions. They may not yet be ready for full, independent consent, but are capable of participation.[40] Researchers have found that most adolescents beyond the age of 14 have full decisional capacity.[41] The clinician must individually evaluate each child's and adolescent's capacity. Other professionals (nurses, child psychiatrists/psychologists, social workers) may provide important insight into a particular child's developmental level and ability to comprehend the information presented. As with older individuals, capacity should be judged based on the decision at hand.

Several Canadian provinces have enacted legislation that entitles children to make their own healthcare decisions. In British Columbia, the clinician must be convinced that the child understands the risks and benefits of healthcare and has taken reasonable steps to conclude that the care is in the child's best interest; New Brunswick requires two physicians to make a similar assessment.[42] Public policy in Great Britain has also moved in this direction; children have been granted the right to receive appropriate information, to express their views, and to grant or withhold consent — provided that they are considered to be capable by the clinician who is acting in good faith. British policy makers assert that the assessment of capacity should be based on functional ability, not on age. All children of school age should be presumed capable.[43]

Some have suggested that the mature adolescent should have the right to refuse life-sustaining treatment, even when this decision is opposed by the parents.[44] Others have suggested caution in evaluating and accepting capacity in the adolescent.[45] Some studies indicate that younger adolescents tend to think in terms of short-term and hedonistic needs, and that until they develop a higher cognitive maturity level, they will be disinclined to comply with an uncomfortable course of treatment.[46] Chronically or acutely ill adolescents demonstrate high rates of illness-related emotional distress. Striving to become autonomous with their own identities apart from family, they face impediments to these goals of normal adolescent development. Hospitalized and isolated from peers, they may regress to earlier stages.[47] They suffer from depression, family problems, anxiety, and other emotional disorders at rates exceeding peers and younger children or adults with similar disorders.[48] A study of adolescents in a pediatric renal clinic reported that 49 percent of the subjects suffered from a major emotional disorder related to their illness.[49]

Several specific categories of minors who are assumed to be capable, unless other circumstances are involved, are defined below:

1. *Emancipated minor.* This category includes minors who are married or who are not subject to parental control. They may be self-supporting and living on their own. Definitions vary from state to state. In most states, this category includes college students and military personnel. Minors who are pregnant or married are often considered emancipated and able to consent for themselves and their children.

2. *Mature minor.* Adolescents have a right to participate to varying degrees, appropriate to their age and maturity, in decisions about their healthcare. This definition also varies according to jurisdiction. Courts have occasionally absolved clinicians and hospitals from liability and accepted the older minor's consent when medical care was rendered without parental consent.

3. *Statutory Adult.* In some states, a minor can give consent for medical or mental health services involving diagnosis or treatment of venereal or other contagious disease, birth control, pregnancy, substance abuse, or out-patient mental health treatment.

E. Decision Making for the Incapacitated Patient

1. Advance Directives

The prospective, plan-of-care approach would recommend anticipating when a patient may become incapable in the future, discussing the patient's values and preferences, and possibly suggesting formal written directives or appointment of a healthcare proxy. This discussion is appropriate for out-patient, primary-care clini-

cians as well as clinicians in the acute-care hospital setting. It is appropriate for inclusion in the standard medical history interview.

Advance directives theoretically allow capable patients to plan for future medical situations in which they would no longer be able to make decisions for themselves. They would define how others are to decide for them. Since the mid-1970s, there has been growing support for the importance of advance directives in healthcare. State legislatures enacted law providing for and defining advance directives. The federal Patient Self-Determination Act (PSDA) required medical institutions to ask about and give information to patients about advance directives.[50] Several landmark court cases seemed to reinforce the value of patients defining "clearly and convincingly" their treatment wishes at the end of life.[51] Advance directives may denote specific instructions for decisions in specific circumstances, usually written as a "living will," but some states also allow witnessed oral directives, or appointment of a decision maker, a "healthcare proxy," "healthcare power of attorney," or "durable power of attorney for healthcare."

1. *Living wills.* Living wills may give instructions on limiting, withholding, or withdrawing treatment, or instituting or continuing certain treatments when certain conditions are met. Living wills may be simple "boiler-plate" documents, often described as examples in state law, or more complex, extremely detailed documents. Forms have been developed by physicians and ethicists, medical organizations, lay organizations, and bar associations.[52] As clinical experience with living wills has grown, it has become apparent that, while the documents may in some cases simplify decision making, they do not resolve difficult clinical situations in many cases. Patients have often defined decisions for specific clinical situations without input from clinicians, resulting in ambiguous or illogical direction. In many states, a living will is not activated until a patient is "terminally ill" or permanently unconscious, the definition of which is often a source of conflict between clinicians and family. While there may be very detailed descriptions of clinical situations, often the patient's specific current situation is not included, or "reading between the lines" creates conflict. They may be seen as vague or imprecise.[53] The document is often not avail-

able. Recent studies suggest that living wills often do not affect a patient's treatment.[54] In some jurisdictions, the document may not be effective if the patient is pregnant or restricts certain treatments, for example, artificial hydration and nutrition.

2. *Durable power of attorney for healthcare.* The capable patient appoints, in a written document, a surrogate decision maker, who the patient expects would make the same decision the patient would in a given clinical situation. Appointing a surrogate avoids potential conflict when there is uncertainty about who has authority to make decisions, when there is family conflict about a decision maker, when there is no family, or when the patient is in a relationship that would not normally be recognized by statute as giving the other person decision-making responsibility. Ideally, the surrogate is well acquainted with the patient's philosophy and values, in general, about life and the end of life, and the patient and surrogate may even have had conversations about clinical situations that may arise. The surrogate's responsibility begins when the patient is not capable, and does not require a determination of terminal illness or permanent unconsciousness. However, as discussed below, whether a surrogate has been appointed by the patient or defined by statute, it is possible that proxy decisions may not be the decisions that the patient would have made. Unfortunately, many patients do not appoint a surrogate before they became incapacitated; do not have family to act as surrogate; or may not have discussed their healthcare preferences with their surrogate.[55]

2. Who Makes the Decision?

Surrogate or proxy decision makers must be moral as well as legal representatives of the incapacitated patient's interests. They fall into four major groups:

1. *Designated proxies.* The patient may have previously, voluntarily designated a proxy, in a living will or durable power of attorney for healthcare.
2. *Family members.* The family is usually very concerned with the patient's interests, is aware of the patient's values and goals, and generally has the "highest and most loving" motives.[56] Most people would prefer to have decisions made on their behalf by a relative rather than a stranger. All surrogates, including clinicians and judges, may be biased by their own values and interests. Family members who are motivated by love may be better able to compensate for such biases. The New Jersey Supreme Court suggests that family members "provide for the patient's comfort, care and best interest" and "treat the patient as a person, rather than a symbol of a cause."[57]

3. *Institutional committees.* Committees have been established in a variety of circumstances, both formal and informal, as decision makers or advisors to decision makers. New York State has a system of volunteer committees for the mentally ill who have no family.[58] Some institutional ethics committees require routine review of some categories of surrogate decisions (such as withholding/withdrawing life-sustaining therapy). Committees may be cumbersome, of variable quality, and unaware of the patient's specific values and goals.

4. *The courts.* The courts are often cumbersome, adversarial, unfamiliar with the patient's goals, and usually strongly dependent on the physician's viewpoint. According to the New Jersey Supreme Court: "Courts are not the proper place to resolve the agonizing personal problems that underlie these cases. Our legal system cannot replace the more intimate struggle that must be borne by the patient, those caring for the patient, and those who care about the patient."[59] However, they may be useful as a last resort when other modes fail to resolve a conflict — for instance, when surrogates are not acting in good faith, or when decisions of the surrogates cannot be considered by a reasonable person to be consistent with the patient's wishes or best interest. In these sorts of situations, the courts may be better suited to choose appropriate surrogates than to make decisions about patient care.[60] For patients who have no identifiable surrogate (either family member or previously appointed, for example, patient QR), the courts will quickly grant permission for acute care or emergency issues. However, for ongoing care decisions, including placement, it will probably be necessary, in most situations, to apply through the courts for a guardian to make decisions for the patient. This process may be very time-consuming. The guardian

often has no prior knowledge of the patient or the patient's values. In many circumstances, the court will often be unwilling to consider withdrawal of life-sustaining therapy.

Most states have defined a hierarchy of decision makers for the incapacitated patient. The Virginia Health Care Decisions Act recognizes the following surrogates in order of priority when the patient has not made an advance directive for a surrogate:
1. A guardian or committee for the patient,
2. The patient's spouse,
3. An adult child of the patient,
4. A parent of the patient,
5. An adult brother or sister of the patient, and
6. Any other relative of the patient in descending order of blood relationship.[61]

Problems may arise when the legally determined proxy has a potential conflict of interest, (for example, the separated but not yet divorced spouse) or when the ethically more suitable proxy has no legal standing (such as a long-term significant other or partner). In many cases, the proxy can amicably be transferred by mutual agreement to a more appropriate party. At times, there is conflict among surrogates of equal standing, for example, adult children. Some states allow the majority to rule, while others require a consensus. Mediation may be helpful. In some circumstances, when equal numbers are in opposition, some states will allow the physician to select the surrogate; others require court intervention. Even when there is a recognized surrogate or majority agreement among surrogates, one individual may demand a role in decision making. Some jurisdictions, for example the Veterans Administration Health System, will allow a "close friend" who has "shown care and concern for the patient's welfare and is familiar with the patient's activities, health and religious beliefs and values" to act as a surrogate. In some states, the patient's physician may assume decision-making authority, sometimes with the ethics committee.

The powers of the surrogate may be limited in some jurisdictions, not permitting withdrawal of life-sustaining treatments, withdrawal of artificial hydration and nutrition, termination of pregnancy, sterilization, or electroconvulsive therapy. In some states, the patient is not allowed to select his or her healthcare provider as a surrogate.[62]

3. How Is the Decision Made?

Several standards have evolved legally and ethically.
1. *The substituted-judgment standard.* This standard allows the patient's own values and definition of well-being to shape healthcare decisions. In some cases, the patient has previously expressed a prior directive or an opinion about the situation he or she is now in. This may be verbal or, preferably, written (a living will). Ideally, the proxy decision maker arrives at the same decision the patient would, if competent.
2. *The best-interest standard.* English common law gave the government the authority and obligation to protect the incapacitated. In addition, a long history of medical paternalism ("what I think is best for you") evolved into the concept of the proxy decision maker who considers what will be best for the patient and who avoids doing the patient harm (benefits versus burdens). The proxy decision maker should consider relief of suffering, preservation and restoration of function, and the quality and extent of the life sustained. This standard is intended to be applied to patients who have never been competent (such as children or patients with severe retardation) or when the patient has never expressed a specific opinion, or his or her opinion is not known. The proxy decision maker should promote the welfare of the "average" patient. In the courts, the application of the best-interest and substituted-judgment standards has not always been clearly defined, and scholars debate terminology.
3. *Other standards.* The professional standard (in which the physician decides) may subject patients to decisions that conflict with their own values. Or, if there are no clear standards, patients may be subjected to over- or undertreatment.

Making decisions for another is not the same as making decisions for oneself. In the latter case, the capable patient can refuse all types of treatment. The proxy, however, has to operate within the defined standards.

Although proxy decision making is becoming more recognized and endorsed, it has also become apparent through a number of empiric studies that there are limitations in its day-to-day application.

Proxies and patients often have not discussed in meaningful detail the issues and values that the proxy would need to make a decision as the patient expected. Families are often quite unreliable at assessing the patient's quality of life, and such assessments often include biases (for example, biases about elderly patients' functional status). Finally, proxies are not accurate in predicting patients' preferences for life-sustaining treatment. In fact, some researchers have found that a proxy's selection of therapy is not much better than random chance.[63] Surrogates often misunderstand their role and base decisions on their own preferences, rather than what the patient may have wanted. Emanuel and Emanuel have proposed several options to improve decision making: revision of the justification for and expectations of proxies to honor families' "good-faith" decisions based on patients' best interests, use of more comprehensive documentation of advance-care planning, or development of community-based standards for terminating care of incapable patients.[64]

F. The Questionable Surrogate

The clinician should take reasonable care to ensure that the surrogate's decisions are motivated by respect for the patient's interests and values. The clinician is the patient's advocate and has a duty to the patient and to no other person in the interim.[65] Families or other surrogates may have other agendas that do not include the best interest of the patient. Take, for example, the Philip Becker case.[66]

Philip was a mildly retarded 12-year-old with Down syndrome. He could communicate verbally, was educable, could dress himself, had good motor and manual skills, and took part in school and Boy Scout activities. At age 12, he was diagnosed with a cardiac defect, which, if corrected, was compatible with a normal life span and quality of life. If uncorrected, he would suffer progressive distress and eventual death. Although Philip had never lived at home, his parents refused the surgery. They were concerned with the care that would be available to him as he aged, and did not want him to be a burden on the other children in the family. The court upheld the family's refusal.

There is some debate about how much consideration should be given to the impact on the family of the patient's care. Some would exclude these considerations entirely, while others would suggest the importance of considering the impact on family finances, emotional health, other children, and stress.[67]

The surrogate's role may be shaded by issues of inconvenience to themselves, financial obligations, prior emotional conflicts or guilt, religious beliefs, or disinterest. In the case of LM at the beginning of this chapter, was LM's husband's role as surrogate invalidated by his relationship with another woman? Was he no longer able to make reasonable decisions for his wife? In many situations, property or large inheritances are at stake. How much of a role might these factors play in the surrogate's decision? Do they automatically call the surrogate's validity into question? Some surrogates have standing under law, but in fact may not be the best surrogate for the patient. The husband who has been estranged from his wife for 10 years, but not divorced, is still her legal surrogate; however, an adult child of the patient may be much closer to the patient. Just as the patient may be incapable of making decisions, surrogates also, for exactly the same reasons, may be incapable.[68]

When the clinician has cause to question the surrogate's capacity, believes a decision is not consistent with the patient's wishes or best interest, or believes that the surrogate has a major conflict of interest, that clinician has an obligation to pursue the matter. This might involve further discussions with the surrogate, participation of other professionals, consultation, legal counsel, or, if the concern is not resolved, intervention by the court. In the question of whether a surrogate is impaired, most agree that the burden of proof rests with those who question the surrogate's decision.[69]

G. Ethical and Legal Dimensions of Landmark Cases

In Re Quinlan, 1976 (New Jersey). The parents of Karen Quinlan, a young woman in a persistent vegetative state due to barbiturate-alcohol intoxication, petitioned the court to allow withdrawal of mechanical ventilation, based on the patient's previous statements about life-prolonging therapy.[70]

Supt. of Belchertown State School v. Saikewicz, 1977 (Massachusetts). The court allowed the withholding of chemotherapy from Mr. Saikewicz, a severely mentally retarded 76-year-old, with leukemia, based on the best interest of the patient (although the court used *substituted-judgment* terminology).[71]

Rogers v. Okin, 1979 (Massachusetts). The court allowed patients committed to a state mental institution to refuse psychotropic medications. The court was persuaded that "although mental patients do suffer at least some impairment of their relationship to reality, most are able to appreciate the benefits, risks, and discomfort that may reasonably be expected from receiving psychotropic medication."[72]

Cruzan v. Director, Missouri Department of Health, 1990 (U.S. Supreme Court). Nancy Cruzan was in a persistent vegetative state following an auto accident. Her parents petitioned to have her feeding tube removed, based on her values and general lifestyle. The patient had never made explicit statements about a situation similar to hers at the time. Missouri courts had ruled that there was no "clear and convincing evidence" to prove Nancy's desires. The U.S. Supreme Court upheld the Missouri decision, holding that states may establish safeguards to protect against abuses, as well as to sustain the person's own previously established values and preferences.[73]

In re A.C., 1990 (District of Columbia). A patient with terminal cancer gave birth by cesarean section at 26 weeks' gestation under a court order, in spite of the objections of her family, physicians, and her court-appointed attorney. There was some confusion and conflict as to whether the patient was capable of making her own decision. In overturning the original decision for surgery, the court ruled that substituted judgment should have been used to determine what the patient's own wishes would have been. The court held that the "right of bodily integrity belongs equally to persons who are competent and persons who are not. . . . To protect that right against intrusion by others . . . we hold that a court must determine the patient's wishes by any means available, and must abide by those wishes unless there are truly extraordinary or compelling reasons to override them. When the patient is incompetent, or when the court is unable to determine competency, the substituted judgment procedure must be followed."[74]

Florida Department of Health and Rehabilitative Services v. Benito Agrelo, 1995 (Florida). Benny, a 15-year-old boy who had undergone two liver transplants (the first, five years previously) began to experience side-effects from his immunosuppression and other medications, resulting in hallucinations and severe headaches. He stopped taking his medications against the advice of his physicians but with his family's support. A team of police and social workers carried him from his home strapped to a stretcher to the hospital for treatment. In the hospital, he continued to refuse treatment. Three days later, a circuit court judge ruled in favor of Benny, saying that quality of life was a personal decision.[75]

V. ETHICS GROUNDING

The guidelines on capacity are based on the principle of *respect for persons.* The capable patient's right to participate actively in medical decision making is based on the principle of *autonomy*— the right to be self-governing. However, when the patient is no longer or has never been capable, his or her personhood still must be respected. When others must make decisions for the incapacitated patient, the principles of *beneficence* (provision of benefits and the balancing of benefits and harms) and *nonmaleficence* (not inflicting harm) should prevail.

VI. STATEMENTS BY AUTHORITATIVE BODIES

The President's Commission for the Study of Ethical Problems in Medicine and Biomedical and Behavioral Research states,

> For patients to participate effectively in making decisions about their health care, they must possess the mental, emotional and legal capacity to do so. . . . Decision-making capacity is specific to a particular decision and depends not on a person's status or on the decision reached, but on the person's actual functioning in situations in which a decision about health care is to be made.[76]

The American College of Physicians has stated,

> All adult patients are considered competent to make decisions about medical care unless a court declares them incompetent. In clinical practice, however, physicians and family members usually make decisions for patients who lack decision making capacity, without a formal competency hearing in the courts. This clinical approach can be ethically justified if the physician has carefully determined that the patient is incapable of un-

derstanding the nature of the proposed treatment, the alternatives, the risks and benefits, and the consequences of it.

When a patient lacks decision making capacity (that is, the ability to receive and express information and to make a choice consonant with that information and one's values), an appropriate surrogate should make decisions with the physician. Ideally, surrogate decision-makers should know the patient's choices and values and act in the best interests of the patient. If the patient has designated a proxy, as through a durable power of attorney for health care, that choice should be respected. When patients have not selected surrogates, standard clinical practice is for family members to serve as surrogates. Some states designate the order in which family members will serve as surrogates, and physicians should be aware of legal requirements in their state for surrogate appointment and decision making. In some cases, all parties may agree that a close friend is a more appropriate surrogate than a relative.

Physicians should take reasonable care to assure that the surrogate's decisions are consistent with the patient's preferences and best interests. When possible, these decisions should be reached in the medical setting by physicians, appropriate surrogates, and other caregivers. Physicians should emphasize that decisions be based on what the patient would want and not on what the surrogates would choose for themselves. If disagreements cannot be resolved, hospital ethics committees may be helpful. Courts should be used when doing so serves the patient, such as to establish guardianship for an unbefriended, incompetent patient; to resolve a problem when other processes fail; or to comply with state law.[77]

The Council on Judicial and Ethical Affairs (CEJA) of the American Medical Association states,

If an incompetent patient is to receive medical treatment, a reasonable effort should be made to identify the presence of an advance directive. When such a patient lacks a documented advance directive . . . physicians should defer to state law to identify a surrogate decision maker. In the absence of state law, the patient's family, or persons with whom the patient is closely associated such as close friends or domestic partners, should become the surrogate decision maker. In the case when there is no family, but there are persons who have some relevant knowledge of the patient, such persons should participate in the decision-making process. In all other instances, a physician may wish to utilize an ethics committee to aid in identifying a surrogate decision maker or to facilitate sound decision making.

When there is evidence of the patient's preferences and values, decisions concerning the patient's care should be made by substituted judgment. This entails considering the patient's advance directive (if any), the patient's values about life and how it should be lived, how the patient constructed his or her identity or life story, and the patient's attitudes towards sickness, suffering, and certain medical procedures.

In some instances, a patient with diminished or impaired decision-making capacity can participate in various aspects of health care decision making. The attending physician should promote the autonomy of such individuals by involving them to a degree commensurate with their capabilities. Factors that should be considered when weighing the harms and benefits of various treatment options include the pain and suffering associated with treatment, the degree of and potential for benefit, and any impairments that may result from treatment. Any quality of life considerations should be measured as the worth to the individual whose course of treatment is in question, and not as a measure of social worth. One way to ensure that a decision using the best interest standard is not inappropriately influenced by the surrogate's own values is to determine the course of treatment that most reasonable persons would choose for themselves in similar circumstances.[78]

With regard to decision-making capacity in children, the CEJA has concluded:

Determination of . . . [decision making capacity] must be based on an evaluation of the patient's ability to understand, reason and communicate. In general, adolescents 14 and above appear mature enough to make decisions about their medical care, but [capacity] must be evaluated on a case by case basis.[79] Parents and physicians are in the best position to demonstrate a child's ability to understand, reason and communicate. They are most familiar with the child's maturity level and reasoning skills. Moreover, a physician may have a history with the child and be able to judge the child's present ability to participate in decisions affecting his or her health as well as the child's independence of thought and freedom from family pressure.[80]

The American Geriatrics Society, with regard to treatment decisions for incapacitated elderly patients without advance directives states:

Position 1

Except in cases of obvious and complete incapacity, an attempt should always be made to ascertain the patient's ability to participate in the decision making process. . . .

Position 2

It should not be assumed that the absence of traditional surrogates (next-of-kin) means the patient lacks an appropriate surrogate decision maker. A nontraditional surrogate, such as a close friend, a neighbor, a close member of the clergy, or others who know the patient well, may, in individual cases, be the appropriate surrogate. Health professionals should make a conscientious effort to identify such individuals. . . .

Position 3

After a conscientious effort has failed to identify an appropriate surrogate, a group of individuals who care for the patient may appropriately determine treatment goals and design a humane care plan to meet those goals. . . . The standard of decision making regarding treatment should consider any present indications of benefits and burdens that the patient can convey, and should be based on any knowledge of the patient's prior articulations, cultural beliefs if they are known, or an assessment of how a reasonable person within the patient's community would weigh the available options. . . . For some particularly

difficult cases, such as where motives might be in conflict, external advice or review should be considered.

Position 4

Patients with long-term incapacity and no surrogate available are best served by having a continuous surrogate. The broader community should ensure that an appropriate guardian is appointed, or that other decision making procedures are followed, as established by laws of each state. . . . [81]

VII. GUIDELINES FOR HEALTHCARE PROFESSIONALS

A. Determining Capacity

A patient is functionally able to make a particular healthcare decision when he or she can do the following:
- Understand the information relevant to the decision,
- Communicate with caregivers about the decision, and
- Reason about relevant alternatives and consequences against a background of personal values and goals.

B. Prior Directives

Capable persons should strongly consider defining prior directives for their care, should they become incapacitated and/or terminally ill, including identifying/appointing a proxy decision maker. Clinicians, families, attorneys, and others should encourage this process. Clinicians should inquire about and document such directives and the proxy when the patient is capable.

C. Decision Making for the Incapacitated Patient

Clinicians have an obligation to implement healthcare decisions for the incapacitated patient that:
- Are consistent with the values and goals of a patient who has lost decision making capacity (substituted judgment); and
- Best reflect the interests of a patient who has never been decisionally capable (best interest).

VIII. CASES FOR FURTHER STUDY

Case 1: The Unbefriended

LR is a 58-year-old male who was brought to the emergency room after being found in his rented room unconscious and in a pool of blood. Prior to arrival at the hospital he required resuscitation with aggressive fluids and CPR (cardiopulmonary resuscitation). In the emergency room, he continued to require aggressive CPR. He was noted to have lower gastrointestinal bleeding. Review of his history revealed diabetes, chronic hypertension, and chronic alcohol abuse. The landlord reports that he has no known family. He has rented a room with him for five years. The landlord's mother, however, knows the patient well. There is no known advance directive.

The patient was admitted to the ICU, unresponsive, on mechanical ventilation, with pharmacologic support for blood pressure and frequent blood product transfusion. After several days, the patient had not improved neurologically. A CT (computed tomography) scan showed marked hypoxic-ischemic injury. Neurological consult felt the prognosis for meaningful recovery was poor. Urine output had been poor, and the medical team requested the local magistrate to grant permission for placement of appropriate lines to begin renal dialysis. Permission was also given for colonoscopy. In the meantime, the social worker had been in touch with the landlord and his mother. The latter had known the patient for five or six years and felt that he would not want to be maintained in this condition. She agreed to be his guardian if necessary. Petition for guardianship was begun through Social Services. The clinical team asked the Ethics Consultation Service to review the case. The consult service agreed with proceeding to have the potential guardian appointed. They also suggested that given the patient's poor prognosis that it would be reasonable to write a medical, DNR (do-not-resuscitate) order, in case the patient should acutely change. Finally, it was recommended, after discussion with the team, that if the patient were to deteriorate, that additional or escalated aggressive care would be withheld. Several days later, the magistrate approved a request for tracheostomy. The patient's neurological condition had not improved.

The patient however, weaned off the ventilator, and moved to the ward. The new team was appraised of the previous plan of care and its rationale by the Ethics Consultation Service. Approximately one week later, the patient was again requiring high concentrations of oxygen, and the medical team felt he might be infected. He continued receiving regular hemodialysis. The decision was made not to treat him with antibiotics and not to place him back on the ventilator. The social worker reported that it would be several more weeks before the guardian was approved.

Four days later, the medical team contacted the Ethics Consultation Service again to report that the patient had deteriorated and asked for advice on how to proceed.

Do you agree with the approach taken to this point for this incapacitated patient without a surrogate? How would you proceed at this point?

— Ethics Consultation Service, University of Virginia Health System.

Case 2: The Case of Arlene A

Arlene A (AA) is a 38-year-old woman who was admitted to the emergency department at the University of Virginia following an overdose of tricyclic antidepressants. She had checked into a local motel the day before and was discovered by a housekeeper at 13:00 the following afternoon. She was unconscious and lying in a prone position with a suicide note. The note asked her family to forgive her for any inconvenience that she might have caused, stated that she loved them all, and requested that they please take care of her cat. While conducting a room search, rescue personnel discovered a partially full bottle of imipramine (a tricyclic antidepressant).

Rescue personnel noted that AA was unresponsive to verbal and painful stimuli. She was transported to the emergency room. She was dusky and had dried vomit on her face. The cardiac monitor revealed a sustained sinus tachycardia (rapid cardiac rhythm) with a wide QRS complex (indicating some ventricular dysfunction). She was intubated and placed on mechanical ventilation; a nasogastric tube was placed and gastric lavage was performed. Neurological exam revealed intact gag and corneal reflexes, marked clonus (repetitive muscle spasms), and unresponsiveness to verbal or painful stimuli. She had one generalized tonic/clonic seizure while in the emergency room. Her cardiac rhythm progressed to sustained ventricular tachycardia. She was started on intravenous lidocaine and norepinephrine infusions and transferred to the medical intensive care unit.

The patient's head CT scan was normal. AA subsequently developed persistent fevers, and her chest X-ray showed pulmonary infiltrates. She was diagnosed with an aspiration pneumonia, probably resulting from the inhalation of vomit. Blood cultures were positive for *Staphylococcus aureus*. All invasive catheters were replaced, and a course of antibiotic therapy was begun. AA's condition worsened. She developed adult respiratory distress syndrome, leading to progressive difficulties in maintaining adequate ventilation and oxygenation. Her lungs became increasingly stiff, requiring high-pressure mechanical ventilation. She developed subcutaneous emphysema and bilateral pneumothoraxes, which required chest tube placement. Because she was becoming increasingly difficult to ventilate, she was pharmacologically paralyzed and sedated. The pulmonologists gave her a grim prognosis. They considered it doubtful that she would survive to discharge, or ever be weaned from the ventilator. AA's prior medical history is significant for schizoaffective disorder, borderline personality anxiety disorder, and four suicide attempts.

AA's father visits daily. He lives several hours away and cares for his wife, who is bedridden and suffers from advanced Alzheimer's disease. He tells the staff that AA lives alone and is unemployed. She has been in psychotherapy for many years and has battled emotional problems for most of her adult life, with little benefit from therapy or medications. He says, "She has tried so hard, but nothing has helped." AA's two brothers live in New York and California. They call frequently to inquire about their sister.

AA's physicians have discussed in detail her condition and grim prognosis with her father and brothers. AA's father and brothers have requested that no further chest tubes be placed, and that no resuscitative efforts be made in the event of cardiac arrest. The family and healthcare team agree that a DNR order is medically indicated, and it is written in AA's chart.

Because the treatment team and family members would like AA's input if possible, they decide to discontinue paralysis and sedation in hopes that AA will regain consciousness. AA slowly awakens and is found to be neurologically intact. She is oriented to person and place and recognizes her father. At first, she indicates no memory of the recent suicide attempt. Later that day, she expresses alarm and dismay at being alive and demands (by mouthing words) that the ventilator be turned off. The medical resident develops a good rapport with her over the next two days and discusses her situation with her in depth. She firmly maintains her wish to die. She pleads with him to "let her go" and specifically requests that the ventilator be turned off. She refuses any further psychiatric treatment or medications and offers to be an organ donor.

The psychiatric consultant who is following the case has learned from AA's previous treating psychiatrist that she is suffering from borderline personalty disorder, rather than a severe depressive episode. She has a history of schizoaffective disorder and has had only marginal response to antidepressants in the past. The psychiatric consultant finds no evidence of current psychosis or delirium. AA is alert and oriented, and capable of answering questions by indicating "yes" or "no" with a nod of the head and by mouthing words. The consulting psychiatrist writes the following note in the chart: "Answers 'yes' when asked if she is feeling depressed. Answers 'yes' if asked if she wants ventilator disconnected. Says 'yes' she understands she will probably die if this happens. She states that she wants to die no matter what her physical condition. The consulting psychiatrist suggests, but does not write in the chart, electroconvulsive therapy followed by a course of antidepressants.

The treatment team believes that AA is competent and capable of making her own decisions. Discussions with her and her family members yield the consensus that she has rejected a future on the ventilator and that the most humane course is to respect her wishes and let her die as comfortably as possible. The consulting psychiatrist believes that she is clearly aware of what she is requesting and of the consequences; that the humane course is probably to withdraw treatment; but, be-

cause she has been suicidal, she cannot be allowed to make this decision. Furthermore, because of her suicide attempt, to allow the ventilator to be turned off would be tantamount to assisted suicide.

AA's brothers, John and Richard, have made arrangements to travel to Charlottesville. John is in complete agreement with his father's desire to respect AA's wishes, even though he does not want AA to die. He states that he knows what she has been through most of her life, and he wants her to be at peace. Richard understands AA's desire to be taken off the ventilator, but he now states that he does not agree with suicide. He wants to see his sister and knows that she may die soon, even with continued mechanical ventilation. Both brothers agree, however, to respect AA's wishes. They will both be arriving within a few days.

On 6 December, AA's father and the clinical team jointly request an ethics consultation. AA's father wants more people involved in the decision-making process. He wants to honor his daughter's request, but does not want the burden of being the sole decision maker.

As the ethics consultant, how would you proceed?

— Ethics Consultation Service, University of Virginia Health System.

Case 3: You Can't Go Home

JT is a 49-year-old male admitted to the emergency room after vomiting for several days. He presented with moderately severe dehydration and shock. His blood pressure was low. He was resuscitated with large volumes of intravenous fluids. His urine output was quite low, and a Foley catheter was placed in his bladder to monitor urine output. A nasogastric tube (NG tube) was inserted to drain gastrointestinal secretions. An abdominal X-ray suggested a small bowel obstruction. He was transferred to a surgical ward where vigorous fluid therapy was continued. His diagnosis was recorded as "severe dehydration, shock, and probable small bowel obstruction, for observation and possible laparotomy." He was not allowed to receive any food or liquid by mouth.

Within 24 hours, JT was feeling much better. He was making adequate amounts of urine, suggesting that there had been no insult to his kidneys from his dehydration and shock. His vomiting had stopped, although he still had the NG tube draining his stomach. The volume of drainage was relatively small. He still had not taken anything to eat or drink. He wanted to leave the hospital because he felt better.

The surgical resident was called, and discussed the patient's situation with him. There was still the possibility that JT had a partial bowel obstruction. Also, he had not had a trial without the NG tube, he had not taken liquids, and he still needed to have his renal function monitored to ensure complete recovery. JT still demanded to leave. The intern discussed the situation with the patient's wife, who agreed with the patient.

The couple was moderately unsophisticated and of lower socioeconomic status. The physician appraised the patient as "mildly retarded" and noted that he did not feel the patient was able to make appropriate decisions for his care. The physician contacted the psychiatric liaison service, who suggested obtaining a temporary detaining order from the court to require continued hospitalization for the patient. The hospital administrator was called. The special justice was contacted, who issued the order. The hospital administrator, however, felt uncomfortable with the situation and called the Ethics Consultation Service. The ethics consultants — a pediatrician and social worker — and the sheriff with detaining order in hand arrived on the ward at the same time.

After initial discussion with the resident, the consultants, the resident, and the patient's nurse met with JT and his family (his wife, his married son, and his daughter-in-law). The resident explained again the medical problems and the risks of leaving the hospital at that time (recurrence of vomiting, dehydration, and shock — possibly with life-threatening consequences). JT said he understood all of this information, but he felt much better. He explained that he must get home that evening to be with his elderly mother, who was afraid to be alone and would be angry with him if he was not there. Various alternative arrangements were suggested for the mother's care, but none of the family members believed that the alternatives were acceptable. The ethics consultants' impression was that JT was unsophisticated, but clearly understood the issues at hand. In addition, his wife and son also understood and agreed completely with the patient.

The patient and family agreed that if the patient left that evening, he would be in contact with his private physician immediately if the symptoms recurred.

As the ethics consultant involved in this case, what would you recommend at this point?

— Ethics Consultation Service, University of Virginia Health System.

IX. STUDY QUESTIONS

1. What is the difference between decisional capacity in the medical context and legal competence?

2. How does a "sliding-scale" determination of capacity relate to risk-benefit assessment? How does one apply the sliding scale in determining a patient's capacity to make decisions regarding treatment?

3. Differentiate between substituted judgment and best interest as standards for surrogate decision making. Which one takes precedence logically and ethically?

4. What would you do if you believed that an incapacitated patient's surrogate decision maker:

A. Was not using substituted judgment as the criterion for decision making and was in clear conflict with the patient's known values?

B. Was not acting in the patient's best interest, given the inability to apply the substituted-judgment standard?

5. Consider case 2, "The Case of Arlene A." What do you think of the consulting psychiatrist's opinion that because the patient had been suicidal, she should not be allowed to make the decision to disconnect the mechanical ventilator? What do you think about the psychiatrist's subsequent opinion that to withdraw the ventilator would be assisted suicide?

NOTES

1. J.F. Drane, *Clinical Bioethics: Theory and Practice in Medical-Ethical Decision Making* (Kansas City, Mo.: Sheed & Ward, 1994), 155.

2. A.R. Jonsen, M. Seigler, and W.J. Winslade, *Clinical Ethics: A Practical Approach to Ethical Decision in Clinical Medicine* (New York: MacMillan, 1982), 57-8.

3. L.H. Roth, A. Meisel, and C.W. Lidz, "Tests of Competency to Consent to Treatment," *American Journal of Psychiatry* 134 (1977): 279-84.

4. President's Commission for the Study of Ethical Problems in Medicine and Biomedical and Behavioral Research, *Making Health Care Decisions*, vol. 1 (Washington, D.C.: U.S. Government Printing Office, 1982), 57.

5. C. Elliott, "Competence as Accountability," *The Journal of Clinical Ethics* 2, no. 3 (Fall 1991): 167-71; E.H. Morreim, "Impairments and Impediments in Patients' Decision Making: Reframing the Competence Question," *The Journal of Clinical Ethics* 4, no. 4 (Winter 1993): 294-307; B.C. White, *Competence to Consent* (Washington, D.C.: Georgetown University Press, 1994); T. May, "Assessing Competency Without Judging Merit," *The Journal of Clinical Ethics* 9, no. 3 (Fall 1998): 247-57.

6. *Bartling v. Superior Court,* 163 Cal. App.3d 186, 209 Cal. Rptr. 220 (1984).

7. G.J. Annas, *Judging Medicine* (Clifton, N.J.: Humana Press, 1988), 317-22.

8. See note 4 above, pp. 57-62.

9. P.S. Appelbaum and T. Grisso, "Assessing Patients' Capacities to Consent to Treatment," *New England Journal of Medicine* 319 (1988): 1635-8.

10. See White, note 5 above, pp. 154-83.

11. Ibid., 174.

12. Ibid., 167.

13. E.G. Howe, D.S. Gordon, and M. Valentin, "Medical Determination (and Preservation) of Decision-Making Capacity," *Law, Medicine & Health Care* 19 (1991): 27-33; L. Ganzini et al., "Depression, Suicide, and the Right to Refuse Life-Sustaining Treatment," *The Journal of Clinical Ethics* 4, no. 4 (Winter 1993): 337-40; M.A. Lee, "Depression and Refusal of Life Support in Older People: An Ethical Dilemma," *Journal of the American Geriatrics Society* 38 (1990): 710-4; H.J. Bursztajn, "From PSDA to PTSD: The Patient Self-Determination Act and Post-Traumatic Stress Disorder," *The Journal of Clinical Ethics* 4, no. 1 (Spring 1993): 71-4; L. Ganzini et al., "Is the Patient Self-Determination Act Appropriate for Elderly Persons Hospitalized for Depression?" *The Journal of Clinical Ethics* 4, no. 1 (Spring 1993): 46-50.

14. L. Ganzini et al., "Pitfalls in Assessment of Decision-Making Capacity," *Psychosomatics* 44 (2003): 237-43.

15. See Bursztajn, note 13 above.

16. W. Davis and A. Ross, "Making Wishes Known: The Role of Acquired Speech and Language Disorders in Clinical Ethics," *The Journal of Clinical Ethics* 14, no. 3 (Fall 2003): 164-72; A. Braunack-Mayer and D. Hersh, "An Ethical Voice in the Silence of Aphasia: Judging Understanding and Consent in People with Aphasia," *The Journal of Clinical Ethics* 12, no. 4 (Winter 2001): 388-96.

17. See note 1 above, pp. 152-4.

18. J. Drane, "The Many Faces of Competency," *Hastings Center Report* 15 (1985): 17.

19. See May, note 5 above.

20. See note 3 above.

21. D.M. High, "Surrogate Decision Making: Who Will Make Decisions For Me When I Can't?" *Clinics in Geriatric Medicine* 10 (1994): 445-62.

22. P. Finucane, C. Myser, and S. Ticehurst, "Is She Fit to Sign, Doctor?: Practical Issues in Assessing the Competence of Elderly Patients," *Medical Journal of Australia* 159 (1993): 400-3.

23. B.A. Lustig, "Competence," in *Encyclopedia of Bioethics,* ed. W.T. Reich (New York: Simon & Schuster MacMillan, 1995), 447.

24. L.J. Markson et al., "Physician Assessment of Patient Competence," *Journal of the American Geriatrics Society* 42 (1994): 1074-80; T. Grisso and P.S. Appelbaum, "Comparison of Standards for Assessing Patients' Capacities to Make Treatment Decisions," *American Journal of Psychiatry* 152 (1995): 1033-7; L.M. Cohen, J.D. McCue, and G.M. Green, "Do Clinical and Formal Assessments of the Capacity of Patients in the Intensive Care Unit to Make Decisions Agree?" *Archives of Internal Medicine* 153, no. 21 (1993): 2481-2485.;

25. "McArthur Competence Assessment Tool," in T. Grisso and P.S. Appelbaum, *Assessing Competence to Consent to Treatment* (New York: Oxford University Press, 1998), 101-26 and appendix 1; "Hopkins Competency Assessment Tool," in J.C. Holzer et al., "Cognitive Functions in the Informed Consent Process: A Pilot Study," *Journal of the American Academy of Psychiatry and Law* 25 (1997): 531-40; "Aid To Capacity Evaluation," *www.utoronto.ca/jcb/_ace/ace.html;* "Mount Sinai Capacity Assessment Tool," in M.T. Carney et al., "The Development and Piloting of a Capacity Assessment Tool," *The Journal of Clinical Ethics* 12, no. 1 (Spring 2001): 17-23; H.R. Searight, "Assessing Patient Competence for Medical Decision Making," *American Family Physician* 45 (1992): 751-9.

26. M. Freedman, D.T. Stuss, and M. Gordon, "Assessment of Competency: The Role of Neurobehavioral Deficits," *Annals of Internal Medicine* 115 (1991): 203-8.

27. J.S. Janofsky, R.J. McCarthy, and M.F. Folstein, "The Hopkins Competency Assessment Test: A Brief Method for Evaluating Patients' Capacity to Give Informed Consent," *Hospital and Community Psychiatry* 43 (1992): 132-6.

28. L.J. Fitten, R. Lusky, and C. Hamann, "Assessing Treatment Decision-Making Capacity in Elderly Nursing Home Residents," *Journal of the American Geriatrics Society* 38 (1990): 1097-104.

29. C.C. Marson et al., "Assessing the Competency of Patients with Alzheimer's Disease under Different Legal Standards: A Prototype Instrument," *Archives of Neurology* 52 (1995): 949-54.

30. See Howe et al., note 13 above.

31. M. Plumb and J. Holland, "Comparative Studies of Psychological Function in Patients with Advanced Cancer," *Psychosomatic Medicine* 39 (1997): 264-76.

32. M.D. Sullivan and S.J. Youngner, "Depression, Competence, and the Right to Refuse Lifesaving Medical Treatment," *American Journal of Psychiatry* 151 (1994): 971-8.

33. M. Lee and L. Ganzini, "Depression in the Elderly: Effect on Patient Attitudes toward Life-Sustaining Therapy," *Journal of the American Geriatrics Society* 40 (1992): 983-8.

34. Ibid.

35. M.B. Gerety et al., "Medical Treatment Preferences of Nursing Home Residents: Relationship to Function and Concordance with Surrogate Decision-Makers," *Journal of the American Geriatrics Society* 41 (1993): 953-60.

36. See Lee, note 13 above, p. 713.

37. See note 32 above, p. 977.

38. Ibid.

39. J.C. Fletcher et al., "Ethical Considerations in Pediatric Oncology," in *Principles and Practice of Pediatric Oncology,* ed. P.A. Pizzo and D.G. Poplack (Philadelphia, Pa.: J.B. Lippincott, 1989), 309-20; N.M.P. King and A.W. Cross, "Children as Decisionmakers: Guidelines for Pediatricians," *Journal of Pediatrics* 115 (1989): 10-6; S.L. Leikin, "Minors' Assent or Dissent to Medical Treatment," *Journal of Pediatrics* 102 (1983): 169-76; S. Leikin, "The Role of Adolescents in Decisions Concerning Their Cancer Therapy," *Cancer* 71 (1993): 3342-6.

40. W.G. Bartholome, "Care of the Dying Child: The Demands of Ethics," *Second Opinion* 18 (April 1993): 25-38; J.A. Deatrick et al., "Correlates of Children's Competence to Make Healthcare Decisions," *The Journal of Clinical Ethics* 14, no. 3 (Fall 2003): 152-63.

41. D. Brock, "Children's Competence for Health Care Decision-making," in *Children and Health Care: Moral and Social Issues,* ed. L. Kopelman and J. Moskop (Boston, Mass.: Kluwer Academic, 1989); R.H. Nicholson, "Can Children Permit Research?" *Medical Research with Children: Ethics, Law and Practice* (New York: Oxford University Press, 1986).

42. E. Kluge, "Informed Consent by Children: The New Reality," *Canadian Medical Association Journal* 152 (1995): 1495-7.

43. P. Alderson and J. Montgomery, *Health Care Choices: Making Decisions with Children* (London: Institute for Public Policy Research, 1996).

44. M.T. Derish and K. Vanden Heuvel, "Mature Minors Should Have the Right to Refuse Life-Sustaining Medical Treatment," *Journal of Law, Medicine & Ethics* 28 (2000): 109-24.

45. M. Oberman, "Minor Rights and Wrongs," *Journal of Law, Medicine & Ethics* 24 (1996): 127-38.

46. G.M. Ingersoll et al., "Cognitive Maturity, Stressful Events and Metabolic Control Among Diabetic Adolescents," in *Emotion, Cognition, Health and Development in Children and Adolescents,* ed. E.J. Susman, L.V. Feagans, and W.J.

Ray (Hillsdale, N.J.: Erlbaum, 1992), 121-32.

47. See note 39 above.

48. Ibid.

49. B.M. Korsh et al., "Non-Compliance in Children with Renal Transplants," *Pediatrics* 61 (1978): 874.49-1.

50. Patient Self Determination Act of 1989, S. 1766, 101st Cong., 1st Session. 1989.

51. *Cruzan v. Director,* Mo. Dep't of Health, 497 U.S. 261, 290 (1990); *In re Martin,* 538 NW2d 399; Mich. 1995; *Conservatorship of Wendland,* California Supreme Court 28 P.3d 151; 2001.

52. L.L. Emanuel and E.J. Emanuel, "The Medical Directive: A New Comprehensive Advance Care Document," *Journal of the American Medical Association* 261 (1989): 3288-93; Aging with Dignity, "Five Wishes," *www.agingwithdignity.org.*

53. A.S. Brett, "Limitations of Listing Specific Medical Interventions in Advance Directives," *Journal of the American Medical Association* 266 (1991): 825-8; A Fagerlin and C.E. Schneider, "Enough: The Failure of The Living Will," *Hastings Center Report* 34 (2004): 30-42; A. Meisel and K.L. Cerminara, "Advance Directives," in *The Right to Die: The Law of End-of-Life Decisionmaking* (New York: Aspen, 2004), 7.01, 7-7- 7-11; J.M. Teno, "Advance Directives: Time to Move On," *Annals of Internal Medicine* 141 (2004): 113-7.

54. M.D. Goodman, M. Tarnoff, and G.J. Slotman, "Effect of Advance Directives on the Management of Elderly Critically Ill Patients," *Critical Care Medicine* 26 (1998): 701-4; R.S. Morrison et al., "The Inaccessibility of Advance Directives on Transfer from Ambulatory to Acute Care Settings," *Journal of the American Medical Association* 274 (1995): 478-82; J.M. Teno et al., "Do Advance Directives Provide Instructions that Direct Care?" *Journal of the American Geriatrics Society* 45 (1997): 508-12.

55. N. Karp and E. Wood, *Incapacitated and Alone: Health Care Decisions for the Unbefriended Elderly* (Washington, D.C.: American Bar Association Commission on Law and Aging, 2003).

56. *In re O'Connor,* 72 N.Y.2d 517, at 533, 531 N.E.2d 607 at 615 (1988).

57. *In re Jobes,* 108 N.S. 394, at 415, 529 A.2d 434 at 445 (1987).

58. S.S. Herr and B.L. Hopkins, "Health Care Decision Making for Persons with Disabilities: An Alternative to Guardianship," *Journal of the American Medical Association* 271 (1994): 1017-22.

59. *Jobes,* 529 A.2d at 451.

60. B. Lo, F. Rouse, and L. Dornband, "Family

Decision Making on Trial: Who Decides for Incompetent Patients?" *New England Journal of Medicine* 322 (1990): 1228-32.

61. *Code of Virginia,* sec. 54.1-2986.

62. See note 43 above; Department of Veterans Affairs, Veterans Health Administration, "VHA Informed Consent For Clinical Treatments and Procedures," *VHA Handbook* 1004.1, 2003.

63. E.J. Emanuel and L.L. Emanuel, "Proxy Decision Making for Incompetent Patients: An Ethical and Empirical Analysis," *Journal of the American Medical Association* 267 (1992): 2067-71; R.F. Uhlmann, R.A. Pearlman, and K.C. Cain, "Physicians' and Spouses' Predictions of Elderly Patients' Resuscitation Preferences," *Journal of Gerontology* 43 (1988): M115-M121; A.E. Meier, M. Mullvihill, and B.E. Cammer Paris, "Substituted Judgment: How Accurate are Proxy Predictions?" *Annals of Internal Medicine* 115 (1991): 92-8; D.P. Sulmasy et al., "The Accuracy of Substituted Judgments in Patients with Terminal Diagnoses," *Annals of Internal Medicine* 128 (1998): 621-9; M.A. Lee et al., "Do Patients' Treatment Decisions Match Advance Statements of Their Preferences?" *The Journal of Clinical Ethics* 9, no. 3 (Fall 1998): 258-62.

64. See Emanuel and Emanuel, note 52 above.

65. "American College of Physicians Ethics Manual. Part 2: The Physician and Society; Research; Life-Sustaining Treatment; Other Issues," *Annals of Internal Medicine* 111 (1989): 327-35.

66. *In re Phillip B,* 92 Cal. App. 3d 796, 156 Cal Rptr. 48 (1979).

67. G.E. Hardart and R.D. Truog, "Attitudes and Preferences of Intensivists Regarding the Role of Family Interests in Medical Decision Making for Incompetent Patients," *Critical Care Medicine* 31 (2003): 1895-900; J. Blustein, "The Family in Medical Decisionmaking," *Hastings Center Report* 23 (1993): 6-13; J.L. Nelson, "Taking Families Seriously," *Hastings Center Report* 22 (1992): 6-12; Meisel and Cerminara, see note 53 above, pp. 4-70; L.F. Ross, *Children, Families, and Health Care Decision-Making* (New York: Oxford University Press, 1998).

68. S. Van McCrary, W.L. Allen, and C.L. Young, "Questionable Competency of a Surrogate Decision Maker under a Durable Power of Attorney," *The Journal of Clinical Ethics* 4, no. 2 (Summer 1993): 166-8.

69. B. Lo, "Caring for Incompetent Patients: Is There a Physician on the Case?" *Law, Medicine & Health Care* 17 (1989): 214-20.

70. *In Re Karen Quinlan, an Alleged Incompetent,* 70 N.J. 10, 355 A.2d 647 (1976).

71. *Supt. of Belchertown State School v. Saikewicz,* 370 N.E. 2d 417 (Mass. 1977).

72. *Rogers v. Okin,* 478 F. Supp. 1342 (1979), 643 F.2d 650 (1st Cir. 1980).

73. *Cruzan v. Director, Missouri Dept. of Health,* 573 A.2d 1235, at 1246 (D.C. Ct. App. 1990).

74. *In re A.C.,* 497 U.S. 261 (1990).

75. *Florida Dept. of Health and Rehabilitative Services v. Benito Agrelo,* as reported by A. Driscoll, "Teen Shunned Medication," *Miami Herald,* 21 August 1994, 1A.

76. See note 4 above, p. 55.

77. American College of Physicians, "Ethics Manual: Fourth Edition," *Annals of Internal Medicine* 128 (1998): 576-94.

78. American Medical Association, Council on Ethical and Judicial Affairs, "Surrogate Decision Making," in *Code of Medical Ethics: Current Opinions with Annotations* (Chicago, Ill.: AMA, 2002), pp. 210-2, ¶ 8.081.

79. American Medical Association, Council on Ethical and Judicial Affairs, "Confidential Care of Minors," in *Code of Medical Ethics: Current Opinions with Annotations* (Chicago, Ill.: AMA, 2002), pp. 136-7, ¶ 5.055.

80. American Medical Association, Council on Ethical and Judicial Affairs, "The Use of Minors as Organ and Tissue Donors," in *Code of Medical Ethics: Current Opinions with Annotations* (Chicago, Ill.: AMA, 2002), pp. 58-9, ¶ 2.167.

81. These are four of nine positions from American Geriatrics Society Ethics Committee, "American Geriatrics Society Position Statement: Making Treatment Decisions for Incapacitated Elderly Patients Without Advance Directives," *http://www.american geriatrics.org/products/ positionpapers/ treatde.shtml,* accessed 1 June 2005.

10

The Process of Informed Consent

Robert J. Boyle

CASE HISTORIES

AB is a 35-year-old woman who seeks a surgeon's advice about a mass in her breast. Physical exam and mammography are compatible with carcinoma of the breast. During the initial office visit, the physician presents the patient with this information and discusses with her the current controversy about surgical management of breast cancer — including questions about whether to perform radical mastectomy, modified radical mastectomy, lumpectomy, with or without chemotherapy, and with or without radiation therapy. He presents to her his recommendation based on his clinical experience and his interpretation of the literature. He provides her with patient education materials about breast cancer and the various options. He recommends that she discuss the matter with her husband and family and return in one week.

The patient returns with her husband, and they and the surgeon decide to have a lumpectomy performed as soon as possible. The patient's concerns center on the risk of recurrent disease and the disfigurement of the more invasive procedures. The patient is referred to the breast clinic, where the nurse coordinator provides her with additional information about the disease, the planned procedure, what will be done, what the scar will look like, how she will feel after the surgery, what concerns other patients have, and so forth. AB is admitted to the hospital the morning of the procedure, is interviewed and examined by an anesthesiologist, and is asked to sign a consent for the surgery by the surgical resident.

CD is a 65-year-old man who is transferred from his local hospital to the University Medical Center for evaluation and treatment of a possible cerebral aneurysm. He is seen immediately by a neurosurgeon, whom he has never met before, who states that the patient requires a cerebral arteriogram. The radiologist who is to do the procedure follows along quickly; he discusses the procedure, the risks, and alternatives — all in moderate detail — and asks the patient if he has any questions. The patient at this point is overwhelmed and asks no questions. Shortly before the procedure, a resident asks the patient to read and sign the standard consent form.

I. INTRODUCTION

This chapter continues the discussions of disclosure (chapter 8) and capacity (chapter 9) as a foundation for the shared decision-making process that is expected in contemporary clinical encounters. *Informed consent* refers to legal rules regarding clinicians' interactions with patients, to ethical doctrine rooted in respect for autonomy that promotes the patient's right to self-determination, and to a process whereby clinicians and patients interact to select an appropriate course of medical care.[1] Informed consent is expected to improve the care of patients by increasing the bond of trust, facilitating autonomy by providing choices, and by increasing patients' participation.[2]

Prior to initiating medical or surgical treatment or enrolling subjects into research protocols, clinicians are required ethically and legally to seek consent and to ensure that this consent is informed. As a legal requirement, the burden of ensuring informed consent lies with the physician. However, the ethical standard must recognize informed consent as shared decision making involving the patient, physician, nurse, family, and all those with an ethical interest in the patient. The informed-consent process is typically recognized in the patient's signature of the consent document prior to surgery. However, it must be recognized that this, in fact, represents only one segment of a much broader process. Decision making involves not only high-risk surgical procedures, but also low-risk diagnostic testing in the physician's office and prescribing medication. Decision making may involve a one-time discussion between clinician and patient, a series of discussions in the office prior to hospital admission, or a long-term relationship between clinician and patient.

The mechanics of informed consent for human research protocols have been carefully defined and detailed by governmental and institutional regulation. This area of informed consent is not discussed specifically in this chapter.

II. HISTORY OF THE CONCEPT OF INFORMED CONSENT

Informed consent is a relatively new concept in medicine. As noted in chapter 8, the Hippocratic Oath does not mention a physician's obligation to converse with patients. The duty was to "follow that system of regimen which according to my ability and judgment I consider for the benefit of my patients."[3] Other Hippocratic writings, in fact, spoke against disclosure. In the ancient Greeks' view, cooperation between physician and patient was important, not for the sake of sharing decision-making burdens, but for the sake of friendship that, in turn, led to trust, obedience, and then to cure.

In the Middle Ages, conversation with patients was intended to comfort, reassure, and induce patients to take the cure. Obviously with what was available to medicine at that time, the choices and results were limited.

By the eighteenth century, physicians were advocating that the public become more enlightened about medical matters. However, this enlightenment did not extend to involving parties in shared decision making. Rather, the intent was to bring patients into common cause with the physician against disease and suffering and foster acceptance of the physician's authority.

Nineteenth-century English physician Thomas Percival, in his treatise *Medical Ethics; or A Code of Institutes and Precepts, Adapted to the Professional Conduct of Physicians and Surgeons,* urged physicians to be attentive to the patient's welfare, treating the patient with "attention, steadiness and humanity." However, he did not mention the patient's right to liberty of choice. He recommended care when the patient opposed treatment, not out of concern for the patient's rights, but because of the potential medical complications of using force. He wrote, "the prejudices of the sick are not to be condemned or opposed with harshness" because such behavior might create "fear, anxiety and watchfulness," which could be a detriment to the patient's recovery.[4]

Percival's *Medical Ethics* became the basis for the first code of ethics of the American Medical Association (AMA) in 1847.[5] Oblivious to the issue of informed patients, it asserted that doctors "have a right to expect and require that their patients should entertain a sense of the duties which they owe to their medical attendants." Patients' "obedience . . . should be prompt and implicit."[6]

The doctrine of informed consent began to evolve in the courts after the turn of the twentieth century. In 1914, Justice Benjamin Cardozo wrote, "Every human being of adult years and sound mind has a right to determine what shall be done with his own body."[7] The case involved a patient with a uterine growth. She gave consent for an examination under anesthesia, but specifically refused to authorize any additional surgery. When the physician found a tumor, he removed it without the patient's consent. Infection followed the surgery, gangrene set in, and the patient eventually suffered serious long-term morbidity.

In 1957, the courts began to define the legal requirement for consent. In *Salgo v. Leland Stanford, Jr., University Board of Trustees,* the court declared that uninformed consent is not true consent: "A physician violates his duty to his patient and subjects himself to liability if he withholds any facts necessary to form the basis of an intelligent consent by the patient to the proposed treatment."[8] The ruling emphasized disclosure, however, and not the right of the patient to make the decision.

The AMA's code evolved into shorter statements that provided little insight into the respect required of physician-patient interactions. The 1957 code, now called the *Principles,* stated, "The prime objective of the medical profession is to render service to humanity with full respect for both the dignity of man and the rights of patients."[9]

The accompanying *Opinions* of the AMA's Council on Ethical and Judicial Affairs (CEJA) provided three s1pecific instructions with respect to disclosure and consent:

1. A surgeon is obligated to disclose all facts relevant to the need and performance of the operation;
2. An experimenter is obligated, when using new drugs or treatments, to obtain the "voluntary consent" of the person; and
3. Investigators involved in clinical investigations primarily for treatment must "make relevant disclosure and obtain the voluntary consent of patients."[10]

The first provision was added to comply with malpractice law, and the other two to comply with congressional legislation on the conduct of research.[11]

By 1980, the *Principles* had changed minimally. However, the *Current Opinions of the Judicial Council* did address the issue of informed consent: "The patient's right of self-decision can be effectively exercised only if the patient possesses enough information to enable an intelligent choice. The patient should make his own determination on treatment. Informed consent is a basic social policy. . . . Social policy does not accept the paternalistic view that the physician may remain silent because divulgence might prompt the patient to forgo needed therapy. Rational, informed patients should not be expected to act uniformly, even under similar circumstances, in agreeing to or refusing treatment."[12]

The forces and "social policy" that shaped the doctrine of informed consent at this time included the civil liberties revolution, the movement for consumer rights and advocacy, media coverage of medical issues, and consumers who were better informed about treatments and alternatives.

III. OBSERVATIONS OF PRACTICE

In a 1980s observational study of physician-patient interactions in a university medical center, Lidz and colleagues noted:

1. Great variety in what doctors told patients, what patients learned from other sources, what patients understood, and how decisions were made.
2. Great variety in the ways in which decisions were made from close conformity with the legal model to almost no resemblance to the legal model.
3. Informing and consenting often took place over time, and the greater the degree of patient participation in the process, the more this was so.
4. In general, the physician was clearly the dominant actor in terms of making decisions about what treatments, if any, a patient was to have.
   a. The doctor's ordinary role, in practice, was to decide what was to be done and to inform the patient of that decision, along a spectrum running from an "order" at one end, to a neutral disclosure of alternatives at the other end.
   b. The patient's ordinary role, in practice, was to acquiesce to the physician's recommendation.[13]

Lidz and colleagues concluded that "disclosure" does not typically occur. Rather, patients learn various bits of information — some relevant to decision making, some not — from doctors' and nurses' efforts to obtain compliance and from "situational-etiquette" conversations held because "that's what humans do." Patients do not make "decisions"; instead, doctors make "recommendations" to patients. "Consent" does not exist. Instead, these authors found "acquiescence," the absence of "objection," or occasionally a "veto."[14] In this and an earlier study they found that when patients are given information about their treatment and treated as if they had decision-making authority, they act in a passive manner.[15] When asked, most patients are happy with the amount of information that they receive. When they said they wanted information to make treatment decisions, they often acted as if they would rather have the doctors decide, because of doctors' technical expertise and commitment to the best interest of the patients. Patients felt they were unequal to the task of making medical decisions.

In response to a survey conducted in the 1980s by Harris and Associates, only 10 percent of the patients interviewed saw themselves as having an active role in decision making; 43 percent of the public and 58 percent of physicians described informed consent as informing patients about their condition and recommended treatment. However, while 43 percent of the public closely associated the term with permission or consent to treatment, only 26 percent of physicians interpreted it in that manner. Of physicians, 47 percent described informed consent in terms of explaining treatment risks, while only 8 percent of the public mentioned this aspect. Even fewer physicians (14 percent) included the discussion of alternative treatments in informed consent.[16]

Recent studies disagree as to whether there has been significant change. Sulmasy and colleagues interviewed patients who reported that physicians explained procedures 90 percent of the time, explained risks 86 percent of the time, asked permission 98 percent of the time, but explained alternatives only 53 percent of the time. 64 percent of these patients, felt the physician had done an excellent job in explaining what the procedure would be like, versus only 10 percent of patients who said the physician did a poor or fair job. Likewise, 54 percent felt the physician had done an excellent job in explaining the risks, and only 13 percent a fair or poor job.[17] However, in a videotape study of both primary care physicians and surgeons, Braddock and colleagues found that informed decision making was often incomplete.[18] They noted that only 9 percent of decisions met their quite reasonable criteria for completeness. Basic decisions (for example, obtaining a laboratory test) were more often informed (17 percent) than more complex decisions (0.5 percent) (for example, consent for a procedure). Discussion of the nature of the intervention occurred most frequently (71 percent) and assessment of the patient's understanding least frequently (1.5 percent). Uncertainties and alternatives were also rarely discussed.

In actual practice, there is a wide variation in what is understood and carried out as "informed consent." Many clinicians believe that the process of informed consent is an externally imposed requirement that is necessary to protect them from lawsuit. Others resent the pressures to describe in detail the possible complications or alternative methods of therapy when evidence exists that patients forget most of what they are told, they often ask no questions, and most accept the clinician's recommendations. Still others consider informed consent as no more than a hospital form to be signed.[19]

McNutt suggests that "shared" decision making is a misnomer that emphasizes clinicians making choices for patients. He suggests that the important issues are how the clinician informs patients about the consequences of their choices and how they help patients use the information to make choices. He describes a view of decision making that places the patient in the role of pilot and the clinician in the role of navigator. He concludes the goal should be to make decision making difficult, not easy: to make sure patients understand the uncertainties and risks. "The ideal is not to reduce decisional conflict, but to maximize it."[20]

IV. ELEMENTS OF INFORMED CONSENT

Valid informed consent requires the presence of multiple, interrelated elements:
- Threshold elements (preconditions)
  1. Capacity (to understand and decide)
  2. Voluntariness (in deciding)
- Information elements
  1. Disclosure (of material information)
  2. Recommendation (of a plan)
  3. Understanding (of disclosure and recommendation)
- Consent elements
  1. Decision (in favor of a plan)
  2. Authorization (of the chosen plan).[21]

A. Threshold Elements

1. Capacity
Valid consent requires a capable decision maker, as described in chapter 9.

2. Voluntariness
Voluntariness implies exercising choice that is free of coercion or other forms of controlling influences by other persons. Beauchamp and Childress note, "control over another person is necessarily an influence, but not all influences are controlling."[22] In a broad context, influence may include both positive and negative influences: acts of love, threats, education, lies, manipulative suggestions, emotional appeals, bedside vigil, and so forth.

Beauchamp and Childress define three categories of influence: coercion, persuasion, and manipulation. *Coercion* occurs when one person intentionally uses an actual threat of harm or force to influence another (for example, the threat of abandonment or refusal to do procedure X if procedure Y is not agreed to as well). With *persuasion,* a patient is convinced to consent through the merits of reasons advanced by another person. With their recommendation of a plan of care, clinicians almost always persuade the patient to some degree toward one choice based on physicians' knowledge and expertise. If a patient refuses or is uncertain about a procedure or treatment that offers significant benefits to the patient, the clinician has an obligation to continue to inform and work with the patient. How intense the activity becomes determines when it becomes a negative influence. *Manipulation* represents attempts to influence that are neither coercion nor persuasion. Here the influence usually occurs with informational manipulation — playing with the data to change a person's understanding. Here the model begins to overlap with the disclosure element.

In fact, rarely, if ever, is a patient entirely free from various pressures. "Fully voluntary choice" is an ideal. We make decisions in a context of competing needs, familial interests, legal obligations, persuasive arguments, religious beliefs, and so forth. However, if pressure from a clinician, family member, religious group, or others is difficult for the patient to resist, valid informed consent does not occur. For example, a patient who is pressured by members of his or her religious group to refuse treatments, or a potential bone marrow or organ donor who is badgered by the potential recipient and his or her family to proceed with donation, would present challenges to the voluntary element of consent. Consent must be a situation in which there are "no strings attached."

Clinicians have a responsibility to be aware of situations when voluntariness is threatened. Others involved with the patient have a responsibility to refrain from coercion, even subtle coercion, and to allow the patient to make his or her decision freely.

B. Information Elements

1. Disclosure

The clinician is obligated to disclose to the patient or surrogate the information necessary to make an informed judgment. The disclosure should include information on the following:

1. The nature of the therapy,
2. The purpose,
3. The risks and consequences,
4. The benefits,
5. The probability that the therapy will be successful,
6. The feasible alternatives, and
7. The prognosis if the therapy is not given.

The clinician is not required to list every possible risk. Patient CD, in the case history given at the beginning of this chapter, seemed overwhelmed by the amount of information presented to him in a brief period of time.

The legal doctrine of informed consent defines two standards of disclosure: the *professional standard* and the *reasonable-person standard.* These standards have been criticized as either too clinician-centered or too vague to be useful for clinical care. The professional standard requires that the physician disclose only what other physicians would disclose in a similar situation. Although some states still hold this standard, many believe that this paternalistic, physician-centered approach undermines patients' autonomy.[23] Cases such as *Canterbury v. Spence* have led some states to adopt a reasonable-person standard. In *Canterbury,* a surgeon failed to disclose risks of neurologic injury following a laminectomy, describing them as "not any more [risky] than any operation."[24] The court concluded that, although the likelihood of injury was relatively low, the potential severity of harm (paralysis and loss of function) required more elaborate disclosures to be made. The ruling allowed the jury to decide whether the informed-consent requirement was violated. If an "average, reasonable person" would decline to proceed with treatment in the face of fully disclosed risks, the physician who fails to make appropriate disclosures can be liable for any injuries that follow the treatment provided.

The reasonable-person standard, while defined in the legal framework in some jurisdictions, has been criticized as impossible to satisfy. What the reasonable person needs to know depends very much on the patient's particular circumstances at the time. It does not provide the clinician much assistance in defining what must be disclosed. From this discussion has evolved the *subjective standard,* which requires the clinician to disclose whatever information is material to the particular patient, in a particular situation or context. If patients have a right to make idiosyncratic choices, they may need information that would not be considered significant by the profession, or the average person.[25] A concert pianist might certainly prefer much more information about risks of hand surgery than another patient who was about to undergo the same procedure. Some patients may require the kind of detail that is listed in a drug package insert before agreeing to a particular course of medication.

In the usual case, the risks and benefits that most "average reasonable patients" would prefer to have explained should be explained. The clinician is not required to list every possible, extremely rare, or theoretical risk. To do so may be counterproductive to the entire decision-making process. The severity of the risk must also be considered. For example, the risk of paralysis associated with a laminectomy (Canterbury), although only 1 percent, should be disclosed, whereas it may not be necessary to disclose the risk of a hematoma following venipuncture.

If communication is effective and the patient is truly a partner in the process, then the extent of disclosure should be apparent from the questions and concerns of the patient, the patient's situation, and so forth. The clinician's judgment about what to disclose is still important, but that judgment should be based on the physician's interaction with the patient, and not on a predetermined script.

Brody has proposed a model — *transparency* — for disclosure in informed consent not based on previous standards. The clinician discusses why the proposed treatment is recommended over the alternatives, the patient is allowed to ask questions suggested by the disclosure of the clinician's reasoning, and those questions are answered to the patient's satisfaction. Disclosure is adequate when the clinician's basic thinking has been rendered transparent to the patient. The clinician engages in the typical thought process involved in the management of patients, only he or she does it aloud in language understandable to the patient.[26]

Feld suggests four elements of risk that the clinician and patient should consider:
1. The nature of the risk,
2. The seriousness of the risk,
3. The probability the risk will occur, and
4. The imminence of the risk (peri-procedure or years later.) The more serious or probable the risk, the more disclosure is required.[27] Quan-

tity is not necessarily quality. Overwhelming the patient with frightening numbers may not accomplish the goal.

Some have suggested that detailed disclosure of risks may promote anxiety in the patient. However, multiple studies have found that either the anxiety is minimal for most patients or that the patients are willing to accept the anxiety in order to have thorough disclosure.[28]

The case of *Moore v. Regents of the University of Califor*nia presented a different issue related to disclosure.[29] Mr. Moore was diagnosed with a rare leukemia. His physician recommended a splenectomy, and Moore consented to the procedure. The physician obtained portions of the spleen and eventually established a patented cell line, with a potential market value of several billion dollars. The physician requested that Moore continue to see him periodically for checkups, at which time additional blood, skin, bone marrow, and sperm were collected (some of which were to be used for research). The California Supreme Court eventually concluded that Moore had no property interests in his excised spleen, but the court did recognize that the physician had failed to disclose his research interest in the spleen and subsequent samples. The court concluded that doctors have a duty to inform patients of research interests deriving from treatment, that a person's consent to treatment requires complete information, and that the physician has a duty to disclose all information that is relevant to a patient's decision, including research or economic interests.

According to Veatch: "The implications [of this evolution] are enormous. It means that, in principle, no professional can determine what to disclose to a patient by introspecting about what he or she would want to know in that circumstance. It also means that the question cannot be answered by turning to one's colleagues or examining what is normally disclosed in similar circumstances. If the principle of autonomy is the foundation of the informed consent doctrine, then patients will have to be told whatever they reasonably want to know, even if it is not normal practice for that information to be disclosed."[30]

The controversy among the U.S. Centers for Disease Control and Prevention (CDC), Congress, and numerous professional societies about informing patients of clinicians' human immunodeficiency virus (HIV) status adds another element to this discussion. How much is the clinician obligated to tell the patient about personal issues that may place the patient at increased risk? *Behringer v. The Medical Center at Princeton* explored the status of someone who was both an HIV-positive patient and a surgeon. As a patient, the surgeon had the same right to privacy as anyone else, and improper disclosures of his condition led to liability for the hospital. At the same time, the court upheld the hospital's policy that required him, as a condition of surgical privileges, to disclose his HIV-positive status to patients during the informed-consent process.[31]

In *Hidding v. Williams,* a malpractice action in which the patient agreed to surgery in the absence of informed consent, the court reached two critical conclusions. First, the fact that the patient signed a form for informed consent did not relieve the doctor of liability when he — and the form — failed to disclose significant risks of surgery to the patient. Second, the surgeon's chronic alcohol abuse should have been revealed to the patient; failure to make this disclosure constituted a violation of the requirement of informed consent.[32]

In the future, will physicians be required to disclose other information — such as a history of substance abuse, mental illness, or performance measures such as infection rates or malpractice history — because this information may be material to a patient's decision?[33]

2. Recommendation

It is important in most circumstances that the clinician, having disclosed the necessary information about the proposed therapy and its alternatives, make a recommendation. This is the clinician's area of education and expertise, and this is why the patient seeks care from the clinician. In fact, disclosure of information is often less important than the clinician's recommendation. Recommendations may be far more meaningful to the patient than results of empirical studies.[34] With the recognition of patient autonomy and the progressive development of the concept of informed consent, it is apparent that, at times, the message has been exaggerated. Patients are presented with lists of options and told "it's your decision." Patients may feel lost, abandoned, overwhelmed by the issues, and confused by the uncertainty inherent in treatment decisions. With a shared approach, the patient seeks the clinician's advice, but is free to reject the recommendation, ask for a second opinion, and investigate other alternatives.

Making a recommendation should not be seen necessarily as a violation of voluntariness.

3. Understanding

The information obviously must be disclosed in a manner that a particular patient can understand. Huge amounts of technical information and medical jargon may overwhelm or confuse most patients and would not validly inform them. The clinician should recognize that words may have special meaning or no meaning for the patient. Illness, anxiety, or borderline capacity may also influence understanding. The clinician should confirm that patients understand by asking them to describe in their own words the medical problem and the proposed therapies. The question "Do you understand?" may not provide this validation. This emphasis upon patients' understanding may be especially important in pediatric or geriatric patients, those with limitations of intelligence, or those with negative experiences with the medical system.

In the case history at the beginning of this chapter, the validity of CD's consent should be questioned on the basis of his understanding what was disclosed. Time and repetition may also dramatically improve the patient's understanding. Recent studies support the use of more easily understood statistical references, diagrams and charts, and computer aids to supplement, not replace, the discussion with the clinician.[35]

C. Consent Elements

1. Decision

After consideration and discussion, a process that in many cases may occur over time and with one or several clinicians, the patient makes a decision about treatment or a plan of care. The patient may, at any time, change his or her decision. However, the decision must be in the context of what the alternatives are. For example, if a patient is offered a choice of treating mild hypertension or undergoing further observation, the patient cannot choose what specific drug he or she wants to take; that decision is the physician's.

2. Authorization

The patient must do more than express agreement or comply with a proposal. He or she must authorize a professional to do something through an act of informed and voluntary consent.

V. EXCEPTIONS TO THE REQUIREMENT FOR INFORMED CONSENT

The following exceptions to the requirement for informed consent have been recognized:

1. *Emergency:* when the patient is in a life-threatening situation and unable to consent.
2. *Incapacity:* when the patient is unable to consent; the process must involve a surrogate decision maker.
3. *Patient waiver:* when the patient waives the right to know: "I don't want to know. Just do what you think is best." The physician must be certain that this is, in fact, what the patient wants.
4. *Therapeutic privilege:* when fully informing a patient poses a significant threat to the patient's well-being, not because it will make the patient feel upset or depressed. Therapeutic privilege should be invoked only in rare circumstances. (For a discussion of the concept of therapeutic privilege, see chapter 8.)
5. *National/state waivers:* when the federal or state government waives informed consent for vaccination programs, newborn genetic screening, and so forth.

VI. IMPLEMENTING INFORMED CONSENT

Valid informed consent in our medical system may be difficult to achieve. This is especially so in a tertiary-care center, where care is so specialized. A patient's care may involve many different professionals who have very brief contact with the patient and no opportunity to form a relationship with the patient. (Malpractice studies confirm the problem of lack of patient-clinician relationship.)[36]

Lidz defines two models for informed consent based on different types of medical care:

1. *The event model,* in which the clinician meets the patient, explains the procedure, and obtains the patient's consent and signature (for example, the case of CD).
2. *The process model,* in which the patient and clinician establish individual responsibilities (for example, the case of AB). Several questions may arise with this model: What is the clinician's role — primary clinician or consultant? What is the clinician's area of expertise? What is the anticipated duration of care?[37]

In the process model of informed consent, the patient's problem is defined in dialogue (Katz uses the metaphor of "conversation"[38]) between clinician and patient. Does the patient agree with what the clinician thinks the problem is? They set goals (such as curing the disease or treating the symptoms). Finally, they select appropriate therapy using the elements of information and consent discussed above.

Quill and Brody have suggested that the current approach of many clinicians — to objectively present patients with options and odds but, in an attempt to not overly influence the patient, withhold their experience and recommendation — confuses independence with autonomy, sacrifices competence for control, and discourages active persuasion. They propose an "enhanced autonomy" model involving active exchange of ideas, negotiation of differences, and shared power and influence. They recommend:

1. Clinicians should share medical expertise fully, while they listen carefully to the patients' perspective.
2. Recommendations must consider both clinical facts and personal experience.
3. Clinicians should focus on general goals, not technical options.
4. Disagreements should initiate a process of mutual exchange.
5. Final choices belong to fully informed patients.
6. Clinicians must work to refine and express their own values.[39]

VII. OTHER CONSIDERATIONS

A. Cross-Cultural Issues

While full disclosure and active patient participation in decision making has become the standard for clinical practice in this country, it has also become apparent in multiple studies that there are cultural groups for which this is not the norm and may, in fact, be an intrusion on patients' wishes, expectations, and perceived role. Studies have suggested that older patients prefer to receive less information about their illness and treatment and assume a less active role in making treatment decisions.[40] Another study indicated that elderly Korean-Americans and Mexican-Americans were less likely than elderly African-Americans and European-Americans to believe that a clinician should inform a patient of a terminal illness or involve a patient in decision about life-support technology, and were more likely to believe that the family should make end-of-life decisions.[41] The clinician must approach these situations sensitively, asking patients what they would prefer: to be informed about their illness and involved in making decisions or to have their families handle decisions.[42] Assuming that a patient does not want to be involved is as problematic as forcefully involving an unwilling patient.[43]

B. Children as Decision Makers: Assent/Dissent

The recognition of the progressive capacity of the older child and adolescent to participate in decision making, the desire to enhance the child's autonomy and skill as a decision maker, and the recognition of the child's need to know the diagnosis and proposed treatment have led to an increased role in decision making for the child-patient (see chapter 9). Clinicians and parents have an obligation to involve a child to the extent that the specific child is able — from encouraging participation in decisions (the younger child) to granting full decision-making power (the adolescent over 14 years of age).[44]

The term *assent* was suggested in the mid-1970s by a national commission on human research to distinguish a child's agreement to treatment from a legally valid consent, which can only be given by a competent adult.[45] The American Academy of Pediatrics suggests that *assent* should include at least the following elements:
1. The patient should be helped to achieve a developmentally appropriate awareness of the nature of his or her condition,
2. The patient should be told what he or she can expect with tests and treatments,
3. Clinicians should make a clinical assessment of the patient's understanding of the situation and the factors influencing how he or she is responding (including whether there is inappropriate pressure to accept testing or therapy),
4. Clinicians should solicit an expression of the patient's willingness to accept the proposed care. Regarding this final point . . . no one should solicit a patient's views without intending to weigh them seriously. In situations in which the patient will have to receive medical care despite his or her objection, the pa-

tient should be told that fact, and should not be deceived.[46]

The child's situation influences each of the elements of consent. The clinician must present information in a manner suited to the child's developmental level. Parents should be able to assist, but in some cases they may be too close to the situation to assess the child's status accurately. Other professionals (such as pediatricians, nurses, child psychiatrists/psychologists, or social workers) may provide important insight into a particular child's developmental level and comprehension of the information presented.

Children render the voluntary consent element problematic. The risk of coercion is much higher in the parent-child relationship. Younger children are less likely to assert themselves against their parents; they tend to acquiesce to and attempt to please those in authority, while adolescents may do the opposite. Intervention by the clinician, an outsider, in situations where the family's influence seems excessive may be very difficult. The clinician's relationship with the family and understanding of the family's values and culture, and the family's previous experience with the child's decision making, are important. At times, it may be necessary for the clinician to confront a family with the issue. Chapter 14 discusses in more detail the issues surrounding parents' role and rights in decision making for children of all ages.

Some jurisdictions have given children much broader rights of decision making (see chapter 9). The American Academy of Pediatrics suggests that clinicians seek the assent of the school-age patient as well as informed permission of the parent for procedures such as venipuncture for diagnostic study in a nine year old, psychotropic medication for attention-deficit disorder in an eight year old, or an orthopedic device for scoliosis in an 11 year old. For older children and adolescents, the organization encourages the clinician to seek informed consent from the patient for a pelvic examination in a 16 year old, long-term antibiotics for severe acne in a 15 year old, or diagnostic evaluation for recurrent headache in an 18 year old.[47]

C. The Nurse's Role

The role of the nurse in informed consent is complex, and will become progressively more so as nursing and its collegial relationship with physicians evolves. In Lidz's observational study, nurses obtained the patients' signatures on consent forms, a practice that is rapidly changing. However, probably more significantly, nurses provided a major portion of information about treatment.[48] In fact, in many situations, the nurse spends more time than the physician talking with the patient, either in a formal educational process or in informal bedside conversation. The paradox is that, in our current environment, physicians and not nurses make decisions about treatment. In this role as patient educator, the potential exists for nurses to appear to challenge the traditional authority of the physician. The discussion of risks, which a physician might not have disclosed, may seem to question the physician's recommendation. There is no doubt, however, that the active role of nurses in educating patients certainly furthers the goal of informed consent. The nurse's role includes evaluation of the process of informed consent: the adequacy of disclosure and the patient's understanding, capacity, and voluntariness. Anyone with concerns about an invalid or questionable informed consent should present those concerns to the individual who is primarily responsible for the consent.

D. The Consent Form

The consent form is often the focus of the process, but, in fact, it should only be a written record of a process of disclosure and discussion. A signed form alone does not represent valid consent — legally or ethically.

VIII. ETHICAL AND LEGAL DIMENSIONS OF OTHER LANDMARK CASES

In addition to the cases noted above, a number of others have further expanded the legal doctrine of informed consent.

Natanson v. Kline, in which the physician failed to disclose the risks of radiation therapy, defined the "professional standard."[49] This standard assumes the physician "knows best" about what should be disclosed to the patient.

In *Cobbs v. Grant,* Mr. Cobbs suffered from a duodenal ulcer that required surgery. The surgeon, Dr. Grant, explained the nature of the operation with the patient but did not discuss any of the inherent risks. After surgery, Cobbs developed

abdominal bleeding due to a tear in the splenic artery. He later developed a new ulcer that required further surgery. Finally, he required additional surgery for bleeding due to suture failure. All of these complications were identified subsequently as potential risks from the initial and subsequent procedures. The court reasoned that the surgeon's failure to inform may have constituted a violation of the physician's duty. The patient sought disclosure of information about risks and alternatives that the "reasonable" person would find significant in deciding whether to consent to or refuse treatment.[50]

Mohr v. Williams resulted in a plaintiff's judgment against a physician who had obtained consent to operate on the patient's right ear. After the patient was anesthetized, the physician decided to operate instead on the left ear. The court ruled there was no urgent need to proceed without consulting the patient.[51]

In *Arato v. Avedon,* the Supreme Court of California ruled that the physician was not obligated to disclose statistical life-expectancy information to a patient with pancreatic cancer. In recommending a course of chemotherapy and radiation treatment, none of the treating physicians specifically disclosed the high mortality rate for this type of cancer. The patient ultimately died. The physicians justified the nondisclosure on the grounds that it was medically inappropriate given the patient's anxiety, the risk of depriving any hope of cure, and the problem of predictive data when applied to a specific patient.[52] The patient had been informed that the type of cancer he had was usually fatal.

IX. ETHICAL GROUNDING FOR INFORMED CONSENT

As with capacity, the patient's right to participate actively in medical decision making is based on the principle of autonomy. Individual autonomy must be respected as long as the individual's actions do not infringe on the autonomous actions of others. The person has the right to self-governance — personal rule of the self by adequate understanding, while remaining free from controlling interference by others and from personal limitations that prevent choice. To respect an autonomous agent is to recognize that person's capacities and perspective, including his or her right to hold certain views and to take certain actions based on personal values and beliefs.

In the realm of informed consent, autonomy requires the patient to do more than yield to, express agreement with, acquiesce in, or comply with an arrangement or a proposal.[53]

In tension with the principle of autonomy in informed consent is the traditional clinician-patient relationship in decision making, in which the clinician makes the decision for the patient. In this traditional relationship, the clinician was acting in the patient's best interest and was committed to "doing no harm." Clinicians' decisions were based in good faith on their training and medical knowledge. Indeed, the doctrine of informed consent should not and does not question the clinician's integrity or dedication. One could argue that the traditional clinician-patient relationship in decision making was based on the principle of beneficence, "doing good" for the patient. There is still an element of beneficence in this relationship, but it must be balanced to prevent paternalism. *Paternalism* is defined as "the interference with a person's freedom of action or freedom of information, or the deliberate dissemination of misinformation";[54] "substitution of one person's judgment for another's."[55] Paternalism dictates the view that physicians should assume the entire burden of deciding what treatment any patient in whatever condition should undergo, because only clinicians have the necessary medical information and skill. They are the experts.

The tension between autonomy and beneficence allows us to define the patient's and clinician's roles as compatible with both. The clinician's role is to:
1. Determine the patient's problem, in cooperation with the patient,
2. Determine how the problem can be treated,
3. Determine the risks and benefits of the possible therapy, and
4. Communicate this information to the patient.

The clinician's role is primarily cognitive, medical, and technical.

The patient's role is to use the information in the context of his or her own personal values and subjective preferences to make a decision. The patient's role is primarily affective, personal, and subjective.[56] The patient brings something to the process that the clinician cannot know: an understanding of his or her individual priorities, needs, concerns, beliefs, and fears. The need for informed consent is an acknowledgment that a medical procedure or act is meant to be done "for" and not "to" a person.[57]

X. STATEMENTS BY AUTHORITATIVE BODIES

According to the President's Commission for the Study of Ethical Problems in Medicine and Biomedical and Behavioral Research: "The ethical foundation of informed consent can be traced to the promotion of two values: personal well-being and self-determination. To ensure that these values are respected and enhanced, the commission finds that patients who have the capacity to make decisions about their care must be permitted to do so voluntarily and must have all relevant information regarding their condition and alternative treatments, including possible benefits, risks, costs, other consequences and significant uncertainties surrounding any of this information."[58]

According to the American Hospital Association's *Patient Bill of Rights:*

The patient has the right to obtain from his physician complete current information concerning his diagnosis, treatment, and prognosis in terms the patient can be reasonably expected to understand. . . .

The patient has the right to receive from his physician information necessary to give informed consent prior to the start of any procedure/treatment. Except in emergencies, such information for informed consent should include but not necessarily be limited to the specific procedure/treatment, the medically significant risks involved, and the probable duration of incapacitation. Where medically significant alternatives for care or treatment exist, or when the patient requests information concerning alternatives, the patient has the right to such information.[59]

According to the American Nurses Association's *Code for Nurses:*

Truthtelling and the process of reaching informed choice underlie the exercise of self-determination, which is basic to respect for persons. Clients should be as fully involved as possible in the planning and implementation of their own health care. Clients have the moral right to determine what will be done with their own person; to be given accurate information and all the information necessary for making informed judgments; to be assisted with weighing the benefits and burdens of options in their treatment; to accept, refuse, or terminate treatment without coercion; and to be given necessary emotional support. Each nurse has an obligation to be knowledgeable about the moral and legal rights of all clients and to protect and support those rights. In situations in which the client lacks the capacity to make a decision, a surrogate decision maker should be designated.[60]

The Council on Ethical and Judicial Affairs (CEJA) of the American Medical Association states:

The patient has the right to make decisions regarding the health care that is recommended by his or her physician. Accordingly, patients may accept or refuse any recommended medical treatment.[61]

CEJA also notes:

The patient's right of self-decision can be effectively exercised only if the patient possesses enough information to enable an intelligent choice. The patient should make his own determination on treatment. The physician's obligation is to present the medical facts accurately to the patient or to the individual responsible for his care and to make recommendations for management in accordance with good medical practice. The physician has an ethical obligation to help the patient make choices from among the therapeutic alternatives consistent with good medical practice. Informed consent is a basic social policy for which exceptions are permitted (1) where the patient is unconscious or otherwise incapable of consenting and harm from failure to treat is imminent; or (2) when risk-disclosure poses such a serious psychological threat of detriment to the patient as to be medically contraindicated. Social policy does not accept the paternalistic view that the physician may remain silent because divulgence might prompt the patient to forgo needed therapy. Rational, informed patients should not be expected to act uniformly, even under similar circumstances, in agreeing or refusing.[62]

The American College of Physicians states:

In many medical encounters, when the patient presents to a physician for evaluation and care, consent can be presumed. The underlying condition and treatment options are explained to the patient, and treatment is rendered and not refused. In medical emergencies, consent to treatment that is necessary to maintain life or restore health is usually implied, unless it is known that the patient would refuse the intervention.

The doctrine of informed consent goes beyond the question of whether consent was given for a treatment or intervention. Rather it focuses on the content and the process of consent. The physician is required to provide enough information to allow a patient to make an informed judgment about how to proceed. The physician's presentation should be understandable to the patient, should be unbiased, and should include the physician's recommendation. The patient's or surrogate's concurrence must be free and uncoerced.

The principle and practice of informed consent rely on patients to ask questions when they are uncertain about the information they receive; to think carefully about their choices; and to be forthright with their physicians about their values, concerns and reservations about a particular recommendation.

The physician is obligated to ensure that the patient or, when appropriate, the surrogate be adequately informed about the nature of the patient's medical condition, the objectives of, alternatives to, possible outcomes of, and risks involved with a proposed treatment.[63]

XI. GUIDELINES FOR HEALTHCARE PROFESSIONALS

Decisions in healthcare ultimately rest with capable and informed patients, in a context of shared decision making with clinicians and family. An ethically valid informed consent has seven necessary elements, discussed in section IV of this chapter:

1. Capacity,
2. Voluntariness,
3. Disclosure,
4. Recommendation,
5. Understanding,

6. Decision, and
7. Authorization.

XII. CASES FOR FURTHER STUDY

Case 1: "The Placebo"

Mr. X was a 65-year-old, retired army officer who had been very successful in the military and in teaching and research. He had undergone several abdominal operations for gallstones, postoperative adhesions, and bowel obstructions. He was somewhat depressed because of chronic pain. He had lost weight, had poor hygiene, and had withdrawn socially because it was necessary for him to assume awkward or embarrassing postures to control his pain. He had used Talwin six times a day for more than two years to control the pain, but he had so much tissue and muscle damage that he had trouble finding injection sites. And Talwin may itself be addictive.

Stating that his goal was "to get more out of life in spite of my pain," Mr. X voluntarily entered a psychiatric ward, where his treatment included individual behavior therapy programs, daily group therapy, and so forth. Mr. X reduced his Talwin usage to four times a day, and he insisted that this level was necessary to control his pain. After considerable discussion with their colleagues, the therapists decided to withdraw the Talwin over time without the patient's knowledge by diluting it with increasing proportions of normal saline. Although Mr. X experienced nausea, diarrhea, and cramps, he thought that these withdrawal symptoms were actually the result of Elavil (amitriptyline), which the therapists had introduced to relieve the withdrawal symptoms.

Self-control techniques were continued, and the intervals between injections were increased. Although the patient was aware of the changes in intervals, he was not aware that he was receiving only saline. The therapists justified this deceptive use of a placebo on the grounds of its effectiveness: "We felt ethically obliged to use a treatment that had a high probability of success. To withhold the procedure may have protected some standard of openness but may not have been in his best interests. We saw no option without ethical problems." As a member of this team caring for Mr. X, do you agree with the treatment approach?

— Adapted from a case in T.L. Beauchamp and J.F. Childress, *Principles of Biomedical Ethics,* 3rd ed. (New York: Oxford University Press, 1989), 406-07; the original source is P. Levendusky and L. Pankratz, "Self Control Techniques as an Alternative to Pain Medication," *Journal of Abnormal Psychology* 84 (1975): 165-68.

Case 2: "Terry Adolphson"

The physician is a clinician who must make decisions on the basis of probabilities. Most patients, however, have little experience with this method of decision making and are often unwilling to accept the uncertainty of medicine. If I express doubt that a particular diagnosis or treatment is completely reliable, this doubt may seem to my patient that I am not competent, or haven't been thorough, or don't care. Almost all decisions in medicine are made (whether consciously or not) on the basis of probabilities. When I am quite explicit about this process, it can become — even with sophisticated patients — a time-consuming matter, and the pressures of my schedule, if nothing else, often made me want to pull back from such explanations.

Terry Adolphson, for instance, was a 36-year-old friend with a terrible family history of heart disease: all the male family members on his father's side had died with heart attacks before the age of forty. Terry had recently developed pain in the chest, or angina, suggesting that he too had a serious disease of the coronary arteries, the small blood vessels leading to the heart, a disease that could progress to a heart attack and quite possibly death. Recent articles in the medical literature had suggested that certain patients with angina not only had better pain relief but also lived longer if they had coronary-artery bypass surgery than if they were treated only with medicines. On the other hand, these patients had a definite chance of dying during surgery.

To complicate matters further, even the process of examining Terry to discover whether he had disease in the arteries which should be operated upon required a special examination of the coronary arteries (coronary arteriography). There was a small (usually less than 1 percent) chance of heart attack and even death during such an examination.

As I discussed the situation with Terry, I realized that in order to recommend this single test, I had to review with him some very complicated medical studies. There were, at the time, differences of opinion among leading cardiologists about who should receive coronary bypass surgery, since the studies had not yet shown convincingly that such surgery was advantageous. Two studies of which I was aware had followed for five years patients who had symptomatic and arteriographically proven heart disease. In each study, the patients were randomly divided into two groups. One group had surgery, and the other was treated only with medicine. The studies showed that for blockages in certain coronary arteries there was no real difference in survival between the surgical and nonsurgical groups; in some cases the nonsurgical group even did better. However, for blockages in other coronary arteries — the left main artery, for example — a greater number of patients were alive five years later in the subgroup that chose surgery than in the subgroup that was treated with medicine alone.

Terry and I reviewed the reasons for his undergoing the coronary arteriography and the chances of his dying during the examination. Since there was no reason even to consider the arteriography test unless he was interested in surgery, we went over the studies that seemed to show advantage for the surgical treatment of some patients. We examined what the literature had to say about the statistical chances of dying during the surgery, as well as the chances of surviving with or without the surgery. I realized that I was not merely informing Terry about a complex disease involving complex therapy but also about a method of decision making which, though routine in medical circles, was quite alien to him. Medical science could only report what had happened to groups of other people; these statistical "certainties" could not be translated into an individual certainty — into a reliable prediction for Terry. The discussion was time-consuming and therefore expensive. It took him several days just to absorb the concepts.

My only alternative (on the surface, the easier path) would have been to ignore this reasoning process and tell him: "I, as your physician and friend, recommend that you have this operation. Trust me." But the situation was not at all black and white. It involved not only uncertainties but values. Did Terry wish to take a chance on death resulting from an "unnatural" surgical intervention or on "natural" death as a result of avoiding surgery? Did he wish to risk a smaller chance of dying sooner (with the surgery) or a larger chance of dying in the indefinite future? Although I could interpret the medical information for Terry so that he could understand it, ultimately he had to take responsibility for the decision.

Even so, I did not share with Terry certain more complex uncertainties. I decided not to complicate the discussion further by reminding Terry of the uncertain nature of any statistical analysis. Perhaps even the studies that showed improvement after surgery were the result of coincidence or of some unknown difference between the surgical and nonsurgical groups. A statistical analysis of the studies could tell me there was only a 5 percent chance that the results were due to coincidence, but we could not be 100 percent sure even that the studies were reliable. Nothing seems 100 percent sure in medicine! But Terry had enough uncertainty in his life. I chose to keep my "5 percent probabilities" to myself.

Terry decided, after much thought and consultation, to proceed with the coronary arteriography, and it indeed showed a blockage in those coronary arteries which, the statistics indicated, it would be advantageous to bypass. He had the surgery, but the first nine months after the operation were difficult. Symptoms continued, a repeat coronary angiogram was required, and there was much uncertainty about the wisdom of surgery. Had I initially talked Terry into the surgery by insisting that he trust me, that trust would have been severely threatened by all the unforeseen complications he experienced. Instead, he was able to face his future with some equanimity because he had made a reasonable decision based on adequate, if sometimes frustrating, information.

— Reprinted from D. Hilfiker, *Healing the Wounds* (New York: Pantheon Books, 1985), 64-67.

Case 3: "Whose Choice Really?"

WL is a 22-year-old man who worked as a farm laborer. He is married with one child. The patient first noted a swelling on his left hip about 15 months earlier. It was tender, but caused no impairment in his daily work. Approximately five months ago, he began to experience pain in his left leg and some restriction in its use. Soon thereafter he noted a swelling in his abdomen. He consulted a general practitioner in a nearby town and was referred to a cancer center 300 miles from his home.

Diagnostic evaluation established that he suffered from a bone cancer arising in the ridge of the left hip. The cancer had extended along the pelvic bone and across the middle of the abdomen. Workup for metastases was negative. The extent of the tumor precluded surgical resection. The patient was placed on a protocol of front-line experimental chemotherapy, but within two months there was documented progression of the tumor. With the failure of this regimen, it was no longer realistic to hope that he could be cured. However, physicians believed that alternative chemotherapy might achieve temporary remission of the disease, and the patient was switched to escalating doses of methotrexate.

At this time, the management of his pain became a significant problem. He requires very high doses of morphine and Dilaudid, which are often insufficient to provide adequate pain control, but cause him to slip in and out of a clouded state of consciousness. The fact that he has not yet developed lung metastases and the observation that the tumor is growing slowly has led the clinicians to suspect that he might survive for as long as a year. Given this prospect, physicians are deeply concerned about long-term pain control. Because WL is in relatively constant and often severe pain, he is pressing the staff for more adequate pain management.

There are three options for improving control of the pain. One is to amputate his left leg by performing a hemipelvectomy. This would remove the leg in which intense pain is occurring and reduce the amount of tumor in the abdomen. Substantial pain relief, after surgical recovery, could be expected, although recurrence of pain would be expected with further spread of the disease. Some rehabilitation would be necessary, such as learning to use crutches.

A neurosurgical consultant has suggested two other options. One is to control pain through nerve-block procedures. This would require a series of procedures in which specific nerve roots are exposed to chemicals that impair their ability to conduct pain impulses. The results of each procedure would be used to determine what additional nerve roots might be blocked to achieve additional pain relief. Completion of this process might require several weeks. Although nerve-block procedures carry less than a 10 percent risk of urinary bladder and bowel incontinence, there may be motor weakness in the affected limb.

The neurosurgeon thinks it unlikely that WL's pain could be completely controlled in this way, but it is reasonable to expect a very substantial reduction in WL's need for analgesics.

The other neurosurgical approach involves performing a cordotomy, a procedure that surgically severs nerve tracts responsible for pain conduction. The neurosurgeon believes that the procedure, performed at the level of the 12th thoracic vertebra, is virtually certain to produce complete pain relief. The patient would be able to leave the hospital within a few days after the operation. However, there are side-effects. Although sensation of touch, vibration, and position are preserved, sensation of temperature is eliminated. More importantly, the surgeon estimates an 80 percent chance of urinary bladder and bowel incontinence.

As WL's physician, you are faced with how to manage the process of informed consent. There are significant trade-offs among the options for treatment. How the patient might assess these options would depend on his reaction to the specific benefits and problems associated with each treatment. For example, if complete pain relief were his overriding and exclusive concern, the cordotomy would be the obvious choice. By contrast, if he were hesitant to risk impotence and the loss of bladder function and willing to accept an extended hospitalization away from his family, he might choose to have the nerve blocks. You could remain neutral, helping the patient compare the alternatives and allow WL to make the final choice. On the other hand, you could be more directive.

WL has shown a clear proclivity toward surgical removal of his tumor. Although his doctors explained the uselessness of surgical resection for curing his disease before they initiated chemotherapy, the patient continues to ask frequently about surgery. He seems to view it as a decisive, one-shot approach to the removal of the tumor and the relief of his pain, which does not carry the chronic suffering (nausea, vomiting, and so forth) associated with chemotherapy. WL also has some difficulty understanding how chemotherapy works. He has a common-sense understanding of cutting a tumor out, but the idea of "melting it away" with drugs is confusing, and he has little confidence in this mode of treatment. In preliminary discussions, he seemed to lean toward the hemipelvectomy for these inappropriate reasons, despite the fact that the procedure would be mutilating and would provide only temporary pain control.

A second concern is that WL's preference seems to vary with the intensity of his pain. On several occasions when his pain was especially severe and had persisted for several hours, he said that cordotomy would probably be the best step to take. However, when he had achieved moderate pain relief, he expressed much deeper concern about being rendered impotent and incontinent by the cordotomy. At these times he was also less inclined to undergo the hemipelvectomy. As a result, he seemed to favor a series of nerve blocks. Thus, there is legitimate concern that his choice might reflect how tolerable his pain is on a given day, rather than a careful weighing of the risks and benefits of each option.

You and your team are also concerned about the patient's needs in the coming months before his death and about WL's ability to genuinely appreciate those needs at this time. You believe that his most serious need will be for pain relief. You expect his pain to worsen with time. Only the cordotomy would ensure complete pain control without heavy use of analgesics. If performed, it would reduce the physical drain of pain-related suffering and allow him more quality time to share with his family. The patient's other need is to be reunited with his family. They have little money, and his wife has been unable to visit during this hospitalization. The remaining period before his death is limited, so spending time at home is quite important. Moreover, the patient's degree of suffering might decline if he could be with his wife, child, and extended family. Again, either alternative to the cordotomy would require an additional hospitalization of several weeks. With the cordotomy, he could return to his family within several days.

You wish to respect the patient's choice, but you are concerned about these various impairments of the patient's capacity to make a decision based on his own values and interests. WL is typically very quiet, cooperative, and deeply respectful of the authority of the nurses and physicians, and he could be easily persuaded to undergo the cordotomy with directive and persuasive recommendations. How should you proceed?

— Adapted from T.F. Ackerman and S. Strong, *A Casebook of Medical Ethics* (New York: Oxford University Press, 1989), 14-17.

XIII. STUDY QUESTIONS

1. What is the difference between the "event" model of informed consent and the "process" model of informed consent? What sorts of medical situations would justify either approach?

2. What do you think of Brody's "transparency" model of informed consent? What are its strengths and/or weaknesses?

NOTES

1. J.W. Berg et al., *Informed Consent: Legal Theory and Clinical Practice,* 2nd ed. (New York: Oxford University Press, 2001).

2. E.J. Cassell, "Informed Consent in the Therapeutic Relationship: Clinical Aspects," in *Encyclopedia of Bioethics,* ed. W.T. Reich (New York: MacMillan Free Press, 1978).

3. Hippocrates, *Decorum,* trans. W. Jones (Cambridge, Mass.: Harvard University Press, 1967), 297.

4. T. Percival, *Medical Ethics; or A Code of Institutes and Precepts, Adapted to the Professional Conduct of Physicians and Surgeons* (Manchester, England: S. Russell, 1803) as noted in J. Katz, *The Silent World of Doctor and Patient* (New York: Free Press, 1984), 17.

5. Katz, *The Silent World of Doctor and Patient,* see note 4 above, pp. 16-22.

6. American Medical Association, "Code of Medical Ethics," (adopted May 1847, chapter 1, article 1, section 4), in Katz, *The Silent World of Doctor and Patient,* see note 4 above, p. 21.

7. *Schloendorff v. Society of N.Y. Hospital,* 211 N.Y. 125, 105 N.E. 92 (1914).

8. *Salgo v. Leland Stanford, Jr., University Board of Trustees,* 317 P.2d 170 at 181 (1957).

9. American Medical Association, "Principles of Medical Ethics," (adopted 1957, section 1), in Katz, *The Silent World of Doctor and Patient,* see note 4 above, p. 22.

10. American Medical Association, "Opinions and Reports of the Judicial Council, 1957," in Katz, *The Silent World of Doctor and Patient,* see note 4 above, p. 23.

11. Ibid.

12. American Medical Association, "Current Opinions of the Judicial Council, 1981," in Katz, *The Silent World of Doctor and Patient,* see note 4 above, p. 23.

13. C.W. Lidz et al., "Informed Consent and the Structure of Medical Care," in President's Commission for the Study of Ethical Problems in Medicine and Biomedical and Behavioral Research, *Making Health Care Decisions,* vol. 2 (Washington, D.C.: U.S. Government Printing Office, 1982), 317-410.

14. C.W. Lidz et al., *Informed Consent: A Study of Decision-making in Psychiatry* (New York: Guilford Press, 1984).

15. C.W. Lidz et al., "Barriers to Informed Consent," *Annals of Internal Medicine* 99 (1983): 539-43.

16. L. Harris and Associates, "Views of Informed Consent and Decision-Making: Parallel Surveys of Physicians and the Public," in President's Commission for the Study of Ethical Problems in Medicine and Biomedical and Behavioral Research, *Making Health Care Decisions* (Washington, D.C.: U.S. Government Printing Office, 1982), vol. 1, 17-8.

17. D.P. Sulmasy et al., "Patients' Perceptions of the Quality of Informed Consent for Common Medical Procedures," *The Journal of Clinical Ethics* 5, no. 3 (Fall 1994): 189-94.

18. C.H. Braddock et al., "Informed Decision Making in Outpatient Practice: Time to Get Back to Basics," *Journal of the American Medical Association* 282 (1999): 2313-20.

19. W.S. Edwards and C. Yahne, "Surgical Informed Consent: What It Is and Is Not," *American Journal of Surgery* 154 (1987): 574-8.

20. R.A. McNutt, "Shared Medical Decision Making: Problems, Process, Progress," *Journal of the American Medical Association* 292 (2004): 2516-8.

21. T.L. Beauchamp and J.F. Childress, *Principles of Biomedical Ethics,* 5th ed. (New York: Oxford University Press, 2001): 80.

22. Ibid., 94-5.

23. R.R. Faden and T.L. Beauchamp, *A History and Theory of Informed Consent* (New York: Oxford University Press, 1986), 30-4, 133-8.

24. *Canterbury v. Spence,* 464 F.2d 772 (D.C. Cir. 1972).

25. See note 23 above.

26. H. Brody, "Transparency: Informed Consent in Primary Care," *Hastings Center Report* 19, no. 5 (1989): 5-9.

27. A.D. Feld, "Informed Consent: Not Just for Procedures Anymore," *American Journal of Gastroenterology* 99 (2004): 977-80.

28. M.T. Bowden et al., "Informed Consent in Functional Endoscopic Sinus Surgery: The Patient's Perspective," *Otolaryngology Head and Neck Surgery* 131 (2004): 126-32; D.D. Kerrigan et al., "Who's Afraid of Informed Consent?" *British Medical Journal* 306 (1993): 298-300; A. Moores and N.A. Pace, "The Information Requested by Patients Prior to Giving Consent to Anaesthesia," *Anaesthesia* 58 (2003): 703-7; E. Guadagnoli and P. Ward, "Patient Participation in Decision Making," *Social Science and Medicine* 47 (1998): 329-39.

29. *Moore v. Regents of the Univ. of California,* 51 Cal.3d120, 793 P.2d 479 (1990) (*en banc*).

30. R.M. Veatch, *The Patient-Physician Relation: The Patient as Partner,* part 2 (Bloomington, Ind.: Indiana University Press, 1991), 84.

31. Estate of Behringer v. The Medical Center at Princeton, 249 N.J.Super. 597, 592 A.2d 1251 (1991).

32. *Hidding v. Williams,* 578 So.2d 1192 (La.Ct.App. 1991).

33. B. Spielman, "Expanding the Boundaries of Informed Consent: Disclosing Alcoholism and HIV Status to Patients," *American Journal of Medi-*

cine 93 (1992): 216-8.

34. See note 21 above, p. 80; F.J. Ingelfinger, "Arrogance," *New England Journal of Medicine* 303 (1980): 1507-11.

35. A. Barratt et el., "Use of Decision Aids to Support Informed Choices About Screening," *British Medical Journal* 329 (2004): 507-10; M.J. Green et al., "Effect of a Computer-Based Decision Aid on Knowledge, Perceptions, and Intentions About Genetic Testing for Breast Cancer Susceptibility: A Randomized Controlled Trial," *Journal of the American Medical Association* 292 (2004): 442-52; T. Whelan et al., "Effect of a Decision Aid on Knowledge and Treatment Decision Making for Breast Cancer Surgery: A Randomized Trial," *Journal of the American Medical Association* 292 (2004): 435-41; J. Paling, "Strategies to Help Patients Understand Risks," *British Medical Journal* 327 (2003): 745-8; A.M. O'Connor, F. Legare, and D. Stacey, "Risk Communication in Practice: The Contribution of Decision Aids," *British Medical Journal* 327 (2003): 736-40; L.B. Dunn et al., "Enhancing Comprehension of Consent for Research in Older Patients with Psychosis: A Randomized Study of Novel Consent Procedure," *American Journal of Psychiatry* 158 (2001): 1911-3; R.A. Deyo, "A Key Medical Decision Maker: The Patient: New Decision Making Aids Should Help Patients Make the Decisions," British Medical Journal 323 (2001): 466-7.

36. R.S. Shapiro et al. "A Survey of Sued and Nonsued Physicians and Suing Patients," *Archives of Internal Medicine* 149 (1989): 2190; J.K. Avery, "Lawyers Tell What Turns Some Patients Litigious," *Medical Malpractice Review* 2 (1985): 35; B.M. Ashley and K.D. O'Rourke, *Ethics of Health Care,* 3rd ed. (Washington, D.C.: Georgetown University Press, 2002), 83-85.

37. See note 13 above.

38. See note 4 above, pp. 130-47.

39. T.E. Quill and H. Brody, "Physician Recommendations and Patient Autonomy: Finding a Balance Between Physician Power and Patient Choice," *Annals of Internal Medicine* 125 (1996): 763-9.

40. M. Pinquart and P.R. Duberstein, "Information Needs and Decision-Making Processes in Older Cancer Patients," *Critical Reviews in Oncology/Hematology* 51 (2004): 69-80.

41. L.J. Blackhall et al., "Ethnicity and Attitudes Toward Patient Autonomy," *Journal of the American Medical Association* 274 (1995): 820-5.

42. L.O. Gostin, "Informed Consent, Cultural Sensitivity, and Respect for Persons," *Journal of the American Medical Association* 247 (1995): 844-5.

43. I. Hyun, "Waiver of Informed Consent, Cultural Sensitivity, and the Problem of Unjust Families and Traditions," *Hastings Center Report* 32 (2002): 14-22.

44. J.C. Fletcher et al., "Ethical Considerations in Pediatric Oncology," in *Principles and Practice of Pediatric Oncology,* ed. P.A. Pizzo and D.G. Poplack (Philadelphia, Pa.: J.B. Lippincott, 1989), 309-20; N.M.P. King and A.W. Cross, "Children as Decisionmakers: Guidelines for Pediatricians," *Journal of Pediatrics* 115 (1989): 10-6; S.L. Leikin, "Minors' Assent or Dissent to Medical Treatment," *Journal of Pediatrics* 102 (1983): 169-76; Committee on Bioethics, American Academy of Pediatrics, "Informed Consent, Parental Permission, and Assent in Pediatric Practice," *Pediatrics* 95 (1995): 314-7.

45. National Commission for the Protection of Human Subjects of Biomedical and Behavioral Research, *Report and Recommendations Concerning Research Involving Children* (Washington, D.C.: Department of Health, Education, and Welfare, 1977, DHEW Publication no. (OS)77-0005).

46. See note 43, Committee on Bioethics, American Academy of Pediatrics, pp. 315-6.

47. Ibid., 317.

48. See note 13 above, pp. 363-73.

49. *Natanson v. Kline,* 186 Kan. 393, 104 Cal.Rptr. 505, 350 P.2d 1093 (1960).

50. *Cobbs v. Grant,* 502 P.2d 1 (1972).

51. *Mohr v. Williams,* 95 Minn. 261, 104 N.W. 12 (1905).

52. *Arato v. Avedon,* 5 Cal.4th 1172, 858 P.2d 598 (Cal. 1993).

53. T.L. Beauchamp, "Informed Consent," in *Medical Ethics,* ed. R.M. Veatch (Boston, Mass.: Jones and Bartlett, 1989), 173-200.

54. A. Buchanan, "Medical Paternalism," *Philosophy and Public Affairs* 4 (1978): 372.

55. G. Dworkin, "Autonomy and Informed Consent," in President's Commission for the Study of Ethical Problems in Medicine and Biomedical and Behavioral Research, *Making Health Care Decisions* (Washington, D.C.: U.S. Government Printing Office, 1982), volume 3, 70.

56. See note 15 above.

57. E.J. Cassell and J. Katz, "Informed Consent in the Therapeutic Relationship," in *Encyclopedia of Bioethics,* ed. W.T. Reich (New York:

MacMillan Free Press, 1978).

58. President's Commission for the Study of Ethical Problems in Medicine and Biomedical and Behavioral Research, *Making Health Care Decisions* (Washington, D.C.: U.S. Government Printing Office, 1982), 2.

59. American Hospital Association, *A Patient's Bill of Rights* (Chicago, Ill.: American Hospital Association, 1992).

60. Committee on Ethics, American Nurses Association, *Code for Nurses with Interpretive Statements* (Washington, D.C.: American Nurses Association, 1983), ¶ 1.1, p. 2.

61. American Medical Association, Council on Ethical and Judicial Affairs, "Fundamental Elements of the Patient-Physician Relationship," in *Code of Medical Ethics: Current Opinions with Annotations* (Chicago, Ill.: AMA, 2002): ¶ 10.01, p. 281.

62. American Medical Association, Council on Ethical and Judicial Affairs, "Informed Consent," in *Code of Medical Ethics: Current Opinions with Annotations* (Chicago, Ill.: AMA, 2002): ¶ 8.08, p. 206.

63. American College of Physicians, "Ethics Manual," *Annals of Internal Medicine* 128 (1998): 576-94.

Part 3
Ethical Problems in Particular Cases

11

Treatment Refusals by Patients and Clinicians

Edmund G. Howe

Some of the most agonizing situations in medicine arise when a patient refuses a treatment that seems to be beneficial; others arise when a careprovider refuses to treat a patient in the way that the patient wants.[1]

Patients may have an absolute right to make decisions that are wholly against their own best interests, so long as they are competent to do so. Careproviders may have an absolute right to act in accordance with their own moral views. This chapter will explore ways that patients' and careproviders' competing interests in these difficult situations can be better resolved.

The first section of this chapter will discuss areas in which patients and their surrogates have rights to refuse treatment. The second section will discuss ways in which careproviders can assist patients who refuse treatment. The third section will consider careproviders who refuse to treat patients as they wish to be treated, and will delineate several specific contexts in which careproviders have the ethical justification to do so.

I. FACILITATING PATIENTS' DECISIONS TO ACCEPT OR REFUSE TREATMENT

A. General Principles

Competent patients can refuse treatment even when it is not in their best interest to do so. (Chap-

ter 13 discusses forgoing treatment for incapacitated patients.) The right to make choices for oneself is important for many reasons; one is that patients' and careproviders' views regarding what is best for patients often differ. In one study, for example, patients and surgeons were asked what treatment they thought was best for lung cancer.[2] The patients favored radiation because it would not involve the pain caused by surgery, and they would not risk dying during surgery. Surgeons favored surgery because, statistically, it would give patients a longer life. Obviously, when patients' and doctors' views differ, patients should prevail, since they will bear the consequences. There is evidence that careproviders' views may, in addition, be overly pessimistic.[3]

Careproviders have unique insights to offer patients; for example, the ability to evaluate and integrate disparate medical considerations. Thus, careproviders should respect patients' decisions to refuse treatment, but should also do all they can to ensure that when patients refuse, it is what they really want.

B. Helping Patients Decide Whether to Refuse Treatment

Patients may refuse treatment for many reasons; when patients refuse treatment, careproviders should inquire why.[4] They should not, however, simply ask this directly, but should "soften" the question. They might say, for example, "There are many reasons patients choose to refuse treatment. Most are very sound. May I ask you your reasons?"

Once the patients give the reasons, even if the careprovider believes that the reasons are invalid, the careprovider should not express this immediately, but instead should validate the patient's view prior to pointing out what might be invalid. For instance, a careprovider could say, "I can understand that pain can be unbearable. No wonder you want to refuse treatment," and could then add, "I am sure we can treat your pain. I can tell you why if you like. Do you want me to tell you more?"

In this example, the hypothetical careprovider gave the patient a choice, which offsets the possibility that the patient might perceive the careprovider as trying to be in control, which might prompt the patient to reflexively respond in the opposite way.

It may be insufficient for careproviders to do simply what is right: they may need to do what is right in the right way. No matter what a patient decides, careproviders should attempt to preserve the patient/careprovider relationship.

Careproviders should understand patients' reasons for wanting to refuse treatment, validate their views, and give them choices, because, without a careprovider's intervention, patients may not be able to make the choices that they really want for themselves.

1. Informing Patients of their Options

Legal standards vary from state to state; in many states, careproviders must tell patients what the average reasonable patient would want to know, but laws don't require what is ethically optimal,[5] and this requirement may fall far short of meeting the needs of individual patients.

Careproviders should engage patients in discussion that involves give and take. After sharing information, careproviders can ask, "Would you like to know more?" Sometimes, some patients continue to want more information, compulsively,[6] and may ask questions until they learn of remote complications that frighten them. Careproviders may give them all the information they request unthinkingly. Should this happen, careproviders can tell them that some patients want to know as much as they can, but, for many patients, additional information doesn't help, but frightens them.

Some patients may say that they don't want to hear more. This may be due to denial.[7] Careproviders sometimes believe that legally they must fully inform these patients, but careproviders can, however, respect this denial.

2. Informing Patients When their Families Are Involved

Still more difficult questions arise when patients' families request that the patients not be told that they are going to die.[8] Some now argue that careproviders should respect these family members' requests, if what they request is the common practice in their culture.[9] Most careproviders believe that if patients and families aren't able to acknowledge that a patient is dying, their interactions may become like "torture" for both, as they must then carry on a charade as the patient dies. Careproviders who encounter this situation should consider telling family members about this risk.

Generally, when patients refuse treatment and request that careproviders not tell their families, careproviders respect such requests. But this may include having to carry on a charade; for example, a patient may request that her or his family not know that he or she has a do-not-resuscitate (DNR) order. When this happens, the outcome for the family may be catastrophic: the patient's heart may stop, and the family may call for a code, only to have no one respond.

Careproviders can discuss this possibility with the patient beforehand, and ask him or her if, out of compassion, the family could be told. If the patient won't change his or her mind, careproviders can inform everyone who visits the ward that the ward policy is to respect the wishes of patients who do not want family members told about their DNR orders. Then patients have the option to withdraw their DNR order or tell their family members.

Some individual careproviders don't admit patients to the intensive care unit (ICU) if they have a DNR order, and some ICUs have this policy.[10] There are sound reasons that patients might want to be admitted to an ICU even though they are DNR, so if a careprovider or an ICU has this policy, patients must be informed.[11]

Families of patients who have severe psychiatric illness should not be excluded from information regarding the patients' treatment. As long as the patients' families are emotionally healthy and concerned, their being involved in the patients' treatment often is critical to the patients' doing well.

Careproviders should fully inform patients when a treatment may raise exceptional ethical issues at a future time, such as going on a respirator, having a cardiac pacemaker, or having a feeding tube inserted directly into the abdomen.[12] For example, patients who are placed on a respirator should be told that, at some time in the future, they might be successfully weaned from the respirator.[13] This would be important information to a patient who has quadriplegia who prefers to die by having the respirator removed; if the patient stays on the respirator for some time, he or she may be able to continue to breathe without it when it is removed.

If a patient chooses to refuse further artificial respiration, careproviders should give the patient adequate sedation so that he or she can die without discomfort.[14] Some careproviders morally oppose this practice, because the sedation may decrease the patients' respiratory drive; with the sedation, some patients will die who would otherwise survive. Careproviders who have these moral views should anticipate such situations; they should inform the patient that they may have to withdraw from the patient's care.

C. Specific Situations in which Patients Can Refuse Treatment

1. Jehovah's Witnesses

Patients who are Jehovah's Witnesses can refuse even lifesaving treatment on the basis of their religious views.[15] The main exception to this has been children.[16] The notion here is that children can't yet decide for themselves. Other exceptions have been when young children are solely dependent on a parent or when the patient is pregnant.[17]

Careproviders should know the law in their jurisdiction. They can call a judge or magistrate—they are always on call. When patients who are Jehovah's Witnesses need blood but their need isn't acute, it may be possible to contact surgeons who have agreed in advance to treat these patients without using blood, even though the risk of death is increased. For this to be possible, hospitals must have the names of such surgeons in advance. Improved technology over recent years has reduced the risks of doing procedures without blood.

As an alternative, patients may give their own blood in advance. Examples are lung and heart transplantation, and cardiac surgery can sometimes now be offered to Jehovah's Witnesses without fear of a poor outcome.[18] In single lung transplantation, preoperative measures can indicate with some accuracy whether transfusion will be needed. Another issue is the extent to which these patients should have equal access to organs when there are other potential recipients who don't refuse blood.

Some Jehovah's Witness ministers have special knowledge about alternatives to blood products. When these experts are called in, they can give up-to-date information. On the other hand, when these ministers are brought in, they may do all they can to try to persuade a patient not to accept blood, when careproviders may hope to persuade the patient to accept it. The beliefs of Jehovah's Witnesses patients may vary: some believe that if blood is given over their objection, they haven't violated the tenets of their religion.

Exceptional concerns exist when the patient is a child. Legally, careproviders may have to give blood to a child over the parents' objection. Yet, when procedures aren't necessary to save a child's life, hard questions remain. An example is a teenager who has severe scoliosis and needs surgery. Careproviders who face non-life-threatening situations such as this may want to go to court on behalf of the child. But if a court rules that the child should have an operation, it may destroy the child's relationship with his or her family.

Special problems exist when Jehovah's Witness patients are mature minors. Generally, this concept has been applied when patients are 15 or older, but there is a current consensus that this determination shouldn't be contingent on chronological age. When Jehovah's Witness patients are mature minors, parents may stay constantly by their bedside, and these patients may want to refuse blood only because they do not want to go against their parents. Staff must decide whether to insist the parents leave so they can better determine what the child really wants.

2. Patients Who May Be Incompetent for Other Reasons

Many persons consider it unconscionable for careproviders to call for a competency determination when a patient refuses treatment, but do not question when a patient who is just as impaired accepts treatment. But this response has ethical justification, because a patient who refuses treatment has more to lose.

Careproviders who take the patient's outcome into account are using a "sliding scale." The arguments on behalf of using this scale are presented in chapter 9. Boyle states, "Capacity should be determined, in part, by the importance of the decision at hand."[19] Some, however, argue that this approach violates the principle of equity and allows clinicians too much discretion.[20]

Typically, when a question arises regarding competency, careproviders call for a psychiatric consultation. If the consulting psychiatrist deems the patient competent, careproviders then tend to go along with the patient's preferences.[21] Determinations by psychiatrists, however, may reflect their personal moral bias as well as their psychiatric expertise. This is because the medical determination that a patient has mental capacity cannot be externally verified; that is, there is no independent, objective standard to determine whether it is "correct." In contrast, if a patient has tuberculosis, this can be externally verified in a laboratory. Thus, psychiatrists may differ in regard to what standard they use. This is a hypothetical example:

If a man's wife and children were just killed in a car accident while he was driving, in addition to unimaginable grief, he may think that he was at fault. Suppose he then needs a lifesaving operation, but refuses. He literally knows and can state his alternatives; some psychiatrists may deem him competent on this ground alone, but other psychiatrists might believe that although he *literally* knows his alternatives at this moment, he is profoundly depressed. With this depression, they might argue, he can't truly appreciate the consequences of a decision to refuse treatment.

Further, when psychiatrists use a standard that requires a patient to more deeply understand the consequences of her or his decisions, they may differ on what criteria to use. Some may think that, as in the above case, grief should warrant greater clinical weight. Others might place greater weight on other criteria, such as a patient's inability to sleep. Both the standards chosen and the criteria used may reflect a psychiatrist's own moral views. It is ethically problematic that a decision on whether a patient lives or dies could be based on the moral views of whichever psychiatrist happens to be on call. Therefore, careproviders shouldn't necessarily defer to what a consulting psychiatrist believes. A careprovider may request a second psychiatric opinion. Even if both

psychiatrists agree, the careprovider still may be ethically justified in taking her or his own view to court.

Patients can be delusional in some respects but competent to make decisions in others. Careproviders may assume that if a patient can't literally understand the situation at hand, they have no choice but to refuse to treat the patient until substitute decision making can be arranged. But an "extreme" sliding scale to determine capacity may be best in such cases. For example:

A patient needed cardiac surgery; it was, in fact, the only way he could survive. Yet, after he gave consent, his mental clarity declined, and the surgery was cancelled. Then his cardiac condition precipitously declined; but the surgeons wouldn't do the surgery because they believed that he would die "on the table."

It is especially important for careproviders to consider a patient's context when they try to discern, by looking at an advance directive, whether the patient would have wanted to refuse treatment. Often, when patients state what they want in a directive, they don't have the future circumstances that may beset them in mind. When this happens, careproviders should ask what the patient would have wanted if he or she could have foreseen the circumstances as they happened.

3. Adolescents

Special problems arise when patients are minors or children, as they lack life experience.[22] Careproviders should try to persuade young patients not to refuse treatment when their decision seems clearly against their best interests. This might be conceptualized as "a sliding degree of paternalism," based in large part on the patient's chronological age. For example:

An adolescent had testicular cancer.[23] Although surgery would be lifesaving, he wanted all treatment withheld. What was most important to him was being "sexually normal." His careprovider found another young man who had testicular cancer, had surgery, and had done well. The careprovider persuaded the young man to meet the patient. They met, and the patient agreed to the surgery, and did well.

Spiegel states that all patients need these three things:
- To know a person who has what they have, and has done well;

- To know someone who is experiencing what they are experiencing; and
- To know someone who is knowledgeable about what they are going through.[24]

In many situations when patients feel despair, they can be heartened by meeting others in their same state. For example:

A young child had progeria.[25] Persons with this disorder look aged when they are still children. The patient was introduced to another child who also had progeria. It changed the patient's outlook — and his life.

Trying to persuade patients to "hold off" on refusing life-preserving treatment until they can gain a clearer picture of the range of possibilities is also important for adult patients.[26] When trauma or illness will have permanent effects, the permanent effects may trigger memories of the initial trauma or illness, and can cause ongoing stress.[27] Careproviders should introduce adult patients to persons with the same condition. When patients have spinal cord injuries, for instance, careproviders should try to introduce them to persons who have coped well, such as the late Christopher Reeve.[28]

4. Children and Infants

Parents generally can't refuse treatment for a child when it would be lifesaving. What they can do in other instances may be legally unclear.[29] For example, parents can generally refuse to allow careproviders to withdraw life-sustaining care from a child, even when this care is futile and its burdens are much greater than its benefits. But, in some cases, careproviders should consider taking initiatives on the child's behalf, as in the following case:

Parents refused to allow careproviders to relieve their infant's pain, although the infant was dying. They believed that analgesics were unnatural and against God's will. This choice could legally have been construed as a form of child abuse.[30] In this case, the ethics consultant encouraged the staff to act immediately to relieve the child's pain, after informing the appropriate hospital authorities. The careproviders took the consultant's advice, and the parents chose not to sue.

The careproviders might have chosen to first gain legal permission. When children can't protect themselves, careproviders may be the only persons who protect them, for example:

A child came to a doctor who diagnosed a treatable cancer. The doctor then told the parents what the child needed, but they didn't return for treatment because they believed in herbal treatments. Eventually, they came back to the doctor after their child was gravely ill. But at that point, his cancer was no longer curable.

Sometimes parents will pursue an intervention with one child to help another child. If, for example, a child has a fatal disease, bone marrow from a sibling may save the child's life. Some oppose this, on the ground that it exploits the donating child's vulnerability. Although a "new" child has been conceived for a particular purpose, she or he may not be conceived solely as a means to an end; there is evidence that parents love and value these children for themselves, and that the children find meaning in helping their siblings.[31]

5. Pregnancy

Special problems may arise when a patient is pregnant and refuses treatment,[32] as below:

In Washington, D.C., a woman dying of cancer refused a caesarian section for her 26-week-old fetus. She was near death, and, if she died, it would most likely have increased the risk of death for her fetus.[33] She was ordered by a court to undergo a caesarian section. Both the mother and the fetus died shortly thereafter. On appeal, the court held that a mother should be allowed to refuse treatment, despite the interests of the fetus, but added that there might be rare circumstances when this might not be the case.[34]

In a recent English case, a 29-year-old woman needed a caesarian section to save both her own life and that of her 36-week-old fetus.[35] She didn't care about her own or her fetus's life, but wanted her baby to be born naturally in Wales, in a barn. A caesarian was performed over her objection, but, on appeal, a court held that she had the right to refuse treatment, even if her decision seemed "morally repugnant." This might have been the kind of rare circumstance that the U.S. appeals court had in mind.

An instance in which it may be permissible to override a pregnant mother's refusal of treatment is when, without it, both the mother and fetus will die:

In a recent case in England, a woman who described herself as a born-again Christian was six days overdue and her fetus could not be delivered vaginally, although its elbow was protruding. She refused treatment, and her decision was overridden by the courts.[36]

6. Surrogate Decision Makers' Refusals

The care perspective assigns first priority to the *relationships* between persons. When a surrogate refuses treatment on the patient's behalf, new levels of complexity are added, as the following case exemplifies.

A patient had six months to live. He was in a coma due to an abscess that gave him a blood infection throughout his body (septicemia). With surgery to treat the abscess, he might come out of his coma. His wife said that, under these conditions, he would prefer to die. His parents and siblings believed, however, that he would want the surgery.

The ethics consultants had two options. They could encourage the wife to "stick to her guns," and encourage the patient's family to accept the wife's decision — which, after all, the family was legally required to do — and then urge the family to forgive the wife for her decision, for the sake of the couple's young child. Or the consultants could encourage the wife and family to find a solution that all could accept. The possibility of the second option was particularly important, because the couple's child would suffer if the wife and family were at odds.

The ethics consultants chose to encourage the wife and family members to find a resolution that they could all accept, and they were able to arrive at such a compromise. The patient recovered from the coma, and died six months later, as expected. But his wife and child remained close to his family, much to their benefit.

In some cases, staff may be concerned that a patient's family seeks to keep the patient alive so they can continue to receive the patient's income. Staff may believe that they can support the family while they are investigating their concerns. This may be impossible. Careproviders may have to choose whether they will investigate the family or support them.

II. PATIENTS WHO REFUSE TREATMENT

It is tragic when patients, due to a short-lived, intense feeling, end their lives when this is not what they genuinely want.[37] Jodi Halpern related the following case example.[38]

During Dr. Halpern's psychiatric residency, she encountered a patient who had a treatable illness, but who refused treatment. The patient had had a similar treatable condition years before, and had accepted the treatment and had done well. Between these experiences, however, the patient had gone through an extremely difficult divorce. Halpern suspected that the patient didn't really want to die, but rather was still responding to the very difficult and hurtful divorce. But Halpern couldn't do anything to move the patient to reconsider, and the patient refused treatment, and died.

Patients' requests to refuse treatment may be based on underlying anger; they may feel so angry that, rather than pursue their own interests and live, they would rather die in the hope of "getting even."[39] Careproviders who hope to help patients in this situation may find it useful to consider evidence that patients can better "hear" their careproviders when they feel safe and protected.[40] Some careproviders have had success meeting with patients in their homes when patients won't show up for appointments or answer their phones.[41] Another useful approach is to validate some aspect of a patient's view, which conveys to the patient that, at least to some degree, what he or she feels makes some sense.[42] This approach may help a patient feel less alone, and that the careprovider is an ally.[43]

Patients may refuse treatment because they feel they have "failed." This may have been the case with Halpern's patient. One way that careproviders can validate a patient's view is to point out that no matter how "poorly" the patient may feel that he or she has done, the patient has done better than they might have.

Careproviders who want patients to accept treatment may inadvertently pressure them to do the opposite. That is, careproviders may encourage patients to have hope, when patients may be able to see only the worst-case scenario; patients may then conclude that their careproviders can't or don't understand their situation — and give up. Instead, careproviders might give these patients "permission" to have no hope; they might say, "Why should you get your hopes up? Getting your hopes up may leave you more vulnerable to being disappointed. Leave hope to me if you want. I believe that things could get better."[44] When patients feel safe, careproviders can validate their point of view and, in addition, acknowledge a strength: "I imagine it wasn't easy for you to tell us you wanted to refuse further treatment, especially because you had to do this by yourself."

This may help patients regard their careprovider as an ally;[45] then, together they can explore whether the patient has a strength she or he might want to use. In Halpern's case, the patient had faced a similar situation once before and had overcome it. Halpern might have been able to say: "I know that you had cancer before and somehow found a way to want to continue to live. How did you do that then? Why? How is this different? Can you help me understand?"

Careproviders should suggest not that patients *should* use their strength again, but that they *could*.

A. Being "Present" to Patients

To succeed, careproviders must be emotionally committed to patients.[46] When patients refuse treatment, careproviders may dread to see them.[47] If they feel dread or find that they are trying to avoid a patient, they should talk to colleagues or mental health professionals who can help them not harm their patient in either of these ways.

III. CAREPROVIDERS WHO REFUSE TO TREAT

There are basically three reasons that careproviders refuse to treat patients:

- To benefit patients,
- To be true to their own moral views, or
- To meet the interests of larger numbers of other patients or the interests of the greater society.

Careproviders may refuse to grant patients' requests when they believe that their efforts would be futile. In these situations, careproviders may also believe that they must refuse to treat to preserve their own or their profession's integrity.

A. Careproviders Who Refuse on Behalf of their Patients

Research has suggested that when patients have written advance directives, careproviders may ignore the directives as much as half of the time.[48] They tend to continue to give life-sustaining treatments to younger patients and less than full treatments to older patients, regardless of what the patients have indicated they would want.

Sometimes careproviders refuse to do what the patients say that they want because the careproviders believe that they know more than patients what is best. Often careproviders' underlying beliefs are correct: that what patients *really* want is some other option than the one they are requesting.[49] It is very important in these cases to try to persuade careproviders to meet with patients to see if they can resolve their conflicting views, as the following case illustrates.

The doctor refused to write a DNR order that the patient had requested. The ethics committee, to which a consult was brought, initially believed that it should "overrule" the doctor, and the proposed solution was to meet with the doctor and tell him that he must respect the patient's DNR request. If the doctor refused, the ethics committee would then go to the head of the service, the head of the hospital, and/or to the hospital lawyers, in that order. A committee member suggested that instead of trying to "coerce" the doctor, they should contact an "ethically savvy" physician they knew, who was this doctor's colleague, and ask him to discuss this problem with the doctor "over coffee." This was done, and the colleagues met. The doctor agreed to change his approach, gave the patient the choice, and discussed it with him. But the result was paradoxical: at that point, the patient changed *his* mind.

1. Preventive Ethics

Consultants should consider how conflicts might be prevented. In the case immediately above, for example, educational sessions might be held throughout the hospital.

Sometimes arrangements are made to allow a patient to die, as by disconnecting a patient's respirator. If there is a change of attending, the new attending may oppose the decision,[50] and this may cause patients and their families extreme emotional pain. Careproviders can anticipate changes in attendings and routinely inform them of events like this long before they come to the ward.

2. Collusion with other Careproviders

Careproviders may refuse to treat patients for what they believe is the patients' best interest, and may indicate to patients that they can get treatment if they can find another careprovider who will give them what they request. Then, with or without knowing it, careproviders may act in ways that influence other careproviders to "side" with them. As a result, patients may be unable to acquire the care that they want. This is what happened in the following case.

A child had Werdnig Hoffman's disease, a genetic disorder in young children in which they undergo ascending paralysis of their muscles, much like adults undergo with amyotrophic lateral sclerosis (ALS, or Lou Gehrig's disease). It causes death at a very early age.[51] This child came at 14 months of age to the hospital with pneumonia that was the result of some initial paralysis of her lungs. The patient's careproviders anticipated that, at her next hospital visit, due to greater lung paralysis, the child might need artificial respiration, and an artificial ventilator could be required, which could never be withdrawn.

The ethics committee pursued preventive ethics. It met, and asked, before this occurred, whether the child would be better off if allowed to die, or better off on a ventilator, even though she would live on, most likely, for only a few months. The committee agreed that the child could have a ventilator started in the future, if a pediatric respiratory specialist who was willing to do this could be found. Her careprovider, a pediatric respiratory specialist, called other specialists, but none could be found who would start the child on a ventilator. It seemed odd that some doctors on the ethics committee felt that the ventilator should be started, but no doctors outside the committee could be found who felt the same way. Nonetheless, it happened.

An indication that collusion may be occurring is when all members of one medical specialty take different views than all members of another. For example:

In one case, all of the neonatologists opposed all of the pediatricians in regard to whether a severely impaired neonate's treatments should be withdrawn.[52] The parents, caught in the middle, wanted initially to withdraw care, but, hearing the "other side," felt guilty. Finally, the parents changed their minds. Guilt may have been the primary reason they did.

B. Careproviders Who Refuse to Treat for Moral Reasons

Careproviders should be free to follow the dictates of their moral conscience.[53] Some careproviders are opposed to birth control, and some believe that even giving a patient the name of another doctor who will give her birth control violates their moral view.

The key ethical piece here is that careproviders must make such issues clear to patients in a "timely manner." For example, careproviders who are opposed to giving sedative medications to patients who are discontinuing artificial respiration should tell patients as early as possible that they can't be involved in this.

A more difficult ethical problem is determining when careproviders are morally justified in refusing to treat a patient based on their moral views, as some moral views are skewed or highly idiosyncratic. Thus, careproviders have an obligation to scrutinize their own moral views, even though it may be exceedingly difficult. John Fletcher once thought, for instance, that it was immoral for doctors to tell parents the sex of a fetus when they might use the information to abort the fetus.[54] He contended that even if the law allowed it, careproviders shouldn't do it. But when he and I discussed the issue with a group of women who were lawyers, they strongly disagreed.

When is a moral view sufficiently valid that careproviders should be ethically justified in standing by it? One criterion is that a reasonable, underlying value supports it.[55] In the case of Fletcher's view that careproviders should not tell parents their fetus's sex, this test is met. Careproviders who disclose the sex of a fetus could facilitate sexual discrimination. Discrimination on this basis may be invidious. Thus, this view has a reasonable value to support it, although other reasonable values may oppose it.

One's view might be morally justifiable, but it does not follow that one is justified in trying to impose it on others. The key question then is: Who is most authorized to act when persons have different moral views?[56] Often, reasonable persons differ, and it is unclear whose view is right. When this is the case, the question shifts to: Under these circumstances, how can a decision best be made? Society can delegate decision-making authority to specific institutions and persons. Even if this authority then makes "the wrong decision," over the long run, the process is superior. In general, such decisions should be made by the greater society. In the case of Fletcher's moral opposition to telling parents about the sex of their fetus, thereby possibly facilitating discrimination on the basis of gender, the analysis would be as follows. Society (citizens) should decide whether careproviders should tell parents the sex of their fetus, not John Fletcher, as it is the members of society, after all, who are most affected by the nature of the society in which they live. Society can delegate the making of this decision, whether it does so explicitly or by default. In many cases, society does delegate decisions — by default, through inaction — to careproviders. Careproviders often must decide, when society hasn't spoken, who, among many patients, should receive limited medical resources.

The greatest drawback of accepting society's judgments is that the "majority" may not be concerned about the needs of patients who are the "worst-off." If this is the case, then careproviders may be justified in doing all they can to help patients, even though the body that is discriminating against them is duly authorized to do so. Such an obligation to help the "worst-off" will be described in the final section of this chapter.

Careproviders should ask themselves before they act: Are my actions ethically justified, or am I acting in this way because I have the unchecked power to impose my views on others? If careproviders find that they are acting primarily on the basis of power, it is wrong, as the following case illustrates.

A patient with several medical problems, including advanced dementia, needed dialysis. One of his doctors, a kidney specialist, refused to give him dialysis on the ground that dialysis wasn't "indicated" in this situation. The patient's prior preference was to stay alive unless this posed an undue burden on his wife. His wife desperately wanted him to stay alive. He could still recognize and speak with her, although he needed to reside in a nursing home. The wife arranged for the patient to be transferred to another institution that had assured her that they would give him dialysis. If the doctor had been successful in imposing his own view, it would have been only because he had the power to do so. But society's judgment, expressed through the law, was that the decision should be made by the patient, not the doctor, through his surrogate decision maker.

A more complex example involves patients who are treated for infertility, who may end up pregnant with several fetuses. Then, they may want to have the lives of some of the fetuses ended so that those fetuses that remain will fare much better.[57] Problems may arise if some of the fetuses have genetic problems or if the parents have preferences based on the fetuses' sex. Parents may want the lives of the fetuses with a genetic problem ended, or they may want the lives of some fetuses ended on the basis of their gender, so that they can have a more balanced family. They may, for example, want to have twins, one of which is a boy and the other a girl. Careproviders may refuse to comply with such wishes, for example, when their views may be similar to Fletcher's on the issue.

The assumption initially made should be that society should make this determination, since the parents, more than their careproviders, will be affected by the outcome. The fetuses may be regarded as the worst-off parties in this situation, however, and thus have a special need for protection. Careproviders could refuse to end the lives of particular fetuses and let the parents go to court.[58] Regardless, careproviders have a moral obligation to anticipate their actions, and should inform parents about their views prior to treating them for infertility.

C. When Careproviders Act on Behalf of Society

Our society has fewer resources than patients need and want. When society remains silent on an issue, it may leave careproviders to act as its agent; in this case, careproviders may be given the task of rationing care. An example is when careproviders decide which patients among many will be admitted to the ICU when there are a limited number of beds.

Careproviders who accept this triage role, such that they admit some patients to the ICU but refuse to admit others, serve two masters. When they do this, they are implicitly violating the integrity of the patient/careprovider relationship, as most patients believe that careproviders act solely to serve patients' best interests. Careproviders have two other options:

1. They can tell patients that they have been triaged, and then the patients may have the choice of going to an ICU at another hospital;
2. Careproviders can delegate rationing decisions to others.

In both of these options, careproviders are able to remain fully open with their patients. The second approach may seem particularly disturbing to careproviders, as it leaves decisions about which of their patients can meet their competing needs entirely up to others. This approach is, in essence, managed care.[59]

Careproviders may refuse to treat a patient when they deem that what the patient wants is futile.[60] Three distinctions regarding futility must be made. First, in some illnesses, a particular treatment simply doesn't work. Careproviders are most justified in refusing in these situations. Second is "quantitative" futility, in which the likelihood of success of a treatment is extremely remote.[61] It is more problematic for careproviders to decide on their own to refuse to treat in these cases,[62] as the bases for moral disagreement are greater. When careproviders override patients' values in these instances, the likelihood of offending the patients' sensibilities is greater. For example:

It became clear to patients on one ward that they could receive cardiopulmonary resuscitation (CPR) when their careproviders believed it would be futile if they said they wanted CPR on religious grounds. Patients who wanted CPR for other reasons learned that, if they weren't religious, they should lie. So they did.

Third, there is "qualitative futility," which is the most problematic for careproviders to determine on their own, because their views on what constitutes futile treatment may be just the opposite of the views of their patients or the patients' loved ones. This is illustrated in another case in which John Fletcher was involved.

Careproviders had repeatedly been called to resuscitate a child who, since birth, had a heart problem that caused her heart to periodically stop. This occurred every few months. But its frequency was diminishing, and it was predicted that in a few years she would no longer need to be resuscitated. The child was four, but had, and would always have, a mental age of two.

The child's careproviders believed that it was futile for them to continue to resuscitate her because her mental age would not progress. The parents doted on her, however, and, thus, totally disagreed with the staff. The careproviders asked for an ethics consult, and the committee agreed with the staff. Fletcher always sought to bring patients, careproviders, and others in for a meeting after an ethical consultation to review together what had been done, and he asked all of those at the initial consult to reconvene a month afterward.

The child's heart had not stopped during this time. If it had, she would not have been given CPR, and would have died. The parents at the follow-up meeting expressed their hurt that the ethics committee had agreed with the careproviders that their child should be allowed to die. At the follow-up meeting, the decision was reversed.

IV. PROBLEMS CAUSED BY THE HEALTHCARE SYSTEM

Careproviders can refuse to treat a patient when the institution they work for won't let them, which may be because the patient doesn't have a life-threatening illness and can't afford to pay for treatment.[63] In such situations, the patient's condition may worsen if untreated, and only the careprovider who saw the patient initially can foresee the risks if alternative sources of treatment aren't pursued. Careproviders who find themselves in such situations should strongly consider taking whatever measures they can to prevent foreseeable bad outcomes. They can urge patients to receive treatment elsewhere, even though they can't pay; they can help patients identify signs their condition is worsening, so they can be admitted before it is "too late"; and they can encourage patients to come up with what money they can so they can be admitted for treatment.

Careproviders may be able to help improve the healthcare system; they may be morally obligated to try, because they can see these problems better than others can.[64] If they don't try, the result may be tragic, as it was in the following case.

A patient had aortic stenosis and no medical insurance, but he was retired and had some retirement savings. The patient went to a doctor for treatment, and the doctor said that the patient would need surgery, but that the patient first had to take care of his dental problems, because, if they weren't treated, it would make the surgery more risky.

The patient took care of his dental problems, but then found that the hospital would not give him surgery unless he used his retirement savings to pay for it. Initially, the patient was very concerned how this would affect his future, but, after a few weeks, he "came to terms with it," and began to make financial arrangements so that his remaining retirement savings could be used to pay for the surgery.

The patient was not aware that his condition was worsening while he waited for his retirement savings to become available. While waiting, he became so ill that he could have had surgery on an emergency basis — that is, the hospital would have admitted him before the funds were available because his illness had become life-threatening. But the patient didn't know this, and died before he had the money for surgery.

Hospital systems may not be adequately structured to "foresee" such problems.[65] Careproviders may be better able to do this than others in the system. In the same way that careproviders are in a unique position to help children who need treatment to receive it — even over their parents' objections — only careproviders may be able to anticipate problems when a patient can't afford needed treatment, and their efforts may prevent tragedies such as the one just described.

V. CONCLUSION

Patients who are competent have a legal right to refuse treatment, and this is often what they most genuinely want, even if it differs from what others might choose. Patients' choices should be respected.

Careproviders' freedom to follow their moral views is equally important. As long as their views are reasonable, they should be allowed to follow them. Because careproviders usually have greater power than patients, however, careproviders may unwittingly impose their values on patients, which is a matter of concern. The circumstances under which patients and careproviders should be able to refuse receiving or giving treatment are sometimes murky. This chapter has attempted to provide guidelines for the murky situations that are most likely to arise.

For patients to be able to refuse knowledgeably, they must have adequate information; this requires careproviders to engage in give-and-take with patients until they meet patients' individual needs for information.

Careproviders sometimes should be willing to be paternalistic. The trust patients feel for them and the strength of their relationship may be enough, in many instances, to enable them to persuade patients to more fully consider all of the alternatives.

This chapter has focused particularly on what careproviders can do when a patient has mental capacity and refuses treatment, but this doesn't seem to be what the patient genuinely wants. Careproviders might consider taking exceptional measures to help patients feel safe; to validate patients' views; to teach patients to use skills that they already have; and, above all, to maintain the relationship by continuing being with patients, regardless of what they decide.

Careproviders may refuse to treat patients. In other contexts, careproviders may best help patients by refusing to go along with their requests to refuse treatment; when this is the case, they should not impose their own views, but, rather, use persuasion. Careproviders may refuse to treat patients because they have conflicting moral views. They may be wholly justified in refusing, but additional obligations follow. Patients never should be harmed as a result. Careproviders should anticipate when they might have a moral conflict; it is optimal for careproviders to review their own values in advance to decrease the likelihood that these problems might occur.

Careproviders may also refuse to treat patients because resources are limited and treatment is futile. It may be ethically permissible for careproviders to act as society's agents to preserve resources, but it is ethically problematic for careproviders to refuse to treat a patient solely because it is within their power to do so.

Giving priority to the maintenance of relationships represents a different perspective from one based primarily on the analysis of conflicting moral principles. When conflicts arise, careproviders should seek to ensure that their relationships with patients and patients' families remain intact.[66] If careproviders have done this, when patients or their loved ones leave the hospital, they will feel that one positive aspect of their experience — even if it is the only one — was the caring they felt from their careproviders. The meaningfulness of this relationship to patients and/or their loved ones — and the careproviders — may then extend long into the future.

When "systems" of medical care delivery have flaws that may harm patients, careproviders should do what they can; this may mean taking initiatives to try to eliminate these flaws. Until these flaws are eliminated, careproviders should try to anticipate potential harms to patients, and, having done this, take the action necessary to prevent the harms.

NOTES

1. K.K. Boyd, "Power Imbalances and Therapy," *Focus* 11, no. 9 (August 1996): 1-4.

2. B.J. McNeil et al., "On the Elicitation of Preferences for Alternative Therapies," *New England Journal of Medicine* 306, no. 21 (May 1982): 1259-62; see also, S. Cykert, "Risk Acceptance and Risk Aversion: Patients' Perspectives on Lung Surgery," *Thoracic Surgery Clinics* 14, no. 3 (2004): 287-93; and K.P. Weingart et al., "Patient Expectations of Benefit from Phase I Clinical Trials: Linguistic Considerations in Diagnosing a Therapeutic Misconception," *Theoretical Medicine and Bioethics* 24, no. 4 (2003): 329-44.

3. S. Saigal et al., "Differences in Preferences for Neonatal Outcomes Among Health Care Professionals, Parents, and Adolescents," *Journal of the American Medical Association,* 281 no. 21 (2 June 1999): 1991-7; see, also, J. Brett, "The Journey to Accepting Support: How Parents of Profoundly Disabled Children Experience Support in Their Lives," *Pediatric Nursing* 16, no. 8 (October 2004): 14-8.

4. H. Stevenson, "Wounded by Words," *Lancet* 364, no. 9436 (28 August 2004): 753.

5. N.G. Messer, "Professional-Patient Relationships and Informed Consent," *Postgraduate Medicine Journal* 80, no. 943 (May 2004): 277-83; K. Berger, "Informed Consent: Information or Knowledge?" *Medicine and Law* 22, no. 4 (2003): 743-50; R.M. Veatch, "Abandoning Informed Consent," *Hastings Center Report* 25, no. 2 (March-April 1995): 5-12; and B.C. White and J. Zimbelman, "Abandoning Informed Consent: An Idea Whose Time Has Not Yet Come," *Journal of Medical Phi-*

losophy 23, no. 5 (August 1998): 477-99.

6. D.W. Evans, M.D. Lewis, and E. Iobst, "The Role of the Orbitofrontal Cortex in Normally Developing Compulsive-Like Behaviors and Obsessive-Compulsive Disorder," *Brain and Cognition* 55, no. 1 (June 2004): 220-34; N. Maltby et al., "Dysfunctional Action Monitoring Hyperactivates Frontal-Striatal Circuits in Obsessive-Compulsive Disorder: An Event-Related fMRI Study," *NeuroImage* 24, no. 2 (15 January 2005): 495-503; and P. Thomas and A.B. Cahill, "Compulsion and Psychiatry: The Role of Advance Statements," *British Medical Journal* 329, no. 7458 (17 July 2004): 122-3.

7. T.C. Flynn, "Denial of Illness: Basal Cell Carcinoma," *Dermatology Surgery* 30, no. 10 (October 2004): 1343-4, p. 1344; see, also, S. Stephenson, "Understanding Denial," *Oncology Nursing Forum* 31, no. 5 (September 2004): 985-8; C. Zimmermann, "Denial of Impending Death: A Discourse Analysis of the Palliative Care Literature," *Social Science and Medicine* 59, no. 8 (2004): 1769-80; C. Zimmermann and G. Rodin, "The Denial of Death Thesis: Sociological Critique and Implications for Palliative Care," *Palliative Medicine* 18, no. 2 (March 2004): 121-8; P. Vuilleumier, "Anosognosia: The Neurology of Beliefs and Uncertainties," *Cortex* 40, no. 1 (February 2004): 9-17; and M.W. Ketterer et al., "Men Deny and Women Cry, But Who Dies? Do the Wages of 'Denial' Include Early Ischemic Coronary Heart Disease?" *Journal of Psychosomatic Research* 56, no. 1 (January 2004): 119-23.

8. J.W. Jones, L.B. McCullough, and B.W. Richman, "Family-Surgeon Disagreements Over Interventions," *Journal of Vascular Surgery* 40, no. 4 (October 2004): 831-2; J.M. Teno et al., "Family Perspectives on End-of-Life Care at the Last Place of Care," *Journal of the American Medical Association* 29, no. 1 (7 January 2004): 88-93; T.A. Mappes and J.S. Zembaty, "Patient Choices, Family Interests, and Physician Obligations," *Kennedy Institute Ethics Journal* 4, no. 1 (March 1994): 27-46; F.D. Ferris, C.F. von Gunten, and L.L. Emanuel, "Competency in End-of-Life Care: Last Hours of Life," *Journal of Palliative Medicine* 6, no. 4 (August 2003): 605-13; and J.R. Curtis, "Communicating about End-of-Life Care with Patients and Families in the Intensive Care Unit," *Critical Care Clinics* 20, no. 3 (July 2004): 363-80.

9. M. McDonald, "Dignity at the End of Our Days: Personal, Familial, and Cultural Location," *Journal of Palliative Care* 20, no. 3 (Autumn 2004):

163-70; A. Dula and S. Williams, "When Race Matters," *Clinical Geriatric Medicine* 21 (2005): 239-53.

10. M.Y. Rady and D.J. Johnson, "Admission to Intensive Care Unit at the End-of-Life: Is It an Informed Decision?" *Palliative Medicine* 18, no. 8 (December 2004): 705-11.

11. R.L. Stephens, " 'Do Not Resuscitate' Orders: Ensuring the Patient's Participation," *Journal of the American Medical Association* 255, no. 2 (10 January 1986): 240-1; S.C. Zweig et al., "Effect of Do Not Resuscitate Orders on Hospitalization of Nursing Home Residents Evaluated for Lower Respiratory Infections," *Journal of the American Geriatric Society* 52, no. 1 (January 2004): 51-8.

12. K.A. Bramstedt, "Elective Inactivation of Total Artificial Heart Technology in Non-Futile Situations: Inpatients, Outpatients and Research Participants," *Death Studies* 28, no. 5 (June 2004): 423-33; R.M. Veatch, "Inactivating a Total Artificial Heart: Special Moral Problems," *Death Studies* 27, no. 4 (May 2003): 305-15; and S.L. Mitchell et al., "Clinical and Organizational Factors Associated with Feeding Tube Use Among Nursing Home Residents with Advanced Cognitive Impairment," *Journal of the American Medical Association* 290, no. 1 (July 2003): 73-80.

13. D.C. Chao and D.J. Scheinhorn, "Weaning From Mechanical Ventilation," *Critical Care Clinic* 14, no. 4 (October 1998): 799-817; D.A. Asch et al., "The Sequence of Withdrawing Life-Sustaining Treatment From Patients," *American Journal of Medicine* 107, no. 2 (August 1999): 153-6; S.A. Mayer and S.B. Kossoff, "Withdrawal of Life Support in the Neurological Intensive Care Unit," *Neurology* 52, no. 8 (12 May 1999): 1602-9; N.A. Christakis and D.A. Asch, "Medical Specialists Prefer to Withdraw Familiar Technologies When Discontinuing Life Support," *Journal of Internal Medicine* 10, no. 9 (September 1995): 491-4; K. Faber-Langendoen, "The Clinical Management of Dying Patients Receiving Mechanical Ventilation: A Survey of Physician Practice," *Chest* 106, no. 3 (September 1994): 880-8; and L. Marr and D. Weissman, "Withdrawal of Ventilatory Support from the Dying Adult Patient," *Journal of Supportive Oncology* 2, no. 3 (May-June 2004): 283-8.

14. J.A. Schaler, "Patients Who Refuse Food and Fluids to Hasten Death," *New England Journal of Medicine* 349, no. 18 (30 October 2003): 1777-9.

15. B.M. Zenon, C. Wong, and M. Thomas,

"Meeting the Clinical Challenge of Care for Jehovah's Witnesses," *Transfusion Medicine Review* 18, no. 2 (April 2004): 105-16; D.S. Davis, "Does 'No' Mean 'Yes'? The Continuing Problem of Jehovah's Witnesses and Refusal of Blood Products?" *Second Opinion* 19, no. 3 (January 1994): 35-43; D.R. Migden and G.R. Braen, "The Jehovah's Witness Blood Refusal Card: Ethical and Medicolegal Considerations for Emergency Physicians," *Academic Emergency Medicine* 5, no. 8 (August 1998): 815-24; and D. Maylon, "Transfusion-Free Treatment of Jehovah's Witnesses: Respecting the Autonomous Patient's Motives," *Journal of Medical Ethics* 24, no. 6 (December 1998): 376-81.

16. J.E. Morrison et al., "The Jehovah's Witness Family, Transfusions, and Pediatric Day Surgery," *International Journal of Pediatric Otorhinolaryngology* 38, no. 3 (3 January 1997): 207-13.

17. A.K. Singla et al., "Are Women Who Are Jehovah's Witnesses at Risk of Maternal Death?" *American Journal of Obstetrics and Gynecology* 185 (2001): 893-5.

18. A. Grande et al., "Lung Transplantation in a Jehovah's Witness: Case Report in a Twinning Procedure," *Journal of Cardiovascular Surgery* 44, no. 1 (2003): 131-4, p. 132; see, also, V. Alexi-Meskishvili et al., "Correction of Congenital Heart Defects in Jehovah's Witness Children," *Journal of Thoracic and Cardiovascular Surgery* 52, no. 3 (June 2004): 141-6; and J.W. Jones, L.B. McCullough, and B.W. Richman, "A Surgeon's Obligations to a Jehovah's Witness Child," *Surgery* 133, no. 1 (January 2003): 110-1.

19. See, also, R.J. Gatchel, "Psychosocial Factors That Can Influence the Self-Assessment of Function," *Journal of Occupational Rehabilitation* 14, no. 3 (September 2004): 197-206; V. Raymont et al., "Prevalence of Mental Incapacity in Medical Inpatients and Associated Risk Factors: Cross-Sectional Study," *Lancet* 364, no. 9443 (16 October 2004): 1383-4; L. Ganzini et al., "Ten Myths about Decision-Making Capacity," *Journal of the American Medical Directors Association* 5, no. 4 (July-August 2004): 278-9; R.J. Leo, "Competency and the Capacity to Make Treatment Decisions: A Primer for Primary Care Physicians," *Primary Care Companion to the Journal of Clinical Psychiatry* 1, no. 5 (October 1999): 131-41; and E. Teirnan et al., "Relations Between Desire for Early Death, Depressive Symptoms and Antidepressant Prescribing in Terminally Ill Patients with Cancer," *Journal of the Royal Society of Medicine* 95 (2002): 386-90.

20. K. Lang, "Mental Illness and the Right to Refuse Lifesaving Medical Treatment," *Princeton Journal of Bioethics* 5 (Spring 2002): 48-58.

21. G. Ranjith and M. Hotopf, " 'Refusing Treatment — Please See': An Analysis of Capacity Assessments Carried Out by a Liaison Psychiatry Service," *Journal of the Royal Society of Medicine* 97, no. 10 (October 2004): 480-2; A. Buchanan, "Mental Capacity, Legal Competence and Consent to Treatment," *Journal of the Royal Society of Medicine* 97, no. 9 (September 2004): 415-20; and A. Vellinga et al., "Competence to Consent to Treatment of Geriatric Patients: Judgments of Physicians, Family Members and the Vignette Method," *International Journal of Geriatric Psychiatry* 19, no. 7 (July 2004): 645-54.

22. A. Holder, "Childhood Malignancies and Decision-Making," *Yale Journal of Biology and Medicine* 65 (1992): 99-104. "Holder's search of case law revealed that it has been over 40 years since any court in the United States has allowed parents of a minor to successfully sue a physician for treating their adolescent without their consent, when consent was given by a patient 15 years or over," quoted in L. Badzek and S. Kanosky, "Mature Minors and End-of-Life Decision Making: A New Development in Their Legal Right to Participation," *Journal of Nursing Law* 8, no. 3 (August 2002): 23-9, p. 27. *Belcher v. Charleston Area Medical Center* 422 S.E.2d 827 (W.Va. 1992).

23. G. Jonker-Pool et al., "Male Sexuality After Cancer Treatment — Needs for Information and Support: Testicular Cancer Compared to Malignant Lymphoma," *Patient Education and Counseling* 52, no. 2 (February 2004): 143-50.

24. D. Spiegel, "Mind Matters — Group Therapy and Survival in Breast Cancer," *New England Journal of Medicine* 345, no. 24 (December 2001): 1767-8.

25. H. Livneh, R.F. Antonak, and S. Maron, "Progeria: Medical Aspects, Psychosocial Perspectives, and Intervention Guidelines," *Death Studies* 19, no. 5 (September 1995): 433-52.

26. R. Schulz and S. Decker, "Long-Term Adjustment to Physical Disability: The Role of Social Support, Perceived Control, and Self-Blame," *Journal of Personality and Social Psychology* 48, no. 5 (May 1985): 1162-72; C. Laenger and E. Laenger, "Learning to Eat After Radiation Therapy for Throat Cancer," *Disability and Rehabilitation* 26, no. 11 (June 2004): 683-5.

27. A. Hartkopp et al., "Suicide in a Spinal Cord Injured Population: Its Relation to Functional Status," *Archives of Physical Medical Rehabilitation* 79, no. 11 (November 1998): 1356-61.

28. G. Pickl, "Changes During Long-Term Management of Locked-In Syndrome: a Case Report," *Folia Phoniatrica et Logopaedica* 54 (2002): 26-43.

29. D.S. Diekema, "Parental Refusals of Medical Treatment: The Harm Principle as Threshold for State Intervention," *Theoretical Medicine and Bioethics* 25, no. 4 (2004): 243-64; D. Oppenheim et al., "An Ethics Dilemma: When Parents and Doctors Disagree on the Best Treatment for the Child," *Bulletin of Cancer* 91, no. 9 (September 2004): 735-8.

30. D.J. Higgins, "The Importance of Degree Versus Type of Maltreatment: A Cluster Analysis of Child Abuse Types," *Journal of Psychology* 138, no. 4 (July 2004): 303-4; N. Fost, "America's Gulag Archipelago," *New England Journal of Medicine* 351, no. 23 (December 2004): 2369-70; S.A. Reijneveld et al., "Infant Crying and Abuse," *Lancet* 364, no. 9442 (9 October 2004): 1340-2; C.D. Berkowitz, "Fatal Child Neglect," *Advances in Pediatrics* 48 (2001): 331-61; American Academy of Pediatrics Committee on Bioethics, "Religious Exemptions from Child Abuse Statutes," *Pediatrics* 81, no. 1 (January 1988): 169-71; R.J. Boyle, R. Salter, and M.W. Arnander, "Ethics of Refusing Parental Requests to Withhold or Withdraw Treatment From Their Premature Baby," *Journal of Medical Ethics* 30, no. 4 (August 2004): 402-5; and D.C. Bross, "Medical Care Neglect," *Child Abuse and Neglect* 6, no. 4 (1982): 375-81.

31. W. Packman et al., "Psychosocial Adjustment of Adolescent Siblings of Hematopoietic Stem Cell Transplant Patients," *Journal of Pediatric Oncology Nursing* 21, no. 4 (July-August 2004): 233-48; W. Packman, "Psychosocial Impact of Pediatric BMT on Siblings," *Bone Marrow Transplantation* 24, no. 7 (October 1999): 701-6; see, also, B.J. Culliton, "Court Upholds Refusal to Be Medical Good Samaritan," *Science* 201 (18 August 1978): 596-97. This case is summarized in M.F. Marshall, "Treatment Refusals by Patients and Clinicians," in *Introduction to Clinical Ethics,* 2nd ed., ed. J.C. Fletcher et al. (Hagerstown, Md.: University Publishing Group, Inc., 1997), 123-4. For a recent fictional account, see J. Picoult, *My Sister's Keeper* (New York: Atria Books, 2004).

32. F.A. Chervenak et al., "A Clinically Comprehensive Ethical Framework for Offering and Recommending Cancer Treatment Before and During Pregnancy," *Cancer* 100, no. 2 (January 2004): 215-22; N. Dresner, V. Raskin, and L.S. Goldman, "Refusing to Terminate a Life-Threatening Pregnancy," *General Hospital Psychiatry* 12, no. 5 (September 1990): 335-40; J.J. Finnerty and C.A. Chisholm, "Patient Refusal of Treatment in Obstetrics," *Seminars of Perinatology* 27, no. 6 (December 2003): 435-45; E. Flagler and F. Baylis, "Bioethics for Clinicians: 12. Ethical Dilemmas That Arise in the Care of Pregnant Women: Rethinking 'Maternal-Fetal' Conflicts," *Canadian Medical Association Journal* 156, no. 12 (June 1997): 1729-32; N. Westgen and R. Levi, "Motherhood After Traumatic Spinal Cord Injury," *Paraplegia* 32, no. 8 (August 1994): 517-23; D.M. Dudzinski and M. Sullivan, "When Agreeing with the Patient is Not Enough: A Schizophrenic Woman Requests Pregnancy Termination," *General Hospital Psychiatry* 26, no. 6 (November-December 2004): 475-80; J.H. Coverdale, L.B. McCullough, and F.A. Chevenak, "Assisted and Surrogate Decision Making for Pregnant Patients Who Have Schizophrenia," *Schizophrenia Bulletin* 30, no. 3 (2004): 659-64; R.A. Welch and V. Poullin, "Specific Roles of the Obstetrician-Gynecologist," *Obstetric and Gynecology Clinics of North America* 30, no. 3 (September 2003): 601-15; J.V. Pinkerton and J.J. Finnerty, "Resolving the Clinical and Ethical Dilemma Involved in Fetal-Maternal Conflicts," *American Journal of Obstetrics and Gynecology* 175, no. 2 (August 1996): 289-95.

33. District of Columbia, Court of Appeals, "In re A.C.," *Atlantic Reporter* 573 (26 April 1990): 1235-64; G.J. Annas, "She's Going to Die: The Case of Angela C," *Hastings Center Report* 18, no. 1 (February-March 1988): 23-5; G.J. Annas, "Forced Caesareans: the Most Unkindest Cut of All," *Hastings Center Report* 12, no. 3 (June 1982): 16-7.

34. H. Newnham, "Mother vs. Fetus: Who Wins?" *Australian Journal of Midwifery* 16, no. 1 (March 2003): 23-6, p. 24.

35. *Re S* [1992] 3 WLR 806, 4 All ER 671, cited in Newnham, ibid., p. 25.

36. *St. George's Healthcare NHS Trust v R v Collins, ex parte S* [1998] 3 All ER 673, cited in Newnham, ibid., p. 25.

37. K.A. Bramstedt and A.C. Arroliga, "On the Dilemma of Enigmatic Refusal of Life-Saving Therapy," *Chest* 126, no. 2 (August 2004): 337-9.

38. J. Halpern, *From Detached Concern to*

Empathy: Humanizing Medical Practice (New York: Oxford University Press, 2001).

39. T.J. Banja, R. Adler, and A. Stringer, "Ethical Dimensions of Caring for Defiant Patients: A Case Study," *Journal of Head Trauma and Rehabilitation* 11, no. 6 (1996): 93-7.

40. A.L. Suchman et al., "A Model of Empathic Communication in the Medical Interview," *Journal of the American Medical Association* 277 (1977): 678-82; see generally, A.N. Sabo and L.L. Havens, ed., *The Real World Guide To Psychotherapy Practice* (Cambridge, Mass.: Harvard University Press, 2000).

41. N. Muramatsu and T. Cornwell, "Needs for Physician Housecalls — Views from Health and Social Service Providers," *Home Health Care Service Quarterly* 22, no. 2 (2003): 17-29; "Doctors' Group Cuts Readmissions by Examining Patients in Homes," *Clinical Resources Management* 1, no. 7 (July 2000): 105-7.

42. An example of Byock's approach is this: He cites Cicely Saunders' statement, "we will do all we can to help you live until you die." I. Byock, "Patient Refusal of Nutrition and Hydration: Walking the Ever-Finer Line," *American Journal of Hospital Palliative Care* 12, no. 2 (March-April 1995): 9-13, p. 13; see also, I. Byock and J.S. Twohig, "Expanding the Realm of the Possible," *Journal of Palliative Medicine* 6, no. 2 (April 2003): 311-3; I. Byock, "The Meaning and Value of Death," *Journal of Palliative Medicine* 5, no. 2 (April 2002): 279-88; C.G. Davis et al., "Searching for Meaning in Loss: Are Clinical Assumptions Correct?" *Death Studies* 24, no. 6 (September 2000): 497-540; N. Friedman, "Godot and Gestalt: the Meaning of Meaninglessness," *American Journal of Psychoanalysis* 49, no. 3 (September 1989): 267-80; J.R. Peteet, "Putting Suffering into Perspective: Implications of the Patient's World View," *Journal of Psychotherapy Practice Research* 10, no. 3 (Summer 2001): 187-92; and D.P. Sulmasy, "Addressing the Religious and Spiritual Needs of Dying Patients," *Western Journal of Medicine* 175 (2001): 251- 4.

43. M.M. Linehan, *Cognitive-Behavioral Treatment of Borderline Personality Disorder* (New York: Guilford, 1993); see, also, C. Calarge, N.C. Andreasen, and D.S. O'Leary, "Visualizing How One Brain Understands Another: A PET Study of Theory of Mind," *American Journal of Psychiatry* 160 (2003): 1954-64.

44. V.A. Galloway and S.L. Brodsky, "Caring Less, Doing More: The Role of Therapeutic De-

tachment with Volatile and Unmotivated Clients," *American Journal of Psychotherapy* 57, no. 1 (2003): 32-8.

45. J.M. Curtis, "Determinants of the Therapeutic Bond: How to Engage Patients," *Psychological Reports* 49, no. 2 (October 1981): 415-9.

46. R. Lazar, "Presentness: an Intersubjective Dimension of the Therapeutic," *American Journal of Psychotherapy* 54, no. 3 (Summer 2000): 340-54.

47. L.E. Smeele and C.M. Van der Feltz Cornelis, "Professional Attitudes to Request for Secondary Facial Reconstruction in Patients Who Have Attempted Suicide," *British Journal of Oral Maxillofacial Surgery* 33, no. 4 (August 1995): 228-30; see, also, R.G. Poggi and R. Ganzarain, "Countertransference Hate," *Bulletin of the Menninger Clinic* 47, no. 1 (January 1983): 15-35.

48. K. Covinsky et al., "Communication and Decision-Making in Seriously Ill Patients: Findings of the SUPPORT project. The Study to Understand Prognoses and Preferences for Outcomes and Risks of Treatments," *Journal of the American Geriatric Society* 48, no. 5 (May 2000): S187-93; J.M. Teno et al., "Do Advance Directives Provide Instructions That Direct Care? SUPPORT Investigators. Study to Understand Prognoses and Preferences for Outcomes and Risks of Treatment," *Journal of the American Geriatric Society* 45, no. 4 (April 1997): 508-12.

49. C.E. Schneider, *The Practice of Autonomy* (New York: Oxford University Press, 1998).

50. S. Wear, S. Lagaipa, and G. Logue, "Toleration of Moral Diversity and the Conscientious Refusal by Physicians to Withdraw Life-Sustaining Treatment," *Journal of Medicine and Philosophy* 19, no. 2 (April 1994): 147-9.

51. Y. Sakakilhara et al., "Long-Term Ventilator Support in Patients with Werdnig-Hoffmann Disease," *Pediatric Institute* 42, no. 4 (August 2000): 359-63.

52. E.D. Pellegrino, "The Anatomy of Clinical-Ethical Judgments in Perinatology and Neonatology: A Substantive and Procedural Framework," *Seminars in Perinatology* 11 (1987): 202-9.

53. M.R. Wicclair, "Conscientious Objection in Medicine," *Bioethics* 14, no. 3 (July 2000): 205-27; J.K. Davis, "Conscientious Refusal and a Doctor's Right to Quit," *Journal of Medicine and Philosophy* 29, no. 1 (February 2004): 75-91; and E.M. Spencer, "Physician's Conscience and HECs: Friend or Foes?" *HEC Forum* 10, no. 1 (March

1998): 34-42.

54. J.C. Fletcher, "Is Sex Selection Ethical?" *Progress in Clinical and Biological Research* 128 (1983): 333-48; see also, D.C. Wertz and J.C. Fletcher, "Fatal Knowledge? Prenatal Diagnosis and Sex Selection," *Hastings Center Report* 19, no. 3 (May-June 1989): 21-7.

55. F. Moazam, "Feminist Discourse on Sex Screening and Selective Abortion of Female Fetuses," *Bioethics* 18, no. 3 (June 2004): 205-20.

56. R.M. Veatch and C.M. Spicer, "Futile Care: Physicians Should Not Be Allowed to Refuse to Treat," *Health Progress* 74, no. 10 (December 1993): 22-7; R.M. Veatch, "Who Should Manage Care? The Case for Patients," *Kennedy Institute of Ethics Journal* 7, no. 4 (December 1997): 391-401.

57. M.C. Bush and K.A. Eddleman, "Multifetal Pregnancy Reduction and Selective Termination," *Clinics in Perinatology* 30, no. 3 (September 2003): 623-41; A. Antsaklis et al., "Pregnancy Outcome After Multifetal Pregnancy Reduction," *Journal of Maternal Fetal Neonatal Medicine* 16, no. 1 (July 2004): 27-31; A. Bhide and B. Thilaganathan, "What Prenatal Diagnosis Should Be Offered in Multiple Pregnancy?" *Best Practice and Research: Clinical Obstetric and Gynecology* 18, no. 4 (August 2004): 431-42; and M.I. Evans et al., "Fetal Reduction from Twins to a Singleton: A Reasonable Consideration?" *Obstetrics and Gynecology* 104, no. 1 (July 2004): 102-9.

58. An example is the case of "Baby K," in which a mother's desire to continue treatment for her child who had anencephaly was brought to court. Though the baby's careproviders opposed continuing Baby K's treatment, the court required this. U.S. District Court, E.D. Virginia, Alexandria Division, *In re Baby K* 1; 832 (July 1993): 1022-31. For a different approach than going to court, see D. Inwald, I. Jakobitovits, and A. Petros, "Brain Stem Death: Managing Care When Accepted Medical Guidelines and Religious Beliefs Are In Conflict," *British Medical Journal* 320 (6 May 2000): 1266-7.

59. R.C. Hall, "Ethical and Legal Implications of Managed Care," *General Hospital of Psychiatry* 19, no. 3 (May 1997): 200-8; W.E. Ford, "Medical Necessity and Psychiatric Managed Care," *Psychiatry Clinics of North America* 23, no. 2 (2000): 309-17.

60. S. Bremberg et al., "GPs Facing Reluctant and Demanding Patients: Analyzing Ethical Justifications," *Family Practice* 20, no. 3 (June 2003):

254-61; K.L. Moseley, M.J. Silveira, and S.D. Goold, "Futility in Evolution," *Clinical Geriatric Medicine* 21, no. 1 (February 2005): 211-22; M. Wreen, "Medical Futility and Physician Discretion," *Journal of Medical Ethics* 30, no. 3 (June 2004): 275-8; D.L. Kasman, "When is Medical Treatment Futile?" *Journal of General Internal Medicine* 19, no. 10 (October 2004): 1053-6; and A. Brooks et al., "Emergency Surgery in Patients in Extremis from Blunt Torso Injury: Heroic Surgery or Futile Care?" *Emergency Medicine Journal* 21, no. 4 (July 2004): 483-6.

61. E.F. Wijdicks and A.A. Rabinstein, "Absolutely No Hope? Some Ambiguity of Futility of Care in Devastating Acute Stroke," *Critical Care Medicine* 32, no. 11 (November 2004): 2332-42.

62. R.M. Veatch, "Forgoing Life-Sustaining Treatment: Limits to the Consensus. Part 2," *Kennedy Institute of Ethics Journal* 3, no. 1 (1993): 1-19; R.M. Veatch and W.E. Stempsey, "Incommensurability: Its Implications for the Patient/Physician Relation," *Journal of Medicine and Philosophy* 20, no. 3 (June 1995): 253-69.

63. K. Capen, "Findings of Negligence Followed Communication Lapses in BC Aneurysm Case," *Canadian Medical Association Journal* 156, no. 1 (January 1997): 49-51; H.L. Hirsh, "Patient Abandonment," *Urban Health* 14, no. 3 (March 1985): 36-41; and M.H. Kottow, "Vulnerability: What Kind of Principle is It?" *Medicine, Health Care, and Philosophy* 7, no. 3 (2004): 281-7.

64. T.F. Dagi, "Physicians and Obligatory Social Activism," *Journal of Medical Humanities and Bioethics* 9, no. 1 (Spring-Summer 1988): 50-9.

65. D. Mechanic, "Socio-Cultural Implications of Changing Organizational Technologies in the Provision of Care," *Social Science and Medicine* 54, no. 3 (February 2002): 459-67.

66. J.D. Hess, "Gadow's Relational Narrative: An Elaboration," *Nursing Philosophy* 4, no. 2 (July 2003): 137-48.2

12

Death and Dying

Charles A. Hite and Mary Faith Marshall

I. INTRODUCTION

Three problems face all clinicians who care for terminally ill patients: defining death, relieving suffering and pain, and delivering bad news. This chapter examines how those problems have been addressed in a society in which issues surrounding death and dying are always prominent and increasingly more controversial.

The success of modern medicine in preserving life brought with it a fundamental transformation in our society's attitude toward death. The lifesaving technologies and treatments used to stave off death frequently result in a more agonizing end of life. The power to prolong life too often brings more horror than hope. It is not uncommon for suffering to result from not only the cause of disease, but also from its treatment. The wisdom of our struggle to gain dominion over death is being questioned. Because the process of fighting death often makes life more unbearable, many choose to embrace death and reject life-sustaining technology.

The demographics of death have changed.[1] The median age at death in the United States is now 77 years, while in 1900, life expectancy at birth was less than 50 years. There has been an enormous increase in the number and health of the elderly, so that, by the year 2030, 20 percent of the U.S. population will be over the age of 65.

Of the approximately 2.5 million people who die each year, only 55,000 of them are children, while 80 percent are Medicare beneficiaries.

The cause of death has changed. At the turn of the twentieth century, death typically followed an acute infection or an accident. At the turn of the twenty-first century, the leading causes of death are chronic diseases such as heart disease, cancer, and stroke. As a result, death now is more of a process than an event, unfolding over months or even years.[2]

The place of death has changed. We no longer die among family and friends; more often, we die among strangers. In 1950, 63 percent of Americans died at home. Today, nearly 80 percent take their last breath in a hospital or long-term care facility.[3] This shift in the venue of death has been accompanied by a change in the relationship between patients and doctors. In the not-too-distant past, most patients were seen by a family doctor — a practitioner who had a limited range of options, but who had intimate knowledge of the patient's history and values. Today we live in an age of specialists. In the hospital setting, in particular, highly trained practitioners often have sporadic, fragmented relationships with patients. They may see not the whole patient, but only the particular pathology treated. Their very specialized and technical knowledge is intended to conquer disease and death, and can lead patients to demand treatment and expect cure. Stopping treatment and accepting death can be seen as tantamount to admitting defeat.

Changes in medical technology have fundamentally altered the once-simple act of declaring a person dead. "Ours will go down as the era that reinvented death," says ethicist Nancy Dubler; "the motivation was the ability to transplant organs."[4] Even in cases of massive brain damage, Dubler notes, organ systems can be maintained for days or weeks. But without an intact brain to regulate them, organs will deteriorate and be unsuitable for transplant. The mere beating of the heart and breathing of the lungs have become an inadequate measure of what constitutes life. The evolution of the concept of brain death will be explored in the second section of this chapter.

The paradox of modern medicine, that treatment intended to save life often ends up prolonging the agony of dying, has spurred a national dialogue about how the dying are treated in this country. The hospice movement — with its holistic approach to treating the body, mind, and spirit of the terminally ill — became more entrenched and helped spawn interest by health professionals and the public in the value of "comfort care" or "palliative care" for all seriously ill patients and their families. The growth of the end-of-life movement and the problems it faces is the topic of the third section of this chapter.

While proponents of hospice and palliative care argue the case that pain and suffering at the end of life can be managed if certain precepts are embraced by the healthcare system, the debate over physician-assisted suicide and euthanasia has been the result. Some family members, frustrated by the medical system's inability to relieve the suffering of loved ones, have been moved to take the life of someone close to them. Some physicians have defied the law and acknowledge their assistance in the deaths of a patient. Some states have held referenda on physician-assisted suicide, and one state has legalized its practice. Two controversial court cases about assisted-suicide have reached the U.S. Supreme Court. Although some view the withdrawing and withholding of life-sustaining treatment as "passive euthanasia," a consensus has emerged over the last decade that such a practice is ethical and legal. Ethical problems surrounding the forgoing of life-sustaining treatment are addressed in chapter 13. In sections four and five of this chapter, we examine the history and court cases associated with assisted-sui-

cide in this country, and in section six we look at the system of euthanasia in the Netherlands.

Discussing death and goals of care at the end of life is challenging, even for the most experienced clinician. Physicians tend to be reluctant to bring up the subject of death, and to be overly optimistic about a patient's prognosis. Sections seven and eight of this chapter build on the work of a noted psychiatrist, Robert Buckman, regarding how to talk with patients or family members when disclosing "bad news."

II. DEFINING DEATH

Until the last 30 years or so, determining whether a person was dead was a relatively simple matter. Reflecting an earlier era when most people died at home, popular guidance was available to family members to assist them in the determination of a relative's death. In *The Old Person in Your Home,* William Poe described the signs of death: "The eyes become fixed, with opened pupils which do not respond to light. The heartbeat and breathing cease. The mouth may be open and motionless. The skin turns pale and cold. The skin in contact with the bed may become bluish or purple — liver mortis. After thirty to sixty minutes the limp extremities may become stiff — rigor mortis."[5]

The cessation of breathing and the absence of an audible heartbeat or a pulse have been death-defining criteria throughout most of history. As in all aspects of medicine, some room for error in the diagnosis of death existed in earlier times, especially prior to the advent of the stethoscope. During the Middle Ages, observers occasionally reported evidence that an individual, assumed to be dead, had been buried alive. The discovery of scratch marks on the inside of coffin lids of exhumed skeletons led to such extraordinary precautions as round-the-clock mortuary attendants who frequently assessed their charges for any signs of life, ropes reaching from buried coffins to an above-ground bell that could be heard by cemetery attendants, and speaking tubes leading from coffins to the ground above, so that the cemetery attendant could be summoned should a corpse "awaken."

Modern technology such as the electrocardiogram, which provides an electrical "picture" of heart activity, makes the definition of death via heart/lung criteria essentially infallible. Defining death using the criteria of cessation of heartbeat and breathing, and the absence of a pulse or blood flow is, in essence, a whole-body orientation toward death. This approach to defining death has its roots in Western Judeo-Christian theological tradition. By traditional Jewish standards, death occurred when an individual drew his or her last breath. The Roman Catholic religion, recognizing the soul as encompassed by all of the body, held to the broader heart/lung criteria.[6]

Until recently, American common law also recognized a whole-body definition of death. In 1968, *Black's Law Dictionary* defined death as "the cessation of life; the ceasing to exist; defined by physicians as a total stoppage of the circulation of the blood, and a cessation of the animal and vital functions consequent thereon, such as respiration, pulsation, etc."[7]

The whole-body concept of death, which had historically sufficed as a standard, became inadequate in the 1960s for a number of reasons. The development of intensive care units (ICUs) and their attendant technologies allowed for the biological maintenance of persons who previously would have died by heart/lung criteria. Occasional legal cases begged the question of the timing of death using heart/lung criteria when order of survivorship was at issue.[8]

The capacity of ICUs to temporarily maintain patients who had lost complete brain function fueled a theoretical debate regarding biological death. The advent of organ transplantation accelerated the debate for pragmatic reasons. Patients who had lost total brain function, including neocortex and brain-stem function, could be biologically maintained on artificial life support for only a period of days before all of the other organ systems subsequently failed. The opportunities that patients who were brain dead presented, as potential sources of organs for transplant, occasioned serious reconsideration of the theoretical and legal definitions of death.

In 1968, the Ad Hoc Committee of the Harvard Medical School to Examine the Definition of Brain Death explored this conceptual issue, and subsequently published a report in the *Journal of the American Medical Association* endorsing a whole-brain (versus a whole-body) definition of death.[9] Its criteria for determining brain death included:

1. Coma, demonstrated by total unreceptivity and unresponsitivity to stimuli;
2. Absence of spontaneous breathing, given a normal carbon dioxide range;
3. Absence of reflexes, given the absence of any

neurologically depressant medications;
4. A flat or isoelectric electroencephalogram (picture of the electrical activity of the brain).[10]

During the 1970s, some 20 states passed statutes that adopted the whole-brain definition of death. In 1975, the American Bar Association even went so far as to propose that whole-brain function be the sole criterion for determining death.[11] Although a few states passed statutes based on this recommendation, its future was foreshortened. In 1981, the President's Commission for the Study of Ethical Problems in Medicine and Biomedical and Behavioral Research proposed a Uniform Determination of Death Act, which endorsed both whole-body (heart/lung) and whole-brain definitions of death. The commission's report stated, "An individual who has sustained either (1) irreversible cessation of circulatory and respiratory functions, or (2) irreversible cessation of all functions of the entire brain, including the brain stem, is dead."[12]

The central thesis behind this conceptual orientation was that the failure of other organ systems (including the heart and lungs) inevitably followed whole-brain death within a relatively short period, and that, with the loss of either whole-brain or heart/lung function, the breakdown of all other bodily functions would shortly follow.

The current theoretical and conceptual debate regarding the definition of death centers on brain function alone. The controversy is framed by the level of brain function (whole-brain versus partial-brain) that is necessary to sustain what might be called "life." The conceptual inquiry no longer involves merely biological questions, but includes the philosophical issue of *personhood.*

The evolution of our concept of death was triggered by the existence of patients who are in states of permanent unconsciousness (particularly patients who are in a "persistent vegetative state" or PVS). Patients in a PVS have suffered the permanent loss of higher cortical brain function; their brain stem, which regulates spontaneous vegetative functions such as breathing and sleep/wake cycles and digestion, continues to function. Patients in a PVS are capable of involuntary movements (for example, eye opening or yawning). They lack any mechanism for sensory input or feeling, lack self-awareness or awareness of their surroundings, and are incontinent. Given adequate maintenance care — including feeding and hydration via nasogastric or gastrostomy tubes, frequent turning to prevent bedsores, physical therapy to prevent contractions, and antibiotics to treat pulmonary infections — the patients can live for years or decades.

The intrinsic horror that many in the general public feel about continued biological existence in a state of permanent unconsciousness such as PVS has escalated the debate regarding the definition of death. The question arises whether human life is defined simply in biological terms, or whether its definition extends to personal qualities such as consciousness and self-awareness. No general consensus exists on this issue among philosophers, clinicians, or laypersons. The issue of whether the definition of death should be extended to cover patients who are in a PVS depends on how one personally views life and death. Some argue that the question is pragmatically moot, because maintenance care can be legally and ethically withdrawn from PVS patients, who will then subsequently "die."

Guidelines for the determination of brain death in newborn infants have evolved more slowly than for adults, due to clinical difficulties in making accurate neurological assessments. In infants carried to full term who are less than seven days old, severe neurological injuries may be reversible; the cause of coma is often difficult to establish and may be reversible; and clinical signs (such as fixed and dilated pupils) may be the result of metabolic imbalances, hypothermia, sedative drugs, or other remedial conditions. The American Academy of Pediatrics (AAP) Task Force for the Determination of Brain Death in Children published guidelines in 1987 that preclude the diagnosis of brain death in premature infants or in full-term infants less than seven days old.[13] Most of the criteria for determining brain death in full-term infants are similar to those used for adults.

Determining brain death in anencephalic infants has, as yet, proved to be impossible. Anencephaly is a clinical condition in which an infant's membranous skull and the cerebral hemispheres of the brain are absent. The degree of brain-stem development may vary. Anencephalic infants are generally stillborn or die within a few days after birth.[14] The inability to declare brain death in these infants often poses a difficult problem for parents who wish to donate their anencephalic child's organs, seeing this "gift" as a possibly positive aspect in an otherwise tragic situation.

Patients who have been diagnosed as brain dead but who are being maintained on life supports often pose special problems for family members who may have difficulty conceptualizing the fact that their relative is dead when they see the patient's chest rise and fall from mechanical ventilation and when a cardiac tracing is visible on an electrocardiogram monitor. General clinical wisdom dictates that once the diagnosis of brain death has been made, all artificial life supports should be withdrawn, and the family should be notified that the patient has died.

III. SUFFERING AND COMFORT

Frequently, clinicians who treat terminally ill patients are reluctant to abandon their traditional role of curing the patient and fighting for life. They may be ill-equipped to deal with the complex and idiosyncratic factors that enter into the suffering of patients. They may refuse to recognize that in the care of dying patients, all other goals take a back seat to the relief of suffering. One of the guiding principles of what has come to be called comfort care or palliative care is that physicians and other clinicians no longer accept suffering as a necessary evil.

Eric Cassell, a physician and bioethicist who has written extensively on care for the dying, emphasizes that suffering involves more than pain:

> Suffering occurs when an impending destruction of the person is perceived; it continues until the threat of disintegration has passed or until the integrity of the person can be restored in some other manner. It follows, then, that although it often occurs in the presence of acute pain, shortness of breath or other bodily symptoms, suffering extends beyond the physical. Most generally, suffering can be defined as the state of severe distress associated with events that threaten the intactness of the person.[15]

Such events arise from a variety of factors that go into what makes up a person, Cassell notes. This includes relationships with family and friends, cultural background, sexuality, self-esteem, physical traits, skills and abilities, important memories, and even previous experiences with healthcare providers.

Hospice care has led the way in addressing the suffering of the dying and hopelessly ill. Hospice care not only focuses on alleviating physical pain, but it also addresses the complex and highly personal factors that cause suffering. The modern hospice movement began in 1967 with the founding of St. Christopher's Hospice in England by Cicely Saunders, MD. The cornerstones of hospice treatment, as defined by Saunders, are effective control of pain and other symptoms, care of the patient and family as a unit, an interdisciplinary team approach, the use of volunteers, a continuum of care that includes care at home, continuity of care between different settings, and follow up with family members after the patient's death. Hospice enrollment in the U.S. grew from 1,000 admissions in 1975 to more than 700,000 in 2000.[16]

Hospice care has been a major influence on how traditional medical care addresses the relief of pain, one of the major fears of dying patients. Hospice clinicians established the importance of administering medication on a regular schedule so that there would be "constant control" of "constant pain."[17] Hospice clinicians also pioneered and promoted the use of continuous or intermittent parenteral narcotics and patient-controlled analgesia, and their experience indicates that addiction to pain medication is not a concern in terminally ill patients. The hospice movement has been a leader in responding to the spiritual and social aspects of suffering for the dying. Hospice careproviders recognized the importance of patients' fears of loss of control and loneliness and abandonment.[18]

Despite the great strides made by hospice in developing the precepts of good care at the end of life, the treatment of the vast majority of the dying in America continues to be woefully inadequate. Beginning in the mid-1990s, a series of studies and initiatives sought to identify barriers to treatment of the dying and to suggest methods to improve end-of-life care.

In November 1995, the *Journal of the American Medical Association* published disturbing findings of the Study to Understand Prognoses and Preferences for Outcomes and Risks of Treatments (SUPPORT). The eight-year-study involved 10,000 critically ill patients at five leading medical institutions. The objective of the study was to improve end-of-life decision making and reduce the frequency of a prolonged, painful process of dying. A major intervention of the study was to make sure physicians received estimates of the likelihood of patients' survival, the outcomes of CPR, and functional disability. The study also used specially trained nurses to encourage the use of pain control; promote advance-care planning; improve the understanding of patients' outcomes; and facilitate communication between patients, families, physicians, and hospital staff.[19]

The SUPPORT study only reported that end-of-life care for seriously ill hospitalized patients was poor, even with its interventions to promote better care.

Patients in the study experienced considerable pain: one half of patients who died had moderate or severe pain during most of their final 3 days of life. Communication between physicians and patients was poor: only 41 percent of patients in the study reported talking to their physicians about prognosis or about cardiopulmonary resuscitation (CPR). Physicians misunderstood patients' preferences regarding CPR in 80 percent of cases. Furthermore, physicians did not implement patients' refusals of interventions. When patients wanted CPR withheld, a do-not-resuscitate (DNR) order was never written in about 50 percent of cases.[20]

The SUPPORT study touched off analysis and debate in the healthcare community about what could be done to improve end-of-life care in the U.S. Some critics suggested that an intervention that relied on nurses to facilitate discussion was doomed in a system dominated by physicians. Others claimed that the study revealed the difficulty in having patients make clear choices in an emotionally charged situation in which the prognosis, although grave, was still uncertain. Still others noted that the study pointed out that the culture of the American system of healthcare is geared toward aggressive treatment. Some commentators noted that the study exposed the reticence of physicians to talk with patients about their illnesses and a fundamental ambivalence in American medicine and American culture about the place of death in human life.[21]

In response to the problems identified in the SUPPORT study, the Robert Wood Johnson Foundation awarded major grants in 1997 to two organizations dedicated to improving end-of-life care in profoundly different ways. One grant established the Education for Physicians on End-of-Life

Care (EPEC) Project to develop a standardized core curriculum to train physicians to care for dying patients and their families. EPEC, an initiative of the American Medical Association's Institute for Ethics, focuses on improving physicians' skills in communication, ethical decision making, pain and symptom management, and psychosocial assessment. EPEC uses train-the-trainer conferences and distance learning as mechanisms to expose physicians around the country to the curriculum.

A second grant went to a coalition of more than 80 health and consumer organizations to launch an initiative called Last Acts: Care and Caring at the End of Life. By 2004, Last Acts had grown to a coalition of more than 1,200 national, state, and local organizations. To that point, Last Acts had published several major reports identifying weaknesses and promoting improvement in end-of-life care; it funded 21 community-state end-of-life partnerships and supported the development of hundreds of community-based end-of-life coalitions. Activities of the partnerships and coalitions took place in five broad areas:
1. Expanding reimbursement mechanisms for hospice and palliative care,
2. Improving pain and symptom management,
3. Promoting higher standards for training health professionals in end-of-life care,
4. Educating policy makers and the public about the need for good advance-care planning, and
5. Establishing quality indicators for pain management and palliative care.[22]

A Last Acts task force outlined the precepts and principles of palliative care in a report issued in late 1997. The task force report stated,

Palliative care refers to the comprehensive management of the physical, psychological, social, spiritual and existential needs of patients. It is especially suited to the care of people with incurable, progressive illnesses. . . . The goal of palliative care is to achieve the best possible quality of life through relief of suffering, control of symptoms and restoration of functional capacity while remaining sensitive to personal, cultural and religious values, beliefs and practices.[23]

All clinicians should be familiar with the fundamental precepts of palliative care, the report maintained. These precepts call for respecting patients' goals and choices, using an interdisci-plinary team to provide patients with comprehensive care, and providing support to family caregivers.

A 1997 Institute of Medicine (IOM) report underscored the shortcomings of the American healthcare system in caring for the dying. Too many people experienced needless suffering and distress at the end of life, according to the report, *Approaching Death: Improving Care at the End of Life.*[24] Some suffering was caused when healthcare providers offered care that was clinically inappropriate or even harmful. In other instances, suffering resulted when providers failed to provide palliative or supportive care that was known to be effective, the report said.

Patients with acquired immunodeficiency syndrome (AIDS), cancer, and other chronic, life-threatening illnesses were inadequately treated for pain, despite the existence of prescription opiates or other drugs and interventions that could have relieved their pain, according to the IOM report. It called for reform of burdensome and scientifically outdated drug-prescribing laws. In addition, the authors of *Approaching Death* called for changes in undergraduate, graduate, and continuing education to ensure that healthcare practitioners obtained relevant knowledge and skills to care well for dying patients. Physicians' training focuses on acute illness and heroic rescues with little emphasis on how to assess and manage pain and other symptoms at the end of life, the report claimed. It called for recognizing the emerging field of palliative care as a defined area of teaching, research, and clinical expertise. The report also pointed to an inadequate system of funding healthcare — in which incentives discourage treatment of people with chronic, serious illnesses — as part of the reason for poor end-of-life care in the U.S. It encouraged reform of healthcare financing to reward, rather than frustrate, coordinated systems of care for the seriously ill and dying.[25]

The American public got an up-close look at the movement to improve the problems that surround end-of-life care when the U.S. Public Broadcasting System (PBS) aired a four-part series in September 2000 entitled "On Our Own Terms: Moyers on Dying." In the series, veteran journalist Bill Moyers engaged in intimate interviews with more than a dozen dying individuals and their families, as well as with pioneering health practitioners in hospice and palliative care. The series was watched by an estimated 19 million viewers, and was promoted by more than 70 national, consumer, medical, and professional organizations. As a result, more than 250 local end-of-life coalitions around the country hosted town hall meetings to discuss ways to improve care for the dying.

About the same time, a national initiative designed to promote palliative care programs in hospitals was launched. The Center to Advance Palliative Care (CAPC), funded by the Robert Wood Johnson Foundation, provides healthcare professionals with training, tools, and technical assistance needed to start and sustain palliative care programs. Professionals from hundreds of hospitals and healthcare organizations have attended CAPC national and regional conferences that are designed to provide a core curriculum in palliative care. In the late 1990s, only a handful of hospital-based palliative care programs were in existence. By the end of 2002, more than 800 hospitals in the U.S. provided palliative services to their patients. In 2003, CAPC funded six palliative care leadership centers at hospitals across the country. Interdisciplinary teams from nearly 1,500 hospitals and other healthcare organizations were expected to visit the centers to study palliative care in practice and to establish long-term mentoring relationships.[26]

Proponents of hospital-based palliative care argue that the quality of care provided to the growing population of patients with serious, advanced and complex illnesses must improve. These patients will experience multiple chronic illnesses over a period of years, and need a system of care that can coordinate both the episodic and long-term nature of these illnesses. These are patients that don't fit the criteria for the Medicare hospice benefit, which was developed to care for dying persons with a six-month prognosis and a decision to forgo life-prolonging care. "We need to uncover palliative care from death and dying," states Diana Meier, MD, Director of CAPC and Director of the Hertzberg Palliative Care Institute at Mount Sinai School of Medicine. "Every patient needs this kind of care. The patient does not have to be in the throes of terminal illness and does not have to forgo life-prolonging treatment. Palliative care is optimal medical care for sick people, whether they will live for 10 days or 10 years."[27]

Hospitals are the single most important place for patients to access palliative care, according to CAPC, because the most severely ill patients are found in hospitals, the most money is spent in hospitals, and hospitals are the best place to plan for the next stage of care. Hospitals with palliative care programs report that they help patients transition to more appropriate levels of care, which can reduce the length of stay for many patients, especially those in the ICU. Palliative programs also help hospitals reduce costs by cutting redundant, unnecessary, or ineffective tests and drugs.[28]

Despite growing interest in and the growing number of palliative care programs, major barriers still existed five years after the IOM report called for drastic reform in end-of-life care. A Last Acts "report card," released late in 2002, gave each U.S. state letter grades on eight key elements of end-of-life care and concluded America was doing a mediocre job — at best. The report cited confusing language and bureaucratic hurdles in state advance directive laws and a disturbing decline in average length of stay in hospice to well below the 60 days considered necessary for people to receive maximum benefit. It found that nearly half of the 1.6 million Americans living in nursing homes have persistent pain that is not noticed and is inadequately treated. It concluded that training physicians and nurses about palliative care lagged far behind the needs of the U.S. population; it pointed to state laws that create formidable barriers to adequate pain management; it stated that spiritual and cultural issues for dying patients and families were not being well addressed.

"Changing the way America cares for the dying amounts to no less than a major social change," said Steven Schroeder, MD, President of the Robert Wood Johnson Foundation, which funded a report, "Means to a Better End: A Report on Dying in America Today."[29] He continues, "As this report points out, although we have begun making progress on many fronts, today we find ourselves at a crossroads. We need the dedicated support of policy makers and healthcare leaders to put us on a path to establishing end-of-life care once and for all as an integral part of American medicine." Of the many problems cited in the Last Acts report, and in other studies of end-of-life care, three consistently emerge as being the keys to bringing about fundamental reform:

1. Inadequate treatment of pain,
2. Barriers to hospice care, and
3. Recognizing and addressing cultural differences.

A. Inadequate Pain Treatment

Failure to treat pain has been well documented in the medical literature, in marked contrast to the relief of suffering, one of the core values in healthcare. A 1973 medical journal article that reported on a study of in-patients at two New York hospitals noted that most patients received inadequate pain relief because of physicians' ignorance of effective doses of narcotic analgesics, and their exaggerated fears of the risk of addiction, even in patients who were terminally ill. More than 30 years later, physicians' ignorance of pain relief and unwarranted fear of addiction persists.[30]

Regulatory policies and fear of legal sanction are said to unduly influence physicians' use of opioid analgesics. One critic claims state medical licensing boards have been "co-opted" to help carry out the mission of the federal Drug Enforcement Agency "to root out all physicians who inappropriately prescribe or divert controlled substances, while demonstrating little or no concern for the patient who suffers from undertreatment of their pain because physicians are intimidated by the regulatory scrutiny that attends an aggressive approach to pain management."[31] Some flawed state policies inhibit appropriate relief of pain because they:

• Imply that opiates be used only as a last resort,
• Place limits on prescribing and dispensing,
• Forbid substance abusers from being treated with opiates, or
• Require doctors to use special prescription forms for pain medications.[32]

Many states are taking action to improve laws and regulations regarding pain treatment, including adopting model guidelines on the use of opiates in pain management promoted by the Federation of State Medical Boards. These guidelines accept the medical legitimacy of opiates, reject the amount and length of prescribing pain medication as indicators of good or bad medical practice, and allow physicians to deviate from the guidelines if good cause is shown. Other steps that states can take to create a more favorable environment for pain management include:

1. Require state-supported medical schools and teaching hospitals to have better and more accurate pain management information in curricula,
2. Provide funding and support for cancer pain initiatives,
3. Guarantee Medicaid funding of pain management and palliative care in a variety of settings,
4. Make sure a pain management expert sits on the state medical board, and
5. Encourage professional and trade associations to promote pain management.[33]

Regulatory and licensing agencies as well as professional groups can work to bring about better pain management. In the late 1990s, more than 30 leaders of national nursing organizations endorsed assessing pain as the "fifth vital sign." At about the same time, the Joint Commission on the Accreditation of Healthcare Organizations (JCAHO) released standards for pain assessment and treatment that must be met by hospitals and home care, ambulatory care, and behavioral health facilities.

B. Barriers to the Delivery of Hospice Care

Despite the institution of hospice as a Medicare benefit in the early 1980s, more than one million Americans die each year without receiving the hospice or hospice-type services that could benefit them and their families.[34] There are other indications that hospice has failed to thrive in the U.S. For instance:

• The average Medicare hospice patient's length of stay decreased from 70 days at the inception of the hospice benefit, in 1983, to about 36 days in 2000.
• More than half of hospice patients are enrolled in hospice for less than 25 days, and more than one-quarter stay less than one week.
• From 1998 to 2002, nearly one-and-a-half times as many hospices went out of business annually as opened their doors.
• Statistics indicate that those who eventually receive hospice usually suffer too long from uncontrolled pain and symptoms before they are referred.
• More than 80 percent of people who are eligible for Medicare don't know it offers a hospice benefit.[35]

Inadequate funding has long been cited as a major barrier to the delivery of hospice care. While more than one-fourth of Medicare spending goes toward end-of-life care, spending for the Medicare hospice benefit totals less than 1 percent of Medicare's annual budget. Increasing the per diem reimbursement that hospices receive to manage the care of patients is necessary for hospices to provide all the services patients need; for example, one estimate puts the average per-patient-per-day cost of drugs for hospice patients at $15, while the daily medication allowance in the hospice benefit is $2.48.[36]

Another concern is the six-month prognosis requirement of the hospice Medicare benefit. Physicians who refer patients to hospice must certify that they believe the patient has six months or less to live if the underlying disease follows its expected course. During the 1990s, the federal government instituted antifraud campaigns that required some hospices to repay millions of dollars in reimbursements for patients who outlived the six-month prognosis. As a result, some hospice programs, fearing denial of reimbursement, began denying access to patients who might stay so long that they would bring regulatory scrutiny. The six-month prognosis certification has also led some physicians to delay referring patients to hospice.[37]

Hospices also encounter a number of problems when they try to care for dying persons who reside in a nursing home. Medicare will reimburse nursing facilities for nursing home residents' room and board under the Skilled Nursing Facility (SNF) Benefit. But when nursing home residents with Medicare enroll in hospice, they become responsible for their own room and board costs. This arrangement creates an incentive for terminally ill patients who are discharged from hospitals to choose the Medicare SNF benefit instead of the Medicare hospice benefit. It also creates an incentive for nursing homes to keep residents off the hospice benefit and send them back to the hospital. For nursing home residents who are eligible for both Medicare and Medicaid benefits, Medicare will pay for hospice costs and Medicaid will pay room and board at 95 percent of the nursing home's rate. This forces hospices to pay the remaining 5 percent out of their pockets.[38]

C. The Importance of Culture

The ability to find meaning in illness, suffering, and death is profoundly influenced by the culture of the patient and the culture of caregivers. Changes in the population of ethnic groups in the U.S. make it more likely that health professionals will care for patients and families who have cultural backgrounds different than their own. Good end-of-life care can be compromised when careproviders fail to understand the cultural context of decisions made by patients and families.[39] *Culture* can be defined as "a shared world view and way of living developed by a society and transmitted from one generation to another. Culture evolves over time, influenced by a people's history, environment, social status, religion and experience."[40] Care must be taken to avoid stereotyping the beliefs and values of a cultural group, which can lead caregivers to believe it possible to know what a patient wants or thinks simply because they know what members of the patient's cultural group tend to want or think. A wide variation of beliefs and behaviors may exist within any ethnic or cultural group.[41]

Physicians and other health professionals need to develop appropriate attitudes and skills to navigate an increasingly diverse patient population, which have been called *cultural sensitivity* and *cultural competence*. Careproviders who demonstrate cultural sensitivity are aware of how culture shapes the values and beliefs of their patients, and respectfully acknowledge that differences exist between themselves and their patients. Further, health professionals must be nonjudgmental toward unfamiliar beliefs and practices, and be willing to negotiate when these beliefs and practices create conflict. Health professionals who demonstrate cultural competence have a sound knowledge base about patients' cultural beliefs and also have the skills necessary to communicate with their patients.[42]

Cultural insensitivity can be found in one model of care in Western medicine that emphasizes individual self-determination and total disclosure about illness and treatment options. This approach can be in direct conflict with the values of minority cultural groups, who may consider it bad luck to discuss death, or disrespectful to not have a patient's family involved in making decisions about end-of-life treatment.[43] Careproviders can explore end-of-life cultural influences by using the mnemonic "ABCDE" to evaluate patients' and families'

- Attitudes,
- Beliefs,
- Context,
- Decision-making style, and
- Environment.

In this scheme, "A" involves looking at what attitudes an ethnic group in general, and the patient and family in particular, have toward disclosure diagnosis and prognosis. "B" involves assessing the patient's and family's religious beliefs, especially those relating to the meaning of death, the afterlife, and the possibility of miracles. "C" relates to looking at the historical and political context of the patient's and family's lives, including place of birth, refugee and immigration status, poverty, and experience with discrimination or lack of access to care. "D" assesses the decision-making styles held by the ethnic group in general, and the patient and family in particular. "E" refers to religious and community organizations that can help interpret the significance of cultural dimensions of a case.[44]

IV. EUTHANASIA AND PHYSICIAN-ASSISTED SUICIDE

Euthanasia, the intentional taking of another life to promote a "good" or merciful death, can be traced as far back as the ancient Greeks and Romans, who did not believe that all life is precious and should be preserved at any cost. The prevailing belief was that life, without a chance for a meaningful or happy existence, had little value. The Spartans, for example, put deformed infants to death. Athenians permitted the destruction of unhealthy or deformed infants. It was morally acceptable to assist those with an incurable disease, who were in great pain, to end their life.[45]

The moral views of Judaism and Christianity provide the foundation for the modern Western concept of the sanctity of life. Jewish theologians teach that helping terminally ill persons to die is wrong. In the early Christian church, taking a human life in any way was absolutely forbidden. Suffering had meaning; in both Judaism and Christianity, suffering allows the individual to identify with the suffering of others and to share a connection with the larger human community; in this way, persons can transcend pain and derive meaning from suffering. Gradually, the Christian church altered its prohibition against taking life to allow killing in a just war or to lawfully execute a criminal. The guiding principle is that the intentional killing of an innocent human is wrong. An emphasis on *intent* allowed the development of the "doctrine of double-effect," which means that an act that has both good and bad consequences can be carried out, as long as certain conditions are met; in the care of a terminally ill patient who is in terrible pain, for example, this doctrine permits physicians to administer dosages of pain-relieving drugs so large that they might unintentionally hasten the death of the patient.[46]

It is against this background that the debate over euthanasia in modern medical history has occurred. During most of the nineteenth century, physicians generally refused to help incurably ill and dying patients end their lives. Napoleon's physician, for instance, refused the general's request to give a fatal dose of drugs to several mortally ill soldiers who were unable to march and likely to fall into enemy hands. The composer, Hector Berlioz, complained bitterly about the refusal of physicians to end the life of an older sister, who died of breast cancer after six months of excruciating pain:

> My other sister, who went to Grenoble to nurse her, and who did not leave her till the end, all but died from the fatigue and the painful impressions caused by this slow agony. And not a doctor dared to have the humanity to end this martyrdom by making my sister inhale a bottle of chloroform. . . . The most horrible thing in the world for us, living and sentient beings, is inexorable suffering, pain without any possible compensation when it has reached this degree of intensity; and one must be barbarous, or stupid, or both at once, not to use the sure and easy means now at our disposal to bring it to an end. Savages are more intelligent and more humane.[47]

By the turn of the twentieth century, however, physicians and laypersons began to call on the medical profession to relax its rigid stance in the treatment of terminally ill patients and patients with incurable disease. Four therapeutic approaches were identified. The first and second applied to patients who were near death. The third and fourth applied to patients who had painful, incurable illness. These approaches continue to shape the euthanasia debate today; they are:

1. The physician could do everything possible to make terminally ill patients as fulfilled and as free from pain as possible. Nothing could be offered, however, that would hasten death.
2. Physicians could take steps to alleviate suffering, even if they jeopardized the patient's life in the process.
3. The physician could withdraw active therapy

that was simply prolonging the patient's suffering. However, the physician was not to abandon the patient.

4. Physicians had the moral right to terminate purposely the life of a patient who suffered from an incurable and agonizing disease and who wanted to die.[48]

The last approach has dominated the debate in recent years over just how far physicians should go in dealing with the requests of incurably ill patients to end their suffering.

In the 1930s in England, the Voluntary Euthanasia Legalization Society was formed to promote the legalization of painless death. The organization presented a bill to Parliament that proposed allowing euthanasia if the candidate was more than 21 years old and suffered from an incurable disorder that involved severe pain. It required a formal written application, certified by two witnesses, to be sent to a referee who was to review the request and interview the patient. If permission was granted, someone other than the patient's doctor was to carry out the euthanasia.[49]

In the U.S., a group of prominent clergymen who later formed the Euthanasia Society of America proposed that it should be legal for "incurable sufferers to choose immediate death rather than await it in agony." In 1938, the founder and chairman of the group, Charles Potter, a Unitarian minister, said that such a choice was necessary to preserve human dignity. According to Potter, "The problem of euthanasia is one which sooner or later confronts every practicing physician. Perhaps the time has come to forget the Commandment 'Thou Shalt Not Kill,' and listen to Jesus 'Blessed Are the Merciful.' There is no logical argument against euthanasia. Most opposition is based on misunderstanding of the proposed procedure."[50]

In the more than half a century since Potter made that statement, the conflict over euthanasia has continued. In 1988, an article in the *Journal of the American Medical Association* touched off a new round of debate over when, if ever, to hasten a patient's death.

A. "Debbie's" Case

In early 1988, an unsigned article in the *Journal of the American Medical Association* presented a first-person account of a gynecology resident who gave a lethal dose of morphine to a 20-year-old woman who was suffering from ovarian cancer. She had not responded to chemotherapy and was being given supportive care only. The resident described an emaciated, hollow-eyed patient suffering from severe air hunger and unrelenting vomiting. "Debbie" had not eaten or slept in two days. Her only words to the resident, who had never seen her before, were, "Let's get this over with."[51]

Response to the article was overwhelming. Although some sympathized with Debbie's plight, few could defend the resident's handling of the situation. Critics said Debbie's case epitomized many of the worst horrors of physicians' participation in euthanasia: the resident had no established relationship with the patient, had made only a cursory review of the patient's chart, had not talked with the patient's treating physician, and had not talked with the patient's family. The resident relied on a quickly formed, personal reaction to Debbie's plight and a vague request from Debbie herself as the basis for taking a life. To some physician-ethicists, this kind of behavior threatened the soul of medicine. According to Gaylin and colleagues, "This issue touches medicine at its very moral center; if this moral center collapses, if physicians become killers or are even merely licensed to kill, the profession — and, therewith, each physician — will never again be worthy of trust and respect as healer and comforter and protector of life in all its frailty. For if medicine's power over life may be used equally to heal or to kill, the doctor is no more a moral professional but rather a morally neutered technician."[52]

Not all cases, however, are as black-and-white as Debbie's. Less than a year after the *Journal of the American Medical Association* devoted a special section to the reaction to Debbie's case, the *New England Journal of Medicine* published an update to a five-year-old article that outlined how physicians should care for hopelessly ill patients. This update urged timely discussion with patients about dying, including the use of advance directives. It urged adjusting the plan of care to suit the needs of each dying patient, including the aggressive use of pain relief. It acknowledged that it is "certainly not rare" for physicians to assist patients in suicide, either by prescribing medication that could be used in an overdose or discussing required doses and methods of administering drugs that could induce death. All but two of the 11 authors agreed, "It is not immoral for a physician to assist in the rational suicide of a terminally ill person."[53]

B. Killing Machine or Compassionate Doctor?

In June 1990, 54-year-old Janet Adkins died in the back of a Volkswagen van in a Michigan campground. The van belonged to Jack Kevorkian, MD, a pathologist who publicly promoted the idea of assisted suicide. Kevorkian invented a "suicide machine" that allowed patients to deliver a lethal dose of medication into their bloodstreams by simply throwing a switch. Adkins was newly diagnosed as having Alzheimer's disease, but she was in excellent health at the time of her death. She had known Kevorkian only briefly. Adkins' death outraged many in the medical community. Critics labeled Kevorkian "Dr. Death," and condemned him for failing to explore adequately other alternatives with a patient he barely knew.

Kevorkian acknowledged assisting in the death of at least 130 patients before April 1999 when he was sentenced to 10 to 25 years in prison on a second-degree murder charge for the death of Thomas Youk. Youk, 52, who had amyotrophic lateral sclerosis (ALS — Lou Gehrig's disease), was shown on CBS's *60 Minutes* in 1998 receiving a lethal injection of potassium chloride from Kovorkian. Prior to the television broadcast, Kevorkian had been in and out of court several times as Michigan courts struck down — but later reinstated — legislation banning assisted suicide. Kevorkian was brought to trial several times for his role in assisted-suicide deaths, but he was never convicted until Youk's case.[54]

Not long after Janet Adkins' death, Timothy Quill, MD, of the University of Rochester wrote about the death of a 45-year-old patient identified as "Diane." Diane had terminal, acute leukemia. She refused treatment that offered her a 25 percent chance of long-term survival, saying she did not want to endure the pain and the loss of dignity and control over her life that would occur with aggressive therapy. Diane told Quill that her desire was to live out her few remaining weeks of life enjoying her family and friends, and asked Quill to provide her with enough medication so she could take a lethal dose when she felt ready to end her life. Quill, who had treated Diane for more than eight years, was convinced she had thoroughly explored and rejected other options, and so gave her the medication.

While some questioned Quill's decision, he has been seen, unlike Kevorkian, as a compassionate, caring doctor who struggled to do what was best for a patient for whom he cared deeply. New York prosecutors declined to seek charges against him, and state medical officials refused to take action against his license to practice. Quill wrote eloquently and movingly about his eight-year relationship with "Diane."[55] He had grown to admire her determination in overcoming personal problems, including the effects of being raised in an alcoholic family and overcoming vaginal cancer as a young woman. In treating her for acute leukemia, he respected the values that went into her decision not to pursue aggressive treatment. He learned about her deep fear that a lingering death would prevent her from enjoying the few months she had left to live. He became convinced that Diane had explored all other options in facing her death and that her decision to choose suicide was well thought-out and rational. He found himself advising her on the amount of barbiturates needed for suicide and writing a prescription, but he felt uneasy in doing so. He wrote, "Yet I also felt strongly that I was setting her free to get the most out of the time she had left, and to maintain dignity and control on her own terms until her death."[56]

While some polls report that two-thirds of the American public consistently support physician-assisted suicide (PAS), there is evidence that this support can vary widely, depending on how questions are worded and the types of choices offered. The best way to understand public opinion might be termed the "Rule of Thirds," according to Ezekiel Emanuel, MD, who, at the turn of the century, conducted a review of survey literature on euthanasia and PAS. In the Rule of Thirds, roughly one-third of Americans said that they support voluntary active euthanasia and PAS under any circumstances. Another one-third oppose these practices no matter what the circumstances. The remaining one-third support euthanasia or PAS in some circumstances, such as those involving extreme pain, but oppose these practices in other circumstances, such as those when patients cite their major reasons as not wanting to be a burden or to preserve dignity. Emanuel terms this segment of the population "the volatile public."[57]

The American public does not seem to make a distinction between voluntary active euthanasia and PAS, according to Emanuel's research.

Roman Catholics and persons who report themselves to be "more religious" are significantly more opposed to euthanasia or PAS, as are African-Americans and older individuals. Having a serious, life-threatening illness does not seem to alter attitudes toward these practices. More than 90 percent of those interviewed said that they see withdrawal of life-sustaining treatment as ethical.

The Council on Ethical and Judicial Affairs (CEJA) of the American Medical Association (AMA) defines euthanasia as "bringing about the death of a hopelessly ill and suffering person in a relatively quick and painless way for reasons of mercy," and PAS as when a doctor "facilitates a patient's death by providing the necessary means and/or information to enable the patient to perform the life-ending act."[58] Both practices have been condemned by the AMA, other professional and healthcare organizations,[59] and a number of ethicists and theologians;[60] however, many physicians and ethicists have proposed or endorsed schemes in which physicians, under certain guidelines, would be allowed to assist patients with suicide.[61] There also are many who would permit physicians to participate in euthanasia.[62]

Arguments favoring euthanasia and PAS focus on two concerns: (1) compassion for the incurably ill who suffer intolerable pain and (2) respect for their human dignity and freedom.[63] These concerns are based on the principle of *beneficence,* to do what is best for the patient, and the principle of *autonomy,* the right of the patient to control treatment.[64] Joseph Fletcher, a pioneer in the field of bioethics, argued that failure to permit or to encourage euthanasia demeans the dignity of persons. People have dignity, he maintained, only if they are able to choose when, how, and why they are to live or to die. "Death control, like birth control, is a matter of human dignity," Fletcher wrote. "Without it persons become puppets. To perceive this is to grasp the error lurking in the notion, widespread in medical circles, that life as such is the highest good."[65]

Opponents of euthanasia and PAS claim that allowing these practices would undermine trust in the patient-physician relationship and lead to the involuntary killing of the handicapped, the poor, or other disenfranchised members of society. They argue that, if physicians were to prescribe adequate pain medication and make sure that patients received necessary comfort care, then there would be no demand for PAS or euthanasia.[66] Edmund D. Pellegrino, an ethicist and physician at Georgetown University, makes these points in an article entitled "Doctors Must Not Kill":

> How can patients trust that the doctor will pursue every effective and beneficent measure when she can relieve herself of a difficult challenge by influencing the patient to choose death? Uncertainty and mistrust are already too much a part of the healing relationship. Euthanasia magnifies these ordinary and natural anxieties.... When the proscription against killing is eroded, trust in the doctor cannot survive.[67]

It is a short way from the need to contain costs to covertly or overtly planned euthanasia for those members of our society who present the greatest economic burdens. At the beginning, some might suggest rationing needed care to retarded or handicapped infants, very old people, or those with fatal, incurable disease like Alzheimer's. Once euthanasia, in any of its forms, is legalized, the temptation to encourage its use, tacitly or overtly, to alleviate one of our most socially vexing problems — the increasing scarcity of healthcare dollars — will be strong. This could be the first step on the slippery slope, which leads inexorably from voluntary to nonvoluntary and involuntary euthanasia.[68]

> Hospice programs or palliative care offer comprehensive alternatives to euthanasia that are more respectful of beneficence and autonomy than killing. They relieve pain and anxiety, prepare the patient for the experience of dying, anticipate the need and value of advance directives, and establish understanding between patient and physician about which life-support measures are acceptable to the patient and which are not.[69]

Objections to euthanasia and PAS have also been raised on religious grounds. Speaking from the Christian tradition, for example, William May and Stanley Hauerwas argue that those who favor euthanasia and physician-assisted death place too much emphasis on avoiding the suffering that is a sometimes necessary part of dying. They both see life as a gift from God that puts obligations on the person who is dying as well as on those who care for the dying person. The Christian prohibition against suicide, Hauerwas maintains, is based on the assumption that our lives are not ours to do with as we please. It is the obligation of caregivers, he adds, to make sure that persons who are dying continue to feel their importance to the larger community. Hauerwas asserts, "The task of medicine is to care when it cannot cure. The refusal to let an attempted suicide die is only our feeble, but real, attempt to remain a community of trust and care through the agency of medicine. Our prohibition and subsequent care of a suicide draws on our profoundest assumptions that each individual's life has purpose beyond simply being autonomous."[70]

May laments that "preoccupation with death has replaced God as the effective center of religious consciousness in the modern world."[71] Those who see death as the absolute evil will view life as sacred, May maintains. Those who see suffering as the enemy will view quality of life as more important than life itself. Like Hauerwas, May believes that society must strike a balance by allowing those near the end of their lives to die, and yet not attempting to solve the problem of suffering by eliminating the sufferer:

Modern culture not only denies the right to die by its often mindless prolongation of life, but, just as seriously, it denies with the same heedlessness the right of the person to do his or her own dying. Since modern procedures, moreover, have made dying at the hands of experts and the machines a prolonged and painful business, emotionally and financially as well as physically, they have built up pressure behind the euthanasia movement, which asserts not the right to die, but the right to be killed.

The euthanasia movement encourages engineering death rather than facing dying. Euthanasia would bypass dying to get one dead as quickly as possible. It proposes to relieve suffering by knocking out the interval between the two states of life and death. The moral impulse behind the movement responds understandably to the quandaries of an age that makes of dying such an inhumanly endless business. However, the movement opposes the horrors of a purely technical death by using techniques to eliminate the victim.[72]

Some proponents of euthanasia and PAS believe that these acts are neither legally nor mor-ally different than withdrawing or withholding life-sustaining treatment. They reject arguments that there is a distinction between actively helping a patient die through administration of drugs and "passively" allowing the patient's death by removing a ventilator.[73] According to Boston College Law School Professor Charles Baron, the potential abuses cited by opponents of euthanasia and assisted suicide — eroding public trust of medicine and exposing the poor and weak to death due to economic considerations — could just as easily occur under the currently accepted "passive" euthanasia of forgoing life-sustaining treatment:

The competent patient should be the final judge of the level of pain, indignity, discomfort, dependency, meaninglessness and anxiety that he or she should have to put up with before giving up on life. When the patient has competently, knowledgeably, and freely decided that it is time to die, he or she should be able to die. He or she should not have to wait for a life-threatening emergency and be put through the charade of being "allowed to die" instead of being assisted in suicide or mercifully put to death. He or she should not have to be put through processes of letting nature take its course which are likely to be horrifying to the patient's family, brutalizing to medical personnel, and undignified (if not painful) to the patient. He or she should be able, where practical, to arrange to die surrounded by loved ones in the most meaningful circumstances possible.[74]

C. "Terminal Sedation" and Forgoing Artificial Nutrition and Hydration

To address intolerable and refractory pain or other symptoms suffered by some patients at the end of life, high doses of opiates, benzodiazepines, barbiturates, neuroleptic drugs, or combinations of these drugs are used to induce what has been termed "terminal sedation." Proponents of the practice argue that drugs are used to render the patient unconscious to relieve suffering, not to intentionally end life. With terminal sedation, life-sustaining treatments such as artificial nutrition and hydration, antibiotics, and mechanical ventilation are withheld or withdrawn because they are seen as prolonging the dying process without contributing to the patient's quality of life. The practice of terminal sedation in cases when suffering is so severe that it cannot be relieved by other means is seen as legally and ethically defensible.[75]

In briefs filed with the U.S. Supreme Court that oppose the practice of PAS, medical, hospice, palliative care, and geriatric groups argue that the practice of terminal sedation is an ethically acceptable alternative because death is not intentionally or directly caused by the physician. Moreover, these groups assure the court that PAS is not necessary to relieve the severe, intractable suffering of some terminally ill patients, because this suffering can be alleviated through terminal sedation. This argument is cited by three justices in their concurring opinions in rejecting a constitutional right to assisted suicide.[76]

However, attorney and ethicist David Orentlicher maintains that terminal sedation amounts to euthanasia, "because the sedated patient often dies from the combination of two intentional acts by the physician — the induction of stupor or unconsciousness and the withholding of food and water. Without these two acts, the patient would live longer before succumbing to illness . . . . It is the physician-created state of diminished consciousness that renders the patient unable to eat, not the patient's underlying disease." Orentlicher asserts that terminal sedation also is more risky than the practice of assisted suicide, because it can be done without the patient's consent or knowledge. Assisted suicide, he argues, at least requires the active participation of the patient.[77]

The practice of allowing a patient to voluntarily refuse food and fluid in the face of very advanced illness has been criticized as a form of suicide. Proponents defend this practice as ethically acceptable, because such patients view continued eating and drinking as measures that prolong life without value. Others claim that this practice amounts to the right of a patient to choose to forgo life-sustaining therapy. It is important for physicians and other clinicians to make sure that a patient's requests to stop eating and drinking do not stem from unrecognized depression.

V. LEGAL GUIDANCE ON PHYSICIAN AID IN DYING IN THE U.S.

The precedent for legalizing PAS in the U.S. was set in the state of Oregon. In November 1994, voters in Oregon narrowly approved a ballot initiative to legalize PAS. Implementation of the Oregon Death with Dignity Act (DDA) was delayed by a court injunction issued shortly after its passage. After months of legal proceedings, the Ninth Circuit Court of Appeals lifted the injunction in October 1997. This followed landmark rulings by the U.S. Supreme Court in June 1997 that held there is neither a constitutional right to nor a constitutional prohibition of euthanasia or PAS. The rulings opened the door for states to craft legislation that allow the practices.

When the Oregon legislature put the DDA before the voters again in November 1997, it was approved by a margin of 60 to 40 percent. The act allows a mentally competent, terminally ill patient to file a written request for medication for the purpose of "ending his or her life in a humane and dignified manner." It contains procedural safeguards, including documentation of the request, a waiting period, referral to a consulting physician, notification of family members, and documentation of the decision-making capacity of the patient. It provides immunity from civil and criminal liability and disciplinary action for doctors and pharmacists who act in good faith.[78]

In the first six years that the Oregon law has been in effect (1998-2004), a total of 171 people used PAS in Oregon. While the number of persons taking lethal medication steadily increased, the number remained small compared to the total number of deaths in Oregon: one-seventh of 1 percent of state residents died by PAS. Terminally ill younger persons were more likely to use PAS than their older counterparts. Rates were higher among those who had been divorced and among those who had higher levels of education. Men and women were equally likely to choose PAS. The rate of use of PAS was significantly higher among patients with ALS, HIV/AIDS, and cancer.[79]

Oregon is the only state that allows PAS; 35 states explicitly prohibit it by statute and nine additional states and the District of Columbia criminalize assisted suicide through the common law.[80] The Florida Supreme Court ruled in 1997 that there was no constitutional right in that state to PAS. Voters in Michigan defeated a referendum in 1998 to legalize PAS, and a similar referendum was defeated in Maine in 2000.[81] In 2001, U.S. Attorney General John Ashcroft challenged Oregon's DDA and issued a directive stating that assisting in suicide was not a legitimate medical purpose within the meaning of the federal Controlled Substances Act. A federal district judge struck down the directive in 2002.[82] The U.S. Department of Justice appealed, but in May 2004, the Ninth Circuit Court of Appeals ruled against Ashcroft and his directive. The directive would have imposed criminal penalties on physicians and pharmacists who knowingly dispensed controlled substances to assist patients planning to commit suicide.

The 1997 U.S. Supreme Court rulings came after groups in the states of Washington and New York challenged laws that banned PAS and were successful in convincing two federal appeals courts that such laws were unconstitutional. Although both appeals courts ruled that terminally ill adults have the right to hasten death with the aid of medications prescribed by their physicians, the courts reached that conclusion by very different routes. Reviewing the arguments of the decisions by the appeals courts lays the groundwork for understanding the reasoning used by justices of the U.S. Supreme Court in finding that there is no constitutional right to nor prohibition of assisted suicide.

On 6 March 1996, the Ninth Circuit Court of Appeals struck down a law in the State of Washington making PAS a felony. In ruling on the case of *Compassion in Dying v. State of Washington,* the court said the law violated the Fourteenth Amendment's guarantee of personal liberty found in the due-process clause. Judge Stephen Reinhardt, in a lengthy majority opinion, said the right of a terminally ill person to choose assisted suicide had the same basis in law as the right of a pregnant woman to choose to have an abortion or the right of a competent patient to refuse life-sustaining treatment. Both of these rights, Reinhardt said, have been upheld by the U.S. Supreme Court in the 1992 decision *Planned Parenthood v. Casey* and the 1990 decision *Cruzan v. Director, Missouri Dept. of Health.* Quoting language from the *Casey* decision, Reinhardt wrote:

Like the decision of whether or not to have an abortion, the decision how and when to die is one of the most intimate and personal choices a person may make in a lifetime, a choice central to personal dignity and autonomy. A competent, terminally ill adult, having lived nearly the full measure of his life, has a strong liberty interest in choosing a dignified and humane death rather than being reduced at the end of his existence to a childlike state of helplessness, diapered, sedated, incontinent.[83]

Reinhardt then turned to the Supreme Court's *Cruzan* opinion, noting it makes clear there is a

. . . due process liberty interest in rejecting unwanted medical treatment, including the provision of food and water by artificial means. Moreover, the Court majority clearly recognized that granting the request to remove the tubes through which Cruzan received artificial nutrition and hydration would lead inexorably to her death. . . . Accordingly, we conclude that Cruzan, by recognizing a liberty interest that includes the refusal of artificial provision of life-sustaining food and water, necessarily recognizes a liberty interest in hastening one's own death.[84]

By concluding that assisted suicide is a fundamental right guaranteed by the U.S. Constitution, Reinhardt made it difficult for state governments to justify any interference with this right. He recognized six interests that could be raised by states in regulating assisted suicide:

1. Preserving life,
2. Preventing suicide,
3. Preventing third parties from unduly influencing an individual to end his or her life,
4. Safeguarding children, family members, and other loved ones who are dependent on persons who wish to commit suicide,
5. Protecting the integrity of the medical profession, and
6. Preventing other adverse consequences that might result if assisted suicide were legal.

After weighing and balancing the individual's constitutional right to assisted suicide against the state's interest to prohibit it, Reinhardt ultimately came down on the side of the individual.

The liberty interest at issue here is an important one and, in the case of the terminally ill, is at its peak. Conversely, the state interests, while equally important in the abstract, are for the most part at a low point here. We recognize that in the case of life and death decisions the state has a particularly strong interest in avoiding undue influence and other forms of abuse. Here, that concern is ameliorated in large measure because of the mandatory involvement in the decision-making process of physicians, who have a strong bias in favor of preserving life, and because the process itself can be carefully regulated and rigorous safeguards adopted.[85]

Less than a month after the Ninth Circuit Appeals Court decision, the U.S. Court of Appeals for the Second Circuit struck down New York laws prohibiting PAS. Judge Robert J. Miner, writing for the majority in the case of *Quill v. Vacco,* refused to declare that the U.S. Constitution gave terminally ill persons a fundamental right to ask for assistance in hastening their deaths by taking medications prescribed by physicians. However, Miner did find that laws prohibiting PAS violated the equal protection clause of the Fourteenth Amendment. He reasoned that, if the state allows citizens to hasten death by refusing life-sustaining treatment, it must also allow similarly situated persons to speed death by taking a prescription for death-producing drugs. Miner wrote:

Withdrawal of life support requires physicians or those acting at their direction physically to remove equipment and, often, to administer palliative drugs which may themselves contribute to death. The ending of life by these means is nothing more nor less than assisted suicide. It simply cannot be said that those mentally competent, terminally ill persons who seek to hasten death but whose treatment does not include life support are treated equally.[86]

The reasoning of both appeals court decisions was attacked by 46 healthcare groups that filed a friend-of-the-court brief urging the U.S. Supreme Court not to legalize PAS. The AMA, the American Nurses Association, the American Psychiatric Association, and 43 other groups acknowledged that many patients do not receive proper care at the end of life, but they argued that physician-assisted death was not a compassionate answer to the problem of inadequate palliative care. The brief also maintained that a patient's right to forgo life-sustaining treatment was fundamentally different from being assisted in suicide.[87]

The importance of the distinction between forgoing life-sustaining treatment and requesting physician aid in dying has been pointed out even by those who favor the legalization of PAS. Franklin G. Miller, who favors voluntary active euthanasia, maintains that there is a distinction between assisting a patient in death and allowing the patient to die after withdrawal of life support:

Comparing the significance of the failure to comply with a refusal of life-sustaining treatment and request for assisted suicide manifests that they are not equivalent. When doctors fail to honor a competent patient's refusal of treatment, the patient becomes subjected to unwanted bodily intrusion. If on life support, the patient forced to endure unwanted treatment becomes a prisoner of medical technology. Out of respect for patient autonomy, doctors are duty-bound to honor informed refusals of life-sustaining treatment by competent patients. A terminally-ill patient who requests assisted suicide, by contrast, is asking for a treatment that lies outside standard medical practice, which includes aggressive palliative care that may risk hastening death but not direct intervention with a procedure that induces death. To deny such a request, for example, because the doctor believes that standard palliative care could relieve the patient's suffering, certainly restricts patient self-determination; but it does not amount to bodily invasion or medical imprisonment. And there remain other ways of hastening death than by physician-assisted suicide: the patient can refuse or refrain from food and water to attempt suicide without medical assistance. Unlike a competent refusal of treatment, a competent request for physician-assisted-suicide does not amount to a moral and legal trump that can compel a doctor's compliance. At most, the patient is free to negotiate assisted suicide with a willing physician. But no doctor has a duty to comply.[88]

There is no compelling liberty interest in a fundamental right to PAS, Miller maintains, because the patient who seeks assisted suicide has alternatives to hastening death. On the other hand, the patient who asks for life support to be withdrawn, or the pregnant woman who asks for an abortion, has no alternatives. In addition, Miller argues that Miner's equal protection argument is undermined by the real differences between forgoing treatment and assisting in suicide. If prohibiting assisted suicide for the terminally ill violates equal protection of the law, then it would also stand to reason that it would be a violation to deny voluntary active euthanasia to terminally ill persons who have no physical capacity to self-administer lethal drugs. Miller identifies other problems with the equal protection argument:

The right to refuse life-sustaining treatment, furthermore, is not limited to terminally-ill patients. The equal protection argument would seem to imply that assisted suicide also should not be limited. Moreover, family members frequently decide to forgo life-sustaining treatments that are judged not to be in the best interests of incompetent patients when their prior wishes are unknown. Would equal protection also support active euthanasia by surrogate decision-making in the best interests of similarly situated patients who are not on life support?[89]

Miller argues that because there is no compelling constitutional protection for the right to assisted suicide, the courts are not the proper vehicles to decide whether to legalize the practice and how it should be regulated. Rather, state legislatures or statewide referendums should decide the issue, Miller believes. In that way, the practice of PAS can be viewed as a policy experiment that can be tested for its benefits and harms.[90]

In its ruling on the two appeals court cases, the U.S. Supreme Court shifted the focus of debate on assisted suicide to state legislatures. With its dissenting opinions, the Court said the right to assisted suicide is not guaranteed in the U.S. Constitution. The rulings, handed down 26 June 1997, upheld New York and Washington state laws that made it a crime for doctors to give lethal drugs to dying patients who want to end their lives. In both decisions, the Court made it clear that states have a number of reasons for banning the practice of assisted suicide — including protecting vulnerable groups in society and preserving the ethics and integrity of the medical profession. But the decisions also left the door open for states to pass legislation that allows assisted suicide when the rights of a terminally ill patient might be seen as outweighing the interests of the state:[91] "Throughout the nation, Americans are engaging in an earnest and profound debate about the morality, legality and practicality of physician-assisted suicide," Chief Justice William H. Rehnquist wrote in the decision in the Washington State case. "Our holding permits this debate to continue, as it should in a democratic society."[92]

In its decision on the New York case, *Vacco v. Quill*, the Court rejected the argument that a ban on assisted suicide violated the Fourteenth Amendment's equal protection clause because it treated two groups of people differently. The Court's opinion, written by Rehnquist, states that there is a fundamental distinction between terminally ill patients who hasten death by withdrawing life support and terminally ill patients must rely on the administration of lethal drugs to hasten death. Rehnquist pointed to a difference in causation and intent. "[W]hen a patient refuses life-sustaining treatment, he dies from an underlying fatal disease or pathology; but if a patient ingests lethal medication prescribed by a physician, he is killed by that medication," Rehnquist wrote. He added that a physician who withdraws life-support may not intend the death of the patient, but rather wants to respect the patient's wishes to refuse what is perceived to be futile or degrading care. A doctor who assists in a suicide, however, clearly wants the patient to die, he said. "By permitting everyone to refuse unwanted medical treatment while prohibiting anyone from assisted suicide, New York law follows a long-standing and rational distinction," Rehnquist concluded.[93]

In the Washington State case, the Court rejected the claim that assistance in suicide is a fundamental right protected by the due process clause in the Fourteenth Amendment. Rehnquist, again writing the main opinion, noted that the Supreme Court, in a long line of cases, has used the due process clause to expand the specific freedoms protected in the Bill of Rights to include rights to marry, to marital privacy, to have children, to use contraception, to direct the education of one's children, and to abortion. But a right to assistance in suicide, Rehnquist wrote, "has no place in our Nation's traditions, given the country's consistent, almost universal, and continuing rejection of the right, even for terminally ill, mentally competent adults." To rule in favor of a right to assisted suicide, Rehnquist continued, "the Court would have to reverse centuries of legal doctrine and practice, and strike down the considered policy choice of almost every state."[94]

Rehnquist dismissed the argument that the Court's opinion in the 1990 case of *Cruzan v. Director, Missouri Dept of Health* — which recognized a constitutionally protected right to refuse lifesaving hydration and nutrition — could be extended to recognizing a liberty interest for a terminally ill patient to hasten death through assisted suicide. The *Cruzan* opinion was grounded in "the common-law rule that forced medication was a battery, and the long legal tradition protecting the decision to refuse unwanted medical treatment," Rehnquist wrote; "The decision to commit suicide with the assistance of another may be just as personal and profound as the decision to refuse unwanted medical treatment, but it has never enjoyed similar legal protection. Indeed, the two acts are widely and reasonably regarded as quite distinct."[95]

The Court also rejected the notion that its decision in *Casey v. Planned Parenthood* — upholding a woman's right to an abortion as being "central to personal dignity and autonomy" — could be interpreted to mean that assisted suicide should also be seen as such a right. The fact that many of the personal rights and liberties protected by the due process clause are grounded in personal autonomy "does not warrant the sweeping conclusion that any and all important, intimate, and personal decisions are so protected," Rehnquist wrote.[96]

VI. THE OUTLOOK ON PHYSICIAN AID IN DYING IN OTHER COUNTRIES

After years of being illegal but tolerated, PAS and euthanasia became legal in the Netherlands in February 2002 after both houses of its Parliament approved legislation that prohibits prosecution, as long as physicians comply with guidelines. The 2002 law formalized a 1994 practice that promised legal immunity to physicians who agreed to participate in a national study of euthanasia and assisted suicide and who followed certain state-mandated requirements.

The criteria that physicians must follow for euthanasia or assisted suicide to be legal in the Netherlands are similar to those in Oregon. The patient must have unbearable and unremitting pain with no prospect of improvement; the patient's request for help to die must be sustained, informed, and voluntary. A second medical opinion must confirm diagnosis and prognosis. All other medical options must have been tried. The termination of life must be carried out with medically appropriate care and attention. The physician must report the death to a government pathologist and state whether the cause of death was euthanasia or assisted suicide.[97]

Dutch researchers have analyzed the rates of euthanasia, PAS, and other decisions to end life for the years 1990, 1995, and 2001. They did this by examining and analyzing death certificates as well as by surveys of physicians. In 1990, approximately 39 percent of all deaths in the Netherlands appeared to be preceded by a medical decision that probably or certainly hastened death. Deaths in this category included not only euthanasia and PAS, but also ending a patient's life without the patient's explicit request, alleviation of symptoms with possible life-shortening effect, and decisions not to treat an illness or disease.[98]

The total percentage of deaths preceded by medical decision grew to just over 42 percent in 1995 and nearly 44 percent in 2001. By far the largest category were decisions to forgo treatment and alleviation of symptoms with possible life-shortening effects, each of which were responsible for slightly more than 20 percent of deaths in 2001. Studies of death certificates indicate that the rate of euthanasia increased from 1.7 percent of all deaths in 1990 (approximately 2,300 persons) to 2.4 percent in 1995 and to 2.6 percent in 2001. The rate of PAS was .2 percent of deaths in 1990 (approximately 300 persons) and remained unchanged in 1995 and 2001. The percentage of deaths attributed to ending a patient's life without strict criteria for euthanasia being fulfilled was .8 percent in 1990 (approximately 1,000 persons) and decreased to .7 percent in 1995 and 2001. In summarizing the trends in the data from death certificates and surveys of physicians', the Dutch researchers conclude:

> The rate of euthanasia and explicit requests by patients for physicians' assistance in dying in the Netherlands seems to have stabilized, and physicians seem to have become somewhat more restrictive in their use. Euthanasia remains mainly restricted to groups other than patients with cancer, people younger than 80 years, and patients cared for by family physicians, who were already frequently involved in 1990. The continuing debate on whether and when physician-assistance in dying may be acceptable and on procedures to ensure transparency and quality assurance seems to have contributed to this stabilization.[99]

Belgium became the second country in the world to legalize PAS and euthanasia in October 2001. Guidelines in the Belgium law are similar to those in the Netherlands. The Northern Territory of Australia passed a law effective in 1996 that allows physicians to prescribe and administer lethal substances to patients who formally requested assistance in ending their lives, but the law was overturned by the Australian Senate in 1997.[100]

VII. TRAINING CLINICIANS TO DELIVER BAD NEWS

Delivering bad news (such as a terminal diagnosis or imminent death to a patient or family member) is universally an unwelcome responsibility. For the current generation of clinicians, the discomfort stems, in part, from the same inexperience with death that typifies the general population. Most medical and nursing students have never experienced a family member's dying at home. Death, for young clinicians, has been "medicalized," as it has for others in our society.

Another reason that clinicians fear delivering bad news is that, as students, they are rarely taught the communication skills and practices that ease the messenger's burden. This lack of training is a clear failing on the part of their teachers and those who develop clinical curricula. Student clinicians, if they are lucky, may encounter during their training a mentor who, through long experience or innate sensitivity, models the careful body language and dialogue, the listening and hearing skills, and the empathy and compassion that are required for the successful delivery of bad news. Too often, a different kind of modeling occurs; for example, medical students may be ordered by harried residents at 3:00 a.m. to call family members (who may be total strangers) and inform them that a patient has just died. Or they may witness a busy attending physician callously inform a patient that he or she has a terminal diagnosis. They may watch while a physician uses medical jargon that the patient does not fully grasp, which ensures a misunderstanding on the patient's part and demonstrates a lack of sincere concern for the patient's reactions, questions, and fears.

Clinicians' qualms about delivering the news of a terminal diagnosis or the death of a family member also stem from myriad other factors. These include the fact that most people have never directly examined or confronted their own feelings and attitudes about death. Also, many clinicians harbor "rescue fantasies" about their patients, or they may too narrowly conceive of their professional roles solely as healers and curers. Such individuals may experience feelings of defeat and failure when their patients become ter-

minally ill or die, because they failed to "save" their patient. They may sense, and often rightly so, that their patients expected (albeit unrealistically) that the medical armamentarium was complete enough to disallow death or disability.

Also, clinicians nurture legitimate concerns about causing their patients pain and distress. Clinicians may fear the reactions that such news might elicit, such as despair, anger, hopelessness, rage, or even legal recourse. Because most clinicians are, by self-selection, compassionate and caring individuals, they empathize with their patients' plight, and cannot help but share in patients' pain and loss.

Delivering bad news, however onerous, remains a professional responsibility of all clinicians. Inherent in this responsibility is the duty to learn and master, to the greatest degree possible, the skills and practices that good messengers possess. Winslade,[101] Buckman,[102] and others maintain that delivering bad news is a skill that can be learned and one that should be an integral part of the clinical curriculum. They emphasize that apart from didactic course work, the most important learning methods involve observing direct interactions between senior clinicians and patients, and that the most instructive element in the entire learning process is the patient.

At the University of Toronto, Robert Buckman and Yvonne Kason have developed a course, "Breaking Bad News," that generated a book with the same title.[103] Buckman maintains that certain communication skills are basic prerequisites to productive encounters during which bad news is delivered to patients. He cites many studies that report that patients' dissatisfaction with clinicians' communication skills outweigh any concerns that they might have about clinical competence.[104] Such sources of dissatisfaction include the appearance that the clinician is not listening to the patient, the use of technical medical jargon, or the appearance of patronizing or "talking down to" the patient.[105] Buckman cites one study that found that patients usually present with between 1.2 and 3.9 major complaints. Unfortunately, physicians generally allow their patients a scant 18 seconds to begin relating their histories before interrupting. An average of 23 percent of patients were allowed to complete their initial statements.[106] As an aid to effective communication between patients and clinicians, Buckman and his colleagues endorse the following listening skills. First, clinicians must prepare to listen by preparing an appropriate setting. This includes:

- Maintaining auditory and visual privacy: taking the patient to a private waiting room, closing the office door, or pulling the curtain around the patient's bed (which offers visual if not auditory privacy).
- Making complete introductions: the clinician should always address the patient first, irrespective of who or how many persons are involved in a meeting; this practice emphasizes the primacy of the patient's importance in the proceedings and is a subtle message from clinician to patient.
- Addressing the patient by the appellation that he or she prefers ("Mrs. Jones" rather than "Mary," or *vice versa*).
- Sitting down, face-to-face, with the patient: if the patient is bedridden, the clinician should find a place to sit so that he or she is not standing above the bed; sitting on chairs, stools, the patient's bed, even a bedside commode (if that is the only seat available) is preferable to literally talking down to the patient from a standing position.
- Asking open-ended, not closed, questions so that the patient is encouraged to voice feelings, fears, and the need for information or support.
- Not interrupting the patient unless necessary.
- Being comfortable with silences: silences often signal that the patient is gearing up to address a painful and/or very important issue.[107]

Once the clinician has set the stage for effective listening, the next step to a successful interaction is to ensure that a complete dialogue occurs between the clinician and the patient. This is facilitated by hearing (not just listening to) what the patient says (or, more important, what the patient doesn't say); by paying attention to how the patient phrases comments and questions; and by paying close attention to body language, since the patient's physical behavior may send a different message than his or her words. For example, the display of denial, indifference, or complete acceptance by the patient may be belied by physical acts such as failure to make eye contact, hand wringing, foot tapping, or other signs of anxiety or distress. Responses such as reiterating the patient's comments, making nonjudgmental observations of behavior, or trying to assess the patient's feelings are important and effective

mechanisms in establishing human connections and assuring the patient that his or her message is being understood. If the patient or family member responds with anger, hostility, or even rage, the clinician must not take this reaction personally: when a patient or family directs blame or invective against the clinician, this response may manifest frustration with the overall situation. The clinician (or messenger) is merely a convenient target.

Delivering the news to family members that a loved one has died can be just as stressful as delivering bad news to a patient; if the death is sudden and unexpected, it may even be more difficult. In general, the same precepts that apply to delivering bad news to a patient apply when dealing with family members. It is important to assess the family members' most recent understanding of the patient's condition. This may provide a general opening to explain that the patient's condition worsened, that attempts to revive the patient (if they were attempted) failed, and that the patient has died. Any euphemisms for death such as "expired" or "passed on" should be avoided. All opportunities to provide support for family members should be made in advance, if possible, including involving a chaplain or counseling services. Providing family members a chance to spend time alone with the dead patient and responding to their requests for information about the circumstances of the patient's death or about the patient's medical condition may be important in alleviating their acute pain and in assisting a healthy grieving process.

Ideally, the news that a family member has died should be given in person. Circumstances do not always allow this, and sometimes tragic news must be imparted over the phone. Buckman has identified some ground rules for this situation that include:

- Always make sure that you know to whom you are speaking.
- Introduce yourself and say what you do, indicating whether you have met the family member.
- Speak slowly and give the relative time to adjust (this is particularly important for phone calls in the middle of the night).
- Let the relative know that you would rather be speaking to him or her in person.
- Precede the news with a warning statement such as, "I am afraid that I have some bad news about your wife."

- If the relative then interrupts to ask whether the patient has died, tell the truth, using a narrative statement such as, "I'm sorry to say that she has died."
- Find out who is with the relative, or who is available to provide support, and suggest that the relative contact this person, and not be alone.
- Offer further contact, such as being available when and if the relative visits the hospital.[108]

VIII. BUCKMAN'S SIX-STEP METHOD FOR DELIVERING BAD NEWS

In their course for medical students, Buckman and his colleagues have developed a six-step protocol to prepare students for effective clinical encounters during which they must be the messengers of bad news:

1. Get off to a good start by:
   - Optimizing the physical context (ensure privacy and a quiet environment if at all possible, make eye-to-eye contact with the patient, sit at the patient's level).
   - Ensuring that all participants who should be at the meeting are there (Whom does the patient want present for support?), and that those whom the patient doesn't want present aren't there; this is another way to assure the patient's privacy and provide psychological support.
   - Making introductions, shaking hands with or touching the patient if he or she is receptive to physical contact; ensure that the patient is always addressed first, both with verbal and physical contact regardless of the presence of others, to reinforce the message that the patient is of primary concern.

2. Find out how much the patient knows about his or her medical condition by using open-ended questions such as, "Can you tell me why Dr. Jones suggested that you see me today?" or "What can you tell me of your understanding of your medical problem?"

3. Find out how much the patient wants to know about his or her clinical situation, by asking such questions as:
   - "If this condition turns out to be serious, are you the kind of person who likes to know exactly what is going on?"
   - "Would you like me to tell you the full details of your condition — or is there

somebody else that you would like me to talk to?"

Remember that cultural traditions may affect not only the patients reception of bad news, but may affect future interactions with the patient and family members. In some Asian cultures, for example, it is considered unkind to deliver the news of a terminal diagnosis directly to the patient. Often when an Asian person is terminally ill, all aspects of treatment are directed by close relatives. The diagnosis of terminal illness is never disclosed to the patient. While such traditions may run counter to the Western cultural ethic of informed consent and respect for autonomy, honoring the conventions and traditions of other cultures should be practiced by clinicians when possible (within the standards of good clinical, ethical, and legal practice), in light of the culturally diverse society in which we practice.

4. Share information according to the patient's needs and desires; make a mutually-agreed upon plan for the future:
   - Decide on a mutual agenda (diagnosis/treatment plan/prognosis/support).
   - Start from the patient's starting point; patients may be in varying degrees of denial, may have misunderstood or forgotten previous information, or may simply need to have details reconfirmed to allay fears of misdiagnosis. Also, remember that what is of primary importance to the patient (loss of hair, for example) may not coincide with clinical priorities.
   - Give information in small chunks; it is difficult for persons under stress to retain information. Patients often relate in subsequent interviews that "Once I heard the word cancer I blocked out everything else that you said."
   - Use English, not "medspeak" or jargon.
   - Check the patient's understanding frequently, by asking such questions as, "Does what I am saying make sense to you?" and by asking the patient to state in his or her own words what you have just said.
   - Reinforce and clarify information frequently.
   - Check your communication level. Speak to an adult patient on adult terms; do not patronize, offer false reassurance, or speak

to an adult as if he or she was a child.

- Listen for the patient's agenda. What are his or her desires in terms of therapy; life goals; important accomplishments prior to death; or fears regarding disability, pain, or loss of dignity?

5. Responding to the patient's feelings:
   - Identify and acknowledge the patient's reaction to bad news. Feelings such as anger, despair, and hostility are common and should not be ignored by the clinician.

6. Planning and follow-through:
   - Make a contract with the patient on a plan of care and follow-through. Establish the patient's priorities about medical treatment as well as plans for the future. When appropriate, discuss advance directives regarding aggressive therapy, an acceptable quality of life, preferences about the circumstances of dying (where, for example), and preferences regarding surrogate decision makers in the event of future incapacity.
   - Remember that the competent adult patient has the right to accept or reject any suggestions.[109]

IX. PROFESSIONAL GUIDANCE

A. Professional Preparation for End-of-Life Care

1. Scientific and Clinical Knowledge and Skills, Including the Following

- Learning the biological mechanisms of dying from major illnesses and injuries
- Understanding the pathophysiology of pain and other physical and emotional symptoms
- Developing appropriate expertise and skill in the pharmacology of symptom management
- Acquiring appropriate knowledge and skill in the non-pharmacological symptom management
- Learning the proper application and limits of life-prolonging interventions
- Understanding tools for assessing patients' symptoms, status, quality of life, and prognosis

2. Interpersonal Skills and Attitudes, Including the Following

- Listening to patients, families, and other members of the health care team
- Conveying difficult news
- Understanding and managing patient and family responses to illness
- Providing information and guidance on prognosis and options
- Sharing decision making and resolving conflicts
- Recognizing and understanding one's own feelings and anxieties about dying and death
- Cultivating empathy
- Developing sensitivity to religious, ethnic, and other differences

3. Ethical and Professional Principles, Including the Following

- Doing good and avoiding harm
- Determining and respecting patient and family preferences
- Being alert to personal and organizational conflicts of interests
- Understanding societal/population interests and resources
- Weighing competing objectives or principles
- Acting as a role model of clinical proficiency, integrity, and compassion

4. Organization Skills, Including the Following

- Developing and sustaining effective professional teamwork
- Understanding relevant rules and procedures set by health plans, hospitals, and others
- Learning how to protect patients from harmful rules and procedures
- Assessing and managing car options, settings, and transitions
- Mobilizing supportive resources (for example, palliative care consultants, community-based assistance)
- Making effective use of existing financial resources and cultivating new funding sources

— Adapted from M.J. Field and C. Cassel, ed., *Approaching Death: Improving Care at the End-of-Life* (Washington, D.C: National Academy Press, 1997), 11.

B. Elements of Quality Care for Patients in the Last Phase of Life

Preamble: In the last phase of life people seek peace and dignity. To help realize this, every person should be able to fairly expect the following elements of care from physicians, health care institutions, and the community.

Elements:

1. The opportunity to discuss and plan for end-of-life care. This should include: the opportunity to discuss scenarios and treatment preferences with the physician and health care proxy, the chance for discussion with others, the chance to make a formal "living will" and proxy designation, and help with filing these documents in such a way that they are likely to be available and useful when needed.

2. Trustworthy assurances that physical and mental suffering will be carefully attended to and comfort measures intently secured. Physicians should be skilled in the detection and management of terminal symptoms, such as pain, fatigue, and depression, and able to obtain the assistance of specialty colleagues when needed.

3. Trustworthy assurance that preferences for withholding or withdrawing life-sustaining intervention will be honored. Whether the intervention be less complex (such as antibiotics or artificial nutrition and hydration) or complex and more invasive (such as dialysis or mechanical respiration), and whether the situation involves imminent or more distant dying, patient's preferences regarding withholding or withdrawing intervention should be honored in accordance with the legally and ethically established rights of patients.

4. Trustworthy assurance that there will be no abandonment by the physician. Patients should be able to trust that their physician will continue to care for them when dying. If a physician must transfer the patient in order to provide quality care, that physician should make every reasonable effort to continue to visit the patient with regularity, and institutional systems should try to accommodate this.

5. Trustworthy assurance that dignity will be a priority. Patients should be treated in a dignified and respected manner at all times.

6. Trustworthy assurance that burden to family and others will be minimized. Patients should be able to expect sufficient medical resources and community support,

such as palliative care, hospice, or home care, so that the burden of illness need not overwhelm caring relationships.

7. Attention to the personal goals of the dying person. Patients should be able to trust that their personal goals will have reasonable priority whether it be: to communicate with family and friends, to attend to spiritual needs, to take one last trip, to finish a major unfinished task in life, or to die at home or at another place of personal meaning.

8. Trustworthy assurance that careproviders will assist the bereaved through early stages of mourning and adjustment. Patients and their loved ones should be able to trust that some support continues after bereavement. This may be by supportive gestures, such as a bereavement letter, and by appropriate attention to/referral for care of the increased physical and mental health needs that occur among the recently bereaved.

— "AMA Statement on End-of-Life Care," *http://www.ama-assn.org/ama/pub/category/ 7567.html.*

X. CASES FOR FURTHER STUDY

Case 1: When Too Much Is Too Little

A 73-year-old man came to the emergency room because of progressive weakness in his left leg. One year earlier, he had noted a sudden weakness in the left lower leg as he was climbing a flight of stairs. He did not seek medical attention at that time, but began to use a cane. Three weeks before his visit to the emergency department, he fell to the floor while attempting to get out of bed. On arising, he had difficulty supporting his weight on his left side. The left-leg weakness subsequently progressed, and he was unable to walk without a walker. He had no other symptoms or medical problems, had an unremarkable family history, and was taking no medication. He was a widower and lived alone. He had worked as a cook in a delicatessen until his recent fall. He smoked approximately 60 packs of cigarettes a year, and drank approximately six glasses of beer a week.

The patient was not in acute distress. He was alert and oriented to person, place, and time, and his speech was fluent. His vital signs were normal, and the general physical examination was unremarkable. Except for a slight left facial droop, the cranial-nerve examination was unremarkable. Vibratory sense was decreased bilaterally over his ankle. He had slightly diminished strength in his left deltoids and biceps and atrophy of the dorsal interosseous muscles in his left hand. He could lift his left leg off the bed for only five to 10 seconds, and the strength in his left gastrocnemius muscle was diminished. Muscle tone was decreased in both legs but much more marked on the left. There were fasciculations of the left vastus medialis and left biceps. Finger-to-nose ataxia was not present. The patient was unable to walk without assistance. He had bilateral Babinski signs and was hyper-reflexive at both knees.

The complete blood count and electrolyte, serum creatinine, and glucose levels were normal. A computed tomographic (CT) scan of the head revealed low attenuation of the right centrum semiovale with associated mass effect.

The patient was admitted to the neurology service. A chest radiograph revealed a density in the right lung apex. Radiographs of the spine showed a possible lytic lesion of the pedicle of the vertebral body of T12. CT scans of the chest and abdomen revealed a 3.5 cm. right-upper-lobe mass abutting the posterior pleural base, without associated hilar or mediastinal lymphadenopathy. The adrenal glands were normal. An MRI scan of the brain showed a large, irregularly marginated, ring-enhancing lesion located in the posterior frontal lobe on the right, with extensive edema and mass effect.

The bone scan and MRI scan of the spine were unremarkable. Treatment with phenytoin and dexamethasone was begun. A biopsy of the lung mass was recommended as a basis for further treatment, but the patient refused additional invasive tests.

The team caring for the patient thought he was "in denial," "very negativistic," and depressed. A psychiatric consultation was obtained to evaluate the patient's mood and capacity to make decisions. The psychiatrist noted that the patient was cognitively intact, reacting appropriately to the diagnosis, and capable of making decisions about treatment. The patient told the psychiatrist that he had watched his wife die of lung cancer two years previously and did not want further diagnostic tests or life-prolonging treatment. He wanted to return home as soon as possible. While discharge planning was under way, the neurology team, as well as the pulmonary and oncology consultants, continued to press for a lung biopsy, and the patient finally agreed to undergo the procedure. The biopsy findings were consistent with non-small-cell lung cancer. Resections of both the primary tumor and the brain metastasis were proposed, but the patient declined surgery and was discharged home on the twenty-first hospital day with 24-hour home healthcare. He was given follow-up appointments at the hospital's neurology and oncology clinics and prescriptions for phenytoin, dexamethasone, and ranitidine.

Three months later, the patient had three grand mal seizures and was brought to the emergency room by his family. He had remained at home in the intervening months and had not kept his follow-up clinic appointments. In the emergency room he was lethargic but arousable. He now had a more prominent left facial weakness, flaccid paralysis of his left arm and severe dysarthria. A CT scan of the head showed that the frontal parietal mass was surrounded by extensive edema, with right subfalcial and uncal herniation. There was an extensive midline shift, with obliteration of both frontal and temporal horns and the right lateral ventricle.

The patient was readmitted to the neurology service, where he was under the care of a new group of house officers and a different attending physician. Intravenous dexamethasone and phenytoin were administered. The patient's son requested that a DNR order be issued on the basis of the patient's prior wishes. The neurology team recommended that the brain lesion be resected, but the family declined on the basis of the patient's prior wishes. The patient was given intravenous fluids and oxygen, and the dexamethasone and phenytoin were continued. A nasogastric tube was inserted, and the patient remained minimally responsive over the next three weeks. Intravenous fluids, phenytoin, dexamethasone, and tube feedings were continued, as were phlebotomies to monitor his electrolyte, glucose, and phenytoin levels. Two subsequent CT scans revealed ongoing brain-stem herniation. The patient removed the nasogastric tube multiple times despite wrist restraints. On the twenty-fifth hospital day, the patient had a cardiopulmonary arrest and died.

— R.S. Morrison and C.K. Cassel, "When Too Much Is Too Little," *New England Journal of Medicine* 335 (1996): 1755-1759.

Case 2: There Isn't An Alternative

Elena Alvarez was a 48-year-old woman who has lived in the U.S. for many years. Originally from El Salvador, her English was very limited. Before her diagnosis with ovarian cancer, she worked as a child-care provider. Her family consisted of a brother and her mother; she lived with her elderly mother who had many health problems of her own. Her disease progressed despite surgery, initial chemotherapy, and a number of attempts at "salvage" chemotherapy. Ms Alvarez spoke openly about her cancer diagnosis with members of the clinic staff, but maintained a complex silence within her family. For many months, she did not name the disease with her elderly mother, preferring to shield her from this information. As her illness progressed, Ms Alvarez's mother eventually learned that her daughter had cancer. However, the severity of the illness was never addressed. One of the nurses commented, "The other thing that Elena said to us when we had this big meeting was that she has not told her mother the truth about her illness. She can't tell her mother the truth about her illness. So I'm sure they haven't had a real honest conversation about what is going on."

From the point of view of her healthcare providers, Ms Alvarez faced many decisions. One said,

Like many of the other patients in our study, she did not experience any sense of choice. In interviews she stated over and over, "You just have to do the treatment, there isn't an alternative. You get treatment to prolong your life and get well, or you let yourself die." Over a nine-month period, she always "*chose*" more treatment. During the informed-consent process for entry into the research, we told the patients that we were studying decision making. Some patients, particularly women, found this perplexing and wondered what we were "really studying," since they did not experience their medical care as including decisions. When discussing her "last" drug, tamoxifen, Ms Alvarez said, "I wait for life. I have the point of view that I am going to be cured. This is going to be my drug. This is going to cure me."

The comments of Ms Alvarez reflect the tension between her beliefs that no choices existed, and the healthcare team's demands that she make decisions. When asked who was the most important person making decisions about her treatment, she answered, "I am," but immediately complained, "Here in this country they don't give you an alternative but to do it alone. . . . In other countries they tell the family and the family has influence. The family decides. Here the patient has to decide for themselves. There is no alternative." She raised two questions: Are there real options, and should the individual patient be shouldered with making decisions alone?

The issue of prognosis was equally complex. Nurse Terry Miller noted, "One of the things that Dr. Ingle and I talked about was, 'When is he going to say that enough is enough?' because this woman is not going to be cured. She is going to die of the disease. Several months ago we sat down with Elena and said, 'It's progressing and we don't know what else we can do for you.' And I asked her at that time, When was she going to know that enough was enough? She told me she would know that when the doctor told her there was nothing left to do." In seeming contradiction to the fundamental assumptions of the autonomy paradigm, Ms Alvarez's physician found it very difficult to discuss the patient's likely prognosis. He explained his frustrations by rehearsing a hypothetical conversation with his patient: "I want to encourage you to keep going with this chemo, but oh, by the way, you're still not going to do well, and you probably only have six months to live. It's kind of hard, and I didn't reiterate that, to tell the truth." The problem was apparent: the doctor was giving the patient mixed messages, and everyone wanted someone else to make the hard decisions. The physician continued, "She lets me make the decisions for her. In Elena's case I'll tell her what I think is best for her, and I tend to push pretty aggressively with Elena. I'm not willing to just sort of like, let her go." The result was a long delay in acknowledgment that further treatment was futile.

The situation of Ms Alvarez was complicated by the need for language interpretation. [The author] was able to observe a long and complicated clinical session, involving the patient, the clinical nurse specialist, oncologist, and social worker. A Spanish language interpreter was also present, since the encounter was foreseen to be important: Would the patient want further salvage chemotherapy for her disease, which had recurred despite numerous interventions (a treatment decision about which she ultimately felt she had no choice)? Although communication is never simple, some elements of failed communication are not overly complex, and were evident in the clinical encounter. Throughout the exchange, [the author] noted many instances in which statements by either the patient or one of the team members were simply not translated. The physician was offering chemotherapy, the nurse was reminding the patient that she mustn't wait until it was too late, meaning that she was too ill to travel, if she wanted to return to her native El Salvador. In this cacophonous five-way exchange, it was difficult to determine what "got through" to the patient, who was weeping softly throughout. As discussed earlier, like many patients, Ms Alvarez appeared to perceive no choice but to follow the physician's option of additional chemotherapy. In later interviews, the physician described the patient's prognosis as extremely poor, regardless of therapeutic endeavors.

But of most interest was the role of the interpreter in placing the clinical session in a certain cultural context. Toward the end of the interview, the interpreter spoke softly with the patient for some time, not volunteering to translate his own remarks for others in the room. Seemingly distressed by the bluntness of the conversation he had just been translating, he ended the exchange by relating a story to Elena; a story suffused with hope: Once the interpreter had known a person with cancer who was told he would only live for two months, and the person was still alive nine years later! Is the interpreter trying to compensate for the teams' lack of sensitivity to a culturally shared (between patient and translator) need to maintain hope? In this type of exchange, which voice captures the patient's attention? The role of the white-coated interpreter, who must appear to the patient as a full member of the team, needs further exploration.

—B.A. Koenig, "Cultural Diversity in Decisionmaking About Care at the End of Life," in *Approaching Death: Improving Care at the End of Life* (Washington, D.C.: National Academy Press, 1997): 363-379.

Case 3: Whose Comfort Are They Managing?

"I am afeard there are few die well that die in a battle,"
said the soldier to Henry V.

And I am afraid that, sadly enough, many of today's battles are being fought in nursing homes, where fewer and fewer die well.

The mounting pressures that permeate medicine — legal issues, finances, time constraints, many others — tend to militate against care and empathy for patients. Too often these days, when some medical professionals strive for comfort and compassion, it's not for the patients — it's for themselves.

My wife's mother died last year at age 90 after four years of declining health. She had lived an active, upbeat life until a year before we finally had to move her from the city of her birth into an assisted-living facility. She spent two years there, and the final two in an excellent nursing home. Gradually, she became so physically incapacitated that she needed round-the-clock care from private aids.

As time passed, speaking coherently became increasingly difficult for her, but, almost to her final hours, she could comprehend most aspects of her daily life. My wife, who saw her nearly every day during those concluding years, was able to understand her mother's thoughts and feelings and to communicate with her, even when nurses, aides, and physicians could not.

A physician whom we knew well took on the care of my mother-in-law and stayed with her until six months before her death, when he retired. Then we turned to a younger doctor, someone who looked after many of the other patients in the nursing home. He came highly recommended and remains well regarded to this day by his patients.

From the start, he seemed to be in a perpetual hurry. On the occasions when he spoke with my wife, he repeatedly labeled his new patient as having "senile dementia," and in our eyes wrote her off as a helpless and hopeless "case."

From our vantage point, he could have done a better job of managing her decline, although I'm not suggesting that there was malpractice of any sort. To us, his care verged on being insensitive and of a quality that one would not wish for anyone's parents when their time comes.

As far as we could tell, he never got to know his patient as more than a bedridden body with "senile dementia." His frequent use of that diagnostic term offended and hurt my wife, however technically correct it may have been. Her mother's former physician had used a phrase my wife had found less denigrating: "the end results of repeated TIAs," an abbreviation for mild strokes. My wife believed, too, that the new doctor thought — incorrectly, in her view — that her mother could not understand much of what was happening to her or what was said in her presence.

The new doctor also seemed to assign much of the responsibility for his patient's care to the nurses, aides, and the physician's assistant. We can't recall his ever asking to meet with my wife to discuss how she thought his patient would wish to die.

Fortunately, the aide hired by my wife to see her mother through the late afternoon and early evening was competent, kind, caring, devoted, and full of common sense.

The most troubling events occurred during the weeks when it became evident that my mother-in-law was dying. Her muscles tightened, perhaps due to the recurrent small strokes, and her joints became twisted. My wife and the aide saw that she was often in pain. She also let my wife know that she was anxious and deeply troubled. To relieve her, the doctor ordered a medication. But the dose was very low and was to be given only at the discretion of the nurses.

As the situation progressed, it became clear to us that my mother-in-law was not receiving enough pain medication. Although I am a doctor and have cared for plenty of patients in my time, some of the shift nurses told my wife that we were mistaken: the pulse rate and breathing pattern, key indicators that they used, showed that she was receiving adequate amounts. They said, too, that they had strong feelings about avoiding overmedication, and they appeared to discount my wife's assessment that, despite the clinical numbers, her mother was fearful and in pain.

We brought in people from hospice care and, after evaluating the patient, they advised round-the-clock intravenous pain medication. Without seeking us out to discuss it, the doctor did not follow their recommendation. A month later, as we continued to press for more medication, he suggested that he and my wife should take the matter to the ethics committee of our nearby hospital.

We never learned why the doctor turned to the ethics committee: whether for legal, moral, or other reasons. In any event, it was another two weeks — two long weeks — before the committee, composed of 15 laypeople, internists, psychiatrists, nurses, members of the clergy, and others, could review our case.

At the hearing, the senior nurse from the nursing home said that some members of her staff felt uncomfortable about giving that much medication to the patient. My wife, speaking movingly and eloquently, stressed that the issue was her mother's comfort, not the comfort of the nurses. My wife suggested that those who felt uncomfortable might want to recuse themselves from her mother's care.

Her mother's doctor told that panel that he depended on the nurses to look after his patients in his absence and thought he should respect their feelings. A lay member of the committee responded that the patient's care — not the nurse's feelings — was his first responsibility. An internist member pointed out that my wife, having looked after her mother for four years, was a far better judge than the nurses and the doctor of whether she was frightened and in pain.

At the end of its hearing, the committee advised unanimously that the patient should be placed on the more intense treatment program recommended by the people from hospice care. Having brought the matter to a head, my mother-in-law's physician now seemed obligated to order the recommended continuous intravenous morphine drip, and he did so. But only after 24 hours went by.

My mother-in-law died about three weeks later. That night, a covering physician, someone whom we did not know, saw her and signed the death certificate. The next day, my wife received a condolence call from the retired physician who had once been her mother's doctor. She has never heard from the doctor in charge of her mother's care.

I do not write this in anger, as an unforgiving tirade about the behavior of a particular doctor. I write it in sorrow that some physicians who work in nursing homes seem not to know how to care for dying patients. They need to realize that pain comes in many forms, emotional as well as physical. They need to understand that relieving pain, and helping a patient die in peace, is more important than not affronting the nurses. They need to listen to the thoughts and concerns of the family. They must learn to grasp, that in the last scene of a life, the patient's comfort comes before the comfort of all the other players.

Why did my wife not encounter similar problems with the first physician? Who can say for sure? Both doctors had to cope with the pressures and challenges of practicing medicine in today's environment. Perhaps by virtue of experience and maturity, the older physician was still up to the task of putting his patient's interest above those pressures, whereas maybe the medical care environment had begun to erode the compassion that had drawn the younger one into the profession.

Going to one's death in fear and anxiety may not be listed in the coding table for reimbursable medical conditions, and it may not rank in urgency with other problems, such as 42 million people without health insurance, medical errors caused by insufficient nursing coverage and dysfunctional information systems, doctors quitting medicine prematurely or to work with for-profit HMOs or Medicare, and the pending implosion of the medical care system. But it touches on the soul of medicine.

— L. Laster, MD, "Whose Comfort Are They Managing?" *Washington Post,* 15 December 2002.

XI. STUDY QUESTIONS

1. What are the criteria for determining brain death? What is the difference between brain death and death as defined by heart/lung criteria? Why can't a premature infant be declared brain dead?

2. Explain the connection between hospice care and palliative care.

3. What are the major barriers preventing widespread use of hospice care?

4. What does Eric Cassell mean when he states that the suffering of the dying is not only physical, but emotional and existential?

5. Is there such a thing as rational suicide?

6. Describe some of the major objections to physician-assisted suicide, both religious and nonreligious.

7. Consider case 1. What, in your opinion, could have been done to bring about a better outcome?

8. Use case 3 to develop a role-play in which

the physician uses Buckman's six-step method to discuss advance care plans with the family of the nursing home patient.

NOTES

1. S.S. Morrison, D.E. Meier, and C. Capello, ed., *Geriatric Palliative Care* (New York: Oxford University Press, 2003), xxi-xxx; Last Acts, "Means to a Better End: A Report on Dying in America Today," November 2002, *http://www.rwjf.org/files/publications/other/meansbetterend.pdf.*

2. Ibid.

3. Ibid.

4. N.N. Dubler and D. Nimmons, *Ethics on Call* (New York: Harmony, 1992), 156.

5. W.D. Poe, *The Old Person in Your Home* (New York: Scribners, 1969), 68.

6. B.A. Brody and H.T. Engelhardt, Jr., *Bioethics: Readings and Cases* (Englewood Cliffs, N.J.: Prentice-Hall, 1987), 377.

7. *Black's Law Dictionary,* 4th ed. rev., (St. Paul, Minn.: West, 1968): 488-9.

8. *Gray v. Sawyer,* 247 S.W.2d 496 (Ky. Ct.App. 1952).

9. Ad Hoc Committee of the Harvard Medical School, "A Definition of Irreversible Coma: Report of the Ad Hoc Committee of the Harvard Medical School to Examine the Definition of Brain Death," *Journal of the American Medical Association* 205 (1968): 337-40.

10. Ibid., 337-8.

11. See note 6 above, p. 378.

12. President's Commission for the Study of Ethical Problems in Medicine and Biomedical and Behavioral Research, *Defining Death* (Washington, D.C.: U.S. Government Printing Office, 1981), 2.

13. American Academy of Pediatrics, Task Force on Brain Death in Children, "Guidelines for the Determination of Brain Death in Children," *Pediatrics* 80 (1987): 298-300.

14. R.E. Behrman and V.C. Vaughan III, *Nelson Textbook of Pediatrics,* 13th ed. (Philadelphia, Pa.: Saunders, 1987), 1299.

15. E.J. Cassell, *Nature of Suffering* (New York: Oxford University Press, 1991), 33.

16. M. Christopher, *State Initiatives in End-of-Life Care* (Washington, D.C. Last Acts, November 2002), 1-8.

17. C.M.S. Saunders, "The Care of the Dying Patient and His Family," in *Ethics in Medicine:*

Historical Perspectives and Contemporary Concerns, ed. S.J. Reiser, A.J. Dyck, and W.J. Curran (Cambridge, Mass.: Massachusetts Institute of Technology Press, 1977), 513.

18. Harvard Medical School Health Publications Group, "A Guide to Hospice Care," *Harvard Health Letter* (September 1994), Special Reprint, First Printing; Ibid., 512.

19. The SUPPORT Principal Investigators, "A Controlled Trial To Improve Care for Seriously Ill Hospitalized Patients: The Study to Understand Prognoses and Preferences for Outcomes and Risks of Treatments (SUPPORT)," *Journal of the American Medical Association* 274 (1995): 1591-8.

20. B. Lo, "Improving Care Near the End of Life: Why Is It So Hard?" *Journal of the American Medical Association* 274 (1995): 1634-1636.

21. D. Callahan, "Once Again, Reality: Now Where Do We Go?: The Lessons of the SUPPORT Study," *Hastings Center Report,* special supp. 25, (1995): S33-S36.

22. See note 16 above, pp.1-10.

23. Task Force on Palliative Care, *Precepts of Palliative Care* (Washington, D.C. Last Acts, December 1997).

24. M.J. Field and C.K. Cassel, ed., *Approaching Death: Improving Care at the End of Life* (Washington, D.C.: National Academy Press, 1997), 1-32.

25. Ibid.

26. The Center to Advance Palliative Care, "FAQ Section: Home Page" *http://www.capc.org,* accessed 20 February 2004.

27. J.E. Brody, "Providing Care, When the Cure Is Out of Reach," *New York Times, Health and Fitness,* 18 November 2003, section F.

28. The Center to Advance Palliative Care, The Case for Hospital-Based Palliative Care, *http://capc.org,* accessed 20 February 2004.

29. Last Acts, see note 1 above.

30. R. Marks and E. Sachar, "Undertreatment of Medical Inpatients with Narcotic Analgesics," *Annals of Internal Medicine* 78 (1973): 173-81.

31. B.A. Rich, "A Legacy of Silence: Bioethics and the Culture of Pain," *Journal of Medical Humanities* 18 (1997): 233-59.

32. *Last Acts Quarterly* 13, no. 3 (2003): 2; see note 1 above.

33. See note 16 above, pp. 6-7

34. B. Jennings et al., "Access to Hospice Care: Expanding Boundaries, Overcoming Barriers," *Hastings Center Report* 33, special supp. (2003):
S3-S59.

35. See note 16 above.

36. Ibid.

37. See note 34 above, S27-S39.

38. See note 16 above.

39. L.M. Crawley et al., "Strategies for Culturally Effective End-of-Life Care," *Annals of Internal Medicine* 136 (2002): 673-9.

40. See note 34 above, S39.

41. M. Kagawa-Singer and L.J. Blackhall, "Negotiating Cross-Cultural Issues at the End of Life: 'You Got to Go Where He Lives,'" *Journal of the American Medical Association* 286 (2001): 2993-3001.

42. See note 39 above, p. 676.

43. L.M. Schmidt, "Why Cultural Issues Must be Recognized at the End of Life," *Care and Caring Near the End of Life* (Washington, D.C.: Last Acts, Winter 2001), 1.

44. See note 41 above, p. 2999.

45. See note 4 above, pp. 1-2; J. Rachels, *The End of Life: Euthanasia and Morality* (New York: Oxford University Press, 1986), 7-19.

46. M.A. Lee et al., "Legalizing Assisted Suicide: Views of Physicians in Oregon," *New England Journal of Medicine* 334, no. 5 (1996): 310-5.

47. S.J. Reiser, "The Dilemma of Euthanasia in Modern Medical History: The English and American Experience," in *Ethics in Medicine: Historical Perspectives and Contemporary Concerns,* ed. S.J. Reiser, A.J. Dyck, and W.J. Curran (Cambridge, Mass.: Massachusetts Institute of Technology Press, 1977), 488.

48. Ibid., 488-90.

49. Ibid., 491.

50. D.C. Thomasma and G.C. Graber, *Euthanasia: Toward An Ethical Social Policy* (New York: Continuum, 1990), 186.

51. "It's Over, Debbie," *Journal of the American Medical Association* 259, no. 2 (1988): 272.

52. W. Gaylin et al., "Doctors Must Not Kill," *Journal of the American Medical Association* 259 (1988): 2140.

53. S.H. Wanzer et al., "The Physician's Responsibility toward Hopelessly Ill Patients: A Second Look," *New England Journal of Medicine* 320 (1989): 848.

54. "Jack Kevorkian to Remain in Prison," *Associated Press,* 2 October 2003.

55. T.E. Quill, "Death and Dignity: A Case of Individualized Decision Making," *New England Journal of Medicine* 324 (1991): 691-4.

56. Ibid., 693.

57. E. Emanuel, "Euthanasia and Physician-Assisted Suicide: A Review of the Empirical Data from the United States," *Archives of Internal Medicine* 162 (2002): 142-52.

58. American Medical Association, Council on Ethical and Judicial Affairs, "Decisions Near the End of Life," *Journal of the American Medical Association* 267 (1992): 2229-33.

59. President's Commission for the Study of Ethical Problems in Medicine and Biomedical and Behavioral Research, *Deciding to Forego Life-Sustaining Treatment* (Washington, D.C.: U.S. Government Printing Office, 1983), 72; American Geriatrics Society Public Policy Committee, "Voluntary Active Euthanasia," *Journal of the American Geriatrics Society* 39 (1991): 826.

60. D. Callahan, "To Kill and to Ration: Preserving the Difference," in *What Kind of Life: The Limits of Medical Progress* (New York: Simon and Schuster, 1990), 221-49; A.J. Dyck, "An Alternative to the Ethic of Euthanasia," in *Ethics in Medicine: Historical Perspectives and Contemporary Concerns*, ed. S.J. Reiser, A.J. Dyck, and W.J. Curran (Cambridge, Mass.: Massachusetts Institute of Technology Press, 1977), 529-35; Gaylin et al., see note 52 above; B. Jennings, "Active Euthanasia and Forgoing Life-Sustaining Treatment: Can We Hold the Line?" *Journal of Pain and Symptom Management* 6 (1991): 312-6; H. Arkes et al., "Always to Care, Never to Kill," *Wall Street Journal*, 27 November 1991, 8; T.D. Sullivan, "Active and Passive Euthanasia: An Impertinent Distinction?" in *Biomedical Ethics*, ed. T.A. Mappes and J.S. Zembaty (New York: McGraw-Hill, 1991), 371-4; R.I. Misbin, "Physicians Aid In Dying," *New England Journal of Medicine* 325 (1991): 1307-11; G.R. Scofield, "Physician-Assisted Suicide: Part of the Problem or Part of the Solution?" *Trends in Health Care, Law & Ethics* 7, no. 2 (Winter 1992): 15-8; A.J. Dyck, "Physician-Assisted Suicide: Is It Ethical?" *Trends In Health Care, Law & Ethics* 7, no. 2 (Winter 1992): 19-22; S.M. Wolf, "Holding the Line on Euthanasia," *Hastings Center Report* 19 (January-February 1989): 13-5; R.A. McCormick, "Physician-Assisted Suicide: Flight from Compassion," *Christian Century* 108, no. 35 (4 December 1991): 1132-4.

61. T.E. Quill, C.K. Cassel, and D.E. Meier, "Care of the Hopelessly Ill: Proposed Clinical Criteria for Physician-Assisted Suicide," *New England Journal of Medicine* 327 (1992): 1380-4; N.S. Jecker, "Giving Death a Hand: When the Dying and the Doctor Stand in a Special Relationship," *Journal of the American Geriatrics Society* 39 (1991): 831-5; H. Brody, "Assisted Death — A Compassionate Response to a Medical Failure," *New England Journal of Medicine* 327 (1992): 1384-8; M. Angell, "Doctors and Assisted Suicide," *Annals of the Royal College of Physicians and Surgeons of Canada* 24, no. 7 (1991): 94-5; C. Cassel and D. Meier, "Morals and Moralism in the Debate over Euthanasia and Assisted Suicide," *New England Journal of Medicine* 323 (1990): 750-2; R.F. Weir, "The Morality of Physician-Assisted Suicide," *Law, Medicine & Health Care* 20 (1992): 116-26.

62. G.I. Benrubi, "Euthanasia — The Need for Procedural Safeguards," *New England Journal of Medicine* 326 (1992): 197-9; J. Rachels, "Active and Passive Euthanasia," in *Biomedical Ethics*, ed. T.A. Mappes and J.S. Zembaty (New York: McGraw-Hill, 1991), 367-70; "Physician-Assisted Suicide and the Right to Die with Assistance," *Harvard Law Review* 105 (1992): 2021-40; E.H. Loewy, "Healing and Killing, Harming and Not Harming: Physician Participation in Euthanasia and Capital Punishment," *The Journal of Clinical Ethics* 3, no. 1 (Spring 1992): 29-34; C.H. Baron, "The Fictional Distinction between Active and Passive Euthanasia and the Danger It Poses to the Civil Liberties of Patients," (paper presented at American Civil Liberties Union Biennial Conference, University of Vermont, 26-30 June 1991); P. Singer, "A Consequentialist Argument for Active Euthanasia," in *Bioethics: Readings and Cases*, ed. B.A. Brody and H.T. Engelhardt, Jr. (Englewood Cliffs, N.J.: Prentice-Hall, 1987),165-9.

63. Dyck, "An Alternative to the Ethic of Euthanasia," see note 60 above, p. 530.

64. E.D. Pellegrino, "Doctors Must Not Kill," *The Journal of Clinical Ethics* 3, no. 2 (Summer 1992): 96-7.

65. J.C. Fletcher, "The Patient's Right to Die," in *Euthanasia and the Right to Death*, ed. A.B. Downing (New York: Humanities Press, 1971).

66. Gaylin et al., see note 52 above; Dyck, "An Alternative to the Ethic of Euthanasia," see note 60 above; Callahan, see note 60 above; see note 58 above; Wolf, see note 60 above; McCormick, see note 60 above; Arkes et al., see note 60 above.

67. See note 64 above, pp. 98-9.

68. Ibid., 100.

69. Ibid., 97-8.

70. S. Hauerwas, *Suffering Presence* (Notre Dame, Ind.: University of Notre Dame Press, 1986),

107.

71. W.F. May, *Physician's Covenant* (Philadelphia, Pa.: Westminister Press, 1983), 67.

72. Ibid., 83-4.

73. See note 62 above.

74. Baron, see note 62 above, pp. 12-3.

75. T.E. Quill and I.R. Byock for the American College of Physicians-American Society of Internal Medicine End-of-Life Care Consensus Panel, "Responding to Intractable Terminal Suffering: The Role of Terminal Sedation and Voluntary Refusal of Food and Fluids," *Annals of Internal Medicine* 132 (2000): 408-14.

76. Ibid. 408-18; D. Orentlicher, "The Supreme Court and Physician-Assisted Suicide — Rejecting Assisted Suicide but Embracing Euthanasia," *New England Journal of Medicine* 337 (1997): 1236-9.

77. Orentlicher, ibid.

78. "Physician-Assisted Suicide: Oregon's Death with Dignity Act," Oregon Department of Human Services, at *http://www.ohd.hr.state.or.us/chs/pas/pas.cfm,* accessed 16 July 2003.

79. R. Leman, "Sixth Annual Report on Oregon's Death with Dignity Act," Oregon Department of Human Services, 10 March 2004.

80. L.O. Gostin, "Deciding Life and Death in the Courtroom," *Journal of the American Medical Association* 278 (1997): 1523-8.

81. See note 57 above.

82. L.F. Wiley, "Assisted Suicide: Court Strikes Down Ashcroft Directive," *Journal of Law, Medicine & Ethics* 30 (2002): 459-60.

83. *Compassion in Dying v. State of Washington,* 79 F.3d 790 (9th Cir. 1996).

84. Ibid., 816.

85. Ibid., 836.

86. *Quill v. Vacco,* 80 F.3d 716, p. 729 (2d Cir. 1996).

87. D.M. Gianelli, "AMA to Court: No Suicide Aid," *American Medical News,* 25 November 1996.

88. F.G. Miller, "Legalizing Physician-Assisted Suicide by Judicial Decision: A Critical Appraisal," *Bioethics Matters* 5, no. 3 (July 1996): insert 1-4.

89. Ibid., 3.

90. Ibid.

91. J. Biskupic, "High Court Allows Ban on Assisted Suicide, Strikes Down Law Restricting Online Speech," *Washington Post,* 27 June 1997, p. A1.

92. *Washington v. Glucksberg,* 521 US 702, p. 753.

93. *Vacco v. Quill,* 521 US 793, p. 808.

94. See note 92 above, p. 723.

95. Ibid., 725.

96. Ibid., 727.

97. R. Cohen-Almago, "Why the Netherlands?" *Journal of Law, Medicine & Ethics* 30 (2002): 95-104.

98. B. Onwuteaka-Philipsen et al., "Euthanasia and Other End-of-Life Decisions in the Netherlands in 1990, 1995, and 2001," *Lancet* 362 (2003): 395-9.

99. Ibid., 398.

100. C. Manuel, "Physician-Assisted Suicide Permits Dignity in Dying," *Journal of Legal Medicine* 23 (2002): 1-21.

101. W. Winslade, "Teaching about Dying," *Choice in Dying News* 1, no. 4 (Winter 1992): 1-6.

102. R. Buckman, *How to Break Bad News: A Guide for Health Professionals* (Baltimore, Md.: Johns Hopkins University Press, 1992).

103. Ibid.

104. Z. Ben-Sira, "The Function of the Professional's Affective Behavior in Client Satisfaction," *Journal of Health and Social Behavior* 17 (1976): 3-11.

105. R.J. Baron, "An Introduction to Medical Phenomenology: I Can't Hear You When I'm Listening," *Annals of Internal Medicine* 101 (1985): 606-11.

106. H.B. Beckman and R.M. Frankel, "The Effect of Physician Behavior on the Collection of Data," *Annals of Internal Medicine* 101 (1984): 692-6.

107. See note 102 above, pp. 44-50.

108. Ibid., 187-8.

109. Ibid., 96-7.

13

The Decision to Forgo Life-Sustaining Treatment When the Patient Is Incapacitated

John C. Fletcher and Walter S. Davis

I. INTRODUCTION

The difficult ethical issues created when a patient decides to forgo life-sustaining medical treatment, discussed in chapter 11 of this text, are compounded and made more complex when (1) the patient is seriously or irreversibly incapacitated; or (2) the patient never had decisional capacity. Ethical problems related to such cases are among the most frequent faced by clinicians, family members, and guardians in critical care settings and long-term care facilities, and the legal battles surrounding these cases have increasingly attracted media and public attention.[1] Indeed, in every decade since the 1960s, there has been at least one or two major legal struggles involving a surrogate seeking to forgo further life-sustaining treatment on behalf of an incapacitated patient. These cases are characterized by a tragic combination of technical uncertainty, pain and suffering, poor quality of life, costly technologies, and the probability of death if the patient is not treated.

This chapter begins by tracing the history of the problem and some of its causes. It then sketches the evolution of ethical and legal norms and describes the types of cases that most frequently arise for clinicians. The evolution of the most salient conceptual issues involved in these cases will be explored, both within and outside the context of the legal cases themselves. Finally, this chapter provides ethical guidelines for clinicians to consider and discusses the reasons for the goals that shape the guidelines.

II. HISTORICAL PERSPECTIVES

A. Early History of Medical Technology

Reiser surveyed the history of medical care for the most hopelessly ill persons, beginning in ancient Greek medicine with Hippocrates and his students.[2] He noted that the main theme in Hippocrates's essay, "Epidemics," is balancing treatment that is intended to benefit patients with the possibility of inflicting harm on them.[3] The Hippocratic medical ethic, widely misunderstood as a simple maxim of "do no harm," is much more complex and integral to the main theme of this chapter. Hippocrates said, "As to diseases, make a habit of two things — to help, or at least to do no harm."[4] Hippocrates also advised students "to refuse to treat those who are overmastered by their diseases, realizing that in such cases medicine is powerless."[5] These ethical concerns are similar to the issues discussed in this chapter, and there is evidence of ancient predecessors of intensive care.

Researchers have found there are records of intensive monitoring of extremely sick persons in ancient Egypt and other civilizations,[6] and Bloom and Lundberg have identified the roots of modern intensive care in many ancient settings.[7] "Rescue" technologies may have begun with Vesalius's (1543) experiment with an animal to maintain breathing with a bellows and tube. Rescue workers in England used this method in the nineteenth century to resuscitate drowned persons. The first tank respirator was invented in 1832. Use of the Drinker/Shaw "iron lung" (1929) in the polio epidemic resulted in the earliest ethical dilemmas of selection and weaning.[8] Technologies to support heart and kidney function came next. Reiser notes that Albert Hyman, in the 1930s, placed a needle electrode into the chest of 43 patients in cardiac arrest and saved 14, but the press condemned his work.[9] Willem Kolff invented the dialysis machine in the 1940s in Holland during the Nazi occupation; selection of patients for dialysis dramatized ethical conflicts and was one of the causes for the "birth of bioethics."

The intensive care unit (ICU) had its origins in England in the mid-nineteenth century, with small rooms next to surgical amphitheaters for extra care in patient recovery, as noted by Florence Nightingale.[10] ICUs for premature infants began in France and spread to many nations. The number of general ICUs to treat acute trauma in adults grew in the years of World War II, especially after the 1942 Coconut Grove fire in Boston. The specialized ICU of today took several decades to evolve.[11] ICU care blossomed in the 1960s, from a place of brief interventions for trauma, to a setting for long-term treatment that has been extended to everyone. With this change came the agenda of ethical and legal concerns that are the main subject of this chapter.

B. Recent History of the Problem

Today, at least three major factors contribute to the high incidence of cases involving the decision to forgo life-sustaining treatment when the patient is incapacitated:
1. The rapid growth of technologies for critical-care medicine and the changing role of physicians, including the expectation that physicians control these technologies,
2. The increasing numbers of incapacitated patients in hospitals and nursing homes, and
3. A cultural demand to use technology to prolong the lives of dying patients.

1. Technology and the Physician's Role

Lewis Thomas, the late medical essayist, told a story of being invited to a county medical association in the 1950s to inaugurate the president-elect. At dinner, the physician-honoree received a phone call. He left, and returned just as the evening was ending. Having missed his own inauguration, he explained to Thomas that his patient, near death for days, had just died. He left the meeting, in his words, because "the family was in distress and needed him." Thomas ended the story, "This was in the early 1950s when medicine was turning into a science, but the old art was still in place."[12]

Thomas's story is in a book by Winslade and Ross that traces the change in the role of the physician in the twentieth century. In the "old art" of medicine, doctors treated the patient in the context of the family. With the "new science," the physician's goal is to diagnose and treat disease processes. The person with the disease is not the center of attention. The physician's task today, the book argues, is to combine the old art and the new science. The authors argue that only the "prepared" patient and family will benefit from the new science and will be able to avoid the harms that can result from inappropriate use of the technologies that are found mainly in large teaching or community hospitals — kidney dialysis, respirators, organ transplantation, chemotherapies, coronary bypass operations, artificial feeding and hydration, and so forth. One of the tasks of an ethics program in a healthcare organization is to prepare members of the community by educating them to be patients and surrogate decision makers in the context of high-technology treatment.

2. Increasing Numbers of Incapacitated Patients

Today, there are many more incapacitated adult patients in the clinical setting than a generation ago. One major cause is the aging of the population; a second is that more patients survive after head trauma, stroke, and alcohol and other substance abuse.

Americans in very large numbers are aging. The fastest-growing age group in America is the population above the age of 85, and those over the age of 65 will soon represent the majority of patients routinely seen by internists.[13] By 2030, when the large baby boom cohort has entered old age, one in five persons (20 percent) will be in the 65-and-older age group.[14] With this phenomenon comes a percentage of patients with diminished capacity due to Alzheimer's disease and other types of dementia. The number of people with severe dementia has increased dramatically in recent years, and, to compound the problem, this cohort has a higher incidence of significant co-morbidities, such as diabetes and heart disease, that predispose them to the intensive care setting at the end of life. In addition to this, there is emerging evidence that patients over 65 who suffer severe trauma have a greater likelihood of dying before discharge from the hospital, despite aggressive trauma management and intensive care.[15] Decisional capacity is therefore an increasingly important issue in hospitals and skilled nursing facilities. Chapter 9 discusses patients' capacity to participate in routine healthcare decisions, a major issue in each clinician-patient encounter.

Concern about incapacity is well justified when the focus is on decision making for patients in the ICU setting. Critically ill patients are more often incapable of communicating. Investigators have found that only 45 percent of the 4,301 seriously ill patients in Phase I of the SUPPORT Study (a two-year prospective observational study) were able to communicate.[16] Decisions to forgo treatment are decisions about death, and that is why these decisions ought to be, and are, so difficult. In the medical-surgical ICUs of two large hospitals in San Francisco, researchers reported that only five of 115 patients were capable of making decisions.[17] In a general medical ICU in a Rochester, New York, community hospital, researchers found that only five of 28 patients could participate in decision making.[18] In the latter two studies, however, family members were available to be surrogates in 90 percent of the cases; thus family members can usually be found to serve as surrogate decision makers.

3. Prolonging Life: What Kind of Life?

Anthropologist Lynn Payer asserts that American medicine is much more aggressive with technology at the end of life than in other cultures.[19] Where Americans die is strong evidence of a cultural shift, despite "halfway" measures: in 1949, half of those who died in the U.S. died at home or at the scene of accidents, and only 49 percent died in hospitals or nursing homes; by 1983, the President's Commission for the Study of Ethical Problems in Medicine and Biomedical and Behavioral Research found that about 80 percent of Americans died in hospitals or nursing homes.[20] Nearly a decade later, the National Center for Health Statistics reported data on deaths in hospitals (61 percent) and in nursing homes (17 percent).[21] There are large variations in specific states.[22]

The findings reported by the SUPPORT investigators provide empirical confirmation of Payer's observation. In Phase I of the study, observers documented shortcomings in communication and on the frequency of aggressive treatment. They also recorded that dying in the hospital was often sad and painful. For example, only 47 percent of physicians knew when their patients desired to avoid cardiopulmonary resuscitation (CPR); 46 percent of do-not-resuscitate (DNR) orders were written within two days of death; 38 percent of patients who died spent at least 10 days in an ICU; and for 50 percent of patients who died in the hospital, family members reported moderate to severe pain at least half of the time.[23]

Phase II of SUPPORT was a controlled trial; 4,804 patients and their physicians were assigned randomly by specialty group to an intervention group (n = 2,652) or to a control group (n = 2,152). For the intervention group, specially trained nurses had multiple contacts with patients, families, physicians, and hospital staff to elicit their preferences, improve understanding of outcomes, encourage attention to pain control, and facilitate advance-care planning and communication. Investigators reported that, as a result of this intervention, there was no improvement in any of the following outcomes:

1. Physician-patient communication (37 percent of control patients and 40 percent of intervention patients discussed CPR preferences),
2. Incidence or timing of DNR orders,
3. Physicians' knowledge of patients' preferences about CPR,
4. Days spent in an ICU,
5. Use of mechanical ventilation,
6. Days comatose before death,
7. Level of reported pain, and
8. Use of hospital resources.[24]

SUPPORT also confirmed that the term "life-sustaining technology" may be misleading. Aggressive measures can rescue some gravely ill patients from certain death. However, these interventions may only prolong the process of dying, cause needless suffering, or maintain a vegetative or profoundly impaired existence that has little benefit to the patient. As gerontologist and bioethicist Jerome Kurent maintains, "there is a tension between our wish to achieve a good death characterized by high quality comfort care versus an increasing tendency to prolong the dying process by providing medically futile care when there is no expectation for meaningful survival."[25] In referring to any life-sustaining technology, the question posed in the title of Daniel Callahan's book, *What Kind of Life?* is always relevant.[26]

4. Quality of Life Questions and Objections to Forgoing Life-Sustaining Treatment

In addition to the above forces producing increasing numbers of these cases overall, there has also been a shift in the source of objections to forgoing life-sustaining treatment and a challenge to our long-held assertions about quality of life as the justification for withholding or withdrawing life-sustaining treatment and technologies. While bioethicists have traditionally approached these cases as "right to die" cases, in which a patient or a surrogate chooses to forgo life-sustaining treatment or technology because death is seen as preferable to the quality of life following a major accident to illness, representatives of the disability community — which we can define as persons living with a significant disability and their advocates — maintain that these cases are really about severely disabled individuals or their surrogates choosing to forgo life with a disability.[27] As a steady stream of cases involving patients with a diagnosis of persistent vegetative state, high-level quadriplegia, or other severe physical and cognitive disabilities has captured public and media attention, disability advocates have weighed in on the side of *not* withdrawing or withholding aggressive care, arguing that the issue is not that patients or their surrogates choose death over a life with a severe disability, but that society does not value the lives of those with disabilities — it is a matter of discrimination. Many disability advocates further assert that bioethicists who argue for a right to die, based on an assumption of autonomous choice, are merely creating a philosophical smokescreen to allow passive, or even active, extermination of those with disabilities that are viewed as too expensive, unpleasant, or emotionally disturbing for society to tolerate.[28]

One such group, which calls itself "Not Dead Yet," in a tongue-in-cheek reference to the black humor of the popular movie *Monty Python and the Holy Grail,* cites a list of studies in the medical literature that point to a pervasive and consistent underestimation by healthcare professionals, and society at large, of the quality of life of individuals with severe disabilities. They call attention to the fact that very little still is known about the actual experience of those with severe neurological impairment such as persistent vegetative state, and that our default assumption should be that patients with these types of severe impairments have some sort of quality of life, and that it is not for those of us on the "outside looking in" to make a judgment that such a life is not worth sustaining.[29] While many bioethicists would counter these assertions with time-honored discussions about autonomy in decisions about medical care, advocacy groups are increasingly making their presence known, not in philosophical discourse in ethics journals, but rather in more active and public ways, in acts of protest and even civil disobedience surrounding high-profile cases followed by the national and international media.

III. CONCEPTUAL ISSUES: THE EVOLUTION OF ETHICAL GUIDELINES FOR CLINICIANS

What norms should guide clinicians in forgoing treatment? And what are the sources of these norms? Ethical guidance for choices to forgo life-sustaining treatment began in ancient Greece and continues to evolve. An older guideline, widely regarded as outworn, is based on a distinction between ordinary and extraordinary or "heroic" treatment. The guideline was that "ordinary treatments" that carry hope of benefit to the patient are obligatory, but "extraordinary treatments" are optional.

A. Futility

In moral debate, *medical futility* can be understood in two senses:

1. In a narrow sense, as physiological futility (that is, when a treatment is ineffective in producing a desired effect, such as using laetrile to treat cancer or administering CPR in the presence of cardiac rupture or severe outflow obstruction), or

2. In a broad sense, as the lack of benefit (that is, even if a treatment might be physiologically effective in a given case, it is futile because it fails to restore consciousness, to prevent total dependence on intensive care, to alleviate suffering, to restore the patient to an acceptable quality of life, or to prevent the patient's dying).

One can immediately see that, if it is used in this second sense, the concept of medical futility is a large tent under which many other disputes can be gathered (such as quality-of-life, rationing expensive end-of-life care, and the issue of who has the authority to make decisions about forgoing treatment).

The literature in clinical ethics on "futility" or "futile care" is large and controversial. After the *Wanglie* decision, there was sharp debate as to how to resolve cases that were seen to involve medical futility.[30] Famous cases included *Baby L,*[31] *Baby K* (see case 2 at the end of this chapter),[32] and other cases involving expensive technology.[33] No consensus about futility has emerged, especially as defined in the broad (second) sense. Physicians' unilateral decisions, especially to withdraw treatments regarded as qualitatively futile, are arguably unethical without a broad consensus in the nation about allocation of expensive resources for critical care. However, the U.S. has neither a political nor an ethical consensus about health policy. We have no consensus about allocation of expensive resources at the end of life, except for organ transplantation.

The literature on futility focuses heavily on resuscitation.[34] Proposals have been made to save money at the end of life by avoiding "futile care,"[35] especially by reducing the incidence of resuscitation for patients with terminal cancer and other poor prognoses.[36] These proposals lack empirical support for the prospect of cost savings. Data from the SUPPORT investigators, expert analysis of Medicare hospital expenditures in the last year of life, and discussion of relatively small economic savings from universal palliative care cast doubt on the prospects of such proposals.[37] Nonetheless, debate about cost savings in critical-care medicine is important, because ICU care is estimated to consume about 1 percent of the U.S. Gross National Product (GNP) or 20 percent of all hospital expenditures.[38] A review article on the history of the do-not-resuscitate order points out that although the concept of the DNR order brought an open decision-making framework to the resuscitation decision and did provide some restraint on the indiscriminate application of CPR to dying patients, there is a surprising lack of training in medical schools and residency programs related to communication with patients and surrogates about DNR decisions, and patients, families, and caregivers continue to inappropriately interpret DNR orders as limitations to treatment other than actual CPR.[39]

Some discussions of futility are also open to criticism because they convey more medical certainty than can be proved, and argue that physicians ought to make unilateral decisions to withhold or withdraw treatment in such a context. Several articles challenge the usefulness of the concept of futility for clinical ethics when it is understood in the broad sense, because it masks so many value judgments.[40] The debate about medical futility can also be a vehicle to "smuggle in" concerns about rationing expensive treatment to the national debate on healthcare reform. Even in the face of disputes about the meaning of futility, some institutions have implemented policies to support and encourage physicians' authority in decisions to withhold treatment in this context.[41]

Stell lucidly explores the historical beginnings and continuing debate about futile treatment.[42] He is critical of defining futility with the concept of lack of benefit. He defines a futile effort in terms of its desired end, due to an "intrinsic defect" (that is, the effort cannot achieve its desired end). He argues that futile efforts, when "undertaken voluntarily and expressing the agent's will, can ennoble the doer and inspire others." In short, futile efforts can have important symbolic meanings for persons, although such expressions clearly have their limits. This issue was clearly part of the dynamics in the Baby K case (*In Re Baby K* — see case 2 at the end of this chapter). One cannot "do" clinical ethics or develop hospital or nursing home policies today without a concept of futility and a strategy for futility disputes.

B. Withholding *versus* Withdrawing: Is It a Distinction with a Difference?

The conventional wisdom was that it was morally harder to withdraw treatment than to withhold it in the first place. For example, in the mid-1970s, a physician wrote: "By not starting a 'routine IV' I am not committed to that modality of therapy. It is easier not to start daily intravenous parenteral fluids than to stop them, once begun — just as it is easier not to turn on the respiratory assistance machine than to turn the switch off, once started."[43]

By the early 1980s, this way of thinking probably was widely shared by clinicians in emergency and critical-care settings. One can question, however, what this physician meant by "easier." If he meant "morally easier," then the claim is open to serious challenge, which the President's Commission did with real effect. In perspective, "easier" likely meant that when resources were virtually unlimited, clinicians felt that more conflict was avoided if they used more technology for the sickest patients. What may feel easier emotionally, however, does not add up to a sound moral judgment.

A preference for withholding treatment was also based on an argument that an important distinction lay between an "act" (leading to death) and an "omission" (leading to death). Withdrawing, in contrast to withholding, was seen as killing the patient. On its face, to act to withdraw appeared to have more moral responsibility attached to it than to omit to act and let the disease take its course.

There are other reasons why it is hard to stop treatments that become marginally beneficial or even futile (for example, loyalty to the patient, gestures aimed toward the family to show that one is doing "everything possible," denial of death, and so forth). A further reason is a misconception, by clinicians or hospital administrators, that the law always requires maintaining life-sustaining treatment.[44] This is untrue in any state, although there are many important variations among states in their laws on forgoing treatment.[45]

Is there a real moral difference — with a sharp bite and a bright line — between withholding and withdrawing treatment? The President's Commission strongly challenged, but did not silence, the conventional wisdom.[46] The commission argued that it ought to be morally harder to withhold any treatment, especially if it has not yet been tried, than to withdraw any treatment that has been tried and has failed to benefit the patient or is physiologically futile. When there is doubt that one or more treatments will benefit a patient, clinicians should consider conducting a brief therapeutic trial. If they know that a treatment is not effective or beneficial, however, there is no moral obligation to continue it.

This point can be reinforced by clarifying the goals of treatment when patients are dying or hopelessly ill. The goals for such patients should shift from prolonging life to providing comfort and relief of suffering. Continuing aggressive treatment, such as mechanical ventilation, may cause discomfort, without producing any compensating benefit for the patient. In caring for dying patients, withdrawing burdensome treatment is just as important as withholding aggressive treatment, such as CPR.[47]

C. The Evolving Spectrum of Neurologic Impairment

While medical technology, especially in the realm of emergency and intensive care, has continued to advance, improving the collective prognosis for patients with serious injury and illness, our understanding of true awareness, and therefore capacity, in patients with severe neurologic impairment remains fairly unsophisticated. We do have a general idea of the major factors that affect outcome and recovery, such as the etiology of the injury, anatomic location, severity, and extent, but the precise interaction and priority of these factors in the overall prognosis remains largely a mystery. New imaging techniques, such as functional magnetic resonance imaging (FMRI) and positron emission tomography (PET), offer the promise of newer and greater understanding of cognition in the injured brain, but we are still far away from a situation in which we are able to predict outcome and functional recovery in these states with enough certainty to help in decision making.

The two most common diagnoses applied to patients with severe cognitive impairment are *coma* and *persistent vegetative state* (PVS). A coma is a profound or deep state of unconsciousness, in which the person is alive, but unable to react or respond to her or his environment. Persistent vegetative state, which can follow a coma, is a condition in which the person has lost cognitive neurological function and awareness of the environment, but retains noncognitive neurological function and a preserved sleep-wake cycle. In 1994, a multi-society task force made up of representatives of the American Academy of Neurology, the Child Neurology Society, the American

Association of Neurological Surgeons, and the American Academy of Pediatrics produced a "Consensus Statement on the Medical Aspects of the Persistent Vegetative State," which states that PVS is "a wakeful unconscious state that lasts longer than a few weeks,"[48] and can be diagnosed according to the following criteria:

- No evidence of awareness of self or environment and an inability to interact with others;
- No evidence of sustained, reproducible, purposeful, or voluntary behavioral responses to visual, auditory, tactile, or noxious stimuli;
- No evidence of language comprehension or expression;
- Intermittent wakefulness manifested by the presence of sleep-wake cycles;
- Sufficiently preserved hypothalamic and brain-stem autonomic function to permit survival with medical and nursing care;
- Bowel and bladder incontinence;
- Variably preserved cranial-nerve reflexes (papillary, oculocephalic, corneal, vestibulo-ocular, and gag) and spinal reflexes.

Despite the comprehensive language of these guidelines and the reliance on largely objective medical criteria, critics argue that decisions about forgoing life-sustaining care in these individuals usually rely upon two problematic assumptions:

- That patients who appear to be in this state have no awareness of themselves or their situation, and
- That the condition is permanent and irreversible.

Both of these assumptions were part of the initial description and definition of the condition put forth by Jennet and Plum in 1972, and continue to be widely held when making the diagnosis of PVS.[49] As noted above, advances in neurological imaging and other technologies are still inadequate to help us clarify these issues, and currently it is possible for those on both sides of the debate to use this uncertainty to support their own assertions about withholding and withdrawing care for these patients.

The reliance upon these two assumptions can also be seen as laying out the agenda for research in the neurosciences. Other terms and diagnoses have been proposed to describe states of severe neurological impairment, including "permanent vegetative state" and "minimally conscious state," but all essentially describe a list of criteria ascer-

tained by clinical neurological examination or specific diagnostic testing. The crucial research question remains: Given certain findings and parameters of neurological impairment, what is the prognosis for recovery of awareness and a return to some level of independent functioning? A 2004 review article found that several simple physical maneuvers strongly predict death or poor outcome in comatose survivors.[50] This meta-analysis involved data from approximately 2,000 patients, was the largest review of this kind to date, and found that the chance of meaningful recovery was very small in patients who lack papillary and corneal reflexes at 24 hours, and have no motor response at 72 hours. The authors of this review point out that the study is intended to provide prognostic information, rather than treatment recommendations, and that actual treatment decisions are best made on an individual basis, incorporating other variables.

D. Advance Directives

A clear, well-considered, and appropriately executed advance directive will obviously be helpful in making decisions about forgoing life-sustaining treatment, but frequently the language of the directive is not specific enough to address the clinical situation at hand. Family members or other surrogates may wish to override the advance directive, with the thought that "this isn't what they meant," and clinicians are often reluctant to strictly honor an advance directive in the face of substantial objections by surrogates.

Bioethicists had great hopes that advance directives would dramatically change decision making about forgoing life-sustaining treatment, but in fact the inherent problems of (1) understanding of options prior to actual morbidity, and (2) the overall vague nature of much of the language used in advance directives continue to limit their usefulness in many cases. Still, for many chronically ill individuals with a fairly comprehensive understanding of their disease process and appropriate treatments, the advance directive can be a useful way of documenting preferences about care at the end of life.

E. Surrogate Decision Making

In addition to the benefits/burdens standard, which is discussed in the next section, legal cases have clarified two standards for surrogate decision making when the patient is incapacitated: (1) substituted-judgment standard and (2) the best-interest standard. The first standard should be used when there is evidence that the patient communicated her or his preferences and values before becoming incapacitated. The second standard should be used by clinicians and surrogates when the patient's views are unknown or unknowable.

1. The Substituted-Judgment Standard

A substituted judgment attempts to approximate the moral choices that a patient would have made if he or she could express these choices. If a patient has been capable of making decisions but is presently incapacitated, clinicians and family should ask, "What would be the patient's preferences, if the patient could speak?" This standard was first clarified in the Clare Conroy case in New Jersey (*In Re Conroy*),[51] and it was described as a "subjective standard." Justice Schreiber wrote:

> We hold that life-sustaining treatment may be withheld or withdrawn from an incompetent patient when it is clear that the particular patient would have refused the treatment under the circumstances involved. The standard we are enunciating is a subjective one, consistent with the notion that the right that we are seeking to effectuate is a very personal right to control one's own life. The question is not what a reasonable or average person would have chosen to do under the circumstances, but what the particular patient would have done if able to choose for himself.

The best evidence decision makers can have is from the patient's own statements, verbal or written. Substituted judgment based on verbal statements played a role in the *Cruzan* case (see case B below), because Nancy Ann Cruzan did not have a written advance directive. The U.S. Supreme Court ruled that Missouri could require "clear and convincing" evidence of a person's prior wishes, such as a written document.

2. The Best-Interest Standard

If the patient's preferences for or against life-sustaining treatment are unknown or unknowable, or if the patient has never been capable, then the clinicians, in consultation with the family or guardian, are morally obliged to shape a plan of care regarded as in the "best interest" of the patient. Best interest, in this context, means "best

medical interest," as evaluated in the framework of the benefits and burdens guideline discussed in guideline 2 below, and illustrated by the Saikewicz case, which is discussed in section V, guideline 2, case C, below.

IV. LANDMARK LEGAL CASES: FORUM FOR ETHICAL DEBATE

In a secular society, court cases are an important forum for debating ethical issues and clarifying legal principles and guidelines for decision making. The ethical issues have mainly concerned questions about the basis for decisions to forgo treatment and questions about who has the moral (and legal) standing to make such decisions for incapacitated patients. Decisions to withdraw treatment (and cause death) are essentially decisions to withdraw life-sustaining *technologies*. In recent years, such cases have often been debated in the context of "medical futility," or, as noted earlier, sometimes as "severe disability" cases. While there are certain themes that run through most of these cases, that is, issues of surrogacy — determining a person's preferences regarding quality of life from past conversations and other undocumented interactions — and debate about medical and psychological aspects of various states of impairment, there are also important differences that underscore the growing need for more precise, meaningful guidelines for dealing with these difficult cases.

In addition to the following cases, another landmark case involving a young woman in a PVS was that of Nancy Cruzan, a case originating in Missouri that was eventually heard by the U.S. Supreme Court (*Cruzan v. Director, Missouri Dept. of Health*).[52] This case is discussed later in this chapter in the context of "guidelines for physicians" in section V, guideline 2, case B, below.

A. *Quinlan:* Withdrawing the Ventilator

Karen Ann Quinlan was the patient in one of the first landmark legal cases involving withdrawal of a ventilator (*In Re Quinlan*).[53] In 1975, Quinlan, a 21-year-old New Jersey woman, suffered severe brain damage from anoxia after an alcohol/drug overdose. Brought to an emergency room, she eventually needed a respirator to breathe and a nasogastric feeding tube. She was not "brain dead," but she was eventually diagnosed as being in a persistent vegetative state.

Several months later, her father asked the court to appoint him guardian to authorize removal of the respirator. He was opposed by her physicians, who argued that maintaining the respirator was "standard treatment," and removing it would be an act of euthanasia because it would cause her death.

A lower court, the local prosecutor, and the state's attorney general agreed with the physicians. The New Jersey Supreme Court, however, granted the request. Her doctors weaned her slowly from the ventilator over a two-month period. To everyone's surprise, Quinlan was able to breathe on her own. She continued in a PVS for 10 more years until her death. About withdrawing the ventilator, the New Jersey Supreme Court's reasoning was: "the State's interest (i.e., in the preservation of life) weakens and the individual's right of privacy grows as the degree of bodily invasion increases and the prognosis dims. Ultimately, there comes a point at which the individual's rights overcome the State's interest."[54]

Quinlan's parents wanted the ventilator stopped, but they never asked that artificial feeding and hydration be withdrawn. Other important legal cases became forums for moral debate about withdrawing artificial feeding and hydration.

B. Herbert: Withdrawing Artificial Feeding and Hydration

In the 1980s, controversy shifted to feeding and hydration by intravenous lines, nasogastric tubes (tubes leading into the stomach by way of the nasal passages), or tubes placed surgically into the gastrointestinal tract. The Clarence Herbert case (*Barber v. Superior Court*)[55] was a legal landmark, because the California court was the first to use the President's Commission's benefits/burdens approach in its decision.

In California in 1982, Neil Barber, MD, and Robert Nejdl, MD, were charged with homicide after they stopped life-sustaining treatment at the request of Herbert's spouse and family. On 26 August 1981, a patient with cancer, Clarence Herbert, had surgery to close an ileostomy. In the recovery room, he stopped breathing and his heart stopped (he had a history of heart problems). He was placed on a respirator. On 27 August, the hospital neurologist diagnosed the patient as severely brain damaged and with a poor prognosis. Dr. Barber recommended to Mrs. Herbert that the

respirator be stopped, and she consented. The respirator was stopped on 29 August. However, the patient did not die, and he began to breathe on his own. The next day, the family signed a consent form and wrote that "all machines [be] taken off that are sustaining life." The nasogastric tube and fluids were stopped on 31 August, and Mr. Herbert died on 6 September from dehydration and pneumonia.

A nursing supervisor, Sandra Bardenilla, was concerned about Dr. Nejdl's decision to stop the air mist after removing the respirator. She believed that, without it, the patient would develop a mucous plug and die. Unable to locate either doctor, she received permission from another doctor to restart the air mist. She was angrily reprimanded by Nejdl, who told her that "patients are taken off respirators so that they will die." Angered, she reported the incident to the district attorney, who brought criminal charges, alleging that forgoing both treatments was part of a conspiracy to kill Herbert to hide malpractice. A hearing and two trials resulted. Finally, the court of appeals found the criminal charges baseless. The court cited the reasoning of the President's Commission, that the main approach to such cases was the proportionality of benefits and burdens of each treatment that sustains life.

Some opponents of removing feeding tubes from hopelessly ill patients claim that it "starves them to death." Richard A. McCormick questioned this reasoning.[56] He compared the impact of the disease on the patient to the smashing of a tree by a hurricane, and feeding and hydration to "propping up" the tree in the aftermath. McCormick doubted that a moral fault can be found in removing props from a smashed tree that will die shortly but is putting forth a few leaves as a result of the props. The damage is irreversible. Further, Lynn and Childress assert that continuing to feed hopelessly ill patients can actually cause harm to them.[57] Such patients typically have little interest in food, and problems from a lack of nutrition can be alleviated by medication. The experience of starving in healthy persons is very different than in patients with an incurable disease.[58]

C. Robert Wendland: A Test-Case for Surrogate Decision Making

In 1993, 42-year-old Robert Wendland, while under the influence of alcohol, lost control of his truck, which then rolled over at a high rate of speed. Wendland suffered a severe traumatic brain injury and was left comatose for approximately 14 months. When he regained consciousness, he remained severely neurologically impaired. His left side was paralyzed, he could not be fed by mouth, and he was incontinent of bowel and bladder. He was able to follow two-step commands with extensive prompting and cueing, and able to draw simple shapes, but he was unable to communicate consistently. Over the next two years, Wendland's feeding tube became dislodged several times. In 1995 Wendland's wife Rose refused to authorize reinsertion of the feeding tube, claiming that her husband would not have wanted it replaced. She cited statements he had made before the accident, which she believed indicated that he would not have wanted to be maintained on tube feedings or other artificial means of life support. Wendland's daughter and brother also recalled these statements and agreed with Mrs. Wendland's decision. The decision not to replace the feeding tube was also supported by the hospital's ethics committee and the county ombudsman for patients, but Wendland's mother opposed this, and sought court intervention to have tube feedings resumed, pending a formal judicial ruling. After a series of lower court rulings and appeals, the California Supreme Court agreed to hear the case in 2001. While the court continued to deliberate, Wendland was hospitalized for refractory pneumonia. After two weeks of essentially unsuccessful treatment, Mrs. Wendland refused further aggressive treatment and asked that he receive palliative care only. He died before the court released its final ruling.[59]

Approximately one month later, the California Supreme Court issued its ruling, which stated that Wendland's tube feedings could not have been discontinued. The court conceded that in some circumstances surrogates could make the decision to withhold or withdraw life-sustaining treatment, but that in a case of a conscious patient like Wendland, a surrogate could do so only if there was "clear and convincing evidence" that the patient wished to refuse life-sustaining treatment, or if withholding such treatment was clearly in the "best interest" of the patient. The court stated that Mrs. Wendland had failed to provide sufficient evidence on both counts.[60]

Although the court indicated that its ruling should only apply to those in a "minimally conscious state," critics warned that the ruling might be interpreted too broadly and applied to other incompetent patients, including those who are terminally ill, or whose families and surrogates agree on withholding or withdrawing aggressive care.[61] The court was also criticized for setting too high an evidentiary standard for surrogates making these decisions, and therefore weakening the role of surrogate decision makers, especially spouses, who are typically the default decision maker in these cases.[62]

It is also important to point out that Robert Wendland, unlike Karen Quinlan and Nancy Cruzan, was not in a PVS. His doctors saw little hope of recovery, but Wendland was able to communicate in some fashion and interact with those around him. This important difference fueled the fire for disability advocates, who maintained that Wendland was an example of a person with severe disabilities whose family, and even society, found intolerable.

D. Terri Schiavo: From the Bedside to the State Legislature

The issue of spousal surrogacy is also at the heart of the Schiavo case, which came to a dramatic close in Florida in the spring of 2005, with the full attention of the international media. Theresa Marie (Terri) Schiavo was 26 years old in 1990 when she suffered a cardiac arrest, due to what doctors believe was a potassium imbalance that may have occurred as the result of an eating disorder. She was resuscitated, but suffered severe anoxic brain injury. For 15 years she had required total care, and received feeding and hydration via a percutaneous endoscopic gastrostomy (PEG) tube. Her husband and legal guardian, Michael Schiavo, was initially hopeful that intensive rehabilitation would assist in Ms Schiavo's recovery, but he became convinced over the years that she would not make significant functional progress and wished to remove her feeding tube and allow her to die. Her parents, Robert and Mary Schindler, opposed this, and maintained that their daughter interacted with her surroundings, and had a better quality of life than Michael Schiavo would concede. The case played out over the years through a complicated series of legal challenges and counter challenges, and became the most highly publicized dispute over withdrawal of life-sustaining treatment in an incompetent patient.[63]

At one point late in 2003, after the Schindlers had lost several attempts to block Michael Schiavo from removing his wife's feeding tube, they appealed to Florida Governor Jeb Bush to intervene. The governor filed a federal court brief in support of the Schindler's efforts to stop the removal of the feeding tube, and ultimately the legislature passed "Terri's Law," which allowed the governor a "one-time stay in certain cases." The Florida State Supreme Court unanimously struck down the law as unconstitutional, but by then the case had become politically charged, with right-to-life groups and disability advocates squaring off against proponents of patient's autonomy and those who believed that Michael Schiavo was serving his wife appropriately as a surrogate decision maker and merely carrying out her wishes.

The Schiavo case is yet another example how states have intervened and played a role in the legal and ethical debates surrounding several of the other cases. In Nancy Cruzan's case, the U.S. Supreme Court acknowledged a state's right to place the burden of proof upon a surrogate to show that the surrogate did, indeed, have evidence from personal and literal knowledge of the patient that pointed to withholding or withdrawing life-sustaining technology, and left it to the states to set their own criteria for evaluating this evidence. In the Wendland case, the State of California found that "clear and convincing evidence" was needed that the patient did not or would not want the disputed treatment before a surrogate could make such a decision.

The court did not rule out allowing a surrogate to make such a decision in some cases, but found that, in Robert Wendland's case, his wife Rose had failed to provide this clear and convincing evidence, and had instead relied upon her own subjective opinion that Wendland would not have wanted his current quality of life to continue. In the case of Hugh Finn, a 44-year-old man with a diagnosis of PVS following a car accident, then-governor James Gilmore of Virginia, where Finn was being cared for in a nursing home, intervened to stop Finn's wife from removing his feeding tube. The Virginia State Supreme Court overruled this intervention, and Hugh Finn died in 1998 after removal of this feeding tube. The U.S. Supreme Court declined to intervene in the Schiavo case three times.

There are three main themes, then, that run through the Schiavo case, each of them shared with one or more of the other major similar cases over the past few decades. The first is the issue of surrogacy. As in the Wendland case, the surrogate decision maker is the spouse, who is seeking to withdraw life-sustaining treatment — feeding via a gastrostomy tube. The parents of the patient oppose this, and are therefore formally challenging the surrogacy of the spouse, another feature that is shared with the Wendland case. In Schiavo, the challenge to Michael Schiavo's surrogacy was based on claims that he received financial gain as a result of his wife's predicament, and would receive even more financial benefit at her death. The Schindlers also charged that Michael Schiavo abused his wife. Rose Wendland's fitness as a surrogate was not questioned; the issue was whether any surrogate had the right to make a decision to withdraw life-sustaining treatments such as tube feedings without specific previous direction from the patient. Robert Wendland ultimately died as a result of recurrent pneumonia, and Rose Wendland was allowed to make the decision not to treat her husband's infection aggressively.

The second issue in the Schiavo case that captured the attention of the media and the public was whether it is reasonable to assume that the condition in which Terri Schiavo found herself — in a PVS — was the situation she wanted to avoid when she said she did not want to be maintained on life-sustaining technologies. This issue also surfaced in the Cruzan case. Some disability advocates saw the decision to stop Ms Shiavo's tube feeding as an indirect method of eliminating a person with severe disabilities, rather than an act of respect for her autonomy.

The third issue highlighted by the Schiavo case was the complex legal question of how, and to what degree, state governments ought to be involved in decisions to forgo life-sustaining technologies. Are states protecting their citizens, or violating privacy concerns, when they seek to block surrogates who would discontinue life-sustaining measures? What features of a case should determine how a state decides on surrogacy issues? Beginning at least as long ago as the Karen Quinlan case, these questions have provided focal points for litigation surrounding end-of-life decisions.

V. GUIDELINES FOR CLINICIANS, WITH CASE DISCUSSIONS

The guidelines recommended below were compiled using documents by the American Medical Association,[64] a task force of the Society of Critical Care Medicine,[65] and interdisciplinary groups for the study of ethical problems in medicine. These groups include the President's Commission,[66] the Office of Technology Assessment of the U.S. Congress,[67] a Hastings Center task force,[68] and an international consensus conference of 33 delegates from 10 nations who worked for two years on this subject.[69]

Four guidelines for clinicians can be adapted from these sources. There appears to be an ethical consensus about guideline 2, which answers the question, "On what basis ought decisions to forgo life-sustaining treatments be made when the patient is incapacitated?" The benefit/burden standard prevails in clinical ethics today, in continuity with older ethical traditions. McCormick explains this standard as follows: "If a proposed treatment will offer no benefit, or the benefit will be outweighed by the burdens, the treatment is morally optional."[70]

Cases posing difficult choices about forgoing life-sustaining treatment can vary factually and in how clinicians interpret them. Duties of disclosure and communication become more difficult in such situations. The cases in this section and those at the end of the chapter illustrate this variety and the potential for misunderstanding. Throughout this section, the guideline is given first, accompanied by a case with discussion to illustrate how the guideline is used.

A. Guideline 1:
Respect Advance Directives

When an incapacitated patient who is terminally ill or in a state of PVS has a living will and/or has appointed a surrogate with a durable medical power of attorney, clinicians and family have moral and legal duties to honor such directives and to share authority with the patient's proxy in decisions to forgo life-sustaining treatment. Statements that persons make in living wills about preferences in the event that they are in a terminal stage of illness are not helpful when they are not yet in that stage. Case A presents a situation in which a patient who is incapacitated wrote personal instructions on a living will, which was not ethically or legally binding unless the patient was terminally ill. The instructions did not anticipate the facts of the medical situation in which the patient's physicians had to make decisions about diagnosis and treatment.

Case A: Do Advance Directives Trump Everything Else?

Ms B, a 70-year-old, single woman with severe hypertension, suffered her first stroke at home, resulting in right-sided hemiplegia (paralysis of one-half of the body). Mrs. N, a widowed sister who lived with Ms B, called the rescue squad. They responded and kept the patient's airway open. Ms B was unable to communicate. On admission to the emergency room, she was intubated and had cardiac arrhythmias. Later that day, in an ICU, she remained intubated and a nasogastric tube was placed to remove gastric secretions and to prevent aspiration pneumonia.

Mrs. N, her only living close relative, brought a properly witnessed living will to the hospital, dated and signed one year earlier by the patient. Ms B had specifically refused CPR and artificial feeding and hydration if "in the opinion of my physicians I cannot be restored to a state of health with the capacity to be in meaningful communication with my loved ones and companions. This communication might be nonverbal, but unless I can meaningfully understand and appreciate it, I prefer to die rather than exist in such a condition. I fear death less than the indignity of dependence and deterioration."

Her physicians tended to view advance directives in terms of the law of the state — that directives became effective when the patient became "terminally ill." In the ICU, Mrs. N objected to intubation and the placement of the nasogastric tube, saying, "That is just what she was talking about. I live with her and know what she meant. You are ignoring me." Ms B had also appointed Mrs. N to hold a durable power of attorney for healthcare decisions.

The physicians persuaded Mrs. N to consent to another computed tomography (CT) scan. Afterward, a neurologist wrote a note that the patient had experienced a large stroke of the dominant hemisphere. Her speech would definitely be affected. It was unclear how much recovery, if any, she would have.

Do a living will and durable power of attorney trump everything else? Some state laws say that the patient's instructions to forgo life-sustaining treatment may only be implemented when the patient is, in the view of two physicians, "terminally ill" and when "death is imminent." How should Ms B's personal instructions be understood?[71]

Advance directives do not trump a benefits/burdens assessment. Ms B's living will ought to be interpreted in the context of her diagnosis and prognosis. It will take time to evaluate the effects of a stroke and develop a plan of care, but treatment cannot proceed unilaterally over Mrs. N's objections. The ethical issues are complex given Ms B's known wishes, her refusal of specific technologies, and Mrs. N's power of attorney. Ms B's views of quality of life and death are known, and Mrs. N has authority to consent or refuse treatment. Meanwhile, the physicians need time to answer these questions: How dependent and impaired will she be? Will she deteriorate? It is not unusual for physicians to decline a family's request to stop treatment. An informative survey on physicians' practices found that

34 percent of a sample of 879 critical-care physicians declined requests by family members to withdraw ventilation, because they believed the patient had a reasonable chance to recover.[72]

If Ms B worsens and becomes terminally ill, the nasogastric tube — even if it was begun to permit feeding, hydration, and administration of other medications during the evaluation period — can ethically be withdrawn; this is true for intubation as well. Mrs. N's agreement is necessary to begin feeding and hydration by the nasogastric tube and for each major step of the case. If she does not agree, the attending physician will be obligated to try to resolve the dispute while continuing to evaluate Ms B's condition and prognosis. There are two acceptable moral options in this case.

1. Continue to treat while establishing a prognosis, assuming that physicians can persuade Ms B's sister that this is the best course.
2. Stop treatment if Ms B's sister can persuade the physicians that this would be her sister's decision if she could make it, regardless of an ambiguous prognosis.

Recognition of Mrs. N's role as surrogate decision maker in this case is a major factor in moral problem solving. Mrs. N felt ignored by the ICU physicians. Clinicians frequently fail to recognize surrogates' authority. Dubler discusses the fragility of the surrogate/proxy-physician relationship.[73] There are similar cases in the literature, but, in these published cases, the patients were more grievously ill than Ms B.[74] Elizabeth Hansot, a faculty member at Stanford University, wrote to a medical journal about physicians' dismissing her role as surrogate in spite of her having a durable power of attorney for healthcare.[75] Dr. Hansot's mother, 87 years old, was a stroke patient like Ms B, but she was in a terminal condition. Hansot reported that despite the fact that her mother had developed an advance directive with her physician, her lawyer, and her offspring, the document was "invisible" when most needed because her mother's physician failed to notify the medical team of its existence. Recalling her harsh interaction with the attending pulmonologist, she said that he challenged her defense of her mother's prior instructions, asking her if she "was an ageist, or an ideologue interested only in abstract principles." After several days, a technician was delegated to extubate her mother, and no physician was present. Gilligan and Raffin presume that Hansot's gender lessened her power in the eyes of male physicians, and they prescribe education.[76]

Another important issue is Ms B's "broad" or nonconforming advance directive. This case occurred in a state with a living will statute that restricts clinicians from honoring the declarant's instructions unless the declarant is diagnosed with a terminal illness or a PVS. Ms B's instructions in her advance directive were broader than the statute permits, in that she directed that treatments be withheld or withdrawn if she suffered irreversible brain damage but was not terminally ill. Her advance directive, as discussed by Alan Meisel, was a "noncon-

forming" type.[77] Should it have been respected? Her physicians believed that the moral limits of their relationship with her were bound only by the legal limits imposed by the state, and that their aggressive plan of care was permitted. However, their interpretation is subject to serious ethical and legal challenge, especially since Mrs. N was on the scene within a few hours of the patient's admission.

A broad advance directive exceeds the narrow scope of most state laws. Is it any the less morally weighty or *prima facie* invalid for that reason? Meisel counsels that nonconforming directives should be "presumed to be valid even in a jurisdiction that has enacted advance directive legislation."[78] He states that "the better view, and the one likely to prevail," is that state legislatures do not create a right to make decisions about treatment in a future situation when they pass statutes regarding living wills or durable power of attorney. Indeed, this right already exists, and the legislation affirms it and provides immunity from legal liability if physicians honor this right, as it did in this particular state. Meisel depicts statutes regarding advance directives as cumulative — intended to "preserve and supplement existing common law and constitutional rights and not to supersede or limit them."[79] Susan Wolf also reasons that "a directive broader than the state statute is not out of bounds."[80] She, like Meisel, argues that common-law rights recognized by judges and constitutional protections, as acknowledged by the U.S. Supreme Court majority in the *Cruzan* decision, also support physicians who honor broader directives.

B. Guideline 2: Use the Benefit/Burden Standard as the Major Guideline

Benefits and burdens can be defined as follows:

1. Treatment *benefits* of two types can increase the well-being of the patient: (a) health benefits — positive and empirically measurable effects in curing, arresting, or relieving the patient's disease, condition, symptoms, and pain; or (b) quality-of-life benefits — improvements in mental status or added days or months of life that are mutually rewarding to the patient and others.
2. Treatment *burdens* of two types can diminish the well-being of patients: (a) when treatment provides no measurable health benefits and entail increased pain, suffering, or debilitation; or (b) when treatment reduces the patient's quality of life.

An ethically sound basis on which to evaluate choices to forgo life-sustaining treatments in incapacitated patients is to assess the benefits and burdens for the patient of each treatment. The following guidelines are suggested:

1. Physicians have a duty to make recommendations to other decision makers based on benefit/burden assessments.
2. Benefits and burdens should be assessed within the framework of the patient's prior expressed wishes or known values, beliefs, and previous decisions about treatment, and a substituted judgment made if possible; if it is not possible, the best-medical interest standard should be followed.
3. Family members are usually the best source of information about a patient's preferences, supplemented by information from other members of the clinical team.
4. When the benefits of treatment are proportionate to or exceed the burdens, it is obligatory to give treatment (unless it is refused by the patient in an advance directive).
5. It is obligatory for clinicians to withhold and strive to withdraw treatment(s) that clearly will harm or are harming the patient.

Cases B and C present complications in using the benefit/burden standard with incapacitated patients. If the patient has no written advance directives and resides in a state with a very high legal standard of evidence for patient preferences, serious problems can arise. Also, if the patient never had capacity to make decisions, the best-interest standard is the preferred approach.

Case B: The Patient's Preferences Are Known but Legally Contested (*Cruzan v. Harmon*)

On 11 January 1983, Nancy Beth Cruzan, then 25 years old, was injured in a single-car accident and was found lying face down in a ditch.[81] She had been thrown approximately 35 feet from her overturned vehicle. A state trooper who first arrived at the accident examined her and found "no detectable respiratory or cardiac function." Paramedics were able to revive her breathing and heartbeat, but she suffered permanent brain damage. In the hospital, a gastrostomy tube was implanted on 5 February 1983 to permit nutrition and hydration, and rehabilitation efforts were begun, but without success. In October 1983, she was transferred to the Missouri Rehabilitation Center in Mount Vernon.

After four years, her parents (as coguardians) asked the hospital administration to end the gastrostomy feedings. Her parents reported that their daughter had made statements to friends that she would never want to be kept alive if she was seriously brain injured. The administration refused the request, and, on 23 October 1987, the Cruzans filed a declaratory judgment action seeking judicial sanction of their instructions. As presented to the Missouri Supreme Court, the medical facts were:

> Ms. Cruzan's respiration and circulation were not artificially supported and are within normal limits. She was oblivious to her environment except for reflexive responses to sound and painful stimuli. She had cerebral cortical atrophy, which is irreversible, permanent, progressive, and ongoing. A spastic quadriplegic, her arms and legs were contracted with irreversible muscular and tendon damage. She had lost all cognitive ability. She could not swallow food or water and will never recover this function. Medical experts testified that she could live for another 30 years in a persistent vegetative state, which was her condition at that time.[82]

In March 1988, a three-day hearing began, at the family's request. Her parents argued that Nancy had a common-law right to be free from unwanted medical treatment as well as state and federal constitutional rights to privacy that protected her right to refuse unwanted medical treatment. Her parents also testified that Nancy had told her housemates that she would not want to continue to live if she could not be "at least halfway normal." Knowing her stated preferences made a substituted judgment possible.

On 27 July 1988, Probate Judge Charles Teel approved the request. On 3 August 1988, Missouri Attorney General William Webster filed a notice that the state would appeal to the Missouri Supreme Court. On 16 November 1988, by a vote of four to three, the Missouri Supreme Court overturned Judge Teel's decision. While recognizing a right to refuse treatment embodied in the common-law doctrine of informed consent, the court questioned whether it applied in this case. The court also declined to read into the state constitution a broad right of privacy that would support an unrestricted right to refuse treatment and expressed doubt that the U.S. Constitution embodied such a right. The court then decided that Missouri's living-will statute embodied a state policy strongly favoring the preservation of life, and that Ms Cruzan's statements to her housemates were unreliable for the purpose of determining her intent. The court rejected the argument that her parents were entitled to order the termination of her medical treatment, concluding that no person can assume the choice for an incapacitated person in the absence of the formalities required by the living-will statute or clear and convincing evidence of the patient's wishes. Further, the majority opinion (written by Judge Edward D. Robertson, r.) based its decision in part on a refusal to engage in "quality-of-life" considerations. Robertson stated, "Were quality of life at issue, persons with all manner of handicaps might find the state seeking to terminate their lives. Instead, the state's interest is in life; that issue is unqualified."[83] The court declared that the state's "interest in life" required that the feeding tube not be removed, even though Ms Cruzan was in a PVS. This decision was appealed by the family to the U.S. Supreme Court (*Cruzan v. Director, Missouri Dept. of Health*).[84]

On 25 June 1990, the U.S. Supreme Court, by a vote of five to four, rendered a decision (written by Chief Justice William H. Rehnquist) with two main parts: (1) the Court "assumed that the United States Constitution would grant a competent person a constitutionally protected right to refuse lifesaving hydration and nutrition"; (2) the U.S. Constitution did not prohibit the State of Missouri from "requiring clear and convincing evidence of a person's expressed decision while competent to have hydration and nutrition withdrawn in such a way as to cause death." The Court held that even though her parents were "loving and caring," Missouri could "choose to defer" only to Ms Cruzan's wishes (which were not written but reportedly oral), and ignore both the parents' own wishes and their views about what their daughter would want.[85]

On 30 August 1990, the Cruzans asked Judge Teel for a second hearing, saying that they had new evidence that their daughter once indicated to three other people that she would rather die than live in a vegetative state. On 17 September 1990, Attorney General Webster said that the state no longer had a "recognizable legal interest" in the case, and asked Judge Teel to drop the state health department and the director of the rehabilitation center from future litigation. Judge Teel dropped the state as a defendant. On 1 November, three former co-workers told Judge Teel that they recalled conversations with Ms Cruzan in which she said she never would want to "live as a vegetable" on medical machines. Her physician, who had opposed removing the feeding tube, termed her life "a living hell" and testified that she should be allowed to die.

On 5 December 1990, Ms Cruzan's court-appointed guardian recommended that the feeding tube be removed so she could die. Judge Teel approved on 14 December. Between 18 December and 24 December, anti-euthanasia groups attempted to stay the court's order and asked state and federal courts for injunctions, which were denied. At one point, some members of the group stormed the clinic in an attempt to reattach the tube. Ms Cruzan died on 26 December, 13 days after the feeding tube was removed.

The U.S. Supreme Court's decision, in effect, affirmed the competent person's right to refuse any life-sustaining treatment, including artificial feeding and hydration. Regarding the incapacitated person, the Court left to the states the choice of whether the legal standard for a substituted judgment would be satisfied if the patient had made only verbal statements. The Virginia Health Care Decisions Act encourages written advance directives and also accepts the validity of prior verbal statements, as do many other states. Weir and Gostin reviewed 50 legal cases about forgoing treatment with incapacitated patients in U.S. state courts. Only four (three in New York and the *Cruzan* case in Missouri) were decided on grounds with such a high standard of evidence of the patient's preferences that the thrust of the benefit/burden standard and prior verbal statements would not be sufficient to resolve the problem.[86] For these reasons, clinicians should be familiar with the law of the state in which they practice.

Case C: The Patient Never Had Capacity

Joseph Saikewicz, at the age of 67, was diagnosed with acute nonlymphoblastic leukemia, at that time (1967) an invariably fatal illness. He has resided at the Belchertown State School, a Massachusetts facility for the mentally retarded, for 40 years. In this era, chemotherapy for this form of leukemia had limited results (that is, short-term remission from two to 13 months in 30 to 50 percent of cases), but much poorer results in patients over 60 years of age. Side-effects were serious: nausea, anemia, and infections. Mr. Saikewicz had never been a capable decision maker. He was severely retarded from birth, with an IQ of 10. He communicated with others by gestures and could not speak except in grunts. He did not understand common dangers and became disoriented when away from his most familiar surroundings.

Officials at the school approached the probate court with the question of whether Mr. Saikewicz should be treated. The court appointed a guardian *ad litem* to consider the relevant issues and to make decisions about his care and treatment. The guardian recommended that "not treating Mr. Saikewicz would be in his best interests" for these reasons: his disease is incurable, treatment would have very serious and painful side-effects that he would neither understand nor be able to put into perspective, and the patient had never been a capable decision maker. This review was upheld by the Supreme Judicial Court of Massachusetts, but the court used a substituted-judgment standard, rather then the argument of the guardian based upon best interests.[87]

The Saikewicz case is important because the court erroneously proposed that a substituted-judgment standard should be used to make the decision. Mr. Saikewicz had never been capable of making any decisions and had no knowable preferences regarding treatment or any other matter. This particular court wanted to avoid even the appearance of quality-of-life reasoning in using the best-interest standard, which was the argument made by the guardian. The court had been deeply divided on the ethical and legal principles relevant to such cases. To use the substituted-judgment standard was erroneous in this case as it should not be used for patients who had never been capable. The only meaningful standard in such cases is the best-interest standard.

There are also famous cases (*Linares* and *Baby K*) in which an ethically defensible decision to forgo life-sustaining treatment is blocked by legal arguments that state law (*Linares*) or federal law (*Baby K*) does not permit the decision explicitly. These cases are presented at the end of the chapter (see cases 1 and 2).

C. Guideline 3: Disclose Poor Prognosis or Futility

If the patient's prognosis is poor or if one or more treatments are futile, physicians have a duty to disclose this assessment, and the reasoning that underlies it, and to recommend to other decision makers that futile treatment should be withheld or withdrawn. The duty to inform falls within the larger scope of duties of disclosing poor prognosis and of limiting medical care when no overall improvement results (see chapter 10).[88]

The following case concerns informing families about poor prognosis or futility (for example before writing DNR orders) or not offering other treatments deemed futile for an incapacitated patient.

Case D: Informing about Poor Prognosis or Futility

On morning rounds outside the room of Mrs. A, a 62-year-old unconscious woman who was dying from ovarian cancer, the healthcare team reached consensus that CPR would be "worse than useless; it would harm her." Her family, large and contentious, had been keeping a bedside vigil, fighting among themselves and the healthcare team about "doing everything" for the patient. The patient's nurse asked the attending physician, "Are you going to speak with the family about DNR?" The attending physician responded, "Do I have a clear duty to speak with them? I ought to be able to write a DNR order, because CPR is not medically indicated. If I do speak with them, they will think I am asking them to 'pull the plug' on their mother. They will want to fight about it. They are burdened enough already without having to hear about this medical decision. Why leave them feeling guilty? It is our job to manage the medical matters." The nurse said, "The hospital policy and state law says that the surrogate decision maker needs to be consulted before the DNR order can be written." The physician replied, "That may be, but we differ about whether informing them will do more harm than good." What should be done?[89]

In the case of Mrs. A, there is a disagreement between a physician and a nurse about disclosure to family members of the reason for a DNR order. The nurse's position is in keeping with the guideline to disclose that a treatment is futile. This guideline reflects respect for the norms of family life and also for shared decision making. But before such disclosure can occur, the family needs help with their inner turmoil and their reasons for fighting with the staff. The physician wants to avoid turmoil by not discussing the DNR order with the family. However, his proposal involves violating the principle underlying the guideline, unless he can defend it on ethical grounds. Is such a defense possible? The only valid argument is that family members were incapacitated as decision makers by their emotional problems, which begs the question about what kind of help is

appropriate. Psychiatric or pastoral help and assessment of the situation is indicated. The higher priority is for the physician to inform the family, in the context of supportive help for them, without unreasonable delay.

CPR and DNR decisions are frequently very difficult choices in critical-care units. After reviewing the recent literature on withholding CPR on medical grounds, Brunetti and Stell advise that the attending physician should decide to forgo CPR only when there is enough information to make an adequately informed judgment that the results will be unfavorable to the patient.[90] Discussions with patients and surrogates regarding CPR should be recorded in the chart. It is also crucial to record the reasons for writing DNR orders in the progress notes of the patient's medical record.

Six steps for writing DNR orders follow:

1. The physician makes a benefit/burden assessment of CPR in the context of the patient's overall prognosis.
2. If the assessment is negative, the physician consults with other members of the healthcare team about the issue and discusses the need for a DNR order.
3. If there is no remaining substantive objection to a DNR order among the team, the physician approaches the patient (if capable) or the designated decision makers (if the patient is incapacitated) and explains a DNR order and why the healthcare team recommends writing such an order.
4. If no substantive objection is made, the physician writes the order in the patient's chart, with the reasons for the DNR order in the progress notes.
5. The DNR order is reviewed regularly, at least every seven days.
6. The DNR order can be revoked if the benefit/burden assessment changes.

D. Guideline 4: In Mediating Disputes with Surrogate Decision Makers, Treat the Patient until the Dispute Is Resolved, Except When Treatment Is Harmful

The fourth and final guideline concerns disputes between clinicians and surrogate decision makers about decisions to forgo life-sustaining treatment. Points 1, 2, and 3 below are well settled in clinical ethics. Point 4 is the least established and is open to further exploration.

If the surrogate of an incapacitated patient demands:

1. *Withholding beneficial treatment that the patient may have wanted.* Clinicians should not acquiesce to the demand. They should strive to resolve the dispute by ethics consultation and other help. Clinicians should put the best medical interest of the patient above all other

considerations. The burden of seeking legal action to stop treatment falls on the family in this situation.

2. *Starting clearly harmful treatment.* After good-faith efforts to resolve the disputes by ethics consultation and other help as indicated, with prior institutional approval, physicians should withhold the treatment, even over the objections of guardians or family members.

3. *Continuing clearly harmful treatment.* After using ethics consultation and other help as indicated (see chapter 17) to resolve the dispute, physicians should, with institutional approval, strive to withdraw the treatment, even over the objections of guardians or family members. In these cases, the institution should seek a court's approval for withdrawal of life-sustaining but harmful treatment(s).

4. *Withholding or withdrawing "medically futile" treatments that are not harmful.* How to resolve these disputes continues to be debated in clinical ethics and law (see the *Baby K* case in section VII, case 2, below).

Case E describes a dispute between surrogates and clinicians about forgoing physiologically futile treatment when an incapable patient's prior wishes were unknowable. This case was one of several that led to an amendment in Virginia state law to permit physicians to refuse to provide treatment under such circumstances. Federal court decisions in the *Baby K* case have pre-empted Virginia law in such cases.

Case E: "Code Him Until He's Brain Dead!"

In 1988, a 61-year-old widowed patient with a 30-year history of alcohol abuse and a history of previous strokes was brought to the Emergency Department by the rescue squad from a nursing home.[91] He was unconscious, with a high fever, and cyanotic. He could not breathe on his own and a breathing tube was placed. He had twice been a patient in the hospital for treatment of strokes. He had not spoken or communicated with anyone since his strokes two years earlier. He had no advance directive. He was transferred to the ICU and treated with several antibiotics, and intubated. Physicians were unable to discover the true source of infection.

His three daughters came quickly to the hospital from a neighboring community. One daughter, Pam, was the spokesperson. Physicians in the ICU recommended that a DNR order was appropriate. She objected vehemently and began every discussion about her father's condition with: "Code him until he's brain dead!" She had learned the term "Code him" in a previous admission (one year prior) of her father to the hospital

for treatment of a stroke. On that occasion, a resident had approached her to discuss a DNR order and made the statement, according to Pam, that her father's condition was "hopeless." She refused the DNR order. At the time, the state law was that no life-sustaining treatment could be withheld or withdrawn without concurrence of surrogate decision makers. Her father survived. She stated, "The doctors were wrong before and they can be wrong now; code him until he's brain dead!"

The daughters said that their father had never made his wishes clear about what he wanted done in this kind of situation, and that they had never talked about this issue with him before his strokes. They did discuss his history of alcohol abuse and said that he had been abusive to them as children. They had never had a good relationship with him. They described a process of "coming together" around his care in the nursing home, and that they believed that he responded to them and heard them, although there were no data to support this impression. ICU physicians requested an ethics consultation, which began on the night of the patient's admission.

The sisters were staunchly opposed to any suggestion of withholding or withdrawing treatment. They made a religious argument, saying, "Where there is life there is hope." They also said, "When God decides to take him, we will accept it, but we will not accept any human decisions to end his life." They insisted that "everything be done." Physicians recommended continuing to search for the cause of his infection, treatment with antibiotics, but no cardiac resuscitation if an arrest occurred.

During a week of "stand-off" between the family and healthcare team, the ethics consultation continued. The consultant arranged several meetings between physicians, nurses, social workers, and family. The patient had not responded to treatment and became steadily worse. His physicians and nurses stated further treatment was "futile." Also, other patients who could benefit more from intensive care were being denied the bed. The clinicians recommended to the daughters that the breathing machine be removed and, if his heart stopped, that he be allowed to die without massaging his chest or restarting his heart by electroshock. They needed to write a DNR order. Pam objected, saying again, "You are asking us to murder our father. This is our belief. We want him coded [resuscitated] until he is brain dead!" In desperation, a physician turned to a nurse and said, "Do we have to take this? What can physicians and nurses do when the law gives the family the upper hand in a dispute like this? What can we do about our own ethical position of not inflicting torture on this hopelessly ill patient? And what about the injustice to other patients?"

The resources of a clinical ethics program (see chapter 17) clearly are needed, but may be ineffective in disputes about medical futility in incapacitated patients. In such disputes, the surrogates tend to mistrust anyone connected with the healthcare organization (HCO).

Following "Code Him" and similar cases, the Virginia General Assembly was persuaded to amend the Virginia Health

Care Decisions Act in 1992. The amendment stipulates that physicians are not required to prescribe or render treatment that the physician determines to be "medically or ethically inappropriate."[92] The law requires that a good-faith effort be made to transfer the patient to the care of another physician. In Maryland, as well, the state legislature amended its Health Care Decisions Act to support the authority of physicians not to render "medically ineffective treatment," which the legislature defined as that which, "to a reasonable degree of medical certainty, will neither prevent nor reduce the deterioration of the health of a patient, nor prevent the impending death of a patient."[93]

Bridging between state law and hospital policy, the University of Virginia Health Sciences Center amended its DNR policy in 1992 to permit physicians to write a DNR order over a surrogate's objection when CPR clearly would be harmful or physiologically futile. This step is a last resort. All efforts to resolve the dispute must have failed, including an offer of ethics consultation, as well as unsuccessful efforts to transfer the patient to the care of another physician. At the time the DNR policy was amended, the hospital required consultation by the attending physician with the chair of the ethics committee, who could assemble an *ad hoc* group to consider the situation. That requirement has now been made an option in a current and revised policy.

The policy was first used in 1993 in a case of a 53-year-old woman with multi-system organ failure, whose husband and family opposed a DNR order. The chair of the ethics committee convened an *ad hoc* group to meet with the attending physician and others. They developed a plan, and a DNR order was written. The patient died eight days later.

Later a dispute arose between the hospital's billing department and the family. Risk management at the University of Virginia believes that aggravation over billing was the primary causation for an ensuing suit. The patient's total bill was approximately $105,000, and her insurance paid for all but about $2,000. The family, already bitter over the outcome of the case, received repeated bills with a final notice that the unpaid bill would be turned over to a collection agency. They turned the letter over to their attorneys, who sought and received the medical record. Within the record was a report from the Ethics Committee chairperson about the consultation and recommendations supporting writing a DNR order.

In the context of this unresolved grievance and the wake of court decisions in the *Baby K* case, the family's attorneys filed two lawsuits: one against the hospital in federal court alleging a violation of the federal "anti-dumping" law, the Emergency Medical Treatment and Active Labor Act (EMTALA), and the other in state court alleging a violation of the Health Care Decisions Act. This second case (*Cindy Bryan v. Rector and Visitors of the University of Virginia*) is discussed in chapter 17, because it named members of the ethics committee and oth-

ers. The suit in the state court was dismissed. The federal appeals court upheld a lower court's dismissal of the EMTALA charge, stating that "emergency treatment" presumed by EMTALA was not in question, as the patient had received stabilizing treatment for almost two weeks.[94]

In some instances, the use of the benefit/burden guideline has been blocked by arguments that no law exists to permit withdrawing treatment (see *Linares,* in section VII, case 1, below) or that federal law does not permit forgoing treatment under emergency conditions (see *Baby K,* in section VII, case 2, below). In both situations, and when it is unclear that treatment would be harmful to the patients, it is advisable for the HCO to seek legal guidance for its actions. The hospital's attorney in the *Linares* case acted irresponsibly in arguing that it was the family's duty to seek a legal resolution of the case, rather than placing the burden on the hospital itself.

Recommendations for action to implement guideline 4 are outlined in table 13.1.[95]

VI. ETHICAL REASONS FOR CLINICIANS TO SUPPORT GUIDELINES

The ethical problems in these cases are caused by clinicians' conflicting moral obligations to patients. On the one hand are obligations to sustain life and benefit patients. On the other hand are obligations not to harm or unduly burden patients for unsound reasons.

Different ethical views about forgoing life-sustaining treatment compete and contend in our society. The prevailing view strives to combine clinical objectivity with respect for the patient's values and preferences. Decisions ought to be made by weighing the best clinical information about the benefits and burdens of each treatment, to that patient, in light of what is known about that patient's preferences and values. An influential report from the President's Commission for the Study of Ethical Problems in Medicine and Biomedical and Behavioral Research took this position.[96] Competing views depend more on other subjective and cultural factors. One view is that the struggle for life should be continued at all costs, out of respect for the sanctity of human life. This view is often expressed in the context of strong religious commitments. Another view, which is less usual, places the highest value on the patient's quality of life, as defined by a society's needs for contributing members. This view would support unilateral, socially approved decisions to withhold or stop all treatment if such qualities were no longer present in the patient.

Guideline 1 (respect advance directives) reflects the duties that are consistent with the principle of respect for persons and the self-determination exercised before persons become incapacitated. These duties also reflect care for the relationships of patients, families, and the larger community. The care shown in planning advance directives strengthens bonds in families and inspires courage to face death with realism. Although children are legally incompetent and their parents are their legally authorized proxy decision makers, several states now have laws that permit proxy decision makers to initiate advance directives on behalf of terminally ill children.[97]

Guideline 2 (use the benefit/burden standard) grows out of claims of the ethical principles of beneficence and nonmaleficence. When clinicians are faced with situations in which harm cannot be avoided, they are still obliged in their actions to attempt to produce a positive ratio of benefits over burdens. The benefit/burden approach to decision making responds to this obligation. This guideline would lead clinicians to avoid harm to a patient and discontinue futile treatments, and to be fair and just in their allocation of expensive treatments. The guideline also places the burden of proof on those who hold that some medical treatments (such as feeding and hydration) have a higher moral requirement than other treatments.

Guideline 3 (disclose poor prognosis or futility) is consistent with other guidelines on truth-telling and informed consent. It is supported by studies that report that the more family members understand the course of a patient's illness and cause of death, the better they can acknowledge their grief and have fewer physical and psychological problems.[98] Full disclosure of clinically relevant information for family members of patients who die tends to promote their mental and physical health in the aftermath of loss and bereavement. Keeping the family abreast of clinicians' decision making is medically and ethically sound, but some clinicians clearly violate this norm — by their own admission.

Asch and colleagues surveyed 879 critical-care physicians. They found that of 713 who withdrew life-sustaining treatment for reasons of futility, 105 (15 percent) did so without the knowledge of the patient or family. Of interest in the context of futility disputes is their finding that 23 (3 percent) withdrew life supports despite the objections of the patient or family.[99] A rule of thumb about what should be disclosed is that if forgoing specific treatments is supported by a consensus in rounds

Table 13.1
Recommendations for Action in Disputes with Surrogates about Incapacitated Patients

Medical opinion	Surrogate evaluation		
	"Worth a try"	"Don't know"	"Not worth it"
Standard treatment; benefits patient	Treat	Treat	Treat; possible legal action by family?
Uncertain	Trial of treatment	Trial of treatment	No treatment
Highly unlikely to work	Trial or transfer	Permissive; no treatment and review	No treatment
No medical benefit; possible harm to patient	Treat and review	No treatment	No treatment
"Won't work"; physiological futility and certain harm to patient	No treatment and notice of public policy about withholding; possible legal action by hospital to withdraw	No treatment	No treatment

Adapted with permission from material presented by Christine Mitchell at the "Bioethics Summer Retreat," 29 June 1994.

by the clinical team, this fact should be communicated to the surrogate by the physician in charge of the case.

Guideline 4 (in mediating disputes with surrogate decision makers, treat the patient until the dispute is resolved, except when treatment is harmful) is the newest and least established guideline for clinicians. This guideline rests on a premise that favors sustaining life while vigorously seeking to resolve the dispute, with attention to the goals of treatment and respect for all parties. The one exception appears when treatment is physiologically futile, and emotional appeals from families to "do everything possible" are demands that clinicians know would harm the patient. Clinicians ought not to consider these demands without real evidence that this would be the clear wish of the patient, and, even then, caution should prevail. The policy of hospitals and nursing homes should state that clinicians are not required to render or prescribe therapy that they know to be physiologically futile or harmful.

Ethics case consultation (see chapter 17) may not be an ideal process to mediate bitter futility disputes, since surrogates tend to mistrust anyone related to an HCO. A better strategy may be to recruit a few well-respected persons from the community as mediators. If attempts fail to resolve such disputes and the surrogate's demands persist, there must be a good-faith attempt to transfer the patient to another facility. Failing transfer, the recommendation is that an HCO should ask a court for approval to withdraw futile treatment. The guideline assumes that an institutional policy permitting the withholding of treatment (especially CPR) under these circumstances is ethically acceptable. The outcome of the *Baby K* case is unusual in that the court order applied to emergency hospital treatment for apnea for an anencephalic infant residing in a nursing home. The outcome of *Cindy Bryan v. Rector and Visitors of the University of Virginia* clarified EMTALA's scope with respect to patients hospitalized for a period of days. Seeking legal relief for ethical problems is a last, but sometimes necessary, resort.

In cases in which the dispute is mainly about a patient's quality of life, respect for the family's wishes should prevail, since families are better situated to evaluate issues related to quality of life. To act unilaterally to withdraw treatment (for example, to turn off a ventilator or to remove feeding tubes) over a family's objections runs contrary to the moral perspective that allows families to be the final interpreters of what quality of life means for their members. Views on quality of life differ greatly among individuals and from family to family. When continuing treatment will clearly involve *harm* to a patient, a clinician's first loyalty is to the patient and to prevent harm.

Guideline 4, section D, on withholding futile or harmful treatments even over family objections, has been shown in one study to be an effective practice.[100] In this study, Massachusetts General Hospital, one of the first institutions to have a patient care ethics committee for intensive care, reported on 20 cases in which clinicians wrote DNR orders, after prolonged attempts to mediate disagreements, over the objections of family members. Brennan described one of these cases in detail.[101] In this same hospital in 1994, physicians decided to write a DNR order and then to wean a patient from a ventilator over her daughter's objection. The patient died and her daughter brought a lawsuit that named, among others, the chairperson of the ethics committee.[102] The jury of a trial court decided in favor of the physicians, defending their decisions on the basis of "medical futility." Capron argues that the trial court did not settle the question of whether society would truly favor health professionals' unilateral decisions to withhold or withdraw life-sustaining treatments over the objections of surrogates, based on the professionals' evaluation of the "worth of the outcome."[103] The decision is being appealed to a higher court. This case, *Gilgunn v. Massachusetts General Hospital,* is also discussed in chapter 17.

Guideline 4, section C, and the recommendations in table 13.1 run counter to the President's Commission's morally inflexible, "fail safe" policy to continue treatment in the context of all types of disputes.[104] This unguarded policy can lead to harm to patients and the demoralization of clinicians. Section C assumes that the approach of the President's Commission is too lenient in permitting families to dictate treatment. The responsibility of physicians to protect patients from harm — even the harm that results from desperate attempts by families to avoid death — is a well-established norm in clinical ethics.

Can futility disputes be prevented? How can the culture that spawns them be changed? Some of the same problems that were identified in the SUPPORT study are at work here. Just as there are many physicians who are uninhibited therapeutic activists in critical care, there are patients and families who, under any circumstances, refuse to "give up," even when massive amounts of resources are involved. They may not feel part of a community that expects treatment to be limited. Lo and Brody each note in reflections on the SUPPORT study that change in the culture of critical care requires fundamental shifts in U.S. healthcare policy, physicians' values, and medical education.[105] These three areas of reform also influence the context of futility disputes. Reform in healthcare policy must precede economic and medical rationing of treatments, and discourage treatment in cases when it would be futile. The values of family practitioners, rather than therapeutic activists, need to be more in evidence in ICUs and critical care. Medical education must emphasize the quality of a "relationship-centered model"[106] and the need to learn the patient's whole story.

VII. CASES FOR FURTHER STUDY

Case 1: The Linares Case

When he was eight months old in September 1988, Samuel Linares swallowed a balloon. His father was with him and responded to the child quickly. He smelled rubber on his breath and tried to revive him, unsuccessfully. He ran with the child to a firehouse where emergency CPR was performed. The child showed no vital signs for at least 20 minutes. He was intubated at the hospital and admitted to the pediatric ICU of Rush Presbyterian Hospital in Chicago and placed on a ventilator. Severe brain damage was diagnosed.

The child did not improve and was diagnosed as being in a PVS. As months passed, his father and mother, Rudy and Tammy Linares, became despondent and requested that physicians stop the ventilator. Neighbors described the parents as devoted to the child. The Linares's financial problems were heavy. Medical bills in the case were estimated to exceed $200,000. Mr. Linares, a 23-year-old laborer, earned about $300 a week. Mrs. Linares was notified in February that she must repay nearly $20,000 that she collected in welfare payments by claiming that she was a single parent.

At this time, the hospital had no ethics committee and offered no ethics consultation. Max Brown, the hospital's attorney, was the most involved person in the case, other than the baby's physicians and nurses. Brown took the position that while Illinois law did clearly permit hospitals to withdraw life supports from patients who are "brain dead" (the Illinois Definition of Death Act), there was no precedent for withdrawing a ventilator in a patient with "minimal brain function." Illinois accepts funds for child protection from the federal government, and, in such cases, the federal "Baby Doe" law applies. This law permits withhold-

ing or withdrawing treatment from infants under one year of age who are in "irreversible coma." Brown, however, did not interpret federal law to permit withdrawal in this case.

After the child was in the ICU for eight months, hospital officials advised the parents to seek a court order authorizing the removal of the respirator. They made an appointment with a lawyer on 28 April 1989 to discuss the matter. On 26 April, they returned to their apartment to find a message on the answering machine from hospital officials that their son was about to be transferred to a long-term care facility about 70 miles away. They had been aware of the hospital's plans, but were shocked that the move was to be made so soon.

Later that day, Mr. Linares entered the ICU with a .357 Magnum pistol. "I'm not here to hurt anyone," he said, as he unplugged his child's respirator, "I just want to let my son die." Within moments, the 16-month-old child's heart stopped. Mr. Linares continued to rock Samuel in his arms for 20 minutes. Then he slid the gun across the floor to the police and collapsed in wrenching sobs. Linares was charged with first-degree murder. Freed on bond, he appeared in Cook County Criminal Court on 18 May.

The child's physician, Gilbert Goldman, said, "There was no ethical difference of opinion here. The physicians agreed that the child was in an irreversible coma and would not recover. There was no medical opposition to removing the ventilator. What we faced was a legal obstacle."

Brown said that he advised the medical staff not to remove the life support. "There is an absence in the law," he said. "I told the medical staff there was a possibility they would face criminal charges. I can't speculate with the careers of doctors and nurses."

The murder charge against Linares was later dismissed by the judge in criminal court, who held that the child's condition was hopeless before the father's action.

— Adapted from S.H. Miles, "Taking Hostages: The Linares Case," *Hastings Center Report* 19, no. 4 (1989): 4; D. Johnson, "Father Speeds Baby's Death as Question of Law Lingers," *New York Times*, 7 May 1989, A26; D.C. Thomasma, "Clinical Care Ethics and Public Policy: Reflections on the Linares Case," *Law, Medicine & Health Care* 17, no. 4 (1989): 335-38.

Case 2: The Case of Baby K

Baby K was born with anencephaly at Fairfax Hospital (hereinafter "the Hospital") in Virginia on 13 October 1992. Anencephaly is a congenital malformation resulting in lack of cerebral hemispheres and with only a brain stem. The infant is permanently unconscious and presumably cannot experience pain. The condition had been diagnosed prenatally. Ms H, the baby's mother, and Mr. K, the baby's father, are unmarried. One year prior to Baby K's birth, Ms H's nine-year-old daughter died in the same hospital of injuries suffered in a motor vehicle accident in which Ms H was driving.

Anencephaly was diagnosed at Ms H's first prenatal and ultrasound examination at six months gestation. Ms H's obstetrician and neonatologist had discussed the option of abortion. They explained that most anencephalic infants die soon after birth, and, if death did not occur, the infant would be permanently unconscious and without feeling. Ms H refused abortion. She requested that the child be treated maximally at birth, because she believes that all human life has value, including that of her anencephalic daughter. She believed that God would work a miracle if it was God's will. Mr. K, the baby's father, disagreed with Ms H about her wishes for treatment.

A cesarean section was needed. Ms H had a general anesthetic and was incapacitated during and after delivery. Physicians intubated Baby K at birth for three reasons: (1) in response to the earlier request of Ms H, (2) to confirm the diagnosis, and (3) to give Ms H a full opportunity to understand the diagnosis and prognosis of anencephaly. The physicians hoped that she would change her mind about treatment upon viewing the infant's condition. She did not change her mind. Physicians discussed a DNR order with Ms H, and she refused. The physicians made many attempts to communicate about the prognosis, and they attempted unsuccessfully to transfer the infant to other neonatal care units and children's hospitals (the clinicians and hospital administrators interpreted that the Virginia Health Care Decisions Act required them to do so).

Physicians asked the ethics committee to meet with Ms H; a three-person team (family practitioner, psychiatrist, and minister) was unsuccessful in resolving the dispute on 22 October 1992. According to the district court, her "treating physicians requested the assistance of the Hospital's Ethics Committee in overriding the mother's wishes." The ethics committee noted that the care was "futile" and advised that the Hospital "attempt to resolve this through our legal system," if, after a waiting period, no change occurred in Ms H's position.[107]

During this period, Ms H contacted the staff of a state agency for protection of the rights of the disabled, which advised the Hospital of its concerns about state and federal nondiscrimination and medical neglect statutes. The Hospital filed a proceeding in federal court in January 1993 to determine the level of care it was obligated to render, and requested appointing a guardian *ad litem*. Having weaned Baby K from the ventilator, physicians transferred her to a nursing home, with an agreement that she could return to the Hospital if breathing problems occurred. After her third admission (3 March 1993), a tracheostomy was performed for placement of a breathing tube, and she was transferred back to the nursing home on 13 April 1993.

Federal Judge Claude Hilton ruled on 1 July 1993 that the Hospital had a duty to provide full medical care (including ventilator support) to Baby K under the Federal Rehabilitation Act of 1973, the Americans with Disabilities Act of 1990 (ADA), and EMTALA. No weight was given to the guardian *ad litem*'s

recommendation that further prolongation of Baby K's dying process was futile and inhumane. The judge made no finding regarding a standard of care for anencephaly or pertaining to the issue of the best interest of the infant.

A key section of the court's ruling was:

The use of a mechanical ventilator to assist breathing is not "futile" or "inhumane" in relieving the acute symptoms of respiratory difficulty which is the emergency medical condition that must be treated under EMTALA. To hold otherwise would allow hospitals to deny emergency treatment to numerous classes of patients, such as accident victims who have terminal cancer or AIDS, on the grounds that they eventually will die anyway from these diseases and that emergency care for them would therefore be "futile."[108]

The U.S. Fourth Circuit Court of Appeals heard arguments on 26 October 1993 in the Hospital's appeal of Judge Hilton's decision. Their two-to-one opinion on 10 February 1994 affirmed the earlier judgment of the trial court. The appeals court examined only one question: Did Congress, in passing EMTALA, provide an exception for anencephalic infants (or anyone else) in respiratory distress? The court found EMTALA's language clear — that is, hospitals are required to stabilize the medical condition creating the emergency. The decision, in effect, informed Congress that it could clarify EMTALA, if it wanted. The dissenting justice argued that EMTALA was passed to prevent "dumping" for economic reasons, and because no treatment for anencephaly existed, there was no legal duty to ventilate the infant on an emergency basis. A key section of the dissent was: "I simply do not believe, however, that Congress, in enacting EMTALA, meant for the judiciary to superintend the sensitive decision-making process between family and physicians at the bedside of a helpless and terminally ill patient under the circumstances of this case. Tragic end-of-life hospital dramas such as this one do not represent phenomena susceptible to uniform legal control."[109]

The Hospital requested an *en banc* hearing with all sitting judges on the Fourth Circuit. The court denied this request. The Hospital, Baby K's father, and the guardian *ad litem* appealed to the U.S. Supreme Court. On 3 October 1994, the Supreme Court declined to review the case without comment regarding its reasons. Congress has made some effort to draft language for federal legislation to clarify congressional intent that EMTALA's requirement for stabilization be "consistent with reasonable medical standards."

Baby K continued to be cared for in a nursing home until she died at the Hospital of cardiac arrest on Wednesday, 5 April 1995, after being vigorously resuscitated.[110] This was her sixth and final admission to the Hospital. She had medical bills of nearly $500,000, which were covered by her mother's insurance and Medicaid. Her hospital bill before her death, nearly

$250,000, had been paid in full by Kaiser Permanente, a health maintenance organization in which Ms H was enrolled in her job as a cafeteria worker before Baby K's birth.

— Adapted from *In Re Baby K*, 832 F.Supp. 1022 (E.D. Va 1993); *In Re Baby K*, 16 F.3d 590 (4th Cir. 1994); M. Tousignant and B. Miller, "Death of Baby K Leaves a Legacy of Legal Precedents," *Washington Post*, 6 April 1995, A1.

VIII. STUDY QUESTIONS

1. Why is the distinction between ordinary and extraordinary treatment considered outworn?

2. Examine the guidance that there is no ethical difference between withholding and withdrawing medical treatment from the perspective of "act" versus "omission."

3. You think that CPR is medically inappropriate for your comatose patient, Mr. R. How do you initiate this discussion with his family/surrogate decision makers? What are the strengths and weaknesses of the following approaches? What is your recommended approach?

A. Ask the family whether they want "everything done" for Mr. R.

B. Ask the family's permission to write a DNR order.

C. Discuss the medical inappropriateness of CPR for Mr. R. Tell the family that this is not an option for treatment, and discuss other treatment plans such as comfort care.

D. Tell the family that you have written a DNR order in Mr. R's chart, as this is your medical prerogative.

4. Consider case B, *"Cruzan v. Harmon."* What are the ethical and legal issues in this case? What are the two major components of the U.S. Supreme Court's decision? Did Nancy Cruzan die on 11 January 1983 (the date of her accident) or on 26 December 1990 (after feeding and hydration had been forgone)?

5. Consider case 1, "The Linares Case." Discuss the clinicians' responsibilities to their patient and his family regarding their approval of removing the ventilator versus the hospital attorney's opposition? Should the clinicians have acted differently?

6. Discuss case E, "Code Him until He's Brain Dead!" in light of Virginia's Health Care Decisions Act. What course of action should clinicians take if this were a current case?

7. Discuss case 2, "The Case of Baby K," and its effects on the guidelines for clinicians in this chapter.

NOTES

1. Local, state, and national experience lies behind this estimate of frequency. Two-thirds (66 percent) of the requests for ethics consultation at the University of Virginia Hospitals concern decisions to forgo life-sustaining treatment. J.C. Fletcher and H. Boverman, "Ethics Consultation at the Medical Center of the University of Virginia," *Newsletter of the Society for Bioethics Consultation* 1, no. 1 (15 July 1988): 3-6; J.C. Fletcher, "Decisions to Forgo Life-Sustaining Treatment," Virginia *Medical Journal* 116 (1989): 462-5. A survey of healthcare professionals in 10 Virginia hospitals was conducted in 1990 to rank the needs that ethics programs in hospitals can meet. The survey also asked respondents to identify the most frequent ethical problems they saw in the hospital. Decisions to forgo life-sustaining treatment was by far the most frequent ethical problem named by 1,541 respondents. Of 22 types of ethical problems identified by respondents as frequent and difficult, 35 percent of all answers referred to forgoing life-sustaining treatment. See E.M. Spencer et al., "Ethics Programs at Community Hospitals in Virginia," *Virginia Medical Quarterly* 119 (1992): 178-9. A study of ethics committees in nursing homes reported that decisions to forgo treatment are the most frequent ethical problem for which such groups are used. See G. Glasser, N.R. Zweibel, and C.K. Cassel, "Ethics Committees in the Nursing Home: Results of a National Survey," *Journal of the American Geriatrics Society* 36 (1988): 150-6. Also, for an excellent "ethical assessment" of the environment of ICUs, see C. Marsden, "An Ethical Assessment of Intensive Care," *International Journal of Technology Assessment in Health Care* 8, no. 3 (1992): 408-18.

2. S.J. Reiser, "The Intensive Care Unit: The Unfolding and Ambiguities of Survival Therapy," *International Journal of Technology Assessment in Health Care* 8, no. 3 (1992): 382-94.

3. Hippocrates, "Epidemics II," in *Hippocrates I*, trans. W.H.S. Jones (Cambridge, Mass.: Harvard University Press, 1923).

4. G.E.R. Lloyed, ed., *Hippocratic Writings* (New York: Penguin Books, 1978), 94.

5. Ibid., p. 103.

6. G. Majno, *The Healing Hand: Man and Wound in the Ancient World* (Cambridge, Mass.: Harvard University Press, 1975).

7. B.S. Bloom and D. Lundberg, "Intensive

Care: Where Are We?" *International Journal of Technology Assessment in Health Care* 8, no. 3 (1992): 379-81.

8. P. Drinker and C.F. McKhann, "The Use of a New Apparatus for the Prolonged Administration of Artificial Respiration," *Journal of the American Medical Association* 92 (1929): 1658-60.

9. See note 2 above, p. 386.

10. F. Nightingale, *Notes on Hospitals,* 3rd ed. (London: Longman, 1863).

11. J.S. Hassett, "Technology's Front Line: The Intensive Care Unit," in *The Machine at the Bedside,* ed. S.J. Reiser and M. Anbar (Cambridge, U.K.: Cambridge University Press, 1984), 95-104.

12. W.J. Winslade and J.W. Ross, *Choosing Life and Death* (New York: Free Press, 1986), 5.

13. H.R. Moody, *Ethics in an Aging Society* (Baltimore, Md.: Johns Hopkins University Press, 1992), 20.

14. F.B. Hobbs and B.L. Damon, "65+ in the United States, P23-190 Current Population Reports: Special Studies," issued in April 1996 by the U.S. Census Bureau, available at *http://www.census.gov/prod/1/pop/p23-190/p23-190.html.*

15. M.D. Grossman et al., "When is Elder Old? Effect of Reexisting Conditions on Mortality in Geriatric Trauma," *Journal of Trauma* 52 (2002): 242-6.

16. SUPPORT investigators, "A Controlled Trial to Improve Care in Seriously Ill Hospitalized Patients," *Journal of the American Medical Association* 274 (1995): 1591-8.

17. N.G. Smedira et al., "Withholding and Withdrawal of Life Support from the Critically Ill," *New England Journal of Medicine* 322 (1990): 309-15.

18. D.K.P. Lee et al., "Withdrawing Care: Experience in a Medical Intensive Care Unit," *Journal of the American Medical Association* 271 (1994): 1358-61.

19. L. Payer, *Medicine and Culture* (New York: Penguin Books, 1988).

20. President's Commission for the Study of Ethical Problems in Medicine and Biomedical and Behavioral Research, *Deciding to Forgo Life-Sustaining Treatment* (Washington, D.C.: U.S. Government Printing Office, 1983), 17-8.

21. National Center for Health Statistics, "Mortality. Part A. Section 1," in *Vital Statistics of the United States,* 1991, (Washington, D.C.: U.S. Government Printing Office, 1996 — DHHS pub. no. (PHS) 96-1101), 380-1.

22. In a personal conversation with the author dated 7 December 1996, Susan Tolle reported: "Figures from the Oregon Health Division Vital Statistics for 1995 are almost evenly divided between three locations: acute care hospitals (32 percent), nursing homes (32 percent), and home (31 percent)."

23. See note 16 above, p. 1594.

24. Ibid., 1596.

25. J.E. Kurent, "Death and Dying in America: The Need to Improve End-of-Life Care," *Carolina Healthcare Business* (January-February 2000): 16.

26. D. Callahan, *What Kind of Life?* (New York: Simon & Schuster, 1990).

27. "Not Dead Yet — The Resistance," at *www.notdeadyet.org,* "Value of Life With a Disability."

28. Ibid.

29. Ibid.

30. M. Angell, "The Case of Helga Wanglie: A New Kind of Right to Die Case," *New England Journal of Medicine* 325 (1991): 511-12.

31. J.J. Paris, R.K. Crone, and F.E. Reardon, "Physicians' Refusal of Requested Treatment: The Case of Baby L," *New England Journal of Medicine* 322 (1990): 1012-5.

32. G.J. Annas, "Asking the Courts to Set the Standard of Emergency Care — The Case of Baby K," *New England Journal of Medicine* 330 (1994): 1542-5.

33. J.J. Paris et al., "Beyond Autonomy: Physicians' Refusal to Use Life-Prolonging Extracorporeal Membrane Oxygenation," *New England Journal of Medicine* 329 (1993): 354-7.

34. L.J. Blackhall, "Must We Always Use CPR?" *New England Journal of Medicine* 317 (1987): 1281-3; J.D. Lantos et al., "The Illusion of Futility in Clinical Practice," *American Journal of Medicine* 87 (1989): 81-4; L.J. Schneiderman, N.S. Jecker, and A.R. Jonsen, "Medical Futility: Its Meaning and Ethical Implications," *Annals of Internal Medicine* 112 (1990): 949-54; T. Tomlinson and H. Brody, "Futility and the Ethics of Resuscitation," *Journal of the American Medical Association* 264 (1990): 1276-80; N.S. Jecker and L.J. Schneiderman, "An Ethical Analysis of Futility in the 1992 American Heart Association Guidelines for Cardiopulmonary Resuscitation and Emergency Cardiac Care," *Archives of Internal Medicine* 153, no. 19 (1993): 2195-8; J.R. Curtis et al., "Use of the Medical Futility Rationale in Do-Not-Attempt-Resuscitation Orders," *Journal of the American Medical Association* 273, no. 2

(1995): 124-8.

35. J.F. Fries et al., "Reducing Health Care Costs by Reducing the Need and Demand for Medical Services," *New England Journal of Medicine* 329 (1993): 321-5; G.D. Lundberg, "American Health Care System Management Objectives: The Aura of Inevitability Becomes Incarnate," *Journal of the American Medical Association* 269 (1993): 2554-5.

36. D.J. Murphy and T.E. Finucane, "Do Not Resuscitate Policies: A First Step in Cost Control," *Archives of Internal Medicine* 153 (1993): 1641-8.

37. J. Lubitz, J. Beebe, and C. Baker, "Longevity and Medicare Expenditures," *New England Journal of Medicine* 332 (1995): 999-1003; E.J. Emanuel and L.L. Emanuel, "The Economics of Dying: The Illusion of Cost Savings at the End of Life," *New England Journal of Medicine* 330 (1994): 540-4.

38. This figure has been constant since the early 1980s. See W.A. Knaus, E.A. Draper, and D.P. Wagner, "The Use of Intensive Care," *Milbank Quarterly* 61, no. 4 (1983): 562; L. Jaroff, "Health: Knowing When to Stop," *Time,* 4 December 1995, 76.

39. J.A. Tulsky, M.A. Chesney, and B. Lo, "How Do Medical Residents Discuss Resuscitation With Patients?" *Journal of General Intern Medicine* 10 (1995): 436-42.

40. S.J. Youngner, "Who Defines Futility?" *Journal of the American Medical Association* 260 (1988): 2094-5; R.D. Truog, "Beyond Futility," *The Journal of Clinical Ethics* 3, no. 2 (Summer 1992): 143-5; R.D. Truog, A.S. Brett, and J. Frader, "The Problem with Futility," *New England Journal of Medicine* 326 (1992): 1560-4; B.A. Brody and A. Halevy, "Is Futility a Futile Concept?" *Journal of Medicine and Philosophy* 20, no. 2 (1995): 122-44.

41. K.A. Koch, B.W. Meyers, and S. Sandroni, "Analysis of Power in Medical Decisionmaking: An Argument for Physician Autonomy," *Law, Medicine & Health Care* 20 (1992): 320-6.

42. L.K. Stell, "Real Futility," *North Carolina Medical Journal* 56, no. 9 (1995): 432-8.

43. *In re Conroy,* 98 N.J. 321, 486 A.2d 1209 (1985).

44. American Medical Association, Council on Ethical and Judicial Affairs, "Withholding or Withdrawing Life-Sustaining Medical Treatments," in *Code of Medical Ethics* (Chicago, Ill.: AMA, 1994), 36-50.

45. Task Force on Ethics of the Society of Critical Care Medicine, "Consensus Report on the Ethics of Forgoing Life-Sustaining Treatments in the Critically Ill," *Critical Care Medicine* 18, no. 12 (1990): 1435-9.

46. See note 20 above.

47. U.S. Congress, Office of Technology Assessment, *Life-Sustaining Technologies and the Elderly,* OTA-BA-306 (Washington, D.C.: U.S. Government Printing Office, July 1987).

48. The Multi-Society Task Force on PVS, "Consensus Statement on the Medical Aspects of the Persistent Vegetative State," *New England Journal of Medicine* 330 (1994): 1499.

49. B. Jennet and F. Plum, "Persistent Vegetative State After Brain Damage: A Syndrome in Search of a Name," *Lancet* 734 (1972): 736.

50. C.M. Booth et al., "Is This Patient Dead, Vegetative, or Severely Neurologically Impaired? Assessing Outcome for Comatose Survivors of Cardiac Arrest," *Journal of the American Medical Association* 291, no. 7 (18 February 2004).

51. See note 43 above.

52. Sources for *Cruzan* case: *Info Trends: Medicine, Law, and Ethics,* Spring 1989, p. 1; *Cruzan v. Harmon,* 760 S.W. 2d 408 (Mo. 1988) (*en banc*); *Cruzan v. Director, Missouri Dept. of Health,* 497 U.S. 261 (1990); E.D. Robertson, Jr., *Personal Autonomy and Substituted Judgment* (Corpus Christi, Tex.: Diocesan Press, 1991); G.J. Annas, "Nancy Cruzan and the Right to Die," *New England Journal of Medicine* 323 (1990): 670-2; M. Gladwell, "Woman in Right-to-Die Case Succumbs," *Washington Post,* 27 December 1990, A3.

53. *In re Quinlan,* 70 N.J. 10, 355 A.2d 647 (1976).

54. Ibid.

55. *Barber v. Superior Court,* 147 Cal. App. 3d 1006, 195 Cal. Rptr. 484 (1983). This account of the case is adapted from B. Steinbock, "The Removal of Mr. Herbert's Feeding Tube," *Hastings Center Report* 13, no. 5 (October 1983): 13.

56. R.A. McCormick, "The *Cruzan* Decision," *Midwest Medical Ethics* (Winter-Spring 1989): 3-9.

57. J. Lynn and J.F. Childress, "Must Patients Always Be Given Food and Water?" *Hastings Center Report* 13 (October 1983): 17-21.

58. P. Schmitz and M. O'Brien, "Observations on Nutrition and Hydration in Dying Cancer Patients," in *By No Extraordinary Means,* ed. J. Lynn (Bloomington, Ind.: University of Indiana Press, 1986), 29-38.

59. B. Lo et al., "Sounding Board: The

Wendland Case — Withdrawing Life Support From Incompetent Patients Who Are Not Terminally Ill," *New England Journal of Medicine* 346, no. 19 (9 May 2002).

60. *Wendland v. Wendland*, 26 Cal. 4th, 519, 28 P.3d 151 (2001).

61. See note 59 above.

62. L.J. Nelson, "Persistent Vegetative State: Reflections on the Wendland Case," *Issues in Ethics* 14, no. 1 (Winter 2003).

63. University of Miami Ethics Programs website, *www.miami.edu/ethics2/schiavo_project.htm*.

64. See note 44 above.

65. See note 45 above.

66. See note 20 above.

67. See note 47 above.

68. Hastings Center, *Guidelines on the Termination of Life-Sustaining Treatment and the Care of the Dying* (Briarcliff Manor, N.Y.: Hastings Center, 1987).

69. J.M. Stanley et al., "The Appleton Consensus: Suggested International Guidelines for Decisions to Forgo Medical Treatment," *Journal of Medical Ethics* 15 (1989): 129-36.

70. See note 56 above.

71. This case was composed for teaching by the faculty at the University of Virginia.

72. D.A. Asch, J. Hansen-Flaschen, and P.L. Lanken, "Decisions to Limit or Continue Life-Sustaining Treatment by Critical Care Physicians in the United States: Conflicts between Physicians' Practices and Patients' Wishes," *American Journal of Respiratory and Critical Care Medicine* 151 (1995): 288-92.

73. N.N. Dubler, "The Doctor-Proxy Relationship: The Neglected Connection," *Kennedy Institute of Ethics Journal* 5, no. 4 (1995): 289-306.

74. S.S. Hall, "The Medical Machine: The Rapps," *Health* (October 1991): 91-102; M.S.D. Bosek, "Ethics from the Other Side of the Bed: A Daughter's Perspective," *Medical Surgical Nursing* 3, no. 4 (1994): 316-18, 334.

75. E. Hansot, "A Letter from a Patient's Daughter," *Annals of Internal Medicine* 125 (1996): 149-51.

76. T. Gilligan and T.A. Raffin, "Whose Death Is It, Anyway?" *Annals of Internal Medicine* 125 (1996): 137-41.

77. A. Meisel, *The Right to Die* (New York: John Wiley & Sons, 1993) and cumulative supplements.

78. Ibid., 26-27.

79. Ibid., 27.

80. S.M. Wolf, "Honoring Broader Directives," *Hastings Center Report* 21, no. 5 (1991): S8-S9.

81. See note 52 above.

82. *Cruzan v. Harmon*, 760 S.W.2d 408, at 411 (Mo. 1988) (*en banc*).

83. Ibid., 420.

84. *Cruzan v. Director, Missouri Dept. of Health*, 497 U.S. 261 (1990).

85. Ibid.

86. R.F. Weir and L. Gostin, "Decisions to Abate Life-Sustaining Treatment for Nonautonomous Patients," *Journal of the American Medical Association* 264 (1990): 1846-53.

87. *Superintendent of Belchertown v. Saikewicz*, Mass. 370 N.E. 2d 417 (1977); the Saikewicz case is also included in T.L. Beauchamp and J.F. Childress, *Principles of Biomedical Ethics*, 4th ed. (New York: Oxford University Press, 1994), 522.

88. Also, for a complete review of studies of CPR as a source of information from which to discuss CPR with colleagues and patients, see an important article by A.H. Moss, "Informing the Patient about Cardiopulmonary Resuscitation: When the Risks Outweigh the Benefits," *Journal of General Internal Medicine* 4 (1989): 349-55. For a review of the subject of in-hospital CPR, see: A.P. Schneider, D.J. Nelson, and D.D. Brown, "In-Hospital Cardiopulmonary Resuscitation: A 30-Year Review," *Journal of the American Board of Family Practice* 6, no. 2 (1993): 91-101.

89. This case was composed for teaching by the faculty at the University of Virginia.

90. L.L. Brunetti and L.K. Stell, *A Physician's Guide to the Legal and Ethical Aspects of Patient Care* (Charlotte, N.C.: Charlotte Area Health Education Center, 1994), 148.

91. Adapted from a case in Ethics Consultation Service, University of Virginia, 1988; J.C. Fletcher and P.J. Eulie, "Code Him Until He's Brain Dead!" in *Ethics at the Bedside*, ed. C.M. Culver (Dartmouth, N.H.: University of New England Press, 1990), 8-28.

92. According to the Virginia Health Care Decisions Act of 1992, Va. Code Ann., sec. 54.1-2990 (Michie 1994): "Nothing in this article shall be construed to require a physician to prescribe or render medical treatment to a patient that the physician determines to be medically or ethically inappropriate. However, in such a case, if the physician's determination is contrary to the terms of an advance directive of a qualified patient or the treatment decision of a person designated to

make the decision under this article, the physician shall make a reasonable effort to transfer the patient to another physician."

93. Maryland Health Care Decisions Act of 1993, Md. Code Ann., Health-Gen sec. 5-601-618 (1993); "Maryland Addresses Right-to-Die Issue with New Surrogate Law," *Medical Ethics Advisor* 9, no. 5 (May 1993): 57-9.

94. *Cindy Bryan v. Rector and Visitors of the University of Virginia,* 95 F.3d 349, (4th Cir. 1996).

95. This table was adapted from material presented by Christine Mitchell, R.N., M.A., at the "Bioethics Summer Retreat," 29 June 1994. Used with permission.

96. See note 20 above, p. 3.

97. L.S. Jefferson et al., "Use of the Natural Death Act in Pediatric Patients," *Critical Care Medicine* 19 (1991): 901-5.

98. J.J. Lynch, *The Broken Heart* (New York: Basic Books, 1977).

99. See note 72 above, p. 291.

100. T.A. Brennan, "Incompetent Patients with Limited Care in the Absence of Family Consent," *Annals of Internal Medicine* 109 (1988): 819-25.

101. T.A. Brennan, "Do-Not-Resuscitate Orders for the Incompetent Patient in the Absence of Family Consent," *Law, Medicine, and Health Care* 14 (1986): 13-9.

102. *Gilgunn v. Massachusetts General Hospital,* a jury trial verdict recorded at Super. Ct. Civ. Action No. 92-4820, Suffolk Co., Massachusetts, 21 April 1995.

103. A.M. Capron, "Abandoning a Waning Life," *Hastings Center Report* 25, no. 4 (1995): 24-6.

104. See note 20 above, p. 247.

105. B. Lo, "End-of-Life Care after Termination of SUPPORT," *Hastings Center Report* 25, no. 6 (1995): S6-S8; H. Brody, "The Best System in the World," *Hastings Center Report* 25, no. 6 (1995): S18-S21.

106. Brody, see note 105 above, p. 520.

107. *In re Baby K,* 832 F.Supp. 1022 (E.D. Va. 1993).

108. Ibid.

109. *In re Baby K,* 16 F.3d 590 (4th Cir. 1994).

110. Ibid.

14

Newborns, Infants, and Children

Robert J. Boyle

CASES

Baby B was the 1,800-gram product of an uncomplicated, full-term pregnancy. At birth he was noted to have multiple congenital anomalies, including a small omphalocele (protrusion of abdominal contents through an opening at the umbilicus), overlapping fingers, scalp defects, and cleft lip and palate. He was transferred by air to the University Medical Center, five hours by car from the family's hometown. Evaluation revealed that the infant had a congenital heart defect, which was causing respiratory distress. The cardiologist reported that the infant had severe pulmonary valve stenosis, which could be easily palliated with a shunt procedure. Physicians also suspected that he had trisomy 13. Infants with trisomy 13 rarely live beyond infancy, and those who do survive have severe developmental delay. Chromosome analysis using bone marrow cells required 24 hours. In the interim, the infant was supported on the respirator. The family was informed by phone about the potential diagnosis. The local pediatrician was also notified so that she could help inform the family and answer their questions. The following day, the diagnosis was confirmed as trisomy 13. The neonatal intensive care unit (NICU) team (attending physician, residents, nurses, social workers) agreed that the most reasonable option was to recommend to the family to discontinue the respirator and to provide only comfort care to the infant. The social worker was to arrange transportation for the family so they could visit the infant and participate in the decision face-to-face.

Baby Doe was the full-term product of an uncomplicated pregnancy. At birth, the infant was noted to have the typical features of Down syndrome (trisomy 21). Shortly thereafter, the infant was also diagnosed as having tracheoesophageal fistula/esophageal atresia, a lesion that would be relatively easily repaired in a newborn. Without repair, the infant would not be able to be fed. The family's obstetrician informed the family that infants with Down syndrome had very delayed development and should be institutionalized. He suggested that the family allow the infant to die. The infant's physician approached the family for permission to transfer the infant to the regional children's hospital for surgery, but the family denied permission for surgery and for transfer. The infant died several days later, after unsuccessful appeals through the state courts.

Baby CD was born at 25 weeks' gestation (15 weeks early) following premature labor. The infant had moderate respiratory-distress syndrome and required a respirator. She was at risk for chronic lung disease, bleeding into the ventricles of the brain, retinopathy of prematurity which may cause blindness, and infection of the bloodstream. A hospital stay of three months was anticipated if there were no severe complications.

The family had read that infants born at this gestation are at increased risk for cerebral palsy and mental retardation. They did not feel that they would be able to handle the burden and educational expense of a child with special needs. They also were concerned that this would have a negative effect on their other child. They asked that the ventilator be discontinued.

EF, an 18-month-old male, was admitted to the local hospital with the diagnosis of croup. During his hospitalization, he was found to have failure to thrive, rickets, iron-deficiency anemia, and probable kwashiorkor (severe malnutrition). When taking the child's medical history, the treatment team learned that his parents were members of a religious sect that required a strict vegetarian diet, to which they had adhered. When clinicians confronted the parents with an explanation of the child's problems, which were caused by the diet, the parents refused to allow further testing and demanded to take the child home immediately.

GH, an 8 year old, was brought to the emergency room by his grandmother, after he became acutely ill while she was caring for him for the weekend. She reports that he had been loosing weight over several weeks and recently vomiting. The day of presentation, he became progressively unresponsive. Initial evaluation strongly suggested diabetic ketoacidosis. The grandmother reported that the child's parents had been taking him to a Christian Science healer for what they thought was probably childhood diabetes. They are strongly opposed to traditional medical care.

I. INTRODUCTION

This chapter examines the particular ethical issues associated with clinical decision making for infants and children. The decision-making processes and guidelines are basically the same as those recommended for decision making in clinical situations involving adults, however, there are significant differences with pediatric patients that require special attention.

Children represent the future of their families, their communities, the nation, and the world. They require special protection because of their immature status. The infant and young child have remarkable reparative and adaptive potential. Their propensity for dramatic and rapid change demands specific and continuing attention. For these reasons, particular ethical questions asked about pediatric patients may be answered differently from the same questions asked about people nearing the normal end of their lives.

The areas of ethical concern particularly related to pediatric patients concern standards for parents and others as surrogate decision makers, the difficulty in establishing specific guidelines for newborn and pediatric issues, the question of moral standing of very young infants, the increase in capacity for decision making with normal intellectual development, children as sources of tissue and organs for their family members and others, the dual responsibility of healthcare professionals who care for infants and children to their patients and to their patients' parents and families, and the inclusion of children in research.

This chapter focuses particularly on the issues associated with newborn infants, because these issues can lead to difficult ethical dilemmas associated with high-technology medical care, quality of life, the authority of parents and others to make decisions for children, and what guidelines should be followed when making these decisions. Any moral precepts or ethical guidelines that can be applied to issues associated with the care of newborns can also be applied to the care of older infants and children, up to the age at which they are considered capable decision makers in their own right.

The issues and guidelines presented in the previous chapters certainly apply to newborns and pediatric patients as well as adults. Specifically, the chapters on capacity, disclosure, informed consent, refusal, death and dying, and forgoing life-sustaining treatment contain material that is related directly to the pediatric patient.

The micro-allocation and macro-allocation of healthcare resources, covered in later chapters, are also critical to pediatric medicine. Healthcare spending for months of neonatal intensive care must be evaluated in relation to underfunded prenatal care, which has been shown to prevent many premature births. Many nurseries have faced the problem of too many babies for their space and nursing personnel, raising critical issues in triage. Care of older, critically ill children in ICUs often presents similar allocation problems. Obtaining funding for acute care of infants and older children is usually not problematic, but, access to routine well-child care, immunization, and care for common childhood illness is often restricted by poverty and underinsurance. Primary care pediatric clinicians also face decisions concerning the proper balance between medical and economic considerations in a managed-care environment. Finally, funding for long-term care, developmental care, physical therapy, speech therapy, home health services, and early intervention services often creates a hardship for families and requires strong advocacy efforts on the part of clinicians.

Much of this chapter focuses on the issues of forgoing life-sustaining therapy in critically ill, malformed, or handicapped neonates and in critically ill older children. Should these decisions ever be made? How are the decisions made? Since these patients are not capable and perhaps never have been capable, the issue of surrogate decision making is central. Who should make decisions? In addition, this chapter addresses the proper role of the parents and others in decision making for children in all clinical situations, relating this general role to decision-making authority in critical-care situations.

II. BACKGROUND AND HISTORICAL ISSUES

The history of providing special consideration to children is a brief one. Infanticide and abandonment were relatively common until the early 1800s. Children in the Middle Ages were considered "chattel" and were put to work as early as age three. Although infanticide was forbidden by church law, it was recognized as only a minor offense. Child labor laws were unknown until the twentieth century, when laws against using children in any manner in the workplace first appeared. Removal of a child from the parents' custody because of flagrant battering was first authorized by a court in 1881, based on a statute protecting animals from cruelty.[1] Death in childhood was common until the advent of antibiotics and universal immunizations after World War II, and before that time children were often considered to be a replaceable resource.

During the early part of this century and particularly since World War II, our culture has paid increasing attention to children's needs. There have been numerous legislative attempts to afford children a safer and better life, and the courts are paying more attention to children and children's issues. Laws requiring universal immunization, access to public health clinics, strictly enforced child labor laws, attempts to ensure children's economic security in divorce, guidelines for state court judges that address decision making by children, and many other activities point to society's continuing emphasis on the interests of children. On the other hand, political decisions concerning allocation of money have often seemed to favor other more vocal and politically astute constituencies than children. Be that as it may, children are now considered to be of significant, if not overriding, value to our society.

III. ETHICAL ISSUES IN THE CARE OF NEWBORNS

Attention to issues of ethical concern related to the care of newborns began in the 1970s, with a dramatic growth in technology and understanding related to the care of critically ill newborn infants. The "premature nurseries" of the 1960s — in which primitive incubators, oxygen, and tube feedings were the extent of the technology available — rapidly evolved into high-tech ICUs (intensive care units) with multisystem monitoring, mechanical ventilators, micro intravenous (IV) lines, routine brain ultrasound, and so forth. Infants who were five weeks premature, had respiratory distress, and weighed three pounds often died in the 1960s, but by the 1970s, these had become straightforward cases, with extremely low mortality and morbidity rates.

In the 1990s, NICUs began using extracorporeal membrane oxygenation (ECMO) heart-lung machines for up to four weeks to support newborns with respiratory failure; for the majority of such patients, the results have been impressively positive. Infants born 15 to 16 weeks early, weighing approximately one pound, now reside for months in the NICU. The dramatic technological advances in adult medical care have been applied to younger and younger patients; these advances include kidney, heart, liver, and bone marrow transplants; cardiac pacemakers; and cardiac surgery techniques. Neonatal heart transplants are now limited only by the short supply of donor hearts.

As has been the case in other areas of medical care, these technological advances have been accomplished without (or with a moderate lag in) philosophical or policy reflection on the use of these technologies — either at the level of the individual patient or at the regional or national level.

IV. SELECTIVE NONTREATMENT OF NEWBORNS

The ethical and medical debate over selective nontreatment of newborns did not become public until the early 1970s. In England, Lorber defined clinical criteria to determine which children with spina bifida were to be treated in his clinic. He believed that his criteria were based on factors that predicted better prognosis.[2] Others in the United States began to question his approach, because many of the children who were untreated did not die, and their outcomes were worse than they would have been with appropriate treatment.

In 1971, bioethicists directed a great deal of attention to a landmark case at the Johns Hopkins Hospital involving an infant with Down syndrome (trisomy 21) who was born with duodenal atresia. The parents decided that they did not want to parent a child with Down syndrome and requested that he be allowed to die. Believing that the parents had the right to make decisions for this child, the hospital agreed to their request. Without a surgical repair, the child could not be fed and was allowed to die of dehydration and starvation.[3]

In a series of articles and commentaries beginning in 1973, pediatricians Duff and Campbell reported on a practice of selective nontreatment at Yale-New Haven Hospital that resulted in the deaths of 43 infants over a period of 30 months. They stated that infants with anencephaly have a "right to die," that some defective infants need to escape a "wrongful life" characterized by cruel treatment in institutions, and that families need to be spared the chronic sorrow of caring for infants with little or no possibility for meaningful lives. The decisions about nontreatment were made jointly by the physicians and parents, with the physicians sometimes yielding to parental wishes.[4]

Also in 1973, Shaw — a pediatric surgeon — wrote that the presence of mental retardation and/or severe physical malformations is an important consideration in deciding whether to treat neonates.[5]

Surveys at that time indicated that many pediatricians and pediatric surgeons agreed with a policy of selective nontreatment of seriously impaired newborns. Researchers who conducted a 1977 survey of Massachusetts pediatricians reported that 54 percent did not recommend surgery for an infant with Down syndrome and duodenal atresia, and 66 percent would not recommend surgery for an infant with a severe case of spina bifida.[6] Researchers who conducted another survey of pediatricians in the San Francisco area reported that 22 percent favored nontreatment for infants who had Down syndrome with no complications, and over half of the respondents recommended nontreatment in cases of Down syndrome with duodenal atresia.[7]

Outside of the U.S., physicians held similar views. A physician in England was accused of "murdering" a patient born with Down syndrome and bowel obstruction by feeding him only water and prescribing large doses of painkiller; the physician was acquitted, having been supported by ranking members of the Royal College of Physicians. In addition, observers in England reported that cardiac surgery routinely performed on nonhandicapped children was withheld from infants with Down syndrome.[8]

These and other reports opened a debate in the ethics and pediatrics literature on the issues of selective nontreatment and "forgoing life-sustaining treatment" in infants in various clinical situations with varying degrees of long- and short-term morbidity.

V. BABY DOE REGULATIONS

In a dramatic shift in 1982, the Reagan administration intervened in response to outcry from right-to-life advocates and advocacy groups for individuals with disabilities over the "Baby Doe" case, described at the beginning of the chapter, which involved forgoing life-sustaining treatment of an infant. Regulations, based on Section 504 of the 1973 Rehabilitation Act, which prohibits discrimination against individuals with handicaps, required that handicapped infants receive all potentially efficacious lifesaving treatment, without consideration of quality of life. The regulations appeared to require maximal treatment in all cases except when treatment was futile because the infant was irreversibly and imminently dying. A "hotline" was set up for individuals to anonymously report instances of nontreatment. "Baby Doe squads" were organized and dispatched to medical institutions where violations had been reported. Hospitals that were found in violation risked loosing their federal funding and federal reimbursements.[9] These regulations were challenged in the courts and eventually were overturned on procedural grounds.

In March 1983, the President's Commission for the Study of Ethical Problems in Medicine and Biomedical and Behavioral Research advocated full treatment for infants with Down syndrome, but the committee also suggested that families and medical teams needed latitude for judgment in complex cases.[10]

The Department of Health and Human Services proposed modified rules, which were finalized in January 1984:

1. All such disabled infants must under all circumstances receive appropriate nutrition, hydration and medication.

2. All such disabled infants must be given medically indicated treatment.

3. There are three exceptions to the requirement that all disabled infants must receive treatment, or, stated in other terms, three circum-

stances in which treatment is not considered "medically indicated." These circumstances are:

a. If the infant is chronically and irreversibly comatose.

b. If the provision of such treatment would merely prolong dying, not be effective in ameliorating or correcting all of the infant's life-threatening conditions, or otherwise be futile in terms of the survival of the infant.

c. If the provision of such treatment would be virtually futile in terms of the survival of the infant, and the treatment itself under such circumstances would be inhumane.

4. The physician's "reasonable medical judgment" concerning the medically indicated treatment must be one that would be made by a reasonably prudent physician who is knowledgeable about the case and the treatment possibilities with respect to the medical conditions involved. It is not to be based on subjective "quality of life" or other abstract concepts.[11]

The Baby Doe rules did identify a role for parents: "Given these requirements and the crucial role of the physician in carrying out these requirements, it must be emphasized that the parents of the disabled infant also play a crucial role in this process, particularly with regard to choices among alternative medical treatments. They too must have assistance and supportive services available during this difficult time and access to current and comprehensive information on the treatment, rehabilitation, and supportive services available for the infant."[12]

The courts heard another case at approximately the same time, involving Baby Jane Doe, who was born with spina bifida and hydrocephalus and whose parents had refused surgery. A "right-to-life" attorney had become aware of the case and filed a petition with the courts. The court refused to grant the U.S. Department of Health and Human Services (DHHS) access to the hospital records. The U.S. Supreme Court eventually ruled that the government had no authority "to give unsolicited advice either to parents, to hospitals or to State officials who are faced with difficult treatment decisions concerning handicapped children."[13]

The federal government continued to pursue the issue. Eventually, after negotiations among hospital associations, physicians' groups, advocates for people with disabilities, and right-to-life groups, Congress passed amendments to the Child Abuse Protection Act.[14] Enforcement was placed in the hands of each state's child protection program. In addition, the rules for implementation of the law suggested, but did not require, the establishment of "infant care review committees" in healthcare institutions.[15] These committees were the seed for the development of hospital ethics committees in many institutions.

Although the original Baby Doe rules were de-emphasized and the government's enforcement power was significantly deflated, these regulations continued to have a significant effect on clinical practice. A 1986 survey of pediatricians found that 60 percent believed that the regulations did not allow for adequate consideration of the infant's suffering. Of the respondents, 33 percent reported that the regulations had altered the care that they provided to infants; 56 percent believed that infants with extremely poor prognoses were being overtreated because of these recommendations. In response to several hypothetical cases, 32 percent of the neonatologists thought that heroic treatment was not in the infants' best interest, but was required by the regulations.[16]

The Baby Doe episode and the unique administrative, judicial, and legislative events that transpired, while extremely unpleasant to many, certainly stimulated discussion and highlighted problems with decision making in some circumstances. Today, the overall effect of the regulations in most nurseries has been tempered, and the process by which such decisions are made has evolved and become more routine; researchers estimate that 65 to 90 percent of deaths in NICUs follow withdrawal of life support.[17] Some court rulings, however, still adhere strictly to the regulations. Likewise, several book-length studies, accounts from parents, and essays by neonatologists have suggested that overtreatment may be a significant problem in some areas of newborn care,[18] but, a 1996 study reported that significant numbers of neonatologists would not recommend lifesaving surgery for an infant born to an HIV-positive mother. The authors concluded that neonatologists may be guilty of discrimination against these infants, based on their estimate of medical condition as well as quality of life.[19]

A survey of New England neonatologists found that while only 31 percent considered treatment at 24 weeks clearly beneficial, at 25 weeks, 75 percent thought it was. When respondents considered the benefits of treatment uncertain, that is, neither clearly beneficial nor futile, 76 percent would follow parental wishes to forgo treatment and allow the infant to die.[20] In response to requests from parents, infants with trisomy 13 and 18 are being offered more aggressive treatment of congenital heart disease and cleft lip and palate and feeding support with gavage and gastrostomy feeding.[21] In the Netherlands, euthanasia of newborn infants has been informally reported, but Dutch physicians described 22 mercy killings of infants with spina bifida from 1997 to 2004.[22]

VI. APPROACHES TO DECISION MAKING

Although neonatologists' approach to treatment of critically ill, malformed, or handicapped newborns has evolved during the past 20 years, the imperiled newborn still presents a special dilemma for the healthcare team. Robert Weir summarized the problem in stark detail:

> The moral decision making process in the NICU is complex. This complexity precludes the selection of any particular persons or groups of persons as automatically the best qualified to make all such decisions. . . . The complicating factors are these: the high stakes involved in decisions, the uncertainty of making proxy decisions for incompetent patients who have never been competent, serious time constraints, maximum emotional stress on parents, occasional disagreements between parents about the morally correct course of action, conflicts of interest (between parents and child, physician and child, parents and physicians), the difficulty of predicting neurologic impairment and future handicaps, inadequate communication of information between parties in cases and the logistical problems in using hospital committees or courts of law.[23]

Weir has identified five basic options for approaching the problem:
1. *Treat all nondying neonates.* Paul Ramsey suggests that clinicians have no moral right to choose that some live and some die when the medical indications for treatment are the same. He and others see no role for judgments about quality of life.
2. *Terminate the lives of selected nonpersons.* How one defines personhood becomes critical. This option has no application to critically ill older children, because they are by definition "persons."
3. *Withhold treatment according to parental discretion.* The traditional role of parents is emphasized. Parental rights are strongly supported. Consideration is given to the emotional, financial, and other effects of the infant's condition on the parents and family.
4. *Withhold treatment according to projections about quality of life.* Considerations about quality of life were specifically prohibited in the Baby Doe regulations, and others have criticized the approach as subjective.
5. *Withhold treatment judged not in the child's best interest.* Defining the child's best interest often overlaps with considerations about quality of life.[24]

Although Weir's discussion specifically addresses newborns, his concepts can be easily adapted to decisions that affect older children, as well.

VII. MORAL STATUS OF THE INFANT

Some have argued that the newborn, especially the handicapped or extremely premature newborn, may not have the same moral and legal protection as the older child or the adult. They find it problematic to define birth as the point at which to draw a major, moral distinction between a fetus with very limited rights and the newborn infant. Is the newborn morally closer to the unborn fetus than to an adult? Tooley concludes that the infant cannot be considered a person because it lacks advanced brain function until at least three months of age. The infant has no self-consciousness, ability to suffer, or sense of the future.[25] Engelhardt softens this view by concluding that newborns are not persons in the strict sense, but are persons in a deeply held social and cultural sense.[26] Others believe that infants have value, based on a relational view that results from interpersonal bonding, affection, and care by parents and other adults.[27]

What role does our society's acceptance of abortion, especially for fetuses with handicapping conditions, influence our judgments about newborns when they are born extremely prematurely or with handicapping conditions? Conversely, Mahowald describes the "premium baby" mentality, a result of reduced family size, contraception, abortion, and antenatal diagnosis.[28] This may be compounded by the psychological and financial costs of in-vitro fertilization and other technology-assisted pregnancy techniques used by some of these parents.

Why does the older child have a deeper value both to parents and to society? Parental refusal of treatment for a five-year-old who has been hit by a car who has severe head trauma and risk of neurological impairment would be quickly challenged, but many individuals tolerate requests for nontreatment of at-risk, extremely preterm infants. Some people believe that, with time, the parent and family have formed a more personal relationship with the older child, have invested emotionally and psychologically in the child, and have had rewarding two-way interaction with the child.

In an interesting anthropological review of maternal-infant attachment in the context of infanticide over the centuries, Daly and Wilson note that maternal (and probably paternal) bonding entails at least three distinct processes that proceed over widely variable time courses. First, in the immediate postpartum period, the mother assesses the quality of the child and the quality of the present circumstances. Many mothers experience an initial indifference to the infant. In the second stage, which usually begins during the following week, the mother feels that the baby is wonderful; this feeling grows over the next several weeks as the baby begins to smile and respond, and an individualized love is established. The third phase continues over several years with a gradual deepening of love. In earlier times, mothers demonstrated a growing disinclination to abandon or damage older children (such as in times of famine).[29] When a child is not attractive at birth or is removed from the parents' presence for days to weeks, the process of deepening love is affected to some degree.

Blustein describes the neonate as "not born into the family circle so much as outside it, awaiting inclusion or exclusion. The moral problem the family must confront is whether the child should become part of the family unit."[30] It is not unusual for parents to delay naming a child who may die, or to refer to the infant as "it."

Ross notes that respect for the person is "owed to all individuals on the basis of the individual's personhood (and developing personhood) ... proportionate to the actualized capacities of the individual and his or her potential to attain full personhood."[31]

It seems unreasonable in our culture to argue that newborns do not have moral worth. In fact, most of the arguments both for and against nontreatment are couched in terms that respect the moral worth (of whatever degree) of these infants. It is problematic, however, that, as some propose, that infants' moral worth is variable, dependent on acceptance by family, rather than on any innate social or legal character.[32] Worth may change over time, and therefore result in different decisions for the same infant prior to birth than at one week of age. Decisions made in the delivery room for an infant who may have a risk of developmental delay prior to its birth and prior to its being seen by parents, become much more difficult when the six month-old infant has confirmed severe delays.

VIII. DECISION MAKERS

Weir proposes that proxy decision makers for infants must meet the following criteria (which are also generalizable to critically ill older children):
1. Relevant knowledge and information about medical facts, prognosis, and family setting;
2. Impartiality;
3. Emotional stability;
4. Consistency: the process should end with the same result in similar cases.[33]

Our legal system has traditionally recognized parental autonomy as parents' authority to make decisions about treatment for their children. During the "Baby Doe period," when parental decision making was challenged, many authoritative groups, ethicists, and the courts strengthened and validated the parental role. Parents' authority to make decisions about treatment is considered part of the power that society grants parents in other important matters regarding their children, such as housing, clothing, nutrition, schooling, and religious upbringing. Parents are recognized as having a moral responsibility for the care of their children, and they should be in a position to judge what is best for their infant — in most cases. Buchanan and Brock have defined several reasons for this stance.
- Parents are generally most knowledgeable and interested in their children and most likely to do the best job for them,
- The family usually bears the consequences of the choices that are made,

- Children learn values and standards within their families, and different values and standards may lead to different healthcare choices.[34]

Parents need unbiased, full disclosure of information pertaining to their infant's diagnosis, prognosis, and options for treatment. Unfortunately, a variety of factors complicate this process. Many infants in neonatal units have been transported there from their hospital of birth. This may be a distance of a few city blocks or several hundred miles. In some cases, the parents may only briefly or never see the infant before he or she is transported. The infant's mother may be ill herself or may be recovering from anesthesia. It is extremely important for the family to see their infant and communicate face-to-face with the healthcare team whenever possible.

Families who are faced with the birth of an infant with unexpected life-threatening problems face major emotional issues. The perinatal period has been recognized as extremely sensitive for both parents. They have expected the birth of a full-term, healthy infant; instead they are faced with tragedy. They may be emotionally devastated, and they grieve the loss of the normal infant that they expected. Denial, anger, depression, fear, and even disgust often overwhelm them. Parent-infant attachment suffers in this setting.

Some clinicians feel strongly enough about the right of the parents to make decisions that they would not override the parents' decisions, even when the clinicians disagree. They believe that parents are the best possible proxies, because parents face the prospect of long-term, emotionally and financially draining treatment of a seriously handicapped child. The validity of this viewpoint is discussed below. Shaw and colleagues reported in 1977 that most pediatricians and pediatric surgeons believe that selective nontreatment is appropriately a matter of parental discretion.[35]

Most clinicians believe that the parents' role is not unlimited, however. The parents' decision must benefit the well-being of the child. Most of the time this occurs; however, when a decision is made that reflects not the child's best interest but other interests (for example, in the cases of Baby Doe and Baby CD presented at the beginning of this chapter), the parents' decision should be questioned. It is not unusual for the court to intervene, if necessary, overriding the parents' authority by proving them unable to protect a child's health or welfare. Parents are not legally at liberty to refuse consent for life-sustaining treatment. Courts usually overturn the decisions of parents who are Jehovah's Witnesses when they refuse blood for their children. Likewise, parents who are Christian Scientists have been prosecuted for refusing or denying care for their children. The courts have seen the need to protect the best interests of such children.

According to Fost, "The history of childhood is one that does not support idyllic notions of parents as decision makers for their children."[36] Whitelaw and Thoresen state, "The statistics on non-accidental injury and sexual abuse indicate that parents' wishes for their children are not necessarily always in the child's best interest."[37]

Families may be unwilling to accept emotionally the "less-than-perfect child." They may be overwhelmed with the prospects of chronic medical care, financial burdens, educational challenges, potential harm to other children in the family, and so forth. Dellinger and Kuszler assert, "It is naive to posit an identity of interest between infant and parent [in all situations]. Parents guard their own interests, those of the family as a unit, and those of current and future siblings — all of which may be gravely threatened by the newborn."[38] According to Weir: "In promoting their own psychological and financial interests, protecting their chosen life-style and other children at home, some parents cannot make impartial judgments."[39]

The current emphasis on autonomy in informed consent means there has been some attempt to apply these concepts to parental decision making. The distinction between *informed consent* and *proxy or substituted consent* is often overlooked. Parents provide the latter. Legal and moral grounds for requiring informed consent are stronger than those for substituted consent. Mahowald states, "The parents' right to decide about their infant's treatment is legally less binding than their right to decide about their own treatments."[40]

Bartholome suggests that the language of "consent" should be replaced by the language of "permission" with regard to parental decision making, in order to better distinguish what persons may do for themselves from what they do on behalf of another. He sees the parents' role as a *duty*, rather than as a *right*. Parents have a duty to ensure that necessary medical care is provided to their child:

Parental permission for interventions into children's lives must not be seen as the unconditional right to demand or refuse a particular intervention because it is a proper exercise of parental authority over the lives of children. That children are largely dependent, at least for a time, on their parents is to be affirmed, but that dependency does not warrant the second-class social standing implied by a parental right of "consent" in decisions affecting the health care of their children.[41]

Weir also raises the problem of consistency when parents are the sole decision makers: "If birth-defective neonates sometimes live or die merely on the basis of parental discretion, the decisions in these cases may adhere to no ethical principles or criteria generally acceptable by other persons . . . there exists virtually no possibility for consistency from case to case."[42]

IX. THE CLINICIAN'S ROLE AS ADVOCATE

Physicians, nurses, and other professionals who care for children have traditionally seen themselves as advocates for their patients. They have a responsibility to promote the child's best interest and to seek intervention if a dilemma cannot be resolved. Beauchamp and Childress reflect this point of view: "Our view is that physicians have a primary responsibility to the patient. . . . The physician ought to act in the patient's best interests, even if it is necessary to seek a court order to authorize surgery, blood transfusion or the like. Other familial interests, such as avoiding the depletion of family resources, should not be considered until a certain threshold is reached, viz., when significant patient interests would not be served by continued treatment or by particular treatment."[43] Bartholome defines clinicians' social roles and relationships with their child-patients as ones that impose "legal and ethical duties and obligations which exist independently of any parental wishes, desires and/or 'consentings.' "[44] Participants in a conference sponsored by the New York Academy of Medicine concluded that "professionals must maintain an independent obligation to protect the child's interests."[45] Others have suggested that clinicians have some insight into a community standard of best interest for the individual patient.[46]

Some have taken this argument to the point of suggesting that physicians should be the deci-

sion makers in these cases, because they have the requisite medical knowledge and insight and are seen as advocates for their patients. However, physicians are not completely objective either. They may have their own biases about treatment or nontreatment of handicapped children, and they may have a conflict of interest relating to nursery census, outcome statistics, and so forth.

Ramsey is convinced that neither parents nor physicians are the best proxies. Instead, he suggests that any decision about the possible termination of an individual's life should be made by a disinterested party.[47] Using this approach, the Baby Doe deliberations and the President's Commission suggested that hospital or unit-based committees address these treatment decisions. Many hospitals set up such committees, not as decision-making bodies, but with advisory or review responsibility. As decision-making bodies, committees have a tendency to be formalistic, slow-moving, and cumbersome, but, they can be useful when there is conflict among the decision makers or when various parties to a decision request outside assistance.

X. THE PROCESS OF DECISION MAKING

The most realistic and functional approach to decision making about treatment of an imperiled newborn is similar to the approach discussed in earlier chapters — a shared process that involves the surrogates (the parents) and the clinicians involved in the infant's care. The clinician's role is to diagnose the infant's condition — seeking consultation as needed — and to present the diagnosis, prognosis, options for treatment, and recommendations, when appropriate, to the family. This process of communication and disclosure should provide the family with insight into all of the issues involved in the child's care. The family can then bring their values, goals, and preferences to the discussion, and ideally all can reach a decision. Involvement of all of the members of the caregiving team (rather than parents and physicians alone) ensures a more open process. This model, although occasionally difficult to achieve, can be considered the basic model for decision making in all pediatric medical care, and, more broadly, for all medical care for individual patients. King adapts Brody's "transparency" model described in chapter 10 to the neonatal intensive care setting.[48]

XI. BASIS FOR DECISION MAKING

What criteria should be used as a basis for decision making for imperiled newborns? Should any consideration be given to the quality of life, long-term outcome, degree of handicap, or family burden?

A. Medical Indications

Ramsey uses an approach that emphasizes medical indications. He contends that there is an obligation to use treatment that is medically indicated, as long as the patient is not dying. He argues that decision makers should avoid making judgments about the quality of life because such judgments violate the principle of equality of life.[49]

The Baby Doe rules took a similar stance. Clinicians were required to provide treatment for infants in all cases except when the infant is permanently comatose, or when treatment will not correct other life-threatening conditions, or when treatment is virtually futile and inhumane. The commentary that accompanied the regulations said that it is a discriminatory act under the law to withhold surgery to correct an intestinal obstruction in an infant with Down syndrome, when the decision to withhold is based upon the future mental retardation of the infant and there are no medical contraindications to the surgery. However, withholding of treatment from an infant with anencephaly would not constitute a discriminatory act, because the treatment would be futile and would only prolong the act of dying. Furthermore, withholding certain treatments from a severely premature and low-birthweight infant on the grounds of reasonable medical judgment concerning the improbability of success or risks of potential harm to the infant would not be in violation. Even the Baby Doe rules involved some consideration beyond life as an absolute, taking into account the issues of futility and burdens and benefits of treatment.

B. Quality of Life

"Quality-of-life" terminology carried negative connotations in the Baby Doe era. Quality of life can be defined subjectively; what one clinician sees as a good quality of life may be unacceptable to another professional or to a parent. A family may see the life of a child who is profoundly visually handicapped but with normal intelligence as qualitatively poor. Although many families do not feel burdened with a moderately mentally retarded child, others consider learning disability with normal intelligence unacceptable. Clinicians who work with developmentally impaired children often have a very different appraisal than laypersons of quality of life for this patient population.

However, it may be possible to use quality of life as a basis for decision making when considering more fundamental issues. Richard McCormick proposes a minimal condition for defining "quality": the capacity for experience or social interrelating. If the condition is not met, as with anencephaly, treatment is not required.[50]

Coulter and colleagues have also defined interests that would constitute a "minimal quality of life":

1. Freedom from intractable pain and suffering: mental retardation, paralysis, or cerebral palsy would not be considered physical suffering; dyspnea or intractable physical pain would.
2. Capacity to experience and enjoy life: the ability to enjoy food, warmth, or the caring touch of another; the ability to give or receive love.
3. Expectation of continued life: heroic treatment, when death will likely occur in a few weeks or months, may be cruel.[51]

C. Technical Medical Criteria

Using a technical medical approach (such as Lorber's criteria for treatment of spina bifida or criteria based on gestational age or birthweight), while based on data from populations of patients, still presupposes value judgments about probable results.

D. Nonmaleficence/Best Interest

Jonsen and Garland argue that neonatal intensive care may violate the obligation of nonmaleficence if one or more of three conditions (the converse of Coulter's quality-of-life criteria) are present:

1. Inability to survive infancy,
2. Inability to live without severe pain, and
3. Inability to participate at least minimally in human experience.[52]

Some conclude that using a best-interest standard — weighing benefits and burdens for the particular patient and, in some cases, for the family — represents the mainstream ethical position in the U.S.[53] Weir and Bale suggest eight variables for evaluating "best interest":

1. The severity of the patient's medical condition,
2. The achievability of curative or corrective treatment,
3. The important medical goals in the case (such as prolongation of life, relief of pain, or amelioration of disabling conditions),
4. The presence of serious neurologic impairments,
5. The extent of the infant's suffering,
6. The multiplicity of other serious medical problems,
7. The life expectancy of the infant, and
8. The proportionality of treatment-related benefits and burdens.[54]

However, quality of life is still involved in the considerations, and the various approaches overlap and complement one another. Brock's discussion reflects this approach:

A narrowly constrained role for quality of life considerations is inevitable if competent patients, or incompetent patients' surrogates, are to be free to decide whether a life-sustaining treatment and the life that it makes possible are on balance a benefit or excessively burdensome. Using this standard, the infant's prospects in relatively few cases will be so poor that it is reasonable to hold that continued life is clearly not in its interests. The clearest cases are probably when its life will be filled with substantial and unrelievable suffering and when the infant has suffered such severe brain damage as to preclude any significant social or environmental interaction. Other cases of very severe disabilities are more controversial and problematic, in part because of the wide variation in the weight adult patients give to such considerations and the fact that infants do not yet have preferences or values of their own.[55]

Clinicians who care for critically ill infants and children have always had both a short-term and a long-term focus to outcome and care. A child's day-to-day survival and survival to discharge have always been interpreted in light of long-term issues of development and the child's ability to perform in school and function in soci-

ety. The child's interests likewise have this short-term and long-term focus. Buchanan and Brock describe these as "current interests" and "future-oriented or forward-looking interests." The current interests of infants are expressively experiential and functional: they are interests in achieving pleasure and in avoiding pain and discomfort. Developmental interests are especially prominent among the forward-looking interests: interests in the development of agency (having the capacity necessary for being an agent), opportunity, and human relationships.[56]

Robertson expresses concern about how quality-of-life criteria are currently being defined for infants, especially extremely low-birthweight infants, particularly when decisions are made before birth or early in the hospital course, when it is virtually impossible to identify those infants who will have the extremely poor quality of life described above.[57]

Another difficult issue in this benefit-burden analysis has to do with benefits and burdens to parties other than the infant, especially the family and, in some circumstances, society. Some, including the President's Commission in 1983,[58] argue that the burdens of caring for and raising a severely impaired child (often over a lifetime), the difficulties of providing an education, the financial burden of chronic medical care, and the effects on normal siblings should all be considered in benefit-burden analysis. According to Silverman, "Parents of a badly damaged baby often resent the implied demand that their family is required to pass a 'sacrifice test' to satisfy the moral expectations of those who do not have to live, day by day, with the consequences of diffuse idealism. It is easy . . . to demand prolongation of each and every new life that requires none of one's own . . . resources to maintain that life later."[59] He has proposed abandoning the term "best interests" and adopting Veatch's concept of a "standard of reasonableness." How far the technology is pursued to accomplish a reasonable end should be "defined by those most directly affected by the decisions — the parents." The concept of "well-being" includes physical function, but should extend into the areas of social, occupational, religious, aesthetic and other aspects of life.[60] Others focus on the burden on society, the expense of caring for the handicapped, the burden of additional numbers of children who require special education, and so forth. Ross, using the concept of "constrained parental autonomy," suggests a model where the parents are guided by the child's well-being, but they would not be obligated to disregard all personal interests of themselves or other children in order to fulfill the child's needs and interests.[61] The model allows sensitivity to the parent and family situation, but it also balances the short- and long-term needs of the child.

The New York Academy of Medicine conference reached the following conclusion:

> Although parents may have legitimate concerns about the effect of treatment decisions on themselves and their other children, the desire to avoid emotional, financial or other hardships cannot justify the denial of clearly beneficial medical care to an ill or injured child. . . . If parents are unable or unwilling to provide essential medical treatment, healthcare professionals should first assure that social counseling and supports are made available to the family to assist them. If the parents remain unwilling to consent to the needed medical treatment, then we must utilize legal mechanisms to ensure social support or supervision to provide those treatments which are clearly in the best interests of the child.[62]

These issues are rarely considered in proxy decisions for adult patients. As this is the case, why should we accept this stance for infants and children? According to Beauchamp and Childress:

> Proxies should not confuse quality of life for the patient with the value of that patient's life for others, and they should not refuse treatment that would be in the incompetent patient's interests in order to avoid burdens to the family or costs to society. Instead . . . the incompetent patient's best medical interests, defined in terms of his or her personal welfare, generally should be the decisive criterion for a proxy, even if these interests conflict with familial interests.[63]

If decisions are soundly based on what is truly in the best interest of the child, treatment should rarely, if ever, be forgone because of the burdens the infant's continuing existence would place on others. On the other hand, it is insensitive to deny the effects of these burdens. Caregivers have an obligation to assist the family, by all possible means, to prevent such burdens (assistance with funding, insurance, educational opportunities, parent support groups, diagnosis-specific information, and so forth). In fact, one of the major criticisms of the Baby Doe regulations was that the Reagan administration required care, but little was done to develop and fund adequate programs for the infants who survived.

Diekema raises multiple concerns about the difficulty applying the concept of "best interests":

- It may be difficult to define, especially when the child's life is not threatened.
- It is inherently a question of values.
- The nature of interests are often complex, including medical, emotional, and psychological issues for the patient.
- It is not clear that the best interest of the child should always be the sole or primary consideration in decisions.

He proposes evaluating decisions based on the "harm principle." Decisions that are life-threatening or pose serious and likely harm to the child should be questioned. In addition, any proposed treatment should be assessed for efficacy in preventing serious harm, as should any risks and burdens associated with the treatment.[64]

Clinicians may be influenced by other factors in considering withholding or withdrawing care. Chiswick warns against being overly influenced by the following:

1. The frustration of caring for an infant on a long-term basis;
2. The appearance of the infant, who may be relatively wasted, with skin lesions and the narrow head of prematurity;
3. A lack of family involvement;
4. A biased impression of prognosis.[65]

XII. CERTAINTY/UNCERTAINTY

Pediatricians — especially neonatologists, geneticists, and developmentalists — have developed a large and constantly updated literature on prognosis, both for survival and morbidity, for most of the common neonatal conditions that might lead to questions about nontreatment. This body of information allows better-informed disclosure to families and better-informed decision making by all of those involved in the care of an infant. For example, 60 to 70 percent of premature infants who develop hemorrhage in the ventricles of the brain but who do not require a shunt to treat hydrocephalus do quite well neurodevelopmentally. Even infants whose bleeding involves the cortex of the brain do not necessarily have mental retardation, although they usually have some element of cerebral palsy. For extremely premature infants who survive beyond four days of age, the overall mortality is equivalent to much more mature preterm infants. Premature infants who are born 12 to 14 weeks early usually have a long-term (two-to four-month) requirement for oxygen, possibly on a respirator; but, of those who survive beyond the first one to two weeks, the vast majority have clinically normal pulmonary function by six to 12 months of age. On the other hand, infants born with severe perinatal asphyxia — who in the first 24 hours of life have seizures that are difficult to control, transient renal and myocardial failure, and flaccidity — have a high rate of mortality in the immediate newborn period; those who survive have at least a 90 percent chance of severe neurodevelopmental impairment, approaching McCormick's criterion for lack of potential for human relationships.

Valid disclosure and careful decision making require that clinicians have current and accurate data available regarding an infant's condition. However, data do not solve all of the problems of prognostication. Interpretation of the data may differ from clinician to clinician, and from parent to parent. A 60 percent survival rate may sound hopeful to some, but sound dismally poor to others. Some may insist that their infant will be one of the 5 percent to survive, or one of the 10 percent who will not be severely neurologically impaired. Some may demand to continue treatment until the prognosis is certain. Decision makers must still make judgments about how much of a burden an infant will be required to bear to possibly be the one survivor out of 20; they must weigh the relatively low burden of tube feedings against the higher burden of surgeries and ventilators.

Rhoden describes several strategies for approaching decisions that must be made in the absence of sufficient information to make the prognosis immediately:[66]

- *Wait until certain:* continue treatment until the patient is actually dying or comatose. Letting one patient die who would have had a tolerable life would be worse than saving one whose life would be devastated. Err on the side of life. Rhoden believes that this approach pays insufficient attention to suffering, especially of the nonsurvivors; that it is governed

by technology rather than by using technology as a tool; and that it sees parents only as onlookers. Evaluation of the approach would have to define the number of infants who would need to be treated for each additional survivor.

- *Statistical prognosis:* use statistical cutoffs and aggressively treat all those selected. The cutoffs may be based on epidemiologic studies using birthweight or gestational age, and may be defined by professional groups or governmental policy. Fewer will live with handicaps, but the few who die may die slowly. This approach sacrifices some potentially normal infants. Decision making is psychologically easier, because it is a "go-by-the-book" approach. It appears to be more "objective." Withdrawing therapy is not an issue. Several European countries have taken this approach with premature infants of a specific birthweight.

- *Individualized prognosis:* decide for each infant using the available data, the present condition, and a benefit-burden analysis. This approach allows a role for the family in decision making. It also can be a source of confusion, uncertainty, error, and agony. However, Rhoden believes that this is justified, given the tragic nature of the situations. Fischer and Stevenson have applied this strategy in their NICU at Stanford and make suggestions for its application in other settings.[67] The American Academy of Pediatrics has endorsed this approach, as well.[68]

There are few, if any, absolute certainties in medical prognostication. Therefore, it is unreasonable to expect or await situations in which issues are completely defined. Beauchamp and Childress summarize the issue:

In cases of incompetent patients, including seriously ill newborns, we should begin with the normal presumption in favor of the prolongation of life. Decision makers should then work diligently to determine the patient's actual interests. Judgments about the best interests of seriously ill newborns must be made by considering the prospective benefits and burdens as objectively as possible, in light of the patient's condition. . . . Although the possibility of error is substantial, it is no greater than in many other judgments in medicine.

Because of potential error in diagnosis, prognosis, and judgments about the patient's interests, the normal obligation to preserve life dictates erring on the side of sustaining life, at least in cases of serious doubt about the available evidence.[69]

XIII. SPECIFIC CLINICAL ISSUES

A. Extremely Premature Infants

Infants who are born at a gestational age of 26 or more weeks or who weigh greater than 800 grams have mortality rates of 10 to 25 percent, with serious morbidity rates of 15 to 20 percent in the survivors. Based on this information, most neonatal physicians believe that aggressive treatment for this population is the standard of care. Infants of lower birthweight or gestational age pose real problems related to the uncertainty of their prognosis for survival and morbidity; necessity for prolonged, very expensive care; questions about quality of life; and the effects on family members during the hospitalization and in the future. (See, for example, the case of Baby CD presented at the beginning of this chapter.) Mortality, at 23 weeks, based on compiled national data, varies from 70 to 90 percent (mean 85 percent); at 24 weeks mortality is 20 to 70 percent (mean 66 percent); at 25 weeks mortality is 25 to 53 percent (mean 40 percent). Studies of neurodevelopmental outcome at age 30 months in survivors at these gestations report an incidence of severe cerebral palsy of 10 to 12 percent and severe disability including blindness, deafness, severe cerebral palsy, or significant mental retardation of 25 percent; 49 percent had no disability. In this same population studied at six years of age, outcomes were similar, although significant numbers of children who were listed as severely affected earlier had now progressed to mild or minimal disability, and some mildly or moderately affected were later classified as severe. Also of importance is the observation that severity of outcome did not correlate with lower gestational age, whereas mortality clearly did.[70]

The ethical problems begin even before delivery, when attempts to plan care are frustrated by an inability to predict exact gestational age accurately. Obstetrical estimates may be two to three weeks less than actual age. These differences may have major implications for mortality and morbidity. Risks change following delivery, depending on initial condition, response to therapy, and postnatal age. For infants who survive their first 96 hours, overall mortality rates fall to 10 to 20 percent. Parents should be properly informed before birth about potential mortality and risks, and also about the uncertainties that exist until an infant is born and evaluated. After birth, parents should be allowed to participate in decisions about their infant's care, and clinicians should give parental choices more weight as the uncertainty of survival and outcome increases.

There is a growing consensus on guidelines for approaching decisions about this population. For infants less than 23 weeks or 500 grams at birth, the presumption should be against resuscitation, unless the parents request full support and the infant is potentially viable. For older or larger infants, the presumption should be in favor of resuscitation, unless the parents request no aggressive care and the infant is in poor clinical condition.[71] Ideally, experts with sufficient experience to assess an infant should be present at its delivery. These infants usually require immediate tracheal intubation and ventilation. Parents should be informed that the infant will be constantly evaluated, and that any decision to resuscitate does not mean that aggressive care cannot be withdrawn if a negative prognosis seems likely.[72] The Canadian Pediatric Society in 1994 recommended against treatment for infants under 23 weeks, recommended that parents be given the option of treatment for babies at 23 to 24 weeks, and strongly recommended continued treatment for babies born at 25 or more weeks of gestational age.[73] The American Academy of Pediatrics/American Heart Association have guidelines that suggest that withholding resuscitation for infants with confirmed gestation of less than 23 weeks is reasonable. They also describe a process for ongoing counseling and communication with families.[74]

Several high-profile legal cases have highlighted the controversies in this area. In *State v. Messenger*, Dr. Messenger, a dermatologist, and his wife, who was in preterm labor at 25 weeks, had discussed their wishes that no resuscitation be performed at birth.[75] The neonatologist believed that the infant should be assessed and, if vigorous, supported. At birth, a physician's assistant resuscitated the baby, who was described as lifeless and cyanotic. Following resuscitation, the infant was taken to the NICU in poor condition. The father denied permission to treat the infant with surfactant (a natural material that coats the alveoli and prevents collapse of the lungs) or to place central arterial and IV lines. The neonatologist believed that the infant had improved somewhat after adjusting the respirator. The family asked to be left alone with the infant. The parents then removed the baby from the ventilator and held him. He was pronounced dead approximately 75 minutes later. The father was charged with manslaughter. The treating neonatologist testified that, given the patient's situation, she would have backed the parents' decision if she had been consulted. A jury later found the father innocent. They believed that the parental choice was in the child's best interest. This case highlights the need for effective communication between clinician and parents.

In *HCA v. Miller,* the mother developed premature labor at 23 weeks gestation.[76] Attempts were made to stop labor, but had to be discontinued due to evidence of infection. The mother's obstetrician and a neonatologist counseled the parents that the infant had little chance of being born alive, and, if she did survive, would probably suffer severe impairments. The parents decided they wanted no heroic measures performed at birth. Nursing staff, other neonatologists, and hospital administration were uncomfortable with the decision and met with the parents. The clinicians asked to evaluate the baby before making a decision about treatment. The parents continued to refuse. At birth, the baby weighed 615 grams, began breathing, and cried spontaneously. The baby was placed on a ventilator and taken to the NICU. The parents apparently never again objected to the treatment of the baby. However, at several days of age, the infant suffered a severe intracranial hemorrhage and developed hydrocephalus, requiring a ventricular shunt. The child at age seven years was unable to walk, talk, feed herself, or sit on her own. She had severe cerebral palsy, mental retardation, blindness, and seizures. The family sued the hospital for battery and negligence. The jury awarded the family approximately $60 million. The decision was overturned on appeal to the level of the Texas Supreme Court. The court concluded that a decision about resuscitation could not be reasonably made before birth and before an assessment by the physician. The initial decision was seen as confirming the rights of parents to refuse care for infants of this gestation. It should be noted, however, that the Texas Supreme Court's decision was limited to the initial resuscitation in "emergent circumstances,"

and it should not be interpreted as interfering with other decisions to withdraw or withhold life-sustaining therapies. The case highlights the importance of providing accurate data when counseling a family, and effective communication among disciplines. While this child's outcome is tragic, as noted above, statistically one would expect this to occur in 10 to 12 percent of surviving infants.

B. Infants with Life-Threatening Congenital Anomalies

Life-threatening congenital anomalies represent a wide spectrum — from a single defect with an extremely poor prognosis such as anencephaly (absence of the cerebral cortex); to a lesion with long-term developmental implications such as meningomyelocele (spina bifida); to cardiac lesions that are life-threatening but relatively easily repaired with excellent long-term prognosis, such as transposition of the great vessels of the heart; to multiple congenital anomalies that require multiple surgical repairs, but present little or no risk of developmental delay or mental retardation, such as the VATER association (vertebral defects, anal atresia, tracheoesophageal fistula with esophageal atresia, and radial and renal anomalies). Therefore, accurate diagnosis and prognostic data are critical for valid decision making. In addition, one or both parents may feel guilty about the defect, the likelihood of the child having an abnormal appearance, or the prognosis of some degree of continuing disability.

C. Infants with Chromosomal Defects

The short-term prognosis for survival of infants with trisomy 13 or trisomy 18 is extremely poor, even when those infants do not have major anomalies. Those who survive beyond the first year of life are extremely mentally retarded. Infants with trisomy 21 (Down syndrome), on the other hand, very often can function in the family setting, attend school, and work in a protected environment. Decisions about treatment for infants with chromosomal defects raise concerns about futile therapy for dying infants and quality of life for those who survive with chronic medical problems and/or mental retardation. (See the cases of Baby B and Baby Doe presented at the beginning of this chapter.) Currently, most clinicians would not recommend or follow a parental request to withhold lifesaving medical treatment for an infant with trisomy 21. The American Academy of Pediatrics has stated that it is not unreasonable to withhold resuscitation when there is a confirmed diagnosis of trisomy 13 or 18. However, some families request aggressive care, including cardiac surgery. These requests should be respected and parent/clinician discussions should focus on the development of a plan of care sensitive to the infant's needs and prognosis.[77]

D. Infants with Severe Birth Asphyxia

Infants with severe birth asphyxia are usually full-term infants who suffer multisystem damage due to lack of adequate oxygen and blood flow before, during, or immediately after birth. Some of these infants survive their multisystem failure; they may have severe central nervous system dysfunction and often require long-term tube feeding, physical therapy, and seizure medication. These patients are later diagnosed as having "cerebral palsy," but early prognostication is difficult for many of them.

E. Infants with Brain Death or Persistent Vegetative State

Most experts agree that the adult parameters for the determination of death by neurologic criteria validly apply to full-term infants older than seven days of age. The immature nervous system makes the determination in younger infants problematic.[78] Ashwal and colleagues have defined guidelines for the determination of persistent vegetative state in children, which allow the same considerations for care as for adults.[79]

F. Infants with Hypoplastic Left Heart Syndrome

Until recently, infants with hypoplastic left heart syndrome, born without a functional left side of the heart, died within several days after birth. First, prostaglandin E became available to maintain patency of the ductus arteriosus and allow blood flow to the body. Second, a series of surgical procedures was developed that palliates the lesion, but the infant still has a significant cardiac defect. The results of such procedures have progressively improved over the past several years. Finally, infant heart transplantation became available; this allows for reasonably good outcomes. However, the child requires lifelong im-

munosuppression, and the supply of donor hearts is extremely limited. Of the candidates, 30 to 50 percent die before receiving their transplants. Whereas families were informed in the past that no therapy was available, options are now available. Most pediatric cardiologists now strongly support surgical repair.[80] However, there is some ongoing debate about whether comfort care alone should still be an option for families.[81]

G. Drug Screening and HIV Testing of Newborns

Screening a newborn infant's stool or urine for drugs has important implications for the baby's mother, because the test also screens the mother for recent drug use. This may violate the mother's privacy. If the information is important for the infant's medical treatment, there may be valid reasons to risk the violation. There is significant controversy about the short- and long-term effects of drug exposure, especially cocaine, on a child; recent studies suggest that the critical issue is the rearing environment of the child.[82] If the test is done solely to identify drug-using parents, the mother's informed consent should be sought. The approach to mother and baby should be supportive, voluntary, and nonpunitive.[83] In some jurisdictions, however, exposure to unprescribed drugs and alcohol must be reported to state agencies.

Likewise, HIV testing of the neonate tests for antibodies acquired across the placenta from the mother, and therefore screens the mother for antibodies. Until recently, there were strong reasons for respecting the mother's privacy; however, early identification of this infection has recently shown to benefit the infant's subsequent health and mortality. This issue has raised heated debate in the arenas of public health, ethics, and legislation.[84] Currently, universal, although not mandatory, screening, preferably of the mother during pregnancy or in labor, is recommended.[85]

H. Healthy Children as a Source of Tissue and Organs

Clinicians have encountered an increasing number of requests to use a child as a source for organ or tissue harvesting (particularly for kidney or bone marrow) for a family member. The risks attending such procedures are relatively well-known, but the possible benefits for the family member who needs the organ donation, for the family, and for the donor child are much more difficult to evaluate. Is there a conflict of interest in the consent process when one of the parents is the recipient of the tissue/organ? Should another party be appointed to attend to the child's interests? Most bone marrow transplant programs accept parental consent as the only permission necessary for sibling donation. In a survey of transplant programs, Chan and colleagues reported that 64 percent think that, when a parent is the recipient, the other parent or both parents together can consent. The remainder of the respondents believe that an independent entity should be involved, either as sole decision maker or working with the parents.[86] Some believe that the child donor should participate in the decision, as developmentally appropriate and, when appropriate, assent to the procedure.[87] Most believe that the benefits to the donor are related to continued emotional bonds to the recipient, increased self-esteem, and prevention of the grief from the death of a sibling or parent. Steinberg would allow donation only when the recipient's death is imminent.[88] For procedures with higher risk to the donor, outside evaluation or even court oversight (including appointment of a guardian *ad litem*) may be warranted.[89]

I. Parental Refusal of Care on Religious Grounds

Should parents be able to refuse needed treatment for their child because of their religious convictions? (See, for example, the cases of EF and GH, presented at the beginning of this chapter.) Presently, different states have different laws concerning this issue. Most states allow overriding the parents' refusal of treatment for their child in a life-threatening situation, but this is not universal. For example, courts usually override decisions by parents who are Jehovah's Witness when they refuse blood transfusions for their child. Some states, however, provide an exemption to neglect statutes for faith healing or spiritual treatment. Even in those situations, when the child's health is in danger, courts have ordered medical treatment. When death has occurred, convictions have been overturned if the parents could be characterized as "well-intentioned."[90] When the child's condition is not life-threatening, the situation may best be approached using the previously described "harm principle." In addition, as the child ma-

tures, disputes may be avoided when the child has the capacity to make an independent decision in light of his or her own religious beliefs.

XIV. STATEMENTS BY AUTHORITATIVE BODIES

A. The American Academy of Pediatrics, 1983

The American Academy of Pediatrics, Committee on Bioethics, in "Treatment of Critically Ill Newborns," stated:

Ambiguities and differences of opinion . . . should not preclude consensus on some ethical principles. The most basic of these principles is that the pediatrician's primary obligation is to the child. While the needs and interests of parents, as well as of the larger society, are proper concerns of the pediatrician, his or her primary moral and legal obligation is to the child-patient. Withholding or withdrawing life-sustaining treatment is justified only if such a course serves the interests of the patient. When the infant's prospects are for a life dominated by suffering, the concerns of the family may play a larger role. Treatment should not be withheld for the primary purpose of improving the psychological or social well-being of others, no matter how poignant those needs may be.

The complexity and importance of these decisions require that they be made with the utmost care. The traditional method of a single physician making such judgments, without exposure to other persons having additional facts, experience, and points of view, may lead to decisions that, in retrospect, cannot be justified.[91]

B. The President's Commission for the Study of Ethical Problems in Medicine and Biomedical and Behavioral Research, 1983

The President's Commission for the Study of Ethical Problems in Medicine and Biomedical and Behavioral Research, in *Deciding to Forego Life-Sustaining Treatment,* stated:

Many therapies undertaken to save the lives of seriously ill newborns will leave the survivors with permanent handicaps, either from the underlying defect (such as heart surgery not affecting the retardation of a Down Syndrome infant) or from the therapy itself (as when mechanical ventilation for a premature baby results in blindness or a scarred trachea). One of the most troubling and persistent issues in this entire area is whether, or to what extent, the expectation of such handicaps should be considered in deciding to treat or not to treat a seriously ill newborn. The Commission has concluded that a very restrictive standard is appropriate: such permanent handicaps justify a decision not to provide life-sustaining treatment only when they are so severe that continued existence would not be a net benefit to the infant. Though inevitably somewhat subjective and imprecise in actual application, the concept of "benefit" excludes honoring idiosyncratic views that might be allowed if a person were deciding about his or her own treatment. Rather, net benefit is absent only if the burdens imposed on the patient by the disability or its treatment would lead a competent decision maker to choose to forego the treatment. As in all surrogate decision making, the surrogate is obligated to try to evaluate benefits and burdens from the infant's own perspective. The Commission believes that the handicaps of Down Syndrome, for example, are not in themselves of this magnitude and do not justify failing to provide medically proven treatment, such as surgical correction of a blocked intestinal tract.[92]

C. The American Academy of Pediatrics, 1984

The American Academy of Pediatrics, in "Principles of Treatment of Disabled Infants," stated:

Discrimination of any type against any individual with a disability/disabilities, regardless of the nature or severity of the disability, is morally and legally indefensible.

These rights for all disabled persons must be recognized at birth.

When medical care is clearly beneficial, it should always be provided. When appropriate medical care is not available, arrangements should be made to transfer the infant to an appropriate medical facility. Consideration such as anticipated or actual limited potential of an individual and present or future lack of available community resources are irrelevant and must not determine the decisions concerning medical care. The individual's medical condition should be the sole focus of the decision.

It is ethically and legally justified to withhold medical or surgical procedures which are clearly futile and will only prolong the act of dying.

In cases where it is uncertain whether medical treatment will be beneficial, a person's disability must not be the basis for a decision to withhold treatment.[93]

D. The American Academy of Pediatrics, 1994

The American Academy of Pediatrics, Committee on Bioethics, in "Guidelines on Foregoing Life-Sustaining Medical Treatment," stated:

The burdens of [life-sustaining medical treatment] may include intractable pain; irremediable disability or helplessness; emotional suffering; invasive and/or inhumane interventions designed to sustain life; or other activities that severely detract from the patient's quality of life. The phrase "quality of life" refers to the experience of life as viewed by the patient, i.e., how the patient, not the parents or health care providers, perceives or evaluates his or her existence. The American Academy of Pediatrics specifically rejects attempts to equate quality of life with "social worth" as judged by others.

Our social system generally grants patients and families wide discretion in making their own decisions about health care and in continuing, limiting, declining, or discontinuing treatment, whether life-sustaining or otherwise. Medical professionals should seek to override family wishes only when those views clearly conflict with the interests of the child.[94]

E. The American Medical Association, 2002

The American Medical Association, Council on Ethical and Judicial Affairs, in "The Use of Minors as Organ and Tissue Donors," stated:

Minors need not be prohibited from acting as sources of organs, but their participation should be limited. Different procedures pose different degrees of risk and do not all require the same restrictions. In general minors should not be permitted to serve as a source when there is a very serious risk of complications (e.g., partial liver or lung donation, which involve a substantial risk of serious immediate or long-term morbidity)... . Minors may be permitted to serve as a source when the risks are low (e.g., blood or skin donation, in which the donated tissue can regenerate and ... anesthesia is not required), moderate (e.g., bone marrow donation, in which the donated tissue can regenerate but brief general or spinal anesthesia is required) or serious (e.g., kidney donation, which involves more extensive anaesthesia and major invasive surgery).

If a child is capable of making his or her own medical treatment decisions, he or she should be considered capable of deciding whether to be an organ or tissue donor. However, physicians should not perform organ retrievals of serious risk without first obtaining court authorization. Courts should confirm that the mature minor is acting voluntarily and without coercion.

If a child is not capable of making his or her own medical decisions, all transplantations should have parental approval, and those which pose a serious risk should receive court authorization. In the court authorization process the evaluation of a child psychiatrist or psychologist must be sought and a guardian ad litem should be assigned to the potential minor donor in order to fully represent the minor's interests.

When deciding on behalf of immature children, parents and courts should ensure that a transplantation presents a "clear benefit" to the minor source, which entails meeting the following requirements:

a. ideally, the minor should be the only possible source;

b. for transplantations of moderate or serious risk, the transplantations must be necessary with some degree of medical certainty to provide a substantial benefit...;

c. the organ or tissue transplant must have a reasonable probability of success...;

d. generally, minors should be allowed to

serve as a source only to close family members;

e. psychological or emotional benefits to the potential source may be considered, though evidence of future benefit to the minor source should be clear and convincing. Possible benefits to a child include the following: continued emotional bonds between the minor and the recipient; increased self-esteem; and prevention of adverse reaction to death of a sibling.[95]

F. The American Medical Association, 2002

The American Medical Association, Council on Ethical and Judicial Affairs, in "Treatment Decisions for Seriously Ill Newborns," stated:

The primary consideration for decisions regarding life-sustaining treatment for seriously ill newborns should be what is best for the newborn. Factors that should be weighed are: (1) the chance the therapy will succeed, (2) the risks involved with treatment and nontreatment, (3) the degree to which the therapy, if successful, will extend life, (4) the pain and discomfort associated with the therapy, and (5) the anticipated quality of life for the newborn with and without treatment.

Care must be taken to evaluate the newborn's expected quality of life from the child's perspective. Life-sustaining treatment may be withheld or withdrawn from a newborn when the pain and suffering expected to be endured by the child will overwhelm any potential for joy during his or her life. When an infant suffers extreme neurological damage, and is consequently not capable of experiencing either suffering or joy, a decision may be made to withhold or withdraw life-sustaining treatment.

When an infant's prognosis is largely uncertain, as is often the case with extremely premature newborns, all life-sustaining and life-enhancing treatment should be initiated. Decisions about ... treatment should be made once the prognosis becomes more certain. It is not necessary to attain absolute or near absolute certainty before life-sustaining treatment is withdrawn, since this goal is often unattainable and risks unnecessarily prolonging the infant's suffering.[96]

G. The American Academy
of Pediatrics, 1995

The American Academy of Pediatrics, in "Perinatal Care at the Threshold of Viability," stated:

Ethical decisions regarding the extent of resuscitation efforts and subsequent support of the neonate are complex. Parents should understand that decisions about neonatal management made before delivery may be altered depending on the condition of the neonate at birth, the postnatal gestational age assessment, and the infant's response to resuscitative and stabilization measures. Recommendations regarding the extent of continuing support depend on frequent reevaluations of the infant's condition and prognosis.[97]

H. The American Academy
of Pediatrics, 1995

The American Academy of Pediatrics, Committee on Fetus and Newborn, in "The Initiation or Withdrawal of Treatment for High-Risk Newborns," stated:

The following dilemma . . . exists: intensive treatment of all severely ill infants sometimes results in prolongation of dying or occasionally iatrogenic illness; nonintensive treatment results in increased mortality and unnecessary morbidity. The overall outcomes of either approach are disappointing.

A reasonably acceptable approach to this dilemma is an individualized prognostic strategy. In this setting, care is provided for the individual infant at the appropriate level based on the expected outcome at the time care is initiated. In this strategy, the infant is constantly reevaluated, and the prognosis is reassessed based on the best available information in conjunction with the physician's best medical judgment. This approach places significant responsibility on the physician and healthcare team to evaluate the infant accurately and continuously. The family of the infant must be kept informed of the infant's current status and prognosis. They must be involved in major decisions that ultimately could alter the infant's outcome.

The rights of parents in decision making must be respected. However, physicians should not be forced to undertreat or overtreat an infant if, in their best medical judgment, the treatment is not in compliance with the standard of care for that infant.[98]

I. The American Academy
of Pediatrics, 1995

The American Academy of Pediatrics, Committee on Bioethics, in "Informed Consent, Parental Permission, and Assent in Pediatric Practice," stated:

In attempting to adapt the concept of informed consent to pediatrics, many believe that the child's parents or guardians have the authority or "right" to give consent by proxy. Most parents seek to safeguard the welfare and best interests of their children with regard to healthcare, and as a result proxy consent has seemed to work reasonably well.

However, the concept encompasses many ambiguities. Consent embodies judgments about proposed interventions and, more importantly, consent expresses something for one's self: a person who consents responds based on unique personal beliefs, values and goals.

Thus "proxy consent" poses serious problems for pediatric healthcare providers. Such providers have legal and ethical duties to their child patients to render competent medical care based on what the patient needs, not what someone else expresses. . . . The pediatrician's responsibilities to his or her patient exist independent of parental desires or proxy consent.[99]

J. The American Academy
of Pediatrics, 1996

The American Academy of Pediatrics, Committee on Bioethics, in "Ethics and the Care of Critically Ill Infants and Children," stated:

The American Academy of Pediatrics supports individualized decision making about life-sustaining medical treatment for all children, regardless of age. These decisions should be jointly made by physicians and parents, unless good reasons require invoking established child protection services to contravene parental authority. At this time, resource allocation (rationing) decisions about which children should receive intensive care resources should be made clear and explicit in public policy, rather than made at the bedside.[100]

XV. PLAN OF CARE

In the clinical setting, most pediatric cases would benefit significantly from the development of a prospective plan of care. At the beginning of the clinical relationship, whether focused on a specific life-threatening diagnosis or on a less dramatic aspect of care, the clinical team (all of those involved with the care of the child, including — but not limited to — attending physicians, residents, consultants, nurses, and social workers) and the family should begin to consider the important issues related to that child's care. For critically ill infants and children, this approach requires considering the meaning of the diagnosis, seeking appropriate information before and after diagnosis, requesting appropriate consultation and support, identifying possible options, and so forth.

An overall plan of care for infants and children is a goal of the primary-care clinicians from whom these patients receive their everyday medical interventions and advice. To achieve this goal, it is necessary for clinicians to maintain an ongoing relationship with the child and his or her family. Primary-care clinicians can be the source of invaluable knowledge and advice when it is necessary to make critical decisions in a tertiary-care center.

XVI. CONCLUSION

Decision making for imperiled newborn infants and critically ill older children has evolved dramatically over the past 20 years under some unusual pressures. Our society has attempted to dictate rigid standards of care, while, at the same time, it has criticized caregivers for poor outcomes and a lack of respect for parents' wishes. There is no doubt that, at times, specific decisions have been in error with regard to undertreatment or overtreatment, but the reflection and evaluation of past mistakes, while often unpleasant, has benefited individual decision makers and society. Our

society has reached a consensus that it is justifiable, in some circumstances, to withhold or withdraw life-sustaining treatment from severely impaired newborns and children.

Because of the relative frequency and complexity of these issues, clinicians should develop a prospective plan of care that addresses current and potential ethical concerns.

Decisions regarding withdrawing or withholding treatment for children should be based primarily on the best interests of the child, as determined by his or her caregivers and family members. The process should be open — it should involve full disclosure of accurate and complete information, with the provision of consultation as necessary. One or more avenues for review of the decisions and the decision-making process can be invaluable for the family and clinicians.

XVII. CASES FOR FURTHER STUDY

Case 1: "When the Bough Breaks"

Baby John Davis was born 12 weeks prematurely, the product of a gestation complicated by recurrent episodes of premature labor. His mother was hospitalized for six weeks prior to delivery. She and her husband had been married for six years. They had lost four previous pregnancies, all at approximately 10 to 22 weeks gestation. On her doctor's advice, Mrs. Davis quit work early in the pregnancy. Her husband had been out of work for several months. The family lived approximately three hours from the medical center.

Baby John weighed 1,000 grams (2.2 pounds) at birth. He immediately developed respiratory distress syndrome and required mechanical ventilation. He developed a patent ductus arteriosus that did not respond to medical therapy and required a thoracotomy for closure. He developed a pneumothorax (leak of air into the chest cavity) that required a chest tube for drainage.

He is now six months old. He has been mechanically ventilated since birth. His chest X-ray shows extremely severe bronchopulmonary dysplasia, with scarring and emphysema. He has been receiving maximal medical therapy with bronchodilators, antibiotics, and several courses of steroids, but he has shown no improvement over the past month.

John is very developmentally delayed. His physicians believe that this delay was caused primarily by his debilitation from his severe lung disease. However, he had had so many episodes of severe hypoxemia and bradycardia (low heart rate) that he may also have had a neurologic injury. Recently, he requires chronic sedation. Otherwise, he is agitated most of the time due to hypoxia. When John becomes agitated, he becomes even more hypoxic and air hungry.

The attending physicians and house staff all agree that it is very unlikely that John will ever go home. They are also concerned that, because he requires sedation most of the time, he is unable to interact with his environment; thus, his development is falling farther behind. They believe that the time has come to approach John's parents about withdrawing the ventilator. The case is discussed at the weekly "family rounds." Most of the nursing staff is in agreement. However, two of the primary-care nurses who have taken care of him since birth feel that this would be euthanasia.

John's parents initially visited each weekend. However, over the past two to three months, they have visited less frequently. The nurses believe John's parents cannot make an informed decision about their son's care, because they seem to have lost interest in him.

The attending physician requests an ethics consultation about how to proceed. She has asked for help with two questions: Is it ethically justifiable to withdraw the ventilator from this child? Who should participate in the decision?

— Source: This case was modified from the author's clinical experience at the University of Virginia.

Case 2: "Futile Care?"

Baby Tina was born at 38 weeks gestation to a 38-year-old mother. This was her first pregnancy. During the second trimester, an ultrasound suggested a congenital heart lesion and cleft palate. In addition, the infant was smaller than expected for her gestational age. The parents were counseled that these findings may be compatible with a chromosomal anomaly. Amniocentesis was performed, and confirmed a diagnosis of trisomy 18. The family was counseled about the limited life-span of children with this lesion, the cardiac disease, the potential for other significant medical problems, the severe developmental delay and mental retardation in those who survive, and the option of terminating the pregnancy. They elected to continue. On a follow-up visit with the neonatologist, the option of not resuscitating the infant at birth was raised, since many of these infants do not tolerate labor and are compromised at birth. The mother asked that the baby be resuscitated so that they could be with her, if only for a short while, alive. They also asked to speak with the cardiologist about the possibility of repairing the cardiac lesion, either in the newborn period or in the first several months. Some of the medical and nursing staff expressed concern that treating this infant who had a well-described poor prognosis was futile care, and did not think that the team should agree to aggressive care after birth.

The obstetrician and neonatologist requested an ethics consultation about how to proceed. Is the parents' request for aggressive care reasonable in this situation? What options do the staff have?

— Source: This case was modified from the author's clinical experience at the University of Virginia.

Case 3: "It Will Ruin My Life"

Baby Adam was born after 27 weeks of gestation (13 weeks premature), weighing 1,140 grams (2.5 pounds). The gestation had been uncomplicated until the sudden onset of vaginal bleeding, which required an emergency cesarean section. The infant was resuscitated in the delivery room, intubated, and placed on the ventilator. Arrangements were made to transfer the infant to the regional NICU.

The mother was Hispanic; she spoke limited English but seemed to understand it fairly well. The father was a professional with a prosperous practice in the area. The couple had been married for five years, and they had a four-year-old daughter.

When the transport team from the regional center arrived at the referring hospital and was preparing the infant for transport, the father entered the nursery and informed the team that he did not want this infant to live if there was any chance that the child could be retarded. He said that he did not want any [censored] ruining his life. The team reassured him that infants this size usually do very well, and the majority are normal children.

The infant was transported and did well over the next several days. On the third day of the baby's life, a routine head ultrasound revealed a mild, grade-2 intraventricular hemorrhage. When the father visited that afternoon, he was informed of the result of the ultrasound and that infants with grade-2 hemorrhage have approximately the same prognosis as children without hemorrhage. He again told the resident and nurse that he did not want the infant to live if there was a possibility of retardation, and he said that he was opposed to the current treatment. However, he did not pursue the issue that day.

Attempts to reach the infant's mother at the referring hospital were only partly successful. At times, the father answered the phone and would not permit the mother to speak. At other times, the mother answered but told the staff that they should talk to her husband.

Intravenous access became difficult, and a central line was required to continue hydration. The attending physician called the father who again expressed his view about the current treatment and refused permission for the central line. When told that the infant would die without fluid therapy, he confirmed that this was what he intended.

The attending physician discussed the case with the staff and with another attending physician. He called the hospital administrator, who filed a petition with the juvenile court to conduct permission for the procedure. A hearing was held by conference call. On questioning by the judge, the father stated that he was opposed to the procedure because of the risk of infection and pneumothorax. The judge gave permission for the procedure.

How should the staff now proceed? How vigorously should the mother's input be sought? What should be the approach toward the father?

— Source: This case was modified from the author's clinical experience at the University of Virginia.

XVIII. STUDY QUESTIONS

1. Richard McCormick has proposed a minimal condition for defining quality of life: the capacity for experience or social interrelating. How would you define "quality of life"? Would you apply a different standard to a neonate than to a child or an adult? If so, why?

2. The Joint Policy Statement of the American Academy of Pediatrics, "Principles of Treatment of Disabled Infants," says: "Discrimination of any type against any individual with a disability/disabilities, regardless of the nature or severity of the disability, is morally and legally indefensible . . . Consideration such as anticipated or actual limited potential of an individual and present or future lack of available community resources are irrelevant and must not determine the decisions concerning medical care." Do you agree with this statement? How does benefit/burden assessment apply under this guideline?

NOTES

1. S.X. Radbill, "Children in a World of Violence: A History of Child Abuse," in *The Battered Child,* ed. H. Kempe and R.E. Helfer (Chicago, Ill.: University of Chicago Press, 1980).

2. J. Lorber, "Results of Treatment of Meningomyelocele," *Developmental Medicine and Child Neurology* 13 (1971): 279.

3. W.G. Bartholome, "The Child-Patient: Do Parents Have the 'Right to Decide,'" in *The Law-Medicine Relation: A Philosophical Exploration,* ed. S.F. Spicker, J.M. Healey, and H.T. Engelhardt, Jr. (Boston, Mass.: Reidel, 1981), 271-7.

4. R.S. Duff and A.G.M. Campbell, "Moral and Ethical Dilemmas in the Special Care Nursery," *New England Journal of Medicine* 289 (1973): 890.

5. A. Shaw, "Dilemmas of 'Informed Consent' in Children," *New England Journal of Medicine* 289 (1973): 885-90.

6. D. Todres et al., "Pediatricians' Attitude Affecting Decisionmaking in Defective Newborns," *Pediatrics* 60 (1977): 197-201.

7. "Treating the Defective Newborn: A Survey of Physicians' Attitudes," *Hastings Center Report* 6, no. 2 (1976): 2.

8. A. Davis, "All Babies Should Be Kept Alive as Far as Possible," in *Principles of Health Care Ethics,* ed. R. Gillon (London: Wiley, 1994), 629-41.

9. U.S. Department of Health and Human Services, "Interim Final Rule 45 *CFR* Part 84, Nondiscrimination on the Basis of a Handicap," *Federal Register* 48 (7 March 1983): 9630-2.

10. President's Commission for the Study of Ethical Problems in Medicine and Biomedical and Behavioral Research, "Seriously Ill Newborns," in *Deciding to Forego Life-Sustaining Treatment: A Report on the Ethical, Medical, and Legal Issues in Treatment Decisions* (Washington, D.C.: U.S. Government Printing Office, 1983), 197-229.

11. U.S. Department of Health and Human Services, "Nondiscrimination on the Basis of Handicaps: Procedures and Guidelines Relating to Health Care for Handicapped Infants," *Federal Register* 49 (12 January 1984): 622-54.

12. Ibid.

13. *Bowen v. American Hospital Association,* 476 U.S. 610, at 611 (1986) discussed in K. Kerr, "Reporting the Case of Baby Jane Doe," *Hastings Center Report* 14, no. 4 (1984): 7-9.

14. 42 U.S.C. sec. 5103 (1982).

15. 50 *Federal Register* 14893 (1985).

16. L.M. Kopelman et al., "Neonatologists Judge the 'Baby Doe' Regulations," *New England Journal of Medicine* 318 (1988): 677-83.

17. E.B. Pearson, C.L. Bose, and E.N. Kraybill, "Decisions about Futile Treatment in an Intensive Care Nursery," *North Carolina Medical Journal* 56 (1995): 462-6; and S.N. Wall and J.C. Partridge, "Withdrawal of Life Support in the Intensive Care Nursery: Decisions and Practice by Neonatologists," *Pediatric Research* 33 (1993): 30A.

18. American Academy of Pediatrics, Committee on Bioethics, "Ethics and the Care of Critically Ill Infants and Children," *Pediatrics* 98 (1996): 149-52.

19. B.W. Levin et al., "The Treatment of Non-HIV Related Conditions in Newborns at Risk for HIV: A Survey of Neonatologists," *American Journal of Public Health* 85 (1996): 1507-13.

20. J.M. Peerzada, D.K. Richardson, and J.P. Burns, "Delivery Room Decision-making at the Threshold of Viability," *Journal of Pediatrics* 145 (2004): 492-8.

21. Support Organization for Trisomy 13, 18

and Related Disorders, *www.trisomy.org.*

22. BBC News, *newsvote.bbc.co.uk,* 26 January 2005.

23. R. Weir, *Selective Treatment of Handicapped Newborns: Moral Dilemmas in Neonatal Medicine* (New York: Oxford University Press, 1984).

24. P. Ramsey, *Ethics at the Edges of Life* (New Haven, Conn.: Yale University Press, 1978), 155.

25. M. Tooley, "Abortion and Infanticide," *Philosophy and Public Affairs* 2 (1972): 37-65.

26. H.T. Engelhardt, Jr., *The Foundations of Bioethics* (New York: Oxford University Press, 1988), 116-9, 145, 217.

27. W.F. May, "Parenting, Bonding and Valuing the Retarded," in *Ethics and Mental Retardation,* ed. L.M. Kopelman and J.C. Moskop (Dordrecht, Netherlands: Reidel, 1984), 141-60.

28. M.B. Mahowald, *Women and Children in Health Care* (New York: Oxford University Press, 1993), 170.

29. M. Daly and M. Wilson, *Homicide* (New York: Aldine De Gruyer, 1988), 71-2.

30. J. Blustein, "The Rights Approach and the Intimacy Approach: Family Suffering and Care of Defective Newborns," *Mount Sinai Journal of Medicine* 56 (1989): 164-7.

31. L.F. Ross, *Children, Families and Health Care Decision-Making* (Oxford, U.K.: Clarendon Press, 1998), 47.

32. R.J. Boyle, R. Salter, and M.W. Arnander, "Ethics of Refusing Parental Requests to Withhold or Withdraw Treatment from Their Premature Baby," *Journal of Medical Ethics* 30 (2004): 402-5.

33. See note 23 above.

34. A.E. Buchanan and D.W. Brock, *Deciding for Others: The Ethics of Surrogate Decision Making* (New York: Cambridge University Press, 1989).

35. A. Shaw, J.G. Randolph, and B. Manard, "Ethical Issues in Pediatric Surgery: A National Survey of Pediatricians and Pediatric Surgeons," *Pediatrics* 60 (1977): 588.

36. N. Fost, "Parents as Decision Makers for Children," *Primary Care Clinics of North America* 13 (1986): 285-93.

37. A. Whitelaw and M. Thoresen, "Ethical Dilemmas Around the Time of Birth," in *Principles of Health Care Ethics,* ed. R. Gillon (London: Wiley & Sons, 1994), 617-27.

38. A.M. Dellinger and P.C. Kuszler, "Infants: Public Policy and Legal Issues," in *Encyclopedia of Bioethics,* ed. W.T. Reich (New York: Simon &

Schuster MacMillan, 1995), 1214-20.

39. See note 23 above, p. 259.

40. See note 28 above, pp. 169-72.

41. See note 3 above, pp. 271-2.

42. See note 23 above, p. 260.

43. T.L. Beauchamp and J.F. Childress, *Principles of Bioemedical Ethics,* 5th ed. (New York: Oxford University Press, 1983), 137.

44. W.G. Bartholome, "Withholding/Withdrawing Life-Sustaining Treatment," in *Contemporary Issues in Pediatric Ethics,* ed. M.M. Burgess and B.E. Woodrow (Lewiston, N.Y.: Edwin Mellen Press), 17.

45. A.R. Fleischman et al., "Caring for Gravely Ill Children," *Pediatrics* 94 (1992): 422-39.

46. C.H. Rushton and J.J. Glover, "Involving Parents in Decisions to Forego Life-Sustaining Treatment for Critically Ill Infants and Children," *Pediatric Annals* 18 (1989): 206-14.

47. See note 24 above.

48. N.M.P. King, "Transparency in Neonatal Intensive Care," *Hastings Center Report* 22 (May-June 1992): 18-25.

49. See note 24 above.

50. R.A. McCormick, "To Save or Let Die: The Dilemma of Modern Medicine," *Journal of the American Medical Association* 229 (1974): 172.

51. D.L. Coulter, T.H. Murray, and M.C. Cerreto, "Practical Ethics in Pediatrics," *Current Problems in Pediatrics* 18 (1988): 168-9.

52. A.R. Jonsen and M.J. Garland, "A Moral Policy for Life/Death Decisions in the Intensive Care Nursery," in *Ethics of Newborn Intensive Care,* ed. A.R. Jonsen and M.J. Garland (Berkeley, Calif.: University of California, Institute of Governmental Studies, 1976), 176.

53. R.F. Weir, "Infants: Ethical Issues," in *Encyclopedia of Bioethics,* ed. W.T. Reich (New York: Simon and Schuster MacMillan, 1995), 1206-14.

54. R.F. Weir and J.D. Bale, "Selective Nontreatment of Neurologically Impaired Neonates," *Neurologic Clinics of North America* 7 (1989): 807-22.

55. D.W. Brock, "Death and Dying," in *Medical Ethics,* ed. R.M. Veatch (Boston, Mass.: Jones and Bartlett, 1989), 352.

56. See note 34 above.

57. J.A. Robertson, "Extreme Prematurity and Parental Rights after Baby Doe," *Hastings Center Report* 34 (2004): 32-9.

58. See note 10 above.

59. W. Silverman, "Overtreatment of Neonates? A Personal Retrospective," *Pediatrics* 90

(1992): 971-6.

60. W.A. Silverman, "Medical Decisions: An Appeal for Reasonableness," *Pediatrics* 98 (1996): 1182-4; R.M. Veatch, "Abandoning Informed Consent," *Hastings Center Report* 25 (1995): 5-12.

61. See note 31 above, p. 51.

62. See note 45 above, pp. 433-39.

63. See note 43 above, p. 158.

64. D.S. Diekema, "Parental Refusals of Medical Treatment: The Harm Principle As Threshold For State Intervention," *Theoretical Medicine* 25 (2004): 243-64; S. Ashwal et al., "The Persistent Vegetative State in Children," *Annals of Neurology* 32 (1992): 570-6.

65. M.L. Chiswick, "Withdrawal of Life Support in Babies: Deceptive Signals," *Archives of Disease in Childhood* 65 (1990): 1096-7.

66. N.K. Rhoden, "Treating Baby Doe: The Ethics of Uncertainty," *Hastings Center Report* 16 (August 1986): 34-42.

67. A.F. Fischer and D.K. Stevenson, "The Consequences of Uncertainty: An Empirical Approach to Medical Decisionmaking in Neonatal Intensive Care," *Journal of the American Medical Association* 258 (1987): 1929-31.

68. American Academy of Pediatrics, Committee on Fetus and Newborn, "The Initiation or Withdrawal of Treatment for High-Risk Newborns," *Pediatrics* 96 (1995): 362-3.

69. T.L. Beauchamp and J.F. Childress, *Principles of Biomedical Ethics,* 2nd ed. (New York: Oxford University Press, 1983), 132.

70. N.S. Wood et al., "Neurologic and Developmental Disability After Extremely Preterm Birth," *New England Journal of Medicine* 343 (2000): 378-84; N. Marlow et al., "Neurologic and Developmental Disability at Six years of Age after Extremely Preterm Birth," *New England Journal of Medicine* 352 (2005): 9-19.

71. See note 20 above.

72. J. Tyson, "Evidence-Based Ethics and the Care of Premature Infants," *The Future of Children* 5 (1995): 197-213; J.R. Botkin, "Delivery Room Decisions for Tiny Infants: An Ethical Analysis," *The Journal of Clinical Ethics* 1, no. 4 (Winter 1990): 306-11; see note 37 above; see note 51 above, pp. 143-95; R.J. Boyle and J. Kattwinkel, "Ethical Decisions Surrounding Resuscitation," *Clinics in Perinatology* 26 (1999): 779-92; R.J. Boyle and N. McIntosh, "Ethical Considerations in Neonatal Resuscitation: Clinical and Research Issues," *Seminars in Neonatology* 6, no. 3 (2001): 261-9.

73. Canadian Pediatric Society, Fetus and Newborn Committee, Maternal Fetal Medicine Committee, Society of Obstetricians and Gynecologists of Canada, "Management of the Woman with Threshold Birth of an Infant of Extremely Low Gestational Age," *Canadian Medical Association Journal* 151 (1994): 547-53.

74. American Academy of Pediatrics, "Special Considerations," in *Textbook of Neonatal Resuscitation,* 4th ed., ed. D. Braner et al. (Elk Grove Village, Ill.: American Academy of Pediatrics, 2000).

75. *State v. Messenger,* file 94-67694-FY, Clerk of the Cir. Ct. County of Ingram, Mich.; J.J. Paris and M.D. Schreiber, "Parental Discretion in Refusal of Treatment for Newborns: A Real but Limited Right," *Clinics in Perinatology* 23, no. 3 (1996): 573-95; F.I. Clark, "Making Sense of *State v. Messenger,*" *Pediatrics* 97, no. 4 (1996): 579-83.

76. *Miller v. HCA,* 47 Tex. Sup. J.12, 118 S.W.3d 758 (2003); G.J. Annas, "Extremely Preterm Birth and Parental Authority to Refuse Treatment — The Case of Sidney Miller," *New England Journal of Medicine* 351 (2004): 2118-23; J.J. Paris, M.D. Schreiber, and F. Reardon, "The 'Emergent Circumstances' Exception to the Need for Consent: The Texas Supreme Court Ruling in *Miller v. HCA,*" *Journal of Perinatology* 24 (2004): 337.

77. See note 19 above.

78. M.M. Farrell and D.I. Levin, "Brain Death in the Pediatric Patient: Historical, Sociological, Medical, Religious, Cultural, Legal and Ethical Considerations," *Critical Care Medicine* 21, no. 12 (1993): 1951-65; M.A. Fishman, "Validity of Brain Death Criteria in Infants," *Pediatrics* 96 (1995): 513-5; Task Force on Brain Death in Children, "Guidelines for the Determination of Brain Death in Children," *Annals of Neurology* 21 (1987): 616-7; K.J. Banasiak and G. Lister, "Brain Death in Children," *Current Opinion in Pediatrics* 15 (2003): 288-93.

79. S. Ashwal et al., "The Persistent Vegetative State in Children," *Annals of Neurology* 32 (1992): 570-6.

80. H.P. Gutgesell and T.A. Massaro, "Management of Hypoplastic Left Heart Syndrome in a Consortium of University Hospitals," *American Journal of Cardiology* 76 (1995): 809-11; H.P. Gutgesell and J. Gibson, "Management of Hypoplastic Left Heart Syndrome in the 1990s," *American Journal of Cardiology* 89 (2002): 842-6; H.P. Gutgesell, "What if It Were Your Child?" *American Journal of Cardiology* 89 (2002): 856; P.A.

Checchia et al., "Effect of a Selection and Postoperative Care Protocol on Survival of Infants with Hypoplastic Left Heart Syndrome," *Annals of Thoracic Surgery* 77 (2004): 477-83.

81. A.A. Kon, L. Ackerson, and B. Lo, "How Pediatricians Counsel Parents When No 'Best-Choice' Management Exists: Lessons to be Learned From Hypoplastic Left Heart Syndrome," *Archives of Pediatric and Adolescent Medicine* 158 (2004): 436-41; A.A. Kon, "Assessment of Physician Directiveness: Using Hypoplastic Left Heart Syndrome as a Model," *Journal of Perinatology* 24 (2004): 500-4; V.L. Zeigler, "Ethical Principles and Parental Choice: Treatment Options for Neonates with Hypoplastic Left Heart Syndrome," *Pediatric Nursing* 29 (2003): 65-9.

82. D.A. Frank et al., "Growth, Development, and Behavior in Early Childhood Following Cocaine Exposure: A Systematic Review," *Journal of the American Medical Association* 285 (2001): 1613-25; W. Chavkin, "Cocaine and Pregnancy — Time to Look at the Evidence," *Journal of the American Medical Association* 285 (2001): 1626.

83. American Academy of Pediatrics, Committee on Substance Abuse, "Drug-Exposed Infants," *Pediatrics* 96 (1995): 364-8.

84. J.T. Berger, F. Rosner, and P. Farnsworth, "The Ethics of Mandatory Testing in Newborns," *The Journal of Clinical Ethics* 7, no. 1 (Spring 1996): 77-84; D.S. Davis, "Mandatory HIV Testing in Newborns: Not Yet, Maybe Never," *The Journal of Clinical Ethics* 7, no. 2 (Summer 1996): 191-2.

85. Centers for Disease Control and Prevention, "Revised Recommendations for HIV Screening of Pregnant Women," *MMWR Recommendations and Reports* 50 (2001): 63-85; American Academy of Pediatrics, Provisional Committee on Pediatric AIDS, "Perinatal Human Immunodeficiency Virus Testing," *Pediatrics* 95 (1995): 303-7; American Academy of Pediatrics, Canadian Pediatric Society, "Evaluation and Treatment of the Human Immunodeficiency Virus-1-Exposed Infant," *Pediatrics* 114 (2004): 497-505.

86. K.W. Chan et al., "Use of Minors as Bone Marrow Donors: Current Attitude and Management: A Survey of 56 Pediatric Transplantation Centers," *Journal of Pediatrics* 128 (1996): 644-8.

87. R.E. Ladd, "The Child as Living Donor: Parental Consent and Child Assent," *Cambridge Quarterly of Healthcare Ethics* 13 (2004): 143-8; S. Zinner, "Cognitive Development and Pediatric Consent to Organ Donation," *Cambridge Quarterly*

of Healthcare Ethics 13 (2004): 125-32.

88. D. Steinberg, "Kidney Transplants from Young Children and the Mentally Retarded," *Theoretical Medicine* 25 (2004): 229-41.

89. W.J. Curran, "Beyond the Best Interests of the Child — Bone Marrow Transplant among Half-Siblings," *New England Journal of Medicine* 324 (1991): 1818-9; T.E. Williams, "Legal Issues and Ethical Dilemmas Surrounding Bone Marrow Transplantation in Children," *American Journal of Pediatrics Hematology Oncology* 6 (1984): 83-8; G.R. Bungio et al., "Bone Marrow Transplantation in Children: Between Therapeutic and Medico-Legal Problems," *Bone Marrow Transplantation* 4, suppl. 4 (1989): 34-7; A.R. Holder, "Adolescents," in *Encyclopedia of Bioethics,* ed. W.T. Reich (New York: Simon & Schuster MacMillan, 1995), 69-70; American Medical Association, Council on Ethical and Judicial Affairs, "The Use of Minors as Organ and Tissue Donors," *Code of Medical Ethics Reports* 5, no. 1 (1994): 229-43; M. Sheldon, "Children as Organ Donors: A Persistent Ethical Issue," *Cambridge Quarterly of Healthcare Ethics* 13 (2004): 119-22; L.M. Fleck, "Children and Organ Donation: Some Cautionary Remarks," *Cambridge Quarterly of Healthcare Ethics* 13 (2004): 161-6; R.D. Pentz et al., "Designing an Ethical Policy for Bone Marrow Donation by Minors and Others Lacking Capacity," *Cambridge Quarterly of Healthcare Ethics* 13 (2004): 149-55; C. Kim, "Children as Live Kidney Donors for Siblings," *Virtual Mentor, Ethics Journal of the American Medical Association* 5, no. 8 (August 2003).

90. R. Swan, "Faith Healing, Christian Science and the Medical Care of Children," *New England Journal of Medicine* 309, no. 26 (1983): 1639-41; K.H. Rothenberg, "Medical Decision Making for Children," in *Biolaw* 8: 149-73; American Academy of Pediatrics, Committee on Bioethics, "Religious Objections to Medical Care," *Pediatrics* 99 (1997): 279-81; K.S. Hickey and L. Lyckholm, "Child Welfare Versus Parental Autonomy: Medical Ethics, the Law, and Faith-Based Healing," *Theoretical Medicine* 25 (2004): 265-76; R.D. Orr and L.B. Genesen, "Requests for 'Inappropriate Treatment' Based on Religious Beliefs," *Journal of Medical Ethics* 23 (1997): 142-7; W.E. Novotny, R.M. Perkin, and R.D. Orr, "Faith Based Decisions: Parents Who Refuse Appropriate Care for Their Child," *Virtual Mentor, Ethics Journal of the American Medical Association* 5, no.8 (August 2003).

91. American Academy of Pediatrics, Commit-

tee on Bioethics, "Treatment of Critically Ill Newborns," *Pediatrics* 72 (1983): 565-6.

92. President's Commission, see note 10 above, pp. 6-8, 218-9.

93. American Academy of Pediatrics, "Principles of Treatment of Disabled Infants," *Pediatrics* 73 (1984): 559-60.

94. American Academy of Pediatrics, Committee on Bioethics, "Guidelines on Foregoing Life-Sustaining Medical Treatment," *Pediatrics* 93 (1994): 532-6.

95. American Medical Association, Council on Ethical and Judicial Affairs, "2.167 The Use of Minors as Organ and Tissue Donors," *Code of Medical Ethics* (Chicago, Ill.: AMA, 2002), 58-9.

96. American Medical Association, Council on Ethical and Judicial Affairs, "2.215 Treatment Decisions for Seriously Ill Newborns," *Code of Medical Ethics* (Chicago, Ill.: AMA, 2002), 92.

97. American Academy of Pediatrics, "Perinatal Care at the Threshold of Viability," *Pediatrics* 96 (1995): 974-6.

98. See note 68 above.

99. American Academy of Pediatrics, Committee on Bioethics, "Informed Consent, Parental Permission, and Assent in Pediatric Practice," *Pediatrics* 95 (1995): 314-7.

100. See note 18 above.

15

Ethical Issues in Reproduction

Cynthia B. Cohen

I. INTRODUCTION

Reproductive healthcare presents challenging ethical issues, for a variety of values — personal, professional, and social — are at stake when making decisions about sexual health and reproduction. Americans place great weight on respect for individual freedom and privacy and are therefore reluctant to override the personal reproductive choices of individuals. This emphasis on individual autonomy, however, can present reproductive health professionals with difficult ethical questions when patients make decisions about their reproductive health in ways that they believe are misplaced or wrong. Moreover, professionals may find that their attempts to assist couples to bring children into the world or to avoid doing so may come up against societal strictures. Consequently, the provision of reproductive healthcare can at times generate misunderstandings and even conflicts among healthcare professionals, patients, families, hospital administrators, and legislators.

With this in mind, this chapter aims to:
- Assist professionals in reproductive medicine to identify major ethical questions that can arise in the clinical care of patients,
- Provide them with insights into the range of reasonable responses that have been developed to these questions within our society,
- Encourage clinicians to plan to address ethical issues and conflicts that might come to the fore in the clinical setting before they arise, and
- Provide starting points for discussion among those professionally and personally affected by ethical issues that may arise in reproductive decision making, as well as hospital administrators and legislators.

The concept of "reproductive health" was developed in the second half of the twentieth century to frame a comprehensive, integrated approach to services related to reproduction. At that time, these services were highly fragmented and not oriented toward meeting the totality of health issues that arise for patients and healthcare professionals involved in reproductive decisions.[1] To remedy this situation, reproductive health came to be defined more broadly by a United Nations group as having "a satisfying and safe sex life . . . , the capability to reproduce, and the freedom to decide if, when and how often to do so."[2]

Five major areas of reproductive health are captured by this concept:
1. Contraception;
2. Sterilization;
3. Abortion;
4. Pregnancy and childbirth, including prenatal diagnosis; and

5. Reproductive technologies, including pre-implantation genetic diagnosis.

This chapter will consider ethical questions that arise during clinical care in each of these areas, point out some of the issues involved, and present some leading ways of responding to them.

II. CONTRACEPTION

The use of contraceptives is an important aspect of reproductive health, in that it allows people to make decisions about the size and spacing of their family. Approximately two-thirds of women of child-bearing years in the United States want to postpone or avoid pregnancy.[3] Yet studies that cross all socioeconomic groups indicate that only half of the pregnancies in this country are planned.[4] Indeed, the U.S. has one of the highest rates of unintended pregnancies among developed nations.[5] Clearly, both women and men need to be counseled about methods of contraception if they are to create families of a size they believe they can raise responsibly.

Significant ethical issues surrounding the use of contraception center on the following:
- Whether it is ethically acceptable to use contraception to prevent pregnancy,
- Whether it is ethically acceptable to impose contraceptive use on individuals involuntarily, and
- Whether healthcare professionals should keep the fact that patients seek contraceptive measures confidential.

A. Whether Contraceptive Use Is Ethically Acceptable

The use of contraception is generally accepted as an ethical means of planning the spacing of one's children. Many religious traditions permit the use of contraceptive measures, including most Protestant denominations,[6] several branches of Judaism,[7] the Eastern Orthodox Church,[8] and the Buddhist tradition.[9]

These traditions, for the most part, adopt a *companionate view* of marriage and sexuality, maintaining that the primary end of sexual intercourse is the expression of love and enhancement of the unity of marital partners.[10] They look with favor upon having children, but do not generally maintain that procreation is the overriding purpose of sexual intercourse in marriage. Within Ju-

daism, which places great importance on having children, the use of contraceptives is accepted. Indeed, some religious groups maintain that unlimited procreation can be harmful to one or both partners, the well-being of already existing children, and the marital relationship itself.[11] Furthermore, some religious thinkers urge the use of contraception in order to lessen the pressures of overpopulation on a global scale.[12]

Some religious bodies, however, reject the use of contraceptive measures. The Roman Catholic Church, for instance, links the use of contraceptives with the practice of abortion in that it maintains that both impede procreation and are contrary to the good of life.[13] Although the "unitive," or loving end of marriage is as important as the procreative end, the Roman Catholic tradition teaches, the unitive end cannot be fully realized unless intercourse is open to the possibility of procreation.[14]

The use of such contraceptive measures as the "morning after" pill and RU-486 is also condemned within some religious traditions, such as the Roman Catholic and Southern Baptist, albeit on different grounds from those on which other forms of contraception are rejected.[15] Since the application of these sorts of contraceptives prevents the implantation of an embryo, these religious groups view their use as akin to abortion in that they result in the death of an embryo, which they regard as a living human being.

In the legal sphere, having access to and receiving information about contraception has been upheld as a constitutional right by the Supreme Court of the U.S.. In the 1965 case of *Griswold v. Connecticut*,[16] the Court invalidated a state law that prohibited physicians from discussing and prescribing the use of contraceptives, maintaining that the right of privacy, derived from several constitutional guarantees, protected access to contraception by married persons. In *Eisenstadt v. Baird*,[17] a related 1972 case, the Court extended this reasoning to unmarried individuals, holding that they, too, have a constitutionally protected right to obtain contraceptives.

Women who are practicing members of a religious tradition that rejects the use of contraception may ask healthcare professionals for assistance in avoiding pregnancy without the use of contraceptives. In such instances, physicians can inform them about the "rhythm method," which does not involve the use of a physical or chemical barrier to avoid pregnancy or prevent an embryo from implanting, but instead entails abstinence from sexual intercourse for a certain "fertile" period of time during each month. However, physicians have an obligation to inform women that this method is not considered one of the more reliable methods of avoiding pregnancy.

Physicians who are themselves practicing members of a religious tradition that rejects the use of contraception may be unwilling to prescribe contraceptives for patients. Although a physician is not obligated to violate his or her personal convictions, he or she is obligated to respect the values of patients who have different beliefs. There is a long-standing tradition that such physicians should refer patients requesting access to contraceptives to another physician or inform them that contraceptives are available elsewhere.[18]

B. Whether it is Ethically Acceptable to Impose Contraceptive Measures on Individuals Involuntarily

Norplant is an implantable contraceptive comprised of several capsules that gradually release progestin, thereby providing contraception for women for three to five years. It presents an easy vehicle for coercive use, since the only way to remove these capsules, which are implanted beneath the skin, is through surgery by a trained health professional. Some judges have required the use of Norplant as a condition of parole for women convicted of child abuse related to drug abuse.[19] However, such judicial decisions have been overturned in several states on grounds that this amounts to coercive control of the reproductive capacities of women by the state and threatens the dignity and reproductive freedom of women.[20]

In lieu of such coercive measures, legislation was introduced in several states offering financial incentives for the voluntary insertion of Norplant into women on welfare or whose children had been born with conditions related to substance abuse. Such proposed programs were not believed to be coercive in the strict sense, for they did not require the use of Norplant. However, they were deemed to offer an undue inducement to women living in poverty to have the contraceptive implanted and thus to present a subtle form of coercion.[21] In addition, some argued that such programs raised the specter of eugenics, in that the coercive use of contraceptives is frequently directed at the poor, the developmentally delayed, and the mentally ill.[22] Finally, concern was raised that these proposed laws might violate the constitutional right of women to control their own reproductive capacities. As a result of these ethical and legal considerations, the drive to pass these laws subsided.

C. Whether Healthcare Professionals Should Preserve the Confidentiality of Patients Seeking Contraceptive Protection

Some women seek to keep information about their use of contraception confidential. For instance, those who are in an abusive relationship and have little control over whether they become pregnant may seek contraceptive protection while hiding this from their spouse or partner. Healthcare professionals to whom they turn for help may be concerned that these women are at risk of physical and emotional injury and may consequently urge them to report their abusive partners. Some women may reject this proposal out of fear that criminal proceedings against their partner would jeopardize their domestic and economic security. Physicians who see such patients should encourage them to develop an "exit plan" and to contact programs developed by state and private agencies that provide support and assistance to abused women and their children.[23]

Teenagers may also seek contraceptive protection. Proponents of mandatory parental consent for contraception for adolescents argue that this would reduce teenage sexual activity and prevent the spread of sexually transmitted diseases among them. However, the American Academy of Pediatrics[24] and the American College of Obstetricians and Gynecologists[25] recommend guaranteeing confidentiality to adolescent patients who seek contraception. They maintain that it is desirable for teens to involve their parents in such healthcare decisions, but that they should not be coerced into doing so. They point to studies demonstrating that if parental consent for obtaining contraception were required of teenagers, this would not keep them from being sexually active, but would deter them from seeking medical advice and lead to pregnancies and an increase in sexually transmitted diseases among teens.[26] The Supreme Court in 1977 held in *Carey v. Population Services International*[27] that the Constitution protects a minor's right to privacy in obtaining contraceptives.

III. STERILIZATION

Pregnancy and childbirth can pose risks to the health of women. To avoid such risks and to ensure that they will not have additional children, some women elect to be sterilized. The method employed is bilateral tubal ligation, which involves surgery under anesthesia. Some men also choose to undergo surgical sterilization. This is usually carried out by means of vasectomy, a minor surgical procedure. More women than men undergo sterilization annually, even though female sterilization is a more risky procedure. Key factors that affect the choice and timing of sterilization include patient preference, medical assessment of the risks that pregnancy would present, and access to sterilization services.[28]

Sterilization differs from contraception in that it takes away a person's capacity to procreate, whereas contraception intervenes into the sexual process without affecting a person's reproductive system permanently. Should an individual change his or her mind and decide to have additional children after sterilization, techniques are available to attempt to reverse this procedure.

Some significant ethical issues surrounding sterilization center on the following:

- Whether it is ethically acceptable to use sterilization procedures and
- Whether it is ethically acceptable to impose sterilization on individuals involuntarily.

A. Whether Sterilization Is Ethically Acceptable

The use of sterility procedures appears to be generally accepted within the U.S. as an ethical way to curtail permanently one's procreative capacities. Studies indicate that it is the most commonly used method for avoiding having children in the U.S.[29]

Only a few religious bodies have specifically addressed the ethics of voluntary sterilization as a means of family planning. Commentators within the Episcopal tradition, for instance, maintain that sterilization can be justified for several reasons: to limit family growth, avoid conceiving children who would inherit genes associated with serious disease, and counter overpopulation.[30] The Evangelical Lutheran Church mentions it very briefly as a procedure to be considered in order to prevent unintended pregnancies.[31] However, within the Jewish tradition with its emphasis on procre-

ation, both vasectomy and tubal ligation tend to be rejected.[32] The Roman Catholic Church, a leading opponent of sterilization, teaches that this practice is wrong because it eliminates a person's procreative capacities. However, this tradition distinguishes morally between therapeutic and contraceptive sterilization.[33] That is, using the doctrine of double-effect, Roman Catholic ethicists maintain that it is morally acceptable to carry out procedures directed toward preservation of the life and health of a woman, such as the removal of a cancerous uterus, even though this may foreseeably result in her sterilization, because such sterilization is the unintended result of the medical procedure. In contrast, it is wrong, according to this tradition, to engage in sterilization that is directly intended to disable or eliminate a person's procreative capacities.

In some instances, the choice that an individual makes to be sterilized runs contrary to the moral or religious beliefs of the treating physician and he or she is therefore unwilling to carry out this procedure. Although a physician is not obligated to violate his or her personal convictions, the beliefs of the patient should also be respected. Therefore, this physician has an obligation to refer the patient to another physician or to inform the patient that this service is available elsewhere.[34]

When discussing sterilization with patients, it is important that physicians address the permanent nature of the procedure, alternative methods available for avoiding pregnancy, and the patient's reasons for choosing sterilization.[35] Physicians should also explain the details of the procedure, the possibility of failure, and the need to use condoms for protection against sexually transmitted diseases after sterilization. Since patients can experience regret after sterilization, it is important to discuss this and other possible emotional consequences with them beforehand.

B. Whether it is Ethically Acceptable to Impose Sterilization on Individuals Involuntarily

Ethical concerns have increasingly been raised in the past 50 years about sterilization of those in certain vulnerable populations, including those with mental disabilities, in institutions, and minors. These concerns have largely been grounded in the contemporary recognition that the eugenic sterilization of those in such populations that was carried out in the U.S. in the last century was terribly wrong.[36] Tens of thousands of persons were involuntarily sterilized in response to laws in many states authorizing this procedure for those assumed to have inherited such conditions as mental illness, alcoholism, and epilepsy. The Supreme Court, in the 1927 case *Buck v. Bell*, upheld such involuntary sterilization, finding that a Virginia statute authorizing compulsory sterilization of the supposedly "feeble-minded" was constitutional.[37] Although this decision has never been explicitly rejected by the Court, another Supreme Court decision in 1942, *Skinner v. Oklahoma*, overturned a state law permitting sterilization of three-time felons (in this case, a chicken thief was involved) on equal protection grounds.[38] That is, it held that the law unfairly discriminated against criminal defendants while allowing civil defendants to retain their procreative capacities. Moral repulsion at compulsory sterilization gradually came to the fore in this country, especially after the sterilization practices of the Nazis became a matter of public knowledge, and, as a result, state laws authorizing eugenic sterilization were largely repealed in the 1960s.

Federal regulations prohibit the use of federal funds for the sterilization of anyone under the age of 21 and require that a consent form must be signed by a person undergoing sterilization.[39] Several states maintain a presumption against the involuntary sterilization of persons who are mentally incapacitated or decisionally incompetent.[40] The reasoning behind this policy is that those who are mentally disabled and who can serve as parents without the risk of child neglect or abuse should not be deprived of their right to procreate. However, when persons are profoundly mentally disabled and sexually vulnerable, legitimate questions can be raised about whether they should procreate.

The Ethics Committee of the American College of Obstetricians and Gynecologists (ACOG) maintains that before a decision to proceed with sterilization of such persons is made, the following four matters should be addressed:

1. Identification of an appropriate decision maker;
2. Consideration of alternatives to sterilization;
3. Assessment of the best interests of the person who is mentally incapacitated or incompetent; and
4. Current understanding of applicable laws.[41]

The committee urges that an assessment be carried out of the ability of the mentally disabled person to give informed consent to sterilization and that his or her current values and wishes should be taken into account by a surrogate and the physician involved. Multiple assessments and conversations with the person over a period of time may be necessary before a final decision is made by the surrogate about sterilization. Court approval of sterilization for such persons may be required by state law.

IV. ABORTION AND PRENATAL DIAGNOSIS

Since 1973, when the U.S. Supreme Court effectively legalized abortion through the second trimester of pregnancy in *Roe v. Wade*,[42] controversy over this practice has continued unabated. At one end of the spectrum of views are those who argue for an absolute prohibition of abortion, whereas at the other end are those who maintain that a woman has a right to abortion on demand at any time during a pregnancy. In between these two groups stand those who believe that the abortion decision belongs to the pregnant woman, but that the state has a duty to intervene:

1. When the fetus has reached viability or some other stage of development at which they maintain that it gains moral status and
2. When the life and health of a woman would not be jeopardized by the continuation of the pregnancy.

Among the significant ethical issues surrounding abortion are:

- Whether abortion is ethically acceptable,
- Whether prenatal testing and the possibility of abortion should be offered,
- How to address certain ethical questions that arise during the abortion procedure,
- Whether "partial birth" abortion is ethically acceptable, and
- How to address violence at abortion clinics.

A. Whether Abortion Is Ethically Acceptable

When abortion is at issue, two major ethical considerations enter: the moral status of the fetus and the needs and rights of pregnant women. Although great emphasis has been placed on the first consideration, the well-being and rights of the pregnant woman also carry great moral weight. Therefore, these two considerations both need to be reviewed and addressed.

1. Questions Surrounding the Moral Status of the Fetus

The term "moral status" means having moral significance in one's own right; being owed moral consideration by others; having one's needs and well-being taken seriously by others because of certain characteristics one possesses, the sort of being one is, or for other reasons.[43] Clearly, the moral status of the fetus is a key ethical matter that arises when abortion is under consideration. Yet, equally clearly, it is a highly contested issue.

Those who are often referred to as "pro-life" are, for the most part, opposed to abortion at any stage of pregnancy because they maintain that the zygote is an individual human being who is owed protection from destruction.[44] They argue that to end the life of a zygote or fetus is as wrong as to kill a child or adult. The Supreme Court decision in Roe v. Wade to allow abortion, some "pro-life" advocates hold, has led to the devaluation of human life and a "culture of death" in which society is increasingly receptive to other forms of killing, such as euthanasia and infanticide.

Several Protestant groups, for example, the Church of Jesus Christ of Latter Day Saints,[45] oppose abortion, as does the Hindu tradition.[46] Interestingly, although the Roman Catholic view is often characterized as viewing the conceptus as a human being from the moment of fertilization, this is not strictly the case. Instead, the Roman Catholic teaching is that it cannot be known with certainty that the conceptus is a human being, but that doubt about this question should be resolved in favor of the conceptus, since it is a grave sin to risk murder.[47]

Those termed "pro-choice" hold a range of views about the moral status of the fetus. Among these are that:

- The fetus gains moral status at some point after conception when it develops a certain property, such as the primitive streak (the precursor of the spinal cord and nervous system),[48] brain function,[49] organized cortical activity,[50] or consciousness and sentience;[51] or
- The fetus gradually increases in moral status as it develops, achieving full moral status at birth;[52] or

- The fetus has no moral status until it becomes self-conscious, which occurs some time after birth.[53]

When the fetus gains full moral status according to one of these standards, "pro-choice" advocates maintain, abortion is no longer morally permissible. Legalizing abortion under such conditions, they maintain, has averted the tragic deaths of women by means of self-induced or unsafe abortions performed by untrained persons. They want to avoid a return to the era before Roe v. Wade, in which the only way for women to end a pregnancy in this country was to risk their lives and health in "back alley" abortions.

Several religious bodies can be placed within the "pro-choice" camp, in the sense that they maintain that abortion can be justified up to certain stages of pregnancy and under certain conditions. The Jewish tradition, for instance, maintains that neither the fetus nor the embryo has the moral status of an individual human being, but is "like water."[54] Abortion is therefore accepted in most branches of Judaism. Many Protestant groups, such as the Evangelical Lutheran, Episcopal, Methodist, and Presbyterian, maintain that decisions to have an abortion are justified in some instances, although they regard abortion as a tragic choice in those cases.[55]

2. When the Life, Health, and Personal Freedom of the Pregnant Woman Are Put at Risk by Pregnancy

Is the pregnant woman obligated to sustain the life of a fetus, even at risk to her own life, health, or personal freedom? The relationship between the pregnant woman and the fetus is unique. There are no other situations in which a living human being provides the use of his or her body for an extended period by an entity that could itself develop into a human being or that is already a human being. Some argue that in this unique sort of situation, the pregnant woman is not required to sustain the fetus at the cost of her own life, health, or personal freedom.[56] Even if the fetus is taken to have moral status at a very early stage of pregnancy, according to this argument, abortion can be morally justified when it is weighed against the cost to the pregnant woman of continuing to sustain the fetus. Others, however, maintain that when the woman has knowingly and voluntarily become pregnant, she has implicitly consented to the use of her body by the fetus, unless this would lead to her death or serious illness. On this view, abortion should be employed in a pregnancy that has been entered into knowingly and voluntarily only when the woman's life or health is seriously threatened.

Feminist scholars argue that most discussions of abortion reveal a failure to understand the social and sexual situation of women. Because pregnancy occurs within the bodies of women and profoundly affects the course of their lives, the determination of the moral status of the fetus is the responsibility and privilege of the woman who carries it, Susan Sherwin holds.[57] Another feminist scholar, Margaret Little, argues that fetuses are worthy of respect because they are burgeoning human beings; to abort them is to lose something significant and valuable.[58] However, she believes that this in itself does not indicate what sorts of duties and responsibilities pregnant women have to continue to assist a fetus during gestation. Pregnancy has a profound impact on women, she points out, for it brings with it the impending relationship of motherhood, a relationship that fundamentally changes their identity. Women should have the option of declining such a fundamental change in their identity, she argues, by ending a pregnancy.

B. Ethical Issues Surrounding Prenatal Testing and Possible Abortion

As concerns about genetic disease have come to the fore and tests have become available for an increasing number of genes, genetic testing is being offered to a growing number of people, including pregnant women. Tests have been specifically developed to ascertain whether a fetus in the uterus has genes associated with serious disease. Ultrasound imaging is also used to diagnose a number of serious disorders, such as neural tube abnormalities, and certain malformations. Chorionic villus sampling, which can be performed at 10 weeks of gestation, and amniocentesis, which is carried out between the fourteenth to the sixteenth week of gestation, allow the detection of chromosomal abnormalities and genes associated with disease in the fetus.

Some expectant couples proceed with prenatal testing as a matter of course, wanting to confirm their belief that their fetus is not affected by a serious condition. Pregnant women over the age of 35 may seek prenatal testing, since women in the later childbearing years have a higher incidence of giving birth to children with chromosomal disorders. Others employ this procedure because they have a family history of an inheritable genetic disorder. Couples who are opposed to abortion but who have a family history of hereditary disease may also seek prenatal testing in order to prepare to meet the needs of their child, should he or she have a chromosomal disorder or gene-based condition.

Concern has been raised about the practice of prenatal testing when there are no hereditary or medical indications for using it. Some argue that such testing implicitly treats the expected child as a marketable product to be assessed by quality-assurance mechanisms that can be tossed out if it does not measure up to parental standards.[59] However, others see such testing as part of responsible parenthood, for they maintain that it would be wrong knowingly to bring children into the world who would suffer from serious genetic conditions and, in some cases, face an early death.

Couples who receive test results indicating that the fetus has a gene or chromosome of concern will need information and support from their physician. Unfortunately, the degree of severity of the condition involved often cannot be ascertained through prenatal testing. Moreover, little can be done to treat most of the conditions that these tests are designed to detect in children who are born with them. Therefore, many couples who receive prenatal test results indicating that the fetus is affected are faced with the choice of having an abortion or giving birth to a child who may have serious disabilities, and, in some instances, a short life — or else who may have a mild condition that is compatible with a lengthy life. They cannot be sure in advance. When possible, the physician should link such couples with a trained genetic counselor and relevant support groups so that they can gain greater insight into how the condition at issue might affect a future child and how others who have given birth to a child with that condition have addressed their child's needs.

Here, too, the physician's personal values will affect what services he or she is willing to provide to pregnant patients. A physician with moral objections to prenatal testing should inform patients in advance of entering into a physician-patient relationship about those prenatal screening procedures that he or she will and will not provide.[60] Physicians should also be aware that pregnant patients who are not advised by their obstetricians to undergo prenatal testing and who subsequently give birth to a child with a serious condition have sometimes sued their obstetricians for "wrongful life," claiming damages on their own behalf and/or for "wrongful birth,"[61] claiming damages on behalf of their child. The former suits, by and large, have been unsuccessful, but some courts have awarded damages in "wrongful birth" for additional expenses incurred because of the need of the child for special care.

C. Ethical Considerations in Performing an Abortion

Abortion should be carried out only at the request of a woman and only by a healthcare professional who has had training in performing this procedure. Respect for women as persons who are entitled to control their own bodies and reproductive capacities requires that physicians gain their informed consent. The ACOG Executive Board maintains that pregnant women should be fully informed about all the options available, including raising the child, placing the child for adoption, and having an abortion.[62] However, the ACOG Board opposes carrying out the abortion of a healthy fetus that has attained viability (that is, could survive outside the woman's uterus in the judgment of the responsible attending physician) that is being carried by a healthy woman.[63] When abortion is deemed appropriate, the Board maintains, it should be carried out safely and as early as possible. The standard of care is to provide counseling and emotional support before and after the procedure. Medical considerations related to abortion are discussed in a special ACOG Practice Bulletin.[64]

In those instances in which a physician cannot in good conscience carry out an abortion for a woman requesting this, the ACOG policy has been that the doctor should refer the patient to another physician or inform her that abortion is available elsewhere.[65] This, however, is currently a vexed issue; many states have enacted "conscience clause" laws allowing physicians who are morally opposed to abortion to refuse to provide this procedure. Some of those same states, however, have legal provisions requiring hospitals to provide abortions for women in emergency or life-threatening situations. Physicians in such states

who object to carrying out abortions are concerned that they might be asked to provide the procedure for these women if they are the only professionals available and qualified to do so. Yet others point out that if they refuse to perform an abortion for women in such emergency situations, these women could die. No satisfactory way out of this dilemma has emerged.

At times, adolescents who find that they are pregnant may consult with a physician about having an abortion. The Supreme Court has held that minors have a constitutional right to privacy and can end their pregnancy without parental consent, but that it is legally allowable for states to impose parental notification requirements and waiting periods on them.[66] In some states, "judicial bypass" procedures allow judges to waive parental notification at the request of a minor if they find that the adolescent is mature or that notification is not in her best interests. In this last instance, judges usually are concerned that the pregnant minor might be subject to abuse or other danger should her parents learn of her condition.

D. Whether "Partial Birth" Abortion Is Ethically Acceptable

"Partial birth" abortion is a term coined by those who deplore abortion to describe a method of abortion in which a second or third trimester fetus partially exits the womb before the skull is collapsed, leaving a dead fetus to be delivered. The descriptions of the procedure given by those opposed to it are vague, according to the ACOG Executive Board, and do not delineate a specific procedure that is recognized in the medical literature.[67]

In the 1990s, many states enacted legislation banning "partial birth" abortions. These laws were challenged, and in 2000, in the case of *Stenberg v. Carhart*,[68] the Supreme Court held that the Nebraska version was unconstitutional. The Court found that the statute lacked a constitutionally necessary exception for abortion to save the life of the woman and that it could be construed to rule out an accepted medical procedure known as "dilation and evacuation." In 2003, in response to the Court's decision in the Nebraska case, Congress passed the federal Partial Birth Abortion Ban Act, which maintains that partial-birth abortion is never necessary to preserve the health of a woman. This law is currently before the courts.

E. The Problem of Violence at Abortion Clinics

Violence aimed at abortion providers has been decried by those on both sides of the abortion debate. Anti-abortion demonstrators have sometimes established blockades that interfere with the ability of patients and staff to enter abortion facilities. Some among them have engaged in other sorts of harassment, property damage, and even murder. In response, in 1994, Congress passed the Freedom of Access to Clinic Entrances Act, which makes acts of obstruction and interference at places providing abortions and other reproductive services a federal offense punishable by fines and imprisonment. In 2000, the Supreme Court upheld a state statute creating a narrow, eight-foot "bubble zone" around clinics, saying that this imposes a reasonable restriction on the free speech of abortion protesters.[69] Those abortion opponents who have engaged in property damage and murder have been pursued and, when apprehended, have been subject to criminal sanctions.

V. PREGNANCY AND PREIMPLANTATION GENETIC DIAGNOSIS

Many people regard having children as one of the defining experiences of their lives. Yet some women who are eager to have children enter into pregnancy unaware that it can pose the risk of serious illness and, in rare cases, death. Women who begin pregnancy in excellent health may find themselves unexpectedly confronting the risks associated with cesarean section, postpartum hemorrhage, or eclampsia (a disorder of pregnancy that may involve hypertension, acute kidney disease, and insufficient blood supply to the placenta, among other problems). Those who seek to become pregnant should be aware of such risks and should have access to healthcare services that assist them to go through pregnancy and childbirth safely, bringing a healthy child into the world.[70]

A. Maternal-Fetal Relationship

The fetus is no longer predominantly viewed as a part of the pregnant woman, by healthcare professionals, but is coming to be seen as a second patient. This is due, in part, to the development of the prenatal tests discussed above, for they seem to render the fetus a distinct entity in its own right. Yet the fetus, as also observed above, is completely dependent physiologically on the woman who carries it in a way that parallels no other relationship in human experience. Consequently, when a fetus *in utero* appears to be endangered, the path to treating it necessarily goes through the body of the woman who carries it.

Women overwhelmingly appear to view the fetus they intend to bring to term as a being owed protection and nurture. For this reason, they are usually presumed to be the most appropriate advocates for the well-being of the fetus. However, there are some circumstances in which the well-being of the woman and that of the fetus she is carrying may diverge. In such situations, pregnant women and healthcare professionals may disagree about how to proceed because they weigh the risks, benefits, and values at issue differently.

1. When the Pregnant Woman Refuses Procedures or Therapy Intended to Benefit the Fetus

If the life or health of the fetus appears to be at risk, the pregnant woman may be advised by her physician to undergo diagnostic or invasive procedures primarily for the benefit of the fetus. The best known example of this sort of circumstance is when a fetus seems to be in danger of death and a physician urges the pregnant woman carrying it to undergo a cesarean section. Usually, women readily consent to this surgery in these circumstances because they accept that this would benefit the fetus. Some pregnant women, however, are reluctant to undergo a cesarean section for a variety of reasons. They may believe that it would put them at too great a risk, would be "unnatural," would conflict with their religious beliefs, or would be unlikely to assist the fetus.

Although the abortion debate has highlighted questions about whether a fetus is owed the same sort of protections as a living child, when the fetus is intended to be brought to term, it will become a living child and there is good reason to be concerned about its well-being and that of the child it will become.[71] Yet there are also good reasons to respect the pregnant woman as a person in her own right whose health and interests are of concern and importance.

Healthcare professionals who recommend that a pregnant woman undergo certain procedures for the benefit of the fetus have an obligation to present the reasons for their recommendation, to work with her to consider the difficulties that these might entail, and to encourage but not coerce her to proceed when the professional is convinced that the procedures are necessary to preserve the life and health of the fetus and do not involve serious risk for the pregnant woman. An ACOG Committee opinion adds that:

> In interactions with a woman who appears to resist following medical advice that might improve her health or that of her fetus, the obstetrician must keep in mind that medical knowledge has limitations and medical judgment is fallible. . . . great care should be exercised to present a balanced evaluation of expected outcomes for both parties.[72]

Should the patient reject the intervention, the ACOG opinion states, the obstetrician may (1) respect the choice of the patient and not proceed; (2) offer to transfer her to another physician before an emergency situation arises if he or she is unwilling to accede to the patient's decision,; or (3) request court involvement. This last choice has been exercised only on rare occasions. However, if there is insufficient time to transfer the pregnant woman's care to another healthcare professional or go to court, the obstetrician should respect the patient's wishes and not intervene, "regardless of the consequence," the opinion maintains.

In some instances in which pregnant women have refused surgery that they have been advised is necessary to protect the life and health of the child, hospitals and physicians have resorted to the courts to decide whether they should proceed.[73] The prevailing legal position is that a pregnant woman should not be forced to undergo invasive medical treatment, even though such treatment may be considered necessary to preserve the life or health of the fetus.[74] The reasoning behind this view is that it is wrong to require a woman to put her own life and health at risk for the sake of the fetus that she is carrying, much as it is wrong to require one person to give his or her life for another. Even if not legally required, when the risk to the woman of a medical procedure that would be beneficial to the fetus is not great, it is considered incumbent on the pregnant woman to undergo that procedure.

2. When the Pregnant Woman's Behavior May Affect the Health of the Fetus

The misuse of controlled and illegal drugs constitutes a major health risk in the U.S.[75] Substance abuse can have serious adverse effects on the reproductive functions of women and on pregnancy and childbirth.

There are several occasions on which the physician can screen patients for substance abuse, including when taking a history[76] and when patients visit for medical problems that appear to have been exacerbated by substance abuse. ACOG has developed a screening questionnaire for substance abuse that it recommends using universally for all patients, whether they are pregnant or not.[77] In some instances, physicians may find that they have to use indirect evidence and their best judgment to ascertain whether patients may be abusing drugs. If drug testing seems advisable, this should be carried out with the patient's consent. In certain exceptional circumstances, however, such as when patients are unconscious, in a stupor, or obviously intoxicated, they may be tested without their consent in order to direct further medical interventions. Those who are found to be involved in substance abuse should be referred for treatment.[78]

In the second half of the last century, medical researchers came to realize that drug abuse could have a detrimental effect on the fetus. Obstetricians therefore began to advise pregnant women against engaging in the use of alcohol and drugs to protect the health of the fetus. However, pregnant women have at times refused to refrain from such activities after being advised to do so by their physician. This sort of refusal differs from a refusal by a pregnant woman to undergo an invasive surgical procedure in that there is no countervailing personal risk to the woman posed by stopping drug use to weigh against the good of the future child. Therefore, some argue, the moral balance lies in forcing pregnant women who use drugs to stop doing so for the sake of the child.

In a number of isolated instances, judges have jailed pregnant women whom they believed would abuse or neglect their fetuses. In 2001, the Supreme Court struck down a program under which a hospital tested pregnant patients for illegal drug use without their consent and reported patients who refused rehabilitation to law enforcement authorities.[79] The current legal trend maintains that imprisoning or otherwise penalizing women who engage in drinking, smoking, or drug use while pregnant not only entails a major violation of their civil liberties, but also wrongly punishes those who are addicted and cannot stop the relevant behavior at will without treatment.[80]

VI. REPRODUCTIVE TECHNOLOGIES, ALSO REFERRED TO AS "ASSISTED REPRODUCTION"

Millions of couples seek medical assistance every year because they wish to have a child but have difficulties related to conception. The major causes of infertility in women include ovulation disorders, obstruction of the fallopian tubes, pelvic adhesions, and endometriosis; the primary cause of infertility in men relates to the number and quality of their sperm.[81] Physicians vary in their views about when infertility treatment should be recommended, what diagnostic tests should be used and what they mean, and when treatment should be ended.

Some couples who face infertility can overcome this problem through treatment with drugs or surgery. Others, however, may be advised to turn to the use of reproductive technologies. A stunning repertoire of reproductive techniques has been developed to help them. These include, but are not limited to:

- Artificial insemination with husband or by sperm donor. In this procedure, the sperm is inserted into the vagina or uterus of the woman by medical or other (for example, turkey baster) artificial means. It was first carried out in the U.S. by a physician in 1884.
- *In vitro* fertilization (IVF). In its simplest form, this technology involves allowing sperm and egg to join in a laboratory dish (*in vitro*) outside the human body and transferring the resulting embryo(s) by way of the vagina to the uterus of a woman. It was introduced in the United Kingdom in 1978 and was first used in the U.S. in 1981.
- Oocyte donation. This involves obtaining eggs from a donor on behalf of women who cannot produce their own eggs or whose eggs cannot be used for medical reasons, and fertilizing them *in vitro* with sperm. It was introduced in the U.S. 1984.
- Surrogacy. In this arrangement, a woman agrees to undergo pregnancy on behalf of a couple or single person to whom she will give the resulting child to rear. The "surrogate mother" may be artificially inseminated with sperm provided by the male who is the intended father, in which case the child is half hers genetically. Or she may have an embryo developed by means of IVF transferred to her, in which case the intended father and mother

are the genetic parents of the resulting child.
- Intracytoplasmic sperm injection (ICSI). This involves direct injection of a single sperm into an egg in those instances when men have few normal or motile sperm. It first began to be used in the U.S. 1993.
- Reproductive cloning, or somatic cell nuclear transfer. This is a reproductive technology in theory but not in practice. It involves inserting the nucleus of a somatic cell into an enucleated egg, which is then stimulated to develop into an embryo and transferred to a woman's uterus. This procedure has not been carried out successfully, however, and there is almost unanimous opposition to its use among infertility and other medical professionals on grounds that it presents serious dangers to the fetus and any child who might result from this technology.

Among the significant ethical issues surrounding the use of the new reproductive technologies are:
- Whether the use of reproductive technologies is ethically acceptable and
- How to address questions about the meaning of family, parenthood, and certain other questions raised by IVF and its associated techniques.

A. Whether the Use of Reproductive Technologies Is Ethically Acceptable

The new methods of assisted reproduction were initially accepted because they provided a way for those who wanted to be parents to have children in ways that seemed an extension of the usual mode of procreation. Moreover, the resulting children had genes derived from those who would rear them and, by and large, were born into traditionally structured families consisting of a married heterosexual mother and father. However, human intervention into the procreative process has become more complex, technological, and frequent, and the contexts in which the new methods of assisted reproduction are being used are changing today.

The new reproductive technologies facilitate the merger of sperm and egg in ways that are quite disparate from traditional sexual intercourse. Moreover, the sperm and eggs used are not necessarily derived from those who will rear the resulting children. Further, children are being born into a wide variety of family settings that differ from the traditional nuclear family. These novel facets of having children by means of these reproductive technologies are leading people to question whether the intense desire to have children provides sufficient ethical justification to warrant their use.

Some argue that individuals should be free to use these methods of reproduction as long as it does not harm others. Reproductive liberty should be allowed to prevail without state interference unless this would damage those involved in their use, including third parties, or society in general, as when overpopulation looms. This is the view developed by legal theorist John Robertson, among others.[82]

Others respond that the goal of avoiding harm, while laudable, provides an insufficient ethical constraint on the use of methods of assisted reproduction. A position that focuses on individual choice and autonomy to the exclusion of all other considerations except the possibility of harm to others loses sight of significant values relevant to the well-being of the children born as a result of the use of these technologies and the common good. At times, it is necessary to put constraints on individual choices regarding certain uses of reproductive technologies, these respondents argue, in order to safeguard the health of the children born and to preserve basic values at the core of the society into which we bring those children.[83] Is it always a responsible ethical decision to bring children into the world by these technological means? Are there times when we should forgo the use of reproductive technologies?

1. Whether the Use of Reproductive Technologies Is "Unnatural" and therefore Wrong

Probably the chief ethical challenge raised by the new reproductive technologies is that this is "unnatural." Some see procreation as a given process of nature that should always be initiated by the physical union of a man and woman. They maintain that technological intrusions into this process are unnatural and therefore wrong. This is the view of the Roman Catholic Church, which prohibits the use of reproductive technologies because they separate procreation from conjugal union. It teaches that "There is an inseparable connection, willed by God and unable to be broken by man on his own initiative, between the two meanings of the conjugal act: the unitive meaning and the procreative meaning."[84] On this view, procreation must always be the result of sexual intercourse within marriage, the fruit of a loving physical relation between a man and a woman that is not violated by technological intrusions.

Those who disagree with the Roman Catholic position argue that when nature "goes wrong," as it does for many who seek to use reproductive technologies, it is right to attempt to remedy this. They see the use of these technologies as a way of circumventing physical obstacles that prevent the physical union between a man and a woman from resulting in the procreation of children.[85] Certain religious groups, such as the Lutheran, Jewish, Presbyterian, Eastern Orthodox, and Islamic, view most methods of assisted reproduction as ethically acceptable because God has encouraged human procreation. Each act of sexual intercourse, they believe, need not be open to procreation.[86] They teach that it is sufficient that love and procreation are held together within the whole context of the marital relationship.

2. Whether the Use of the New Reproductive Technologies Will Change What We Mean by Family and Parenthood

A related ethical concern is the ethical import of the use of the new reproductive technologies for the meaning of parenthood and the family in our society. As single persons, unmarried heterosexual couples, and homosexual couples have increasingly gained access to these technologies, commentators have expressed concern about whether this would weaken mutual commitment within the family and impinge on the welfare of the resulting children.[87] When procreation takes place in a context other than marriage (as when single women use artificial insemination by donor) or another's body is used to carry a pregnancy to term (as when "surrogate mothers" are employed), this can impinge negatively on the relation between married couples and the significant role of the nuclear family in our society.

Moreover, the use of third parties in reproductive efforts severs the connection between the conceptive, gestational and rearing components of parenthood and leads to confused notions of parentage, critics charge. A child may be genetically related to both, one, or neither rearing parent; may be gestated by a woman with no genetic or subsequent rearing link to the child; and, *ipso facto*, may be reared by parents with no genetic and/or gestational link to hi or her. Indeed, in theory, but rarely in fact, a child might have five different parents: two genetic parents, a gestational parent, and two rearing parents. As a result, a child may not only be confused about his or her "real" parent, but may also find that his or her identity within a family lineage is obscured by these technologies.[88]

To others, however, the use of reproductive technologies mirrors the fact that society has begun to shift away from the nuclear family.[89] They see the development of new sorts of family relationships as a move toward greater equality in a society where homosexual and single persons have historically experienced discrimination. No reliable evidence, they maintain, has surfaced displaying that children born into nontraditional families fare worse than those born into nuclear families.[90]

3. Whether the Use of the Reproductive Technologies Commodifies Procreation and Children

This, in turn, raises the broader question of whether the process of procreating a living child is coming to be viewed as akin to the manufacture of a commercial product. The introduction of payments to third-party donors for their gametes, some argue, risks transforming children into objects of market exchange and diminishing their value as human beings.[91] Moreover, it opens the door to the development of a new economic underclass of women who earn their living by providing body parts and products for those who are economically well-off.

Some maintain that the notion of a "gift" to which the appropriate response is gratitude, rather than money, should be used to model the contribution of those who donate gametes to assist others to reproduce.[92] Payment to gamete donors is prohibited by law in Canada on such grounds, but compensation for expenses and maternity leave is allowed.[93] The American Society for Reproductive Medicine (ASRM) maintains that gamete donors should be paid for their "time, inconvenience, and physical and emotional demands associated with the oocyte donation process."[94]

Others hold that individuals have a right to do what they choose with their bodies and that donors who seek payment for their gametes should be compensated in a way that is commensurate with the degree of effort, risk, and inconvenience entailed by their services. There is agreement on all sides that donors should not be specifically compensated for their gametes, wombs, or babies.

B. Special Ethical Questions that Arise When Clinicians Provide IVF and Related Technologies

In 2002 there were over 400 known assisted reproductive technology clinics in the U.S., 391 of which reported having created 33,141 babies.[95] Yet when this area of reproductive health was first developed and began to spread, the public and members of Congress had little consistently reliable and comparable information about the effectiveness of infertility programs, often leaving the public "vulnerable to both poor quality services and excessive costs."[96] Therefore, in 1992, Congress passed the Fertility Clinic Success Rate and Certification Act, which called for mandatory publication of clinic-specific data about all reproductive procedures employed by assisted reproductive technology programs across the country.[97] It also required that laboratories that handle human gametes develop standards for this. As a result, reports about success rates at individual clinics have been published since 1995. The average success rate of all of these clinics in the most recent set of reports in 2002 was 30 percent.[98]

However, concerns remain about how to ensure that those who provide these various methods of assisted reproduction adhere to ethical standards. Professional organizations within the field of reproductive medicine have established guidelines for carrying out reproductive procedures, but there is no professional or legal requirement that these guidelines must be followed in assisted reproduction programs. This has led some of those who desperately wish to have children and who seek to use some of the reproductive technologies to feel that they are in a vulnerable position, for they have no assurance that they will receive appropriate care.

1. Requiring Evidence of Safety and Effectiveness before Introducing New Treatments into the Clinical Setting

Physicians are often eager to introduce innovations in methods of assisted reproduction into practice. Although the safety and efficacy of many procedures currently in use has been established, at times novel forms of reproductive technology have been offered to patients for which this has not been the case. When there is insufficient evidence of the safety and efficacy of a procedure from research, physicians should offer it to patients only as part of a research project. This means that an institutional review board (IRB) must review the proposed technique and indicate that it meets accepted medical and ethical criteria for introducing innovative forms of treatment. The IRB should certify that patients will be adequately informed about the risks and benefits of the procedure and that patients and any resulting embryos will be protected appropriately from harm that might result.[99]

2. The Need to Improve Informed Consent Procedures

The lack of uniform standards for obtaining informed consent from patients receiving infertility treatment has presented a significant ethical issue. In 1998, the New York State Task Force on Life and the Law conducted an extensive review of IVF consent forms used in that state and concluded that the consent process was widely inconsistent and seriously flawed.[100]

Areas in need of special attention, the task force found, included explanations of the pregnancy rates and experience of individual clinics, the costs of procedures and medications, the health risks to the woman of using drugs to induce ovulation, the risks of multiple pregnancies, and the alternatives to treatment. The task force declared that screening criteria for both patients and donors needed to be discussed explicitly, as should methods for maintaining confidentiality about medical and social information. Others note that patients should be promptly informed when something goes wrong, as when frozen embryos are accidentally thawed or an embryo is mistakenly transferred to the wrong woman. Currently, there is no way of knowing to what extent there are problems related to the adequacy of informed consent for the use of reproductive technologies around the country and whether these are being addressed. Few studies have addressed this question and there are no government regulations or professional supervision of such ethical issues.

3. The Problem of Multifetal Pregnancies

A serious risk of infertility treatment is that a woman will become pregnant with more than one fetus. This can occur when multiple embryos are transferred to a woman undergoing IVF in hopes of maximizing the chances of initiating a pregnancy. Patients agree to allow the transfer of several embryos because they hope that this attempt at a high cost infertility procedure will succeed and spare them from subsequent attempts. Physicians have been sometimes been willing to transfer several embryos to women in hopes of improving the chances that at least one will implant and develop. This, they hope, will enhance the reputation of their program as one with high success rates and will attract future patients. Yet when several embryos implant, creating a pregnancy with two or more fetuses this carries risks of prenatal, neonatal, and maternal morbidity and mortality. The Practice Committee of the American Society of Reproductive Medicine has recognized this serious problem and has therefore issued advisory guidelines on the number of embryos that should be transferred.[101] These numbers vary, depending on the age of the woman and her prognosis. The medical and ethical issues to which multifetal pregnancies give rise should be discussed with patients in advance of treatment so that they can be avoided or overcome.

In those instances in which a multifetal pregnancy has been initiated, fetal reduction to twins, which involves the termination of one or more, but not all, fetuses, is an option. This results in the delivery of fewer infants who have lower risks of preterm birth, morbidity, and mortality. However, this practice bears certain medical risks, such as pregnancy loss and lower birth weight, according to some reports.[102] Further, it raises ethical concerns akin to those raised by abortion. Some patients may find it justifiable to reduce the number of fetuses they are carrying in order to allow some of them to continue to develop and be born. Others, however, may believe that it is ethically unacceptable to terminate an apparently healthy fetus, regardless of the well-being of other fetuses in the pregnancy. Individual patients should be informed about the procedure of fetal reduction and given a choice about how to proceed in these difficult circumstances. Clearly, the preferable option is to avoid such circumstances in the first place by making judicious decisions about the number of embryos that will be transferred.

4. Whether It Is Ethically Acceptable to Employ Certain Unique Financial Arrangements to Address Costs

The cost of employing IVF is staggering for many couples. Although some states require insurers to cover treatment for fertility problems, most patients in those states still have to cover much of the cost of IVF by themselves. A variety of ways of paying for IVF have been developed by assisted-reproduction programs.

Some offer IVF on a "shared-risk" or "warranty" basis, rather than a "fee-for-service" basis. That is, patients pay a higher than usual fee for IVF and, if they become pregnant during a pre-agreed number of attempts, their physician keeps the fee. However, if IVF is not successful, 90 to 100 percent of the fee is returned to the patient. The higher fees are intended to cover the cost of refunds to patients who do not become pregnant.

The advantage of this arrangement is that it leaves patients for whom IVF is unsuccessful with financial resources to pursue other options.[103] Yet this practice can be criticized as exploitative of those with limited income, as it pressures them to invest more money in their treatment than they would ordinarily. Also, it may skew the judgment of physicians who hope to retain the higher than usual payment by leading them to take certain risks. For instance, they may transfer a larger number of embryos than they would otherwise, increasing the likelihood of multifetal pregnancy and its attendant risks to women, fetuses, and future children. This arrangement therefore creates a conflict of interest for physicians that cannot be wholly overcome by an informed-consent rubric with patients who are desperate to have children.

Recently some physicians have invited women seeking IVF treatment to participate in clinical trials of drugs, infertility treatment, or embryo research or else to donate extra eggs or sperm to other couples or to researchers in exchange for a discount that can amount to as much as two-thirds of that treatment.[104] Egg-sharing and related arrangements offers treatment to those who could otherwise not afford it. However, such arrangements can be exploitative of those with limited financial resources because they can pressure them to participate in research or to donate bodily materials at a time when they are especially vulnerable to offers. Moreover, this sort of trade may put women who participate in such research at greater risk of injury than they would have been the case otherwise, since they are engaging in unproven experimentation and treatment.

5. Whether It Is Ethically Acceptable to Employ Pre-Implantation Genetic Diagnosis (PGD)

Pre-implantation genetic diagnosis (PGD) is available at a few clinics in the U.S.. It allows those who are at risk of having children with certain gene-based diseases to avoid doing so. It also enables would-be parents to select certain traits of future children to a limited extent. PGD involves carrying out an IVF cycle, after which one cell is removed from the resulting embryo at the eight-cell stage and is tested for genes and chromosomes related to the condition of concern or to certain characteristics, such as gender. The procedure is usually carried out on more than one embryo in order to increase the chances that at least one will not have the unwanted gene or chromosome. The embryo selected is then transferred to the woman's uterus and, hopefully, will go on to birth. PGD does not guarantee that a couple will have a healthy child, but it does guarantee that their child will not have the condition of concern or, should they engage in tailoring the features of their child, that the child will have the desired trait(s).

Some of those who employ PGD to avoid having a child with a serious gene-based condition view the use of this technique as ethically acceptable because it does not involve abortion of an affected fetus. Instead, embryos that are found to have the gene or chromosome of concern are not transferred to the woman, but are discarded. Some patients, however, view the embryo as a living human being from the moment of conception, and may therefore be unwilling to participate in PGD because it involves the destruction of embryos. Physicians should explain to patients how this procedure is carried out and how it differs from prenatal diagnosis so that they can consider whether its use would raise ethical problems for them.

The use of PGD for nonmedical reasons, such as to select the gender of a future child, raises significant ethical and social concerns. Perhaps the greatest concern is that sex selection, if increasingly employed, would reinforce gender bias within society and lead to gender discrimination against women, the less socially favored of the two sexes in many societies.[105] A further concern is that use of PGD to select some characteristics of children will unjustifiably open the door to control of other features of future children, such as their eye or hair color, thereby resulting in "designer children." Such children may be treated as parental products with no integrity of their own who are mere puppets to be controlled at the will of their progenitors. These children, some maintain, may experience psychological harm in the form of pressure from their parents to conform to the strong expectations they harbor of them, as exhibited by their willingness to invest time, effort, and money to select their gender or other features. However, others argue, we allow parents who reproduce by means of sexual intercourse to have children for reasons that sometimes seem frivolous and outlandish, and there is no reason to prevent those seeking to use PGD from doing the same. Further, they suggest, sex selection, in particular, might provide gender balance in families with more than one child or a preferred gender order among children in families, goals that are not in themselves unethical.

The Ethics Committee of the ASRM has decided that the use of sex selection should not "be prohibited or condemned as unethical in all cases."[106] In contrast, the Institute of Medicine's Committee on Genetic Risk has concluded that sex selection involves a misuse of genetic information and should be discouraged by health professionals.[107]

PGD has also been utilized in instances when couples seek to help an already existing child who faces a serious medical condition by creating another child to donate bodily material to treat the existing child. This has been an extremely controversial use of this technique, for it involves creating a child, not necessarily for its own sake, but clearly for the sake of another child. Indeed, children who are developed for this reason are sometimes referred to as "savior siblings." Some argue that to use PGD for this purpose is to treat children as products who are valued, not in themselves, but for what they can contribute to another child. This, they maintain, violates the Kantian dictum that persons should not be treated as a means only. The use of PGD is banned in a number of countries for this and other reasons. Others, however, respond that the children who are created to help already living children are loved and wanted children who are treated with the same sort of care as already existing children.

VII. CONCLUDING OBSERVATIONS

Reproductive health care can present challenging ethical issues for health care professionals who address the reproductive needs and choices of patients. As the scope of reproductive healthcare practice has gradually expanded to cover not only pregnancy and childbirth, but also the broader aspects of reproductive health, these ethical issues have become more numerous and complex. They include not only those associated with the question of how much moral force should be accorded to individual reproductive decisions, but also those related to social goals, including the scope that should be given to the meaning of parenthood and family and whether the biological processes of reproduction should be augmented when they go awry.

Clinicians in the field of reproductive health care can assure future patients that they are carrying out treatment in ways that are ethically sound by developing inter-program standards that they warrant are followed by professionals at each of their clinics.[108] Such standards would, for example, give attention to specific steps to be followed in obtaining adequate and appropriate informed consent from individuals receiving infertility treatment and those donating gametes, what options will be offered to couples with regard to any embryos remaining after a first attempt at IVF, and how to distinguish treatment that falls within the scope of research and needs IRB review from that which is part of accepted medical care. By their willingness to develop such standards, clinicians will convey to patients that the treatment that they provide adheres to generally accepted ethical and medical requirements and lead patients to feel that they are in safe hands.

ACKNOWLEDGMENTS

The author would like to thank Arthur Leader, MD, of the University of Ottawa, Ottawa, Canada, and Peter J. Cohen, MD, JD, of Georgetown Law Center, Washington, D.C. for their immensely helpful comments about a previous draft of this chapter. Neither of them is responsible for the final version.

NOTES

1. R.J. Cook, B.M. Dickens, and M.F. Fathalla, *Reproductive Health and Human Rights: Integrating Medicine, Ethics, and Law* (Oxford, U.K.: Clarendon Press, 2003), 11-2.

2. United Nations Department of Public Information, *Platform for Action and Beijing Declaration,* Fourth World Conference on Women, Beijing, China, 4-15 September 1995 (New York: UN, 1995), para. 94.

3. American College of Obstetricians and Gynecologists, *Guidelines for Women's Health Care*

(Washington, D.C.: American College of Obstetricians and Gynecologists, 2002), 150.

4. Ibid.

5. Ibid.

6. C.B. Cohen and D.H. Smith, "Bioethics in the Episcopal Tradition," in *Religious Perspectives in Bioethics,* ed. J.F. Peppin, M.J. Cherry, and A. Iltis (New York: Taylor and Francis, 2004), 31-52; R. Groenhout, "Reformed Perspectives in Bioethics," in *Religious Perspectives in Bioethics,* 79-95.

7. H.L. Gordon and M. Washofsky, "Jewish Bioethics," in *Religious Perspectives in Bioethics,* see note 6 above, pp. 131-46.

8. S.S. Harakas, "Eastern Orthodox Bioethics," in *Theological Developments in Bioethics,* ed. B.A. Brody et al., 1988-90, Bioethics Yearbook, vol. I (Dordrecht, Netherlands: Kluwer, 1991), 43-59.

9. D. Keown, "Buddhism and Bioethics," in *Religious Perspectives in Bioethics,* see note 6 above, pp. 173-88.

10. See, e.g., Martin Luther in "Table Talk," in *Luther's Works,* ed. H. Lehmann (Philadelphia, Pa.: Fortress, 1966), vol. 54, 324.

11. C.B. Cohen and M.R. Anderlik, "Creating and Shaping Future Children," in A *Christian Response to the New Genetics: Religious, Ethical and Social Issues,* ed. D.H. Smith and C.B. Cohen (Lanham, Md.: Rowman and Littlefield, 2003), 75-104.

12. Kenneth Vaux, *Birth Ethics: Religious and Cultural Values in the Genesis of Life* (New York: Crossroad, 1989), 1-21.

13. Pope Paul VI, "Humanae Vitae," (1968) in *Why Humane Vitae Was Right: A Reader,* ed. J. Smith (San Francisco, Calif.: Ignatius Press, 1993), 537-57.

14. J.T. Noonan, *Contraception: A History of Its Treatment by the Catholic Theologians and Canonists* (Cambridge, Mass.: Harvard University Press, 1986).

15. Southern Baptist Convention, "Resolution on RU 486, the French Abortion Pill, adopted at the SBC convention 14 June 1994," available at *http://johnstonsarchive.net/baptist/sbcabres.html.*

16. *Griswold v. Connecticut,* 381 U.S. 479 (1965).

17. *Eisenstadt v. Baird,* 405 U.S. 438 (1972).

18. K.E. Powderly, "Fertility Control: Social and Ethical Issues," in *Encyclopedia of Bioethics,* 3rd ed. (New York: Macmillan, 2003), vol. 2, 901-13.

19. J. Forrest and L. Kaeser, "Questions of Balance: Issues Emerging from the Introduction of the Hormonal Implant," *Family Planning Perspectives* 25, no. 3 (1993): 127-32.

20. J. Mertus and S. Heller, "Norplant Meets the New Eugenics: The Impermissibility of Coerced Contraception," *Saint Louis University Public Law Review* 11, no. 2 (1992): 359-83.

21. Board of Trustees, American Medical Association, "Requirements or Incentives by Government for the Use of Long-Acting Contraceptives," *Journal of the American Medical Association* 267, no. 13 (1992): 1818-21.

22. Ibid.

23. American College of Obstetricians and Gynecologists, "Domestic Violence," *ACOG Educational Bulletin* 257 (Washington, D.C.: ACOG, December, 1999).

24. American Academy of Pediatrics, Committee on Adolescence, "Contraception and Adolescents," *Pediatrics* 104 (1999): 1161-6.

25. American College of Obstetricians and Gynecologists, *Health Care for Adolescents* (Washington, D.C.: ACOG, 2003), 25-35.

26. D.M. Reddy, R. Fleming, and C. Swain, "Effect of Mandatory Parental Notification on Adolescent Girls' Use of Sexual Health Care Services," *Journal of the American Medical Association* 288 (2002): 710-4.

27. *Carey v. Population Services International* 431 U.S. 678 (1977).

28. A.P. MacKay et al., "Tubal Sterilization in the United States," *Family Planning Perspective* 33 (2001): 161-5; R.J. Magnani et al., "Vasectomy in the United States," *American Journal of Public Health* 89 (1999): 92-4.

29. American College of Obstetricians and Gynecologists, "Benefits and Risks of Sterilization, Clinical Management Guidelines for Obstetrician-Gynecologists," *ACOG Practice Bulletin* (Washington, D.C.: ACOG, 2003), 46.

30. See Cohen and Smith, note 6 above, pp. 36-7.

31. Evangelical Lutheran Church in America, "Social Statement on Abortion," (1991), available at *www.elca.org/socialstatements/abortion.*

32. See note 7 above, p. 137.

33. J.P. Boyle, *The Sterilization Controversy: A New Crisis for the Catholic Hospital?* (New York, N.Y.: Paulist Press, 1977).

34. American College of Obstetricians and Gynecologists, Committee on Ethics, *Ethics in Obstetrics and Gynecology,* 2nd ed. (Washington,

D.C.: ACOG, 2004), 56.

35. See note 28 above, p. 7.

36. P.R. Reilly, *The Surgical Solution* (Baltimore, Md.: Johns Hopkins University Press, 1991).

37. *Buck v. Bell*, 274 U.S. 200 (1927).

38. *Skinner v. Oklahoma*, 316 U.S. 35 (1942).

39. 42 *Code of Federal Regulations* 50.202.

40. American College of Obstetricians and Gynecologists, Committee on Ethics, no. 73, *Ethical Issues in Sterilization* (Washington, D.C.: ACOG, 1989).

41. American College of Obstetricians and Gynecologists, Committee on Ethics, no. 63, *Sterilization of Women Who Are Mentally Handicapped* (Washington, D.C.: ACOG, 1988).

42. *Roe v. Wade*, 410 U.S. 113 (1973).

43. M.A. Warren, *Moral Status: Obligations to Persons and Other Living Things* (Oxford, U.K.: Oxford University Press, 1997), 3.

44. J.T. Noonan, "An Almost Absolute Value in History," in *The Morality of Abortion: Legal and Historical Perspectives*, ed. J.T. Noonan (Cambridge, Mass.: Harvard University Press, 1972), 1-59.

45. C.S. Campbell, "Authority and Agency: Policies and Principles in Latter-day Saints Bioethics," in *Religious Perspectives in Bioethics*, see note 3 above, 109-30.

46. C. Crawford, "Hindu Bioethics," in *Religious Perspectives in Bioethics*, see note 3 above, pp. 189-210.

47. G. Grisez Germaine, *Abortion: The Myths, Realities and the Arguments* (New York, N.Y.: Corpus Books, 1990).

48. G. Dunstan, "The Moral Status of the Human Embryo," in *Philosophical Ethics in Reproductive Medicine*, ed. D.R. Bronham, M.E. Dalton, and J.C. Jackson (Manchester, U.K.: Manchester University Press, 1988), 2-14.

49. B. Brody, "The Morality of Abortion," in *Contemporary Issues in Bioethics*, 3rd ed., ed. T.L. Beauchamp and L. Walters (Belmont, Calif.: Wadsworth, 1973), 201-10.

50. D. Boonin, *A Defense of Abortion* (Cambridge, U.K.: Cambridge University Press, 2003).

51. B. Steinbock, *Life before Birth: The Moral and Legal Status of Embryos and Fetuses* (New York, N.Y.: Oxford University Press, 1992).

52. R. Green, *The Human Embryo Research Debates: Bioethics in the Vortex of Controversy* (New York, N.Y.: Oxford University Press, 2001); C.A. Tauer, "Abortion: Embodiment and Prenatal Development," in *Embodiment, Morality, and Medicine*, ed. L.S. Cahill and M.A. Farley (Dordrecht, Netherlands: Kluwer, 15), 75-92.

53. M.Tooley, "Abortion and Infanticide," in *Moral Problems in Medicine*, ed. S. Gorovitz, R. Macklin, and A.L. Jameton (Englewood Cliffs, N.J.: Prentice-Hall, 1972), 85-96.

54. L. Zoloth, "The Ethics of the Eighth Day: Jewish Bioethics and Research on Human Embryonic Stem Cells," in *The Human Embryonic Stem Cell Debate*, ed. S. Holland, K.Lebacqz, and L. Zoloth (Cambridge, Mass.: MIT Press, 2001), 95-112.

55. B. Wilding Harrison, "Protestant Perspectives," in *Encyclopedia of Bioethics*, see note 18 above, vol. 1, pp. 35-9; note 6, Cohen and Smith, p. 38 and note 31.

56. J. Jarvis Thomson, "A Defense of Abortion," in *Ethical Issues in Modem Medicine*, 6th ed., ed. B. Steinbock, J.D. Arras, and A.J. London (New York, N.Y.: McGraw Hill, 2003), 483-92.

57. S. Sherwin, *Patient No More* (Philadelphia, Pa.: Temple University Press, 1992).

58. M.O. Little, "The Morality of Abortion," in *Ethical Issues in Modern Medicine*, see note 56 above, pp. 492-500.

59. A. Lippman, "The Genetic Construction of Prenatal Testing: Choice, Consent, or Conformity for Women," in *Women's Prenatal Testing: Facing the Challenges of Genetic Technology*, ed. K.H. Rothenberg and E.J. Thomson (Columbus, Ohio: Ohio State University, 1994): 9-34; Committee on Medical Ethics, Episcopal Diocese of Washington, *Wrestling with the Future: Our Genes and Our Choices* (Harrisburg, Pa.: Morehouse, 1998).

60. J.R. Botkin, "Prenatal Screening: Professional Standards and the Limits of Parental Choice," *Obstetrics & Gynecology* 75, no. 5 (1990): 875-80.

61. A. Allen, "Abortion: Legal and Regulatory Issues," in *Encyclopedia of Bioethics*, see note 18 above, vol. 1, pp. 18-28.

62. American College of Obstetricians and Gynecologists, Executive Board, *ACOG Statement of Policy, Abortion Policy*, reaffirmed September 2000 (Washington, D.C.: ACOG, 2000).

63. See note 61 above.

64. American College of Obstetricians and Gynecologists, "Medical Management of Abortion," *Clinical Management Guidelines for Obstetrician-Gynecologists, ACOG Practice Bulletin* 26 (Washington, D.C.: ACOG, 2001).

65. J. Feder, *The History and Effect of Abortion Conscience Clause Laws* (Washington, D.C.:

Penny Hill Press, 2004).

66. *Hodgson v. Minnesota* 497 U.S. 417 (1990).

67. See note 62 above.

68. *Stenberg v. Carhart* 530 U.S. 914 (2000).

69. *Hill v. Colorado* 530 U.S. 703 (2000).

70. See note 2 above.

71. B. Steinbock, "Maternal-Fetal Relationship: Ethical Issues," in *Encyclopedia of Bioethics,* see note 15 above, vol. 3, pp. 1472-8.

72. American College of Obstetricians and Gynecologists, *Patient Choice in the Maternal-Fetal Relationship,* committee opinion no. 214, April 1999; content revised January 2004 (Washington, D.C.: ACOG, 2004): 34.

73. *In re A. C.,* 573 A.2d 1235 (D.C. App. 1990).

74. L. Nelson, "Legal Dimensions of Maternal-Fetal Conflict," *Clinical Obstetrics and Gynecology* 35 (1992): 738-49.

75. National Institute on Drug Abuse, *National Household Survey on Drug Abuse* (Rockville, Md.: U.S. Department of Health and Human Services, 1990, DHHS publication no. (ADM) 901681).

76. American College of Obstetricians and Gynecologists, *Substance Abuse,* technical bulletin no. 194 (Washington, D.C.: ACOG, 1994).

77. American College of Obstetricians and Gynecologists Committee Opinion, *At-Risk Drinking and Illicit Drug Use: Ethical Issues in Obstetric and Gynecologic Practice,* committee opinion 294 (Washington, D.C.: ACOG, 2004).

78. Ibid.

79. *Ferguson v. City of Charleston,* 121 S. Ct. 1281 (2001).

80. W. Chavkin, "Mandatory Treatment for Drug Use During Pregnancy," *Journal of the American Medical Association* 266, no. 11 (1991): 1556-61.

81. R.W. Rebar and A.H. DeCherney, "Assisted Reproductive Technology in the United States," *New England Journal of Medicine* 350 (2004): 16.

82. J. Robertson, *Children of Choice: Freedom and the New Reproductive Technologies* (Princeton, N.J.: Princeton University Press, 1994).

83. A. Verhey, "On Having Children and Caring for Them: Becoming and Being Parents," in *Christian Faith, Health, and Medical Practice,* ed. H. Bouma, III (Grand Rapids, Mich.: W.B. Eerdmans, 1989).

84. Catholic Church, Congregation for the Doctrine of the Faith, *Instruction on Respect for Human Life in Its Origin and on the Dignity of Procreation: Replies to Certain Questions of the Day,* pub. no. 156-3 (Washington, D.C.: U.S. Catholic Conference, 1987).

85. See note 11 above.

86. Lutheran Church, Missouri Synod, Commission on Theology and Church Relations, Social Concerns Committee, *Human Sexuality: A Theological Perspective* (St. Louis, Mo.: Concordia, 1981); D.M. Feldman, *Health and Medicine in the Jewish Tradition: L'hayyim — To Life* (New York, N.Y.: Crossroads, 1986); S.S. Harakas, *Health and Medicine in the Eastern Orthodox Tradition: Faith Liturgy, and Wholeness* (New York, N.Y.: Crossroad, 1990); F. Rahman, *Health and Medicine in the Islamic Tradition* (New York, N.Y.: Crossroads, 1987).

87. S. Elias and G. Annas, "Social Policy Issues in Noncoital Reproduction," *Journal of the American Medical Association* 225, no. 1 (1986): 62-8; M. Warnock, *A Question of Life: The Warnock Report on Human Fertilisation and Embryology* (Oxford: Basil Blackwell, 1985).

88. National Advisory Board on Ethics in Reproduction, "Report and Recommendations on Oocyte Donation by the National Advisory Board on Ethics in Reproduction (NABER)," in *New Ways of Making Babies: The Case of Egg Donation,* ed. C.B. Cohen (Bloomington, Ind.: Indiana University Press, 1996): 237-320.

89. J. Glover, *Ethics of New Reproductive Technologies: The Glover Report to the European Commission* (DeKalb, Ill.: Northern Illinois University Press, 1989).

90. Canada, Royal Commission on New Reproductive Technologies, *Proceed with Care: Final Report of the Royal Commission on New Reproductive Technologies,* 2 vol. (Ottawa, Ont., Canada: Royal Commission on New Reproductive Technologies, 1993).

91. M.J. Radin, *Contested Commodities* (Cambridge, Mass.: Harvard University Press, 1996).

92. C.B. Cohen, "Parents Anonymous," in *New Ways of Making Babies: The Case of Egg Donation,* see note 82 above, pp. 88-105.

93. Canada, Assisted Human Reproduction Act, 2004, available at *http://www.parl.gc.ca/PDF/ 37/3/~arlbus/chambus/houselbills/govemment/ C-6_3.pd*

94. American Society for Reproductive Medicine, "Financial Incentives in Recruitment of Oocyte Donors," *Fertility and Sterility* 24, no. 2 (2000): 216-20.

95. National Center for Chronic Disease Prevention and Health Promotion, "2002 Assisted Reproductive Technology Success Rates: National

Summary and Fertility Clinic Reports,"
www.cdc.gov/reproductive health/ART02.

96. Senate Report Number 102-452 (Washington: United States Senate Committee on Labor and Human Resources, 1992), 2.

97. 42 U.S.C.A. para. 263a-1 *et seq.* (1997).

98. See note 95 above.

99. C.B. Cohen, "Reproductive Technologies: Ethical Issues," in *Encyclopedia of Bioethics,* see note 18 above, vol. 4, pp. 2298-307.

100. New York State Task Force on Life and the Law, *Assisted Reproductive Technologies: Analysis and Recommendations for Public Policy* (New York, N.Y.: New York State Task Force on Life and the Law, 1998).

101. American Society for Reproductive Medicine, *Guidelines on Number of Embryos Transferred: A Practice Committee Report* (Birmingham, Ala.: ASRM, 1999).

102. American College of Obstetricians and Gynecologists, *Multifetal Pregnancy Reduction,* committee opinion 215, April 1999, revised January 2004 (Washington, D.C.: ACOG, 2004).

103. American Society for Reproductive Medicine, *Ethics Committee Shared-Risk or Refund Programs in Assisted Reproduction, available at http://www.asrm.oriz/Media/Ethics/shared.html.*

104. A. Regalado, "Clinical Trials Offer In-Vitro at a Discount," *Wall Street Journal,* 13 January 2004.

105. D.C. Wertz and J.C. Fletcher, "Fatal Knowledge: Prenatal Diagnosis and Sex Selection," *Hastings Center Report* 19 (1989): 21-5.

106. American Society for Reproductive Medicine, Ethics Committee, "Preconception Gender Selection for Nonmedical Reasons," *Fertility and Sterility* 15, no. 5 (2001), 861-4.

107. L.B. Andrews, J.E. Fullarton, and N.A. Holtzman, ed., *Assessing Genetic Risk* (Washington, D.C.: National Academy Press, 1994).

108. See note 88 above.

16

Healthcare Economics: Integral Aspects of Clinical Ethics

Edward M. Spencer and Ann E. Mills

Ethics distinguishes between desired and desirable goals.
— The American Medical Association,
Economics and the Ethics of Medicine, 1936

I. INTRODUCTION

There is no doubt that economic factors are important in considerations of "justice" for all citizens, but is it reasonable to extend a consideration of economic issues to the care of individual patients and to the clinical and ethical decision makers who are involved in providing these healthcare services? In considering this question, it seems obvious that a patient's income, savings, type and amount of insurance, membership in a particular healthcare program, as well as a clinician's need for appropriate income and need to recover the costs of practice, are important and sometimes critical factors in *all* clinical decision making.

Add to these factors the healthcare institution's need to maintain its viability, the insurer's need to make adequate profit, and, finally, the government's need to maintain a viable political and social climate for its citizens — believed by most to include some attention to healthcare — and it can be appreciated that economic issues may be among the most important considerations that surround healthcare decisions.

In this chapter we explore the relationship between the economics of healthcare in the United States and ethical clinical practice within the healthcare system. A number of important questions direct this inquiry: What is today's healthcare system in the U.S.? How did it evolve and how is it changing now? What are important economic considerations in the present system and how do they affect ethical medical care? What aspects of the system directly or indirectly affect decisions about patient care, and are, therefore, of particular concern for clinical ethics?

In attempting to answer these questions, we consider the following issues:

1. The relevant history and present composition of the healthcare system,
2. The major systemwide changes recently adopted or under active consideration,
3. The economic, social, and ethical considerations affecting the healthcare system of today and the near future, and
4. Conflicts of interest and commitment imposed on healthcare professionals by changes within the system, and appropriate responses to these conflicts.

II. THE U.S. HEALTHCARE SYSTEM TODAY

A. Historical Background

The U.S. has had a healthcare "system" for only a relatively short time. Prior to World War II, healthcare consisted mainly of individual encounters between a physician and patient. Most people completed their lives without an admission to a hospital, and some, particularly the rural poor, had no access to medical care. However, all of the fundamental aspects of today's health industry (physicians, hospitals, adequate training facilities, research, and a fledgling health insurance industry) were in place by the end of the war, with their future development dependent on the development of a system to integrate, manage, and finance all aspects of healthcare.

Although there were attempts to institute national health insurance before and following World War II, it was not until 1965, when the Medicare and Medicaid bills were passed, that federal and state governments became intimately involved in the financing of healthcare. Medicare began as a proposal for limited health insurance for the elderly; during the legislative process, it developed into a more comprehensive package of benefits with coverage of major portions of the costs of hospitalization and physicians' fees. (It did not include a prescription drug benefit.) To ensure passage of the Medicare bill, it was necessary to include payment for hospitals on the basis of their per diem cost per patient and for physicians on the basis of their "usual, customary, and reasonable" fees. In addition, the task of administration of this program, including paying and auditing physicians and hospitals, was given to individual private insurance companies. The choice of the particular insurance company to fulfill the needed administrative work was left to the hospitals and physicians.

Medicaid mandated healthcare insurance for those on welfare and for the medically indigent. The federal government and the states share the costs of this program, with the states maintaining most of the authority to set the specific benefit package offered and to set payment amounts for hospital care and physicians' fees.

As anticipated by many, the adoption of a cost-based, fee-for-service reimbursement system for these programs stimulated increasing use of healthcare resources, with concomitant ballooning of costs. By as early as the 1970s it was obvious that the initial estimates regarding the costs of Medicare and Medicaid were wildly optimistic, and that, rather than stabilizing or decreasing the rate of increase of medical costs, these programs had actually led to a much greater rate of cost increases than had been anticipated.

Several attempts at control costs have been made at the federal level, with limited success. In the 1980s, an example that received a great deal of attention was the institution of diagnosis related groups (DRGs), which mandated one specific payment amount for the total care of a Medicare (or private insurance plan) patient who had a particular diagnosis. The controversial Balanced Budget Act of 1997 further reduced payments to providers through this mechanism (after furious protests from providers, an amended version of the act reinstated some but not all cuts.)

Accompanying the development of federal programs has been an increasing demand from unions and from non-union employees for healthcare benefits. Because expenses for employee healthcare benefits are not taxable for either the employer or the employee, historically this has been a financially appealing way for employers to increase compensation to employees. This is changing as globalization is forcing American employers to become more competitive. (Most industrialized nations other than the U.S. have state-sponsored healthcare programs. And although tax relief is provided in the U.S. for benefits offered to employees, it is still a *cost* to employers, which is ultimately reflected in the price of products and services offered by American companies.) As the costs of coverage continue to mount, more and more employers are trimming benefits, asking workers to pay increased benefits or co-payments, or opting out of offering benefits altogether.[1] Nevertheless, voluntary employer-based healthcare coverage remains the mainstay of our present healthcare system for those under 65.

Another watershed event that is expected to add to anticipated costs is the Medicare Prescription Drug Improvement and Modernization Act, passed in 2003 by Congress and signed into law by President Bush. It is anticipated to cost $395 billion over the next 10 years, and much larger amounts in succeeding decades. (According to the Congressional Budget Office, it will cost more than $1 trillion in the second decade it is in effect.[2])

All of these factors have led to a giant healthcare system with interrelated facets, which consumed 14.9 percent of the gross domestic product (GDP) in 2002, or about $1.6 trillion. The rate of growth of healthcare expenditures, which had slowed somewhat during the late 1990s, began to increase again in 2001 (14.1 percent) and continued to increase in 2002 (14.9 percent). It is projected that by the year 2012 healthcare costs will equal $3.1 trillion, and will consume 17.7 of the country's gross national product.[3] If healthcare spending continues to grow in this manner, it could lead to financial catastrophe.

B. The Present Situation

Observers have described the U.S. healthcare system as irrational, a patchwork, wasteful, and unjust. A closer look at some of the more obvious methods and results of this system will reveal the reasons for these attitudes and the resultant strong sentiment for instituting a method or methods for predictable control.

It is estimated that 47 million people (about 18 percent of the general population) in the U.S. do not have health insurance of any kind and are not members of any group eligible for government-sponsored care.[4] A small percentage of this group is economically secure and able to purchase healthcare directly, but most do not have access to ongoing medical care and receive care in a non-planned, haphazard manner in emergency rooms, free clinics, and physicians' offices. Low-income Americans (those who earn less than 200 percent of the federal poverty level, or $28,256 for a family of three in 2001) run the highest risk of being uninsured.[5]

Little wonder that there have been proposals for systemwide reform by a number of economists, healthcare professionals, and politicians. That the system needs reform is a virtually uncontested conclusion. The best route to reform and its specifics, however, remain the basis of fundamental differences.

The Institute of Medicine (IOM), a part of the prestigious National Academy of Science, began issuing reports with relevance to these issues in 1999. The initial report, *To Err is Human,* focused attention on the number of medical errors occurring in the system and made suggestions as how to prevent them and thereby decrease costs.[6] A second report, *Crossing the Quality Chasm,* looked in more depth at how systemwide changes could improve quality and decrease costs.[7] In addition to making practical recommendations, like incor-

porating evidence-based medicine in medical decision making, as well as the use of information technology, it offered a unique perspective of the healthcare system. The report took the view that the healthcare system and its components are "complex adaptive systems."

A complex adaptive system is a system composed of human beings who have the ability to change both the goals of the system and the system itself. The IOM report suggested that if all components of the system adopt one goal — to continually reduce the burden of illness, injury, and disability, and to improve the health and functioning of the people of the U.S. — then it would naturally follow that the goal would be achieved. While this insight concerning systems and their behavior might very well be helpful on an organizational level or more micro level, on a system-wide level, it is, in our opinion, naïve. It fails to make a realistic or "business" case for incorporating quality considerations, rather than cost considerations, in decision making. Nevertheless, the report set the stage for addressing system wide change.

In 2004, IOM issued a report, *Insuring America's Health,* which contained recommendations concerning the structure and operation of the future healthcare system, as well as a specific timeline to reach the goals set by the IOM.[8] The IOM recommended that by 2010 everyone living in the U.S. should have health insurance. Underlying this "universal insurance" recommendation are four other "principles":

1. Healthcare coverage should be continuous.
2. Healthcare coverage should be affordable to individuals and families.
3. The health insurance strategy should be affordable and sustainable for society.
4. Healthcare coverage should enhance health and well-being by promoting access to high-quality care that is effective, efficient, safe, timely, patient-centered, and equitable.

Few will argue with IOM's goals; however, how to achieve them is and will likely continue to be a matter for controversy. Numerous polls have reported that the U.S. public desires change in the healthcare system. Many individuals polled have articulated a fear of losing health insurance and being financially devastated by one or more illnesses. Most see universal access to healthcare as a positive societal goal and would like to see provision of a universal coverage plan, but are at the same time concerned about the costs involved in guaranteeing access to healthcare for all citizens.

Professional organizations such as the American Medical Association (AMA) and the American Nurses Association (ANA) have, until relatively recently, paid little attention to economic considerations and their relationship to ethical practice. At one time, questions of whether a patient was able to pay for medical care, who was responsible for payment, and whether it was ethical to refuse to treat a patient based on ability to pay, were left to the individual practitioner or healthcare institution to decide. During the past few years, however, these issues have been addressed in professional codes. The AMA's *Principles of Medical Ethics* includes, as Principle IX: "A physician shall support access to medical care for all people,"[9] while the ANA's *Code for Nurses* includes the statement, "The nurse collaborates with other health professionals and the public in promoting community, national, and international efforts to meet health needs."[10] The codes address principles of practice and ethical guidelines for healthcare professions, but there has been little specific guidance as to how the system should be changed to assure better results.

C. Recent Changes

Before looking at major recent changes to the healthcare system, a brief overview of the causes of ever-increasing healthcare costs is in order. The Health Care Financing Administration (HCFA), which was replaced in 2001 by the Centers for Medicare and Medicaid Services, used the following method to simplify consideration of the causes of increased healthcare costs. HCFA divided the increases in healthcare costs into four different categories:

1. General inflation, based on the overall increase in the Consumer Price Index;
2. Population increase;
3. Medical inflation, based on the price increases in a defined "medical market basket"; and
4. Intensity, which refers to new goods and services secondary to new technologies, new procedures, personnel, and other resources.[11]

Consideration of each of these categories separately added to the understanding of the areas that had to be adequately addressed before any major

changes to control costs or enhance quality and efficiency were instituted.

Obviously, no systematic approach to healthcare delivery and financing can control the increase in healthcare costs attributable to general inflation. Institutions and individuals in the healthcare system must buy basic goods and services in the open market and must pay for these goods and services at a rate that is equivalent to that charged other individuals and institutions in the rest of the economy.

It is also true that no changes in healthcare delivery and financing will affect the increase in healthcare costs attributable to population increase. The growing population, particularly in the post-50 age group, which consumes healthcare resources at a greater rate than the rest of the population, will add significantly to the problems of controlling future healthcare costs.

The two causes of increasing healthcare costs that *can* be addressed are medical inflation and intensity of care. To date, much attention has been focused on medical inflation; intensity has been, if not ignored, at least given less attention than it may deserve.

It has been politically popular to suggest that controlling drug prices and decreasing the costs of the bureaucracy that surround healthcare financing (medical inflation) can lead to continuing savings. And indeed, there is merit in this argument. The proliferation of "me too" drugs that are designed to replace those drugs which are about to go off-patent (and hence are marketed as generics) is an increasing cause for concern. "Me too" drugs, in the main, perform the same function as their older counterparts, but slight variations in their chemical compositions or perceived therapeutic use can be the basis for a new patent — and the monopoly prices they command. Direct-to-consumer advertising expands and/or creates demand for these drugs, which may offer little or no benefit over older drugs.[12]

Managed care, which applies management techniques derived from business and industry to healthcare, has been effective in decreasing the bureaucratic inefficiencies that are inherent in the present system, and it has been widely credited for the declining growth in the healthcare costs in the late 1990s. However, few politicians and managed-care representatives have called attention to the fact that the use of new and expensive technologies and techniques (intensity) must be controlled, as well as medical inflation, in order to slow the escalating costs of healthcare.[13] Intensity is starting to be addressed through evidence-based medicine, which we discuss in section III.

Major changes in the financing of the healthcare system that have been or are being considered are:

1. Different models of healthcare plans;
2. A single-payer system;
3. State and local experiments.

Whatever mechanism for the financing of healthcare is instituted, attention to the issues articulated by the IOM (universal access, continuous coverage, affordable for individuals, families and society, and promotion of high quality care) will be necessary to assure that the system instituted is fair and equitable while maintaining, to the extent possible, the desirable characteristics of the former system(s). How to accomplish this is a major question for our society.

1. Healthcare Plans

One type of plan that gained huge recognition in the last two decades is managed care. The concept of managed care is a contractual model of delivery and payment for medical care. Managed-care organizations (MCOs) integrate the different aspects of the system by developing contractual arrangements with each affected sector. MCOs contract with employers and governmental agencies for a certain level of healthcare benefits for employees or recipients of government benefits, thereby providing predictability for healthcare costs. They contract with providers (hospitals, clinicians, nursing homes, home health agencies, hospices, and so forth) for discounted fees for their subscribers or for a capitated rate (each subscriber's total healthcare needs are taken care of in return for one global fee within a specified time frame), thereby assuring providers a certain level of usage. The MCO may act as primary insurer with employers and state agencies.

Although the managed-care model was widely prevalent in the nineties (the proportion of the population enrolled in managed care increased from 13.5 percent in 1990 to more than 30 percent in 2000),[14] it has been declared "dead" by some prominent observers of the healthcare system.[15] Many observers believe that the fatal mistake of managed care was to try and navigate tensions between limited resources and the unlimited expectations of consumers without explaining to the American public what it was trying to do (that is, to control costs.)

Consumer backlash in the late 1990s and early 2000s against managed care, coupled with a tight labor market, forced employers to retreat from many of the cost-containment strategies introduced by managed care. Many believed that economic prosperity, the skepticism of government and corporate dominance, and unparalleled access to information through the internet foretold a new consumer-driven healthcare system.[16] And, to some extent, this anticipation was realized as employers responded to the managed-care backlash. But as employers relaxed access and as MCOs relaxed utilization review, gatekeeping mechanisms, and other forms of cost-control, not surprisingly, costs increased, and, along with increases came premium increases — which, in a global market, cannot be sustained.

By failing to control patients' and potential patients' behaviors and expectations, managed care ultimately failed to control the costs of care. Ominous warnings have come from prestigious watch dog groups like the Kaiser Family Foundation and Health Research and Educational Trust, who report the fourth straight year of double digit growth in employer healthcare related premiums.[17]

But managed-care companies learned from their mistakes. They learned that controlling expectations must be accompanied by choice, and that choice is expensive. They also learned that physicians feel uncomfortable in a cost-containment role. Most physicians want to be patient advocates — not bookkeepers. Thus, insurance companies are beginning to focus on the consumer and are reinventing health insurance with an eye toward segmenting the market. (Some return to managed-care mechanisms can be expected in the short term, as costs continue to increase. But in the same way that employers are moving away from controlling pension plan choices, employers are moving away from controlling their employees' healthcare plan choices.)

Insurance companies have changed their focus from controlling physician behavior to trying to influence the cost-conscious behavior of patients and potential patients through offering different pricing for different products. This strategy offers different patient groups different products based on benefits, networks, and medical management. This includes multiple medical care options, ranging from large preferred provider networks to vertically integrated groups, with varying amounts of co-payments, coinsurance, and deductibles with benefits being either slim or rich. Networks are ranked on breadth and cost-consciousness (and so costs to employees will vary by network) and incentives are embedded in medical management initiatives, to influence patients with chronic diseases to change their behavior toward complying with diet, exercise, and medication therapies.[18]

How this will play out in the future is problematic. Promoting cost-conscious behavior among patients who are the actual consumers of healthcare insurance products may prove to be controversial, especially if patients reject appropriate choices at the expense of their health; on the other hand, it may force people to confront their expectations of the healthcare delivery system.

2. Single Payer

A number of economists, politicians, and physicians have advocated changing the U.S. healthcare system to one in which the government is the only source of payment into the system. Canada has a healthcare system based on this concept. This type of system involves overt rationing and has been difficult to sell to the American public. Also, under this type of system, insurance companies, an important and powerful economic force in the U.S., would no longer have any part in the healthcare payment business. With the public that is worried about the lack of quality of "socialized medicine" and the controls that accompany it, institution of a single-payer system is not politically feasible now, and is likely to remain difficult unless cost increases become unsustainable.

3. State and Local Experiments

A number of states, cities, and other geographical and political entities are attempting major changes in one or more aspects of the healthcare system. For example, the state of Oregon has attempted to address the problem of access to healthcare by legislating universal access for its citizens whose individual incomes are below a certain level. This mandate for access was accompanied by the development of a list of medical problems and treatments, ranked in order of priority, for which the state would or would not pay under the new system. The state legislature passed this overt rationing scheme after several years of

town and community meetings that were designed to educate all of Oregon's citizens about the necessity for such a system. The prioritization of the types of medical interventions for which the state will pay is the responsibility of a diverse citizens' panel that is expected to be responsive to the citizens of Oregon. Implementation of this plan has proven to be more difficult than expected, due to controversies about what was and was not covered (the rationing question). Other states and localities have attempted or are attempting similar interventions or interventions based on the concept of managed care. Another statewide universal access plan for low income residents in Tennessee (TennCare) was abandoned in late 2004, due to major cost overruns that had escalated at an unsustainable rate.

Arguments concerning the direction and scope of additional changes in the healthcare delivery and financing system will certainly continue, but managed care is a prominent model for the delivery system, at least within the public sector. Whether emerging models of healthcare delivery will prove to be responsive to the numerous problems inherent in the system still remains to be seen. Major shifts from differentiated models or managed care toward either a system with greater central control (single payer) or a system driven more by market forces will require a social consensus concerning the proper direction, speed, and specific features of the desired reforms.

III. ECONOMIC, SOCIAL, AND ETHICAL CONSIDERATIONS IN HEALTHCARE REFORM

A. Fundamental Considerations Driving the Debate

Underlying any future debate concerning the effectiveness of managed care and the proper direction for changes are a number of fundamental attitudes and values. Because the federal government seems to have decided to try incremental changes, and because numerous states are attempting statewide reforms, any number of the following individual and societal values and beliefs may affect these attempts at reform.

1. The Current System Is Perceived to Be Unfair

Many see healthcare as a fundamental right, and believe that the government has an obligation to provide healthcare to its citizens in a manner that is fair. Although this concept is popular, it leads to a number of difficult questions, such as the following:

- What is a "fair" method for allocating these fundamental resources?
- Can a system of basic healthcare for all that allows a higher level of care for those who can afford it (two-tiered system) be fair?
- Can one's accumulation of resources be considered a factor in deciding fairness?
- What other factors, if any, should be considered in the development of a fair system?
- Should governmental expenditures on healthcare take precedence over educational expenditures, expenditures for basic services, or expenditures for other services and responsibilities of the government?

2. The Free-Market System Should Be Allowed to Work

Many in our society believe that the free market is the best and fairest way to address economic problems. However, the existing healthcare system is influenced by many "non-free-market" factors, so that a return to a true free-market system is practically impossible.

Supporters of the free-market concept emphasize the importance of the responsibility of individual patients for at least some of the costs of their care, and actively support such reforms as "medical savings accounts," in which a portion of an individual's income could be set aside in a pre-tax account. Medical savings accounts are presently being tried in a number of selected localities as an experiment sponsored by the federal government. Such accounts could be invested at the direction of the owner and the proceeds of the account used to pay medical expenses; or, if the account is not used in this manner, it could be converted to other specified uses. Proponents of the free-market system believe that responsibility for a portion of one's healthcare costs would represent a deterrent to unwise over-use of the system.

Countering this are those that believe that the introduction of medical savings accounts have the potential to destroy the employer-based system of health insurance — especially if medical savings accounts are accompanied by tax incentives. Healthy, affluent workers would have an incentive to opt out of the comprehensive health plans,

thus causing premiums for these plans to rise. The RAND group and the Urban Institute and the American Academy of Actuaries all estimate that premiums for employer-based coverage could more than double if such accounts became widespread.[19]

3. Controlling Development and Use of Technology Will Control Healthcare Costs

The increased use of new techniques and technologies in recent years, as well as the introduction of "me too" and new drugs has been the most important factor in the escalation of healthcare costs, and this issue must be realistically addressed by any healthcare financing plan. If there is to be lasting control of the rapid increases in healthcare costs, this issue must be addressed fully and honestly.

4. Medical Research and Development Will Lead to Greater Efficiency and Lower Costs

Many believe that research will solve most healthcare problems, and will ultimately decrease costs. Research has solved many important healthcare problems, and, in some areas, has led to decreasing costs. Research has also supported dramatic increases in new technologies and new drugs, which have led to major increases in healthcare costs. Whether the benefits afforded by these new technologies and drugs have been or will be worth the costs is a question that is only just beginning to attract attention.

5. Medical Outcome Studies Will Demonstrate the "Best" Treatments and Thereby Increase Efficiency and Lower Costs

The IOM in its report, *Crossing the Quality Chasm,* recommends using the "best practice" or evidence-based medicine studies to determine the "quality" of specific medical treatments. The goal is to develop "practical guidelines" from these studies, which will outline the most acceptable overall treatment protocol for each specific disease entity. Although practice guidelines, derived from appropriate outcome studies, may be of help, they will be difficult to apply to all patients equally. Individual physiological variations, the value judgments of patients and clinicians, judgments about cost-benefit ratios of particular interventions, and possible mistakes in the outcomes studies themselves may make these studies less authoritative than expected. Also, the costs

of good outcome studies, for even common illnesses, may be prohibitive. Like DRGs in the
1980s, practice guidelines may be helpful but are
unlikely to be "the" answer.

6. Increased Spending for Preventive Medicine Will Decrease Overall Costs

Although spending on preventive medicine
may increase the quality of life for many citizens,
it will seldom lead to decreased overall costs in
the healthcare system. Preventive-care interventions, particularly in adults, often help citizens
who have greater healthcare needs to live longer
and consume more healthcare resources. Most individuals agree that this is a benefit to our society, but it does not lead to a systemwide decrease
in costs.

7. Changes in End-of-Life Decision Making Will Decrease Overall Healthcare Costs

Emanuel and Emanuel published an important article, "The Economics of Dying," that challenged the premise that reforms in decisions about
care at the end of life and palliative care will decrease costs. After studying the effects of the use
of advance directives, hospice care, and fewer
high-technology interventions, the Emanuels
found that "cost savings due to changes in practice at the end of life are not likely to be substantial."[20]

8. The Costs of "Futile" Care Are Important Contributors to Overall Healthcare Costs

There is an ongoing debate concerning the
proper definition of "futile" care and the necessity for the system to support such care. It may be
that a consensus in society concerning this issue
would decrease the costs of care for a few individuals at the end of their lives, but, based on the
Emanuels' findings, it is unlikely to make a major
difference in overall costs.

9. Education of Citizens Concerning Rights and Responsibilities Related to Healthcare Decision Making May Lead to Decreased Costs

Regardless of the direction and extent of future changes in the healthcare system and its financing, education of the public will be a necessary condition for changes in the system to be effective and successful. An understanding of the
system and its strengths and weaknesses is a pre-
requisite for the public to use the system well and
efficiently.

B. Problem Areas

Certain diseases place a special economic
burden on affected patients and society. Two conditions of this type are HIV (human immunodeficiency virus) and Alzheimer's disease (AD). Other
conditions that are costly, difficult to control and
treat, and manifest a risk to society may be afforded special consideration in the future; but
AIDS and AD are at present the most well-known
the most feared, and have the greatest potential
for quickly depleting healthcare resources.

1. HIV/AIDS

Issues concerning discrimination in the workplace by an employer or by an insurance provider
against those persons who have HIV/AIDS have
largely been answered by federal legislation and
the courts. In particular, the Americans with Disability Act (ADA) and HIPAA (Health Insurance
Portability and Accountability Act) both afford
protections to those with HIV/AIDS, by preventing on-the-job discrimination and protecting the
privacy of medical records. However, there remain
problems that have to do with the costs associated with the disease, who or which entity pays
for these costs, and how funds available to help
finance the costs of it are managed.

Problems in the private sector generally center on coverage issues. For instance, persons with
HIV/AIDS who do not have group coverage, can
effectively be "priced out" of the market for insurance, as HIV/AIDS is considered "uninsur-
able." Persons with HIV/AIDS, especially those
who work for a small employer, can find their
insurance payout for the disease has been capped
or that they are facing different premiums. In this
section, however, we will primarily look at the
challenges facing the public sector, particularly
Medicaid. Increasingly, those who contract the
disease are low-income persons who qualify for
Medicare or Medicaid or both.[21]

Spending increases for persons with HIV/
AIDS largely reflect the growing number of people
living with the disease who use new drug regimens.
For instance, the current standard of care, "combination antiretroviral therapy," calls for the use
of three or more combinations of expensive
antiretroviral drugs. Price tags for the drugs range
from $10,000 to $12,000 per patient per year. (This
does not include any additional medical expenses
such as doctor's visits, laboratory tests, and drugs
to prevent or treat HIV-related opportunistic in-

fections, et cetera.) It is estimated that there are 850,000 to 950,000 people living with HIV/AIDS in the U.S. today; currently, 42 percent to 59 percent may not be receiving any care at all.

Programs dealing with HIV/AIDS are often badly coordinated, thus making it difficult to get precise and up-to-date information. The Kaiser Family Foundation estimates that in 1998 Medicaid covered 44 percent of the healthcare costs of those living with HIV/AIDS; Medicare covered 6 percent; private insurance covered 31 percent; and 20 percent had no insurance. Those with no insurance may be receiving care from the Ryan White CARE Act or other "safety net" providers. (The Ryan White Comprehensive AIDS Resources Emergency Care Act acts as a payer of last resort for uninsured or underinsured persons living with HIV/AIDS.) Because recent trends indicate reductions in employer-sponsored healthcare plans, these figures probably understate the number of persons living with HIV/AIDS who receive federal or state aid.

Medicaid is generally the second largest item in most state budgets and the one that is growing the fastest. The costs associated with HIV/AIDS pose serious threats to states that already face budget shortfalls, and so many states are revisiting their benefits. In 2003, for instance, 14 states limited the number of prescriptions per month or year. Other problems under Medicaid that may produce ethically problematic outcomes include eligibility requirements for low-income persons, variations in state programs, low payment rates to providers and institutions that have been shown to affect access to care for Medicaid beneficiaries, and different prices paid by different government purchasers for the same medications. Moreover, it is uncertain whether or not there will be a lapse in prescription coverage when the Medicare law goes into effect on 1 January 2006, as it eliminates prescription drug coverage for those who are eligible for more than one coverage, regardless of whether or not they have enrolled in Part D (the new drug benefit.)

2. Alzheimer's Disease

Alzheimer's disease (AD) is another condition for which current and expected future economic considerations generate ethical problems. AD is a degenerative disease of the brain and other nervous system tissue, that leads to a gradually increasing loss of normal cognitive function. The condition is generally associated with aging, because its incidence and prevalence increase dramatically among people over the age of 70. In the U.S., 10 percent of the population over the age of 65 has AD. This prevalence increases with age; approximately 50 percent of 85 year olds have this disease. The direct cause of AD is unknown; there is no cure or means for prevention. Drugs developed to date only slightly ameliorate the symptoms of AD in selected patients, and they are costly. Significant disability accompanies this condition, and individuals with AD require, in most instances, a prolonged period of constant care. The effects of this condition on the patient and the family can be devastating. A patient with advanced AD, who may live for a prolonged period, requires round-the-clock supervision and care. Few family members have the time, or the will, to undertake the care of an afflicted family member, and the responsibility for this care in the home must be shared.[22]

Other facts that show the real and potential economic impact of AD include:

- National direct and indirect annual costs of caring for individuals with Alzheimer's disease are at least $100 billion, according to estimates used by the Alzheimer's Association and the National Institute on Aging.[23] These costs are expected to rise as the disease affects the fastest growing segment of U.S. society.
- Alzheimer's disease costs American business $61 billion a year, according to a report commissioned by the Alzheimer's Association. Of that figure, $24.6 billion covers Alzheimer healthcare and $36.5 billion covers costs related to caregivers of individuals with Alzheimer's, including lost productivity, absenteeism, and worker replacement.[24]
- The average cost for nursing home care is $42,000 per year, but it can exceed $70,000 per year in some areas of the country.[25]
- By 2010, Medicare costs for beneficiaries with Alzheimer's are expected to increase 54.5 percent, from $31.9 billion in 2000 to $49.3 billion, and Medicaid expenditures on residential dementia care will increase 80 percent, from $18.2 billion to $33 billion in 2010, according to a report commissioned by the Alzheimer's Association.[26]

Costs associated with the care of Alzheimer's patients have obvious economic implications, and various agencies are trying to find innovative ways to manage costs effectively. But there are potentially worrisome issues in terms of what we want (a dignified, safe, controlled environment for Alzheimer's patients) versus what we can afford.

IV. ETHICAL PRACTICE

A. Professional Ethics

The traditional professional ethics of medicine has defined the duties of its practitioners in relation to activities that advance the best interest of the individual patient, within the context of a relationship based on mutual respect and trust. Professional ethical mandates of both medicine and nursing have, throughout the history of the professions, advocated a fiduciary duty to the patient. But what does this mean? Does this tradition require unlimited duty to advance a patient's interests, no matter the cost or the magnitude of the expected benefit? Do professionals owe any obligation to society when the obligation to a particular patient is in conflict with the interests of other patients, or society as a whole? These questions are basic to each healthcare professional's conceptualization of the profession of medicine and its ethical obligations.

In spite of the universal recognition of the obligation of the healthcare professional to the patient, there has never been a requirement for unlimited obligation, regardless of cost. Consider how the time of a healthcare professional is allocated. The professional's most valuable asset is often his or her time, and no single patient is allowed unlimited access to this asset. If unlimited access to time were allowed, care could be limited to only one patient. Such a pattern of practice would be unrealistic, and is not expected by patients or other members of society. Honoring the physician-patient relationship involves an obligation to devote adequate time for attention to patient's immediate problem(s), their ongoing health concerns, and to patients as valued persons.

Professional medical decision making exists in a broader social and cultural context. To ignore or downplay any of the aspects of this context is to ignore important data necessary for good decision making. Economic considerations have become an ever-more important aspect of the cultural context of medical care, and therefore need to be addressed in clinical decisions that are associated with case analysis or planning for care.

In what follows we look briefly at some of the ethical concerns raised by the last few years under the managed-care system. Most of these ethical concerns can be characterized as problematic effects on patients from managed care's attempts to control physicians' behavior by interjecting conflicts of interest into the physician-patient relationship. In the newer consumer revolution, we speculate that many potential ethical issues in practice will stem primarily from *conflicts of commitment*.

B. Conflicts of Interest and Managed Care

A *conflict of interest* refers to situations in which one's profession, professional judgment, or professional code is in conflict with other demands or influences that, if acted upon, would compromise professional judgment. An organizational demand that questions one's professional judgment or conflicts with a professional code creates one such type of conflict. Conflicts of interest occur in every part of life, as various roles conflict with others: when professional integrity is at question, when there are professional biases concerning judgment, or when demand for financial rewards, cost-cutting, or greater efficiency challenge one's professional decision making. Having a conflict of interest itself, however, is not unethical. It is only when one acts on that conflict in ways that break acceptable rules for sound medical decisions, that jeopardize professional judgment, or that cause harm that the conflict raises ethical issues.[27]

Managed care sought to control costs by putting physicians in what many viewed as ethically unsustainable positions by pitting individual physicians' (and institutional providers') financial interests against patients' interests. This was done with the use "gatekeeper mechanisms," in which primary-care physicians controlled patients' access to specialized services, and were paid "bonuses" for holding down the costs of specialized care; "capitation," in which the risk that medical care might be more expensive for a designated population was passed on to providers (providers had to absorb losses); "utilization review," in which physicians could be deselected (fired) from plans for overutilization of resources within a given population; and so forth. Many of these mechanisms are still used, especially within populations for which the state and federal governments are responsible. However, they are disappearing within much of the private sector. Below we speculate on problematic outcomes associated with the newer plans and practices.

C. Conflicts of Commitment:
New Plans and New Practices

Conflicts of interest are usually distinguished from *conflicts of commitment,* although they often overlap. For instance, in the managed-care model, a conflict of interest might overlap with a conflict of commitment. An example is a capitated system (conflict of interest) in which a physician is faced with limited resources and the question of how best to allocate those resources over a population of patients who have competing needs (conflict of commitment).

According to Werhane and Doering: "Conflicts of commitment are those sets of role expectations where competing obligations prevent honoring both commitments or honoring them both adequately."[28] As a professional with limited time and resources and a variety of professional demands, one is often faced with conflicting demands of one's profession that are impossible to honor simultaneously. Conflicts of commitment also arise as role conflicts. In a complex society each of us has a number of roles, and inevitably they clash. One simply cannot honor all one's commitments as a parent, spouse, citizen, professional, manager, and employee satisfactorily all of the time. Unlike conflicts of interest, one can neither avoid the existence of conflicts of commitment nor avoid acting on those conflicts — unless one simply abrogates all one's duties altogether.

While an in-depth examination of recent healthcare trends is beyond the scope of this chapter, we have two reasons to speculate that after the "death" of managed care we will see more ethical problems associated with conflicts of commitment than conflicts of interest. The first is the new models of insurance offerings, and second is the changing character of physicians' practices, particularly the growth of "retainer practices" and "luxury care centers."

In the newer models of healthcare delivery, the patient is expected to anticipate future healthcare needs and make choices of benefits appropriately. A physician, then, might be faced with a patient who has made unwise choices. Do these choices, made by the patient, define the physician's relationship with the patient? What obliga-

tion does the physician have to advocate for her or his patient when the physician is facing a variety of other demands?

A "retainer practice" is a practice in which a patient pays the physician a monthly or yearly fee for "access." This fee is over and above whatever the physician is reimbursed by insurance companies for services rendered. Luxury care centers are set up by healthcare institutions to provide services to executives and wealthy overseas "visitors." We discuss conflicts of commitment below in the context of retainer practices, although similar remarks can be made about the growth of luxury care centers.

Practices can be based on a pure retainer model. In this case, nothing is changed in the context of the physician's relationship to his or her population although the physician's relationships to other providers might change. In this model, the physician faces the same conflicts of commitment in terms of allocating resources (albeit greater resources) among the population. Or practices can be "hybrid." Hybrid practices are those in which a physician accepts a limited number of patients who pay for "access," as well as those who don't. In this model, the physician might face serious conflicts of commitment as to her or his obligations toward these two "tiers" of patients.

V. DUTY TO CHANGE THE SYSTEM?

Do clinicians have any obligation to change the healthcare system? If the system is not conducive to providing good medical care for the clinician's patients, then the clinician has an obligation to try to change the system as a part of his or her obligation to patients. But does the clinician have a special obligation as a citizen to change the system to one that he or she believes will be more beneficial for society? An answer to this question is less clear.

It can be argued that clinicians' superior knowledge of the important clinical factors that should be considered in all healthcare decisions makes them uniquely qualified to attempt to improve the system for their patients, for society, and for themselves. Activism in this arena is fraught with difficulty, because it requires a commitment of time and other resources with no guarantees of success. However, many physicians, nurses, and others believe that it is a part of the duty of the professional to try to improve the environment in which decisions about medical care

are made. At a minimum, physicians should have knowledge of the system and its effects on patient care and should educate patients about these issues.

VI. GUIDELINES FOR CLINICIANS

The issues related to ethical practice within the healthcare system are difficult issues. They involve values of clinicians, individual patients, and society in general. There are honest differences in these values, and presently there is no social consensus. Ethical concepts held by individual healthcare professionals, codes of professional societies, policies of healthcare institutions, and laws, court decisions, and commission guidelines are often helpful and should be considered in actual decision making.

The following guidelines are a brief compilation of some of the available information:

1. Clinicians should understand the present healthcare system and its effects on individual decisions about patient care and attempt to transmit this information to their patients.

2. Clinicians should maintain their professional integrity and maintain allegiance to their professional duties. This does not mean that every professional must agree with all of the present tenets of the profession, but that clinicians should be aware of their primary professional duties and attempt to fulfill them. They should continue to be an advocate for the care that reasonably advances the best interest of their patients.

3. Clinicians should be willing to challenge the system when it is in a patient's best interest to do so.

4. Clinicians should understand that the healthcare system competes with other important needs of society (such as education and defense), and that it is the function of society as a whole to decide how and where its resources will be spent. To help in this decision making, each clinician may join in the necessary discussions and clarify any misunderstandings or myths.

VII. FINAL THOUGHTS

Beneficial change in the healthcare system will require attention to all of the problems mentioned above — not just by political and social groups, but by the populace in general. Before lasting, fundamental changes can occur it is necessary to address control of research, a public education program that addresses fundamental assumptions and responsibilities of patients, and a re-emphasis on professionalism in the education of clinicians. It is obvious that economic factors *do* matter in ethical medical care. How they matter now and how they will matter in the future are basic questions that must be addressed. The expectation that the citizens of the U.S. will ever reach complete consensus on these issues is unrealistic; however, it should be possible to introduce methods that will support an ongoing conversation about these matters. This conversation should enable all to have a voice in the decision making, and should lead the way to the development of a working system that will enhance ethical patient care.

NOTES

1. J.C. Robinson, "The End of Managed Care," *Journal of the American Medical Association* 285, no. 20 (May 2001): 2622-8.

2. E. Park et al., "The Troubling Medicare Legislation," Center on Budget and Policy Priorities, *http://www.cbpp.org/11-08-03health 2.htm*, accessed 5 November 2004.

3. Data on healthcare costs is available at the Kaiser Family Foundation website, *http://www.kff.org/insurance/oldmain.cfm*, accessed 8 November 2004; see also K. Levit et al., "Health Spending Rebound Continues in 2002," *Health Affairs* 23, no. 1 (Winter 2004): 147.

4. "The Economic Downturn and Changes in Health Insurance Coverage, 2000-2003," see the Kaiser Family Foundation website, *http://www.kff.org/uninsured/kcmu092704 pkg.cfm*, accessed 4 November 2004.

5. "Health Insurance Coverage in America: 2003 Data Update Highlights," see the Kaiser Family Foundation, *http://www.kff.org/uninsured/profile.cfm*, accessed 4 November 2004.

6. Institute of Medicine, Committee on Quality of Health Care in America, *To Err is Human: Building a Safer Health System*, ed. L. Kohn, J. Corrigan, and M. Donaldson (Washington, D.C.: National Academy Press, 2000).

7. Institute of Medicine, *Crossing the Quality Chasm: A New Health System for the 21st Century* (Washington D.C.: National Academy Press, 2001).

8. Institute of Medicine, Committee on the Consequences of Uninsurance, "Insuring America's Health: Principles and Recommendations,"

2004, *www.iom.edu/uninsured.*

9. American Medical Association, Council on Ethical and Judicial Affairs, *Code of Medical Ethics: Current Opinions with Annotations* (Chicago, Ill.: AMA, 2002), xiv.

10. Center for Ethics and Human Rights, *Code for Nurses* (Kansas City, Mo.: American Nurses Association, 2001), *http://www. nursingworld.org/ethics/chcode.htm.*

11. Health Care Financing Administration, *National Health Expenditures, 1986-2000* (Washington, D.C.: Division of National Cost Estimates, Office of the Actuary, HCFA, 1988).

12. M. Angell, *The Truth about the Drug Companies: How They Deceive and Exploit Us, and What To Do about It* (New York: Random House, 2004).

13. T.A. Massaro, "Impact of New Technologies on Health Care Costs and on the Nations Health," *Clinical Chemistry* 36 (1990); see also L. Baker et al., "The Relationship Between Technology Availability and Health Care Spending," *Health Affairs* Web Exclusives, 5 November 2003.

14. *Health, United States, 2001: Urban and Rural Outlook* (Hyattsville, Md.: National Center for Health Statistics, 2001).

15. See note 1 above.

16. Ibid.

17. Employer Health Benefits 2004 Annual Survey, the Kaiser Family Foundation and Health Research and Education Trust, (2004), *http://www.kff.org/insurance/7148/.* Findings also appear in the September/October issue of the journal *Health Affairs, http://www.healthaffairs. org,* accessed 19 November 2004.

18. See note 1 above; also see J.C. Robinson and J.M. Yegan, "Medical Management after Managed Care," *Health Affairs* Web Exclusives, May 2004, W4-269-W4-280.

19. See note 2 above.

20. E. Emanuel and L. Emanuel, "The Economics of Dying," *New England Journal of Medicine* 330, no. 8 (1994): 540-4.

21. The material from this section is largely drawn from the Kaiser Family Foundation, "HIV/AIDS Fact Sheets,"*http://www.kff.org/hivaids/index.cfm,* accessed 28 November 2004.

22. Alzheimer's Association, "Statistics about Alzheimer's Disease," *http://www.alz.org/AboutAD/statistics.asp#9,* accessed 18 November 2004.

23. Alzheimer's Association, *Medicare and Medicaid Costs for People with Alzheimer's Dis-ease* (Washington, D.C.: Lewin Group, April 2001), 1.

24. R. Koppel, *Alzheimer's Disease: The Costs to U.S. Businesses in 2002* (Washington, D.C.: Alzheimer's Association, 2002).

25. See note 22 above.

26. See note 24 above.

27. P. Werhane and J. Doering, "Conflicts of Interest and Conflicts of Commitment," *Professional Ethics* 4 (1995): 47-82.

28. Ibid., 61.

17

Ethics Services in Healthcare Organizations: Assuring Integrity and Quality

John C. Fletcher and Edward M. Spencer

I. INTRODUCTION

In this chapter we address how to develop and evaluate an effective ethics program in a healthcare organization (HCO). The top priority of such a program is to serve patients, clinicians, and other HCO staff when they have encountered an ethical problem. An HCO's ethics program should assure that ethical problems are addressed appropriately and that the ethical climate of the organization is enhanced by the program. To meet these goals, an HCO needs the following resources:

1. Ethically informed clinicians and healthcare administrators,
2. A well-supported ethics program that addresses patient care and organization ethics, and
3. Consistent, known values of the organization that lead to a positive "ethical climate."

How can an HCO's patients, clinical staff, administration, employees, and the community the HCO represents be assured that these resources are of the highest quality and are an integral part of the organization? We directly address this question in this chapter, even though certain aspects have been addressed previously (the integrity of

organization ethics services in chapter 3, and professional and research ethics issues in chapters 2 and 5). In doing so, we will concentrate on the development of the second resource, an ethics program with services for clinical and organizational ethics. However, these three resources are interdependent and mutually reinforcing, so that a discussion of the development of a quality ethics program necessarily involves considerations of the adequacy (or lack thereof) of the ethical knowledge of the clinical and administrative staff and of the values which define the HCO as an ethical entity.

A. Ethically Informed Clinicians

As discussed in chapters 1 and 2, clinicians must have the knowledge to help patients and others be moral problem solvers in issues concerning patient care. A "clinician" is anyone who interacts with patients and their families within the goals of a plan of care (for example, physicians, nurses, social workers, chaplains, and other healthcare professionals). One of the top priorities of an ethics program is to educate clinicians concerning moral problem solving. Patient care ethics (chapters 6 through 15) and issues of economic and organizational integrity (chapter 3) are two overlapping arenas for this education. Administrators, physician "gatekeepers," case managers, and others also become moral problem solvers in cases where economic issues provoke ethical problems in patient care, or when the fundamental values of the HCO are called into question.

B. Healthcare Ethics Services

We recommend that HCOs, when considering the mechanism(s) responsible for enhancing ethical awareness and addressing specific ethical problems, grow from an "ethics committee" framework to an "ethics program," with services for clinical staff, patients, administrative staff, and the community.

There are crucial differences between an ethics committee and an ethics program. Services are hard to associate with a committee, but not with a program. Committees are more expendable than programs. Committees can be easily abolished by decision of boards or administrators. Ethics programs can be considered as analogous to social work or chaplaincy. The level of social work or chaplaincy services might be reduced for cost savings, but an HCO with no social workers or chaplains would be seen as deficient. Over the past 15 years, ethics programs are gaining status that is similar to these services.

Another reason to aim for an ethics program is that it supports a larger vision than a committee does. Understanding the history and scope of ethics activities and how these connect with an extensive literature, nationally significant cases, and the work of national commissions requires such a vision.

A programmatic direction can reduce resistance, especially by physicians. Physicians tend to understand "ethics" to raise only issues about character or the integrity of professional relationships. Believing that an ethics committee will intrude into these matters, physicians often oppose a committee. A program of "ethics services" or "clinical ethics services" provides a clearer message to counteract this opposition.

As mentioned before (see chapter 1), the important aspects of a complete ethics program are:
1. Ethics education for clinical staff, patients, administrative staff, employees, and community;

2. Policy analysis and development concerning ethical issues of import to the HCO, its patients, and the community it represents;
3. Educated and trained consultants to help with ethical problems and issues at the bedside and the boardroom;
4. Defined methods for evaluation of the activities of the ethics program;
5. For larger and well-functioning programs, research on issues of importance to the clinical ethics and organizational ethics communities.

C. Organizational Values

The values of an organization that define its ethical climate are extremely important in all of its relationships. Values that are shared across an organization support a sense of common purpose and usefulness. They can be the defining factor for morale within the organization and the major influence on the perception of all types of problems (ethical and other) that clinicians and administrators encounter. This set of values helps define the HCO for its community and for all who interact with it. This resource is more fully discussed in chapter 3.

II. THE EVOLUTION OF HEALTHCARE ETHICS COMMITTEES

Leaders of ethics programs need to know the national and local history of ethics committees. Insofar as healthcare ethics committees are an expression of a movement to reform a traditional professional ethics of medicine that often espoused physicians' paternalism and secrecy in the care of patients, their history is deeply linked to reform of the ethics of research involving human subjects. One cannot understand the history of reforms in the ethics of patient care apart from reforms in research or reforms in the education of healthcare professionals concerning the fundamental ethical tenets that formed the basis for their practices.

A. Research Involving Human Subjects

Reform of the ethics of research involving human subjects marks the beginning of contemporary ethics committees. Human subjects research raises large ethical issues of voluntary informed consent and conflicts between moral claims on physicians and scientific claims on researchers, particularly when these roles may both be embodied in one person at different times.

In the early 1970s, federal policy and law mandated the creation of institutional review boards (IRBs), the first type of institutional ethics committee. This reform was a response to serious ethical problems in research involving human subjects, first exposed in the 1960s, when civil rights and other movements had the nation's attention.[1] Controversial research projects such as the following were exposed to moral debate beyond the research community, giving birth to "bioethics":[2]

- Tuskegee (Public Health Service, Centers for Disease Control), 1932-1972;
- Thalidomide and the Food and Drug Administration, 1962;
- Jewish Hospital Cancer Study, 1963;
- Baboon-to-human heart transplant, 1964;
- Willowbrook Hepatitis Study, 1965;
- Beecher article, 1966;
- "Tea Room Trade," 1967;
- Fetal research, 1973.

These studies were widely considered to have exceeded acceptable risks or violated the norms of informed consent. In this period, government slowly became an advocate of "prior group review" by IRBs, as government officials and the public painfully learned that reforms were sorely needed to protect human subjects. Several public scandals in research ethics led to change.

The federal government not only learned slowly from these crises, but had a large blind spot about the ethics of research conducted by its own agencies. This is evident in the long-lived study, begun in 1932, of untreated syphilis in African-American males in Macon County, Alabama (the Tuskegee Study). The study was conducted by the U.S. Public Health Service and the Centers for Disease Control (CDC).[3] Government researchers disguised the diagnosis of syphilis as "bad blood," and described research activities, such as lumbar punctures, as "special treatment." The researchers withheld available treatments from subjects, even after investigators learned in 1943 that penicillin could be used to treat syphilis. It was not until 1972 that the study was finally stopped, after a journalist published a story about it.[4] The terrible moral legacy of this study lives on. Many African-Americans are distrustful of research activities today, especially any concerned with ac-

quired immunodeficiency syndrome (AIDS); they cite "Tuskegee" as the main reason for their distrust and fear.[5]

Reform began with two major steps. In 1966, the U.S. Public Health Service mandated a local process of prior group review of any research project that involved human subjects.[6] Ethics review had to occur before scientific peer review at the National Institutes of Health (NIH) could begin. This was a controversial policy decision. Prior to 1966, researchers had almost total power to design and conduct clinical research, subject to norms of professional integrity and informed consent.[7] It became clear that the research community, acting alone, was not able to protect human subjects. It was necessary for researchers to share the power to involve persons in research with others who had no self-interest in the specific project under consideration.

The U.S. Congress took the second step in 1974, creating a national commission to recommend federal regulations to protect human subjects.[8] This law also required that all institutions and entities supported by federal funds practice prior review through a local IRB. The IRB had to have at least one outside member who was not a scientist and at least one female member. Because the NIH and other government agencies were not subject to the 1966 policy, the new law also applied to them. (The blind spot evident in the history of the Tuskegee study had delayed and hindered reform of research activities within the NIH itself.[9]) This transition to shared decision making — between scientists, their interdisciplinary peers, and the public — took several years, with research scandals exploding along the way.

B. Education of Healthcare Professionals and Other Ethics Committees

In the 1970s, concern turned to improving the education of healthcare professionals in the humanities and ethics, to balance the heavy emphasis on the biological and medical sciences. At that time, few schools had more than occasional lectures on ethical issues. Many schools of medicine and nursing have since changed their curricula and have created new faculty positions in medical humanities and ethics. Today, all U.S. medical schools have some teaching in medical ethics, and many have a separate required course or teach the topic in tandem with another required course.[10]

In addition to IRBs, other types of committees began to focus on different ethical issues in research. In the 1980s, the ethics of research with animals came under scrutiny, due in part to the influence of Singer's argument about "specieism." Singer argued that specieism justifies animal research from a premise that humans are superior in every way to animals, and he linked this view to racism and sexism.[11] Although his argument is foreign to researchers, it contributed to widespread public interest in preventing unnecessary pain and harm to animals in research. Federal law now requires that each HCO that does such research have an ethics committee for prior review of proposed projects with most species of animals.[12]

In the late 1980s, reformers identified the need to develop another form of ethics committee to conduct local investigations of allegations of misconduct and fraud in medical science. Although there is ongoing debate about the definition of scientific misconduct,[13] the tradition of self-regulation today requires impartiality in the investigation of allegations. Also, the federal government now requires a course in research ethics for trainees in the biological and medical sciences who are supported by federal funds.[14]

As a consequence of this history, most teaching hospitals and academic medical centers have at least five types of ethics committees:

1. An IRB for prior group review of research that involves human subjects,
2. A committee for prior group review of proposed animal research,
3. A committee to assist with formal inquiries into allegations of research fraud and education of trainees,
4. An interdisciplinary committee for ethical issues in patient care, and
5. An organizational ethics committee that is concerned with the organization's values and how these values support the ethical climate of the organization.

In addition some have a separate committee to address professional ethics issues. One of the main tasks of ethics programs is to support and nurture the work of these committees.

C. Evolution of Healthcare Ethics Committees

In the late 1970s, healthcare ethics committees began to focus on ethical issues in patient care. Why did these groups emerge? In an important discussion of consensus in clinical ethics, Moreno views healthcare ethics committees as creatures of a period of reform and changing consensus in medical ethics.[15] The cornerstone of traditional medical ethics was an "impregnable" doctor-patient relationship, presumably based upon trust (see chapter 2). The ascendancy of the legal and ethical doctrine of informed consent (see chapter 10) required physicians to respect the freedom and equality of the patient. Moral consensus regarding respect for patients' autonomy, initially framed in the context of research ethics, extended to and transformed the old medical ethics. However, proponents of the new medical ethics also wanted to preserve the beneficence-based duties and professional integrity of physicians. It would have been degrading to the profession to view physicians as mere tools of patients' autonomy. Moreno understands ethics committees as an attempt to promote and "troubleshoot" a new consensus with two key elements: an emphasis on patient self-determination and a continuing defense of physicians' beneficence. The interdisciplinary and community composition of committees and their patient-centered mission confirm Moreno's insights.

The early committees were mainly forums for debate and resources for clinicians with difficult cases. Legal cases such as Karen Ann Quinlan (1976) (see chapter 13) and cases involving handicapped infants such as Infant Doe of Bloomington, Indiana (1982) and Infant Doe of New York (1983) (see chapter 14), sparked widespread debate and drew attention to ethics committees as avenues for conflict resolution. The President's Commission for the Study of Ethical Problems in Medicine and Biomedical and Behavioral Research recommended in 1983 that courts be used only as a last resort to resolve decisions for incompetent patients who required medical treatment.[16] Mindful of these new ethics committees, the President's Commission recommended that HCOs were responsible "to ensure that there are appropriate procedures to enhance patients' competence, to provide for the designation of surrogates, to guarantee that patients are adequately informed, to overcome the influence of dominant institutional biases, to provide review of decision making, and to refer cases to the courts appropriately."[17]

A few states have mandated the creation of healthcare ethics committees. Maryland's law, first passed in 1985 and amended in 1987, requires each licensed hospital and long-term care facility to have a "patient care advisory committee" for guidance on request in cases involving choices to forgo life-sustaining treatment.[18] New Jersey began requiring ethics committees in 1990.[19] Hawaii does not require ethics committees, but recognizes their place in decision making in patient care.[20] Hawaii also gives legal protection to physicians who consult an ethics committee and take their advice. Neither Maryland nor New Jersey provides such a shield for physicians, although Maryland's law provides legal immunity for ethics committee members who make recommendations "in good faith."

An ethics program, or its functional equivalent, is now required of HCOs for accreditation by the Joint Commission on Accreditation of Organizations (JCAHO). In 1991, JCAHO required a "mechanism" for "the consideration of ethical issues arising in the care of patients and to provide education to caregivers and patients on ethical issues in health care."[21] This rule was later reworded to require a "functioning process to address ethical issues" in both patients' rights and organizational ethics.[22] (See appendix 1 for the 2004 standards). JCAHO's involvement has dramatically increased the spread of ethics committees in hospitals. In 1989, approximately 75 percent of U.S. hospitals with more than 200 beds and 25 percent of those with fewer than 200 beds had an ethics committee.[23] By 1992, of all hospitals that responded to a survey by the American Hospital Association, 51 percent had a committee.[24] Today, between 80 and 90 percent of all U.S. hospitals, the number accredited by JCAHO, presumably have an ethics committee. Possibly as many as 25 to 30 percent of nursing homes now accredited by JCAHO have an ethics committee, which represents an increase over the number reported in an earlier national survey.[25]

The needs of ethics committees in nursing homes and hospitals are similar in some important respects, although the physical characteristics of nursing homes and their residents create a "moral ecology" that is somewhat different from hospitals. From this premise, Hoffman and colleagues have created an outstanding written resource for nursing home ethics committees.[26] Home healthcare programs represent a third major type of ethics program; Fry-Revere and colleagues have produced the single best resource for the arena of home healthcare ethics.[27]

III. THE CONDITION OF CLINICAL ETHICS COMMITTEES TODAY

Today, clinical ethics committees are in one of three conditions:
1. In a "failure-to-thrive" condition;
2. Evolving from a "committee" to a "program," with services for patient care issues;
3. Expanding beyond a patient care focus and functioning as a full ethics program throughout the HCO.

To some degree, many of the nation's healthcare ethics committees are failing to thrive.

A. Failure to Thrive

A national survey of healthcare ethics committees in 1988 found that, in their early stage, ethics committees defined their tasks as educating themselves and clinical staff about ethical issues in patient care, developing policy guidelines, and providing consultation services on request.[28] At the time of this survey, the most widely used manual for ethics committees also recommended this threefold mission.[29] We urge a departure from this now narrow definition.

Despite widespread consensus about the tasks of ethics committees, another survey reported that many committees were marginal and were "failing to thrive."[30] This condition, which is still common today, is characterized by the following traits:
• Members are ill educated and untrained for tasks.
• Members feel isolated, vulnerable, and marginal.
• The committee is unsupported by leadership and without a budget.
• The committee's services are unknown to the clinicians who most need them.
• The committee is not consulted for significant ethical problems or is not consulted about preventing these problems.
• Family members and patients are infrequent users.

There are several key causes of this condition. The most weighty, which are not a fault of the committee, are (1) a lack of educational and training opportunities for members and (2) disagreement in the clinical ethics community about the appropriateness of standards for quality and performance of committee services.[31]

Ethics committees began as a voluntary effort in a competitive medical marketplace, without the educational and training infrastructure that would secure their place and development in healthcare. As a result, a weak committee usually does not have the collective will to press an HCO's leaders for stronger support and funding. (The issue of education and training is discussed more fully below.) Also, the bioethics movement and the academic community have not put a high priority on ethics services, as they did on academic endeavors such as teaching and research.

This generic weakness is no secret and is communicated clearly to clinicians. Clinicians' resistance to using committees can be well-grounded in some cases. Clinicians may genuinely lack information about why a committee exists and how it can serve them. In the early "committee" stage, the group can present an unappealing and even threatening face to clinicians. If members do no serious study or training for their tasks, clinicians are right to be concerned that committee deliberations will be thin or out of touch with the clinical ethics and health law literature.

In addition, sensitive clinicians may be concerned about privacy and the rights of patients. Some committees make decisions about difficult cases "behind closed doors" at the request of clinicians who approach the committee without notifying the patient or surrogate decision makers.[32] The committee may not follow or even be aware of standards of due process.[33] The degree of respect for confidentiality and privacy is difficult to judge, but ethics consultants can easily obtain patients' charts without patients' knowledge. Implementation of federal HIPAA (Health Insurance Portability and Accountability Act) regulations in April 2004 has increased all clinicians' (and HCO administrators') attention to issues of confidentiality in medical facilities, by mandating a number of stringent requirements relating to patients' confidentiality.[34] HIPAA obviously increases attention to issues of confidentiality within HCOs, and many ethics committees are involved in developing appropriate confidentiality policies for their institutions. It is assumed that attention to confidentiality in the activities of the ethics program itself will be enhanced by this increased attention throughout the institution but exactly how this will affect ethics consultants is yet to be determined.

Further, clinicians cannot fail to note the paucity of controlled studies showing the benefits of ethics consultation.[35] This lack of good studies has lowered expectations about the work of committees, and may have increased physicians' skepticism about contacting ethics committees in ethically troubling cases.

In addition, physicians may be wary of contacting committees because of potential legal liability. They mistakenly, but understandably, fear that their choices will be legally bound by a committee's recommendation. In HCOs where the ethics committee is weak and marginal, observant clinicians may also see a potential for "ethics disasters" waiting to happen. Poorly led committees or arbitrary decision making are invitations to lawsuits. Lawsuits are a predictable result of violating simple rules of due process or overreaching an educational and advisory role.[36] Six lawsuits in which ethics committees or consultants were named or negatively implicated will be reviewed later in this chapter.

Role conflicts in an organization between the ethics committee, legal officers, and risk managers can cause a committee to become passivie and confused. The committee's role can be displaced by legal and risk-management concerns. Macklin describes a situation in which legal fears undermined a committee's efforts to shape a hospital policy for pregnant women whose beliefs as Jehovah's Witnesses led them to refuse blood transfusions.[37] A committee can abdicate its mission in ethics to risk-management concerns.[38]

As a result of these problems, there is more criticism of ethics committees[39] and of ethics consultation in the context of committees[40] than praise in the literature. Healthcare ethics committees do not enjoy a good reputation. What are the remedies for "failure to thrive"?

B. Strategies for Change

1. Local Strategies: A Programmatic Goal

Various local (institutional) and regional strategies may prove to be effective.[41] The local strategy is to transform the committee's role in the HCO. The goal is to develop the committee into an ethics program that offers services, has its own internal resource persons, and has a budget for operations. The local strategy requires the following steps:

* With support of the HCO leadership, create a work plan that sets as a goal, that the ethics committee will evolve to a new programmatic stage.

- Identify two or more persons in the HCO who desire to make clinical ethics part of their career goals, and invest in their training and education.
- Adopt and implement standards for quality in operation of the committee and its services.[42]
- Adopt and implement standards for education and training of committee members.[43]
- Adopt and implement higher standards for those who provide ethics consultation.[44]
- Develop a capacity for program evaluation and targeted research.
- Join in partnership with others to create a regional or statewide network[45] to support the effort to address the problems of ethics committees.

2. Regional Strategies: Programs for Education and Training in Clinical Ethics

A local strategy will be ineffective without larger regional or statewide strategies. Such larger strategies require the creation of programs for both short-term education and training and long-term education and training.

a. Short-term education and training.[46] The first activity is a conference for education and training of local resource persons, chairpersons, and key committee members. The model is one of brief leadership training, with a time commitment of no more than five or six days.

During the conference, the resource persons develop a plan to create or strengthen their ethics program. The conference gives the HCO an opportunity to select candidates as resource persons and send them to training. The resource persons' assignment is unambiguous: they are expected to develop a plan, return to the HCO, and implement the plan. It is important, of course, that the leadership of the HCO share the same intent for the program as the resource persons. The educational aims of the short-term conference include the following:

- Review the history of healthcare ethics committee and its present situation;
- Review the potential of ethics programs in HCOs with a candid analysis of one's own situation;
- Study the major ethical obligations and problems facing clinicians, patients, and HCOs today, including managed care and economic issues;
- Careful assessment, with the assistance of

guest speakers, of the best examples of the four services of ethics programs (education, policy development, consultation, and targeted research);
- Interaction with clinicians who have benefited from the services of an ethics program and who are articulate about ethical issues;
- Discussions of specific issues in healthcare law (decision making about treatment at the end of life, informed consent, patient capacity, advance directives, and so forth);
- daily seminars on the practical aspects of starting or strengthening an ethics program;
- Participation in several "mock" ethics consultations for practice and reflection (mock consultations are included in appendix 3);
- Consideration of ways one's HCO and ethics program could respond to the "organizational ethics" requirement of JCAHO;
- Sharing with other participants and instructors the elements of a one-year work plan before returning to the HCO.

b. Long-term education and training. The second activity in a regional strategy consists of a long-term education and training program in clinical ethics. Ideally this program should be conducted on a graduate level with qualified faculty. This strategy requires a partnership that consists of the following groups:
- A university-based clinical ethics center with an outreach program and a graduate program offering one or more advanced degrees in clinical ethics,
- Adjunct regional faculty qualified to teach courses,
- A university division of continuing education,
- Regional or statewide bioethics networks,
- HCOs that are willing to share costs with participants whom they sponsor.

Within this partnership, three types of programs can be offered:
1. A program that thoroughly introduces ethics committee members to the content of clinical ethics and the services of an ethics program,
2. A longer program of studies and clinical training that prepares the HCO's resource persons in much more depth than the short conference,
3. A master's level program in clinical ethics for professionals who not only want to serve an HCO's ethics program, but also wish to teach within the region and beyond.

These interdependent local and regional activities will provide the support systems ethics committees need to thrive. Partnerships for education and training need to be created regionally and cooperatively by the professional community in healthcare ethics. The ideal outcome would be accreditation of regional and statewide education and training programs in clinical ethics by the relevant professional societies. Accreditation of education and training programs will help the field of healthcare ethics pass milestones recognized by the larger community and society.

Certification or licensing of individuals to "do" clinical ethics is an unreasonable goal, considering the diverse professional backgrounds of those involved in ethics programs. Certification is unnecessary, because ethics services are not reimbursed in any healthcare system, although the costs of ethics services are allocated in daily patient charges. Ethics services are contributed by the HCO, as are pastoral care and social work. The most important reason to oppose certification is that it would undermine the premise that clinicians are the primary actors in moral problem solving in the clinical setting.

IV. THE SERVICES OF AN ETHICS PROGRAM

With support from the HCO and educational and training opportunities from the clinical ethics community of the region, it is possible to make a transition from the committee stage to a functional ethics program. A full ethics program for an HCO consists of seven components. Four of these are "services" for issues related to patient care (mentioned earlier in this chapter), which can also be developed and extended to organizational ethics. These four services are indicated with an asterisk (*).

1. An interdisciplinary ethics committee[47] that reports to the HCO's governing body, which has a mission statement specifying that it shall provide or oversee the provision of the services outlined below.[48]
2. Education in clinical ethics for the clinicians who serve patients in the HCO and for the community that is served by the HCO.
3. Assistance to the HCO and the community with policy development — on request or at the initiative of the ethics committee.
4. Ethics case consultation, on request, to assist with ethical problems that arise in patient care.

5. Resources for program evaluation and targeted research aimed to prevent ethical problems in the HCO or community that affect patient care.
6. At least two resource persons, selected from clinicians or other professionals in the HCO, to receive advanced education in clinical ethics and to be compensated for time serving the ethics program.
7. A process to address issues in organizational ethics and to offer services in this area that parallel and complement the services described above.

There are no data on how many ethics committees have made a transition to programs that provide all of these services, including organizational ethics, but we know from experience that many have.[49] The four services of clinical ethics are discussed in more detail below. These services can best be organized by a division of labor among members of the ethics program and its resource persons. Even in a small HCO, it is unfair and unrealistic to expect everyone to engage in all services.

A. Ethics Education

It is a commonplace concept that an ethics program ought to provide education for the professional staff and community on issues in ethics and healthcare law. Whether education is a "service" depends on how well it meets the needs of those who participate. By planning good educational events and courses, committee members also continue to educate themselves. Smaller HCOs can increase the effectiveness of their educational program by planning jointly and cooperatively with other HCOs in the region on the most important and costly courses and events. In larger HCOs, such courses can become a routine part of the orientation and continuing education of clinicians. Clinicians need the opportunity to study and discuss basic clinical ethics and healthcare law in their local or regional settings. The framework of a basic course in clinical ethics for healthcare professionals can be adapted from the problem-based typology on which parts II and III of this textbook are based.

Each HCO's ethics committee can also provide an open and inviting forum to which individuals or groups can bring ethical issues for study, debate, and discussion. Maintaining a fair-minded forum requires skills in moderating debate that otherwise can easily be divisive and deteriorate into *ad hominem* comments. Good planning and leadership skills are required. Ethics education must also address major ethical and legal controversies in a timely way. The most critical controversies today include the following:

- Unresolved ethical issues of justice in lack of access to adequate primary and preventive healthcare for a number of U.S. citizens,
- The moral effects of managed-care practices on the clinician-patient relationship,
- The moral and legal debate about physician-assisted suicide,
- The results of the Study to Understand Prognosis and Preferences for Outcomes and Risks Treatment (SUPPORT) study (see chapter 1) and their implications for decisions in critical care and making advance directives,
- Disputes about medical futility and community/regional policy needs,
- Issues of genetic testing in individuals and protection from "genetic discrimination,"
- Confidentiality and privacy issues, particularly in view of on-line medical records,
- Issues raised by pregnant patients, especially regarding refusal of treatments or procedures beneficial for the fetus,
- Clinicians' roles in addressing problems of physical abuse in families,
- The use of chemical or physical restraints in long-term care of the elderly,
- The rights of cultural and religious minorities who reject Western traditions of medicine,
- Alternative forms of healthcare and their place in a plan of care.

An effective ethics program has a long-term and an annual plan for education in clinical ethics for clinicians, patients, surrogates, and the larger community. Regular courses in clinical ethics and healthcare law, combined with special events cosponsored by the HCO and the ethics program, work best. Regular offerings afford the best opportunities to evaluate adult learning. The "easy way out" of education is to rely only on special events and outside speakers.

The following objectives should be incorporated into the plan for an ethics education program:

- Conduct needs assessments among relevant groups.
- Involve members of groups to be served in program planning.
- Attempt to reach the entire HCO community.
- Extend education to the community served by HCO.
- Distribute cases or materials prior to course or event.
- Begin and end sessions on time.
- Use recognized and well-informed teachers.
- Recruit and briefly train small-group discussion leaders.
- Plan for evaluation prior to teaching a course or event.
- Evaluate and communicate findings to participants and leaders.

Parts 1, 2, and 3 of this text can be adapted to create a weekly course for fall, spring, or summer. Another format for small settings is a monthly "ethics lunch" that includes discussion of a previously distributed case. Such a session can be conducted entirely as a group discussion with a summary at the end.

Significant new legal or ethical cases or laws create other opportunities for education. When such a case occurs, in-service education is an excellent format for all staff to raise questions and express their doubts and concerns. The services of policy development and ethics consultation provide other obvious educational opportunities.

B. Policy Development

Assisting clinicians and the HCO to develop policy is a service that also uses skills in education and consultation. A service presumably benefits the persons or groups served. The greatest experiential tests of policies are whether they are understood, are followed, and guide actions in difficult cases. An important distinction ought to be made between policy and guidelines. A *policy* prescribes what should or must be done, assigns responsibilities for decisions and actions, and details procedures to be followed. *Guidelines,* by contrast, only advise or suggest approaches, and allow interpretive latitude to recognize the complexities of clinical situations.

Some policies for an HCO serve as a bridge between federal/state regulations and standards of practice within the institution. Clinicians, surrogates, and patients need specific guidance on such matters. An ethics program serves as a resource for policy study and for drafting proposed guidelines and policies concerning ethical issues. Authorities in the HCO should receive the results of these studies and the recommendations of the ethics committee. Among the issues for which JCAHO requires policy statements and guidelines are:

- The HCO's process for addressing ethical issues in patient care and in organizational life,
- Informed consent to treatment,
- The use of family and/or surrogate decision makers,
- Decisions to participate in research or clinical trials,
- The refusal of medically indicated treatment,
- Advance directives,
- Pain management,
- Decisions to withhold resuscitative services,
- Decisions to forgo life-sustaining treatment,
- Decisions about care and treatment at the end of life,
- Confidentiality of information,
- Privacy and security of patients' property,
- The resolution of complaints,
- The procurement and donation of organs and other tissue, and
- Patients' access to medical records.

Additional issues that require specific policies or guidelines are:

- Jehovah's Witnesses' refusal of blood transfusion,
- Informed-consent practices in the context of human immunodeficiency virus (HIV) testing,
- Maternal-fetal conflicts,
- The status of preexisting do-not-resuscitate (DNR) orders in the context of an operative procedure, including dialysis, and
- Counseling parents who want to donate organs of live-born anencephalic infants.

Leaders in the HCO should refer study of these and other issues to the ethics committee as a first step in developing policies that have a bearing on ethical issues and problems. The committee's work is to draft, debate, and recommend language for such policies and guidelines to the administration and governing body. The HCO's description of the ethics committee's role should recognize the committee's responsibility to recommend specific needs for policy initiatives to the HCO's authorities, rather than only entering the policy arena by request. An ethics committee has no authority to make policy, but it has the standing to recommend new directions for policy and should provide data to support recommendations.

The process of developing policy can be educational for the participants, and members of the ethics committee can serve as consultants and educators for the policy planning group. The steps outlined below can be considered by members of ethics programs serving in this role.

1. *Form a policy design team.* Organize a policy development team with representatives from the ethics committee and representatives of groups who have requested the policy, will need it, and will be most affected by it. Define the need or problem and identify others who should be consulted.
2. *Understand the problem.* Collect necessary information to clarify the issues, focus on relevant values and principles, and study paradigm cases.
3. *Identify policy options.* Be able to offer justifications for each option and practical significance for consideration of policy and guidelines.
4. *Provide feedback to key persons.* Convene representatives from the group(s) most affected by the proposed policy or guidelines. Seek consensus on what would be a policy improvement.
5. *Select among policy alternatives.* Prepare final presentation to key stakeholders, summarizing the need, how the proposed policy was conceptualized, quantitative and qualitative information, criteria for selecting among the options, the proposed policy statement, financial impact (if relevant), and a communications plan.
6. *Implement the policy.* Create an evaluation method, including indicators of the effectiveness of the policy and how data will be collected. Identify who is responsible for the evaluation and establish timelines for regular review.

C. Ethics Case Consultation

A long tradition of medicine encourages requesting consultation[50] for a difficult problem in patient care, so the concept of "ethics consultation" for ethical problems in patient care is not a foreign one. Prior to the institution of formal ethics consultation, physicians had traditionally sought ethical guidance from their peers or trusted clergy advisers,[51] and the founders of some medical humanities and bioethics programs, although not physicians, were expected to consult on difficult cases.[52]

Recently, the scope of Ethics Case Consultation (ECC) services has been widening beyond patient care to include questions concerning organizational values and costs and access to medical care. The range of decision makers who are now concerned with ethical problems also include administrators, case managers, gatekeepers, and so forth. Cases in which practice guidelines and cost-effectiveness strategies impinge on physician-patient relationships will increasingly be subjects for ECC.

1. Models for Ethics Case Consultation

There are three major models for providing ECC (see table 17.1). ECC by an ethics committee, with large variation, is the most prevalent model. In some committees, the chairperson assembles an *ad hoc* team of members and others, depending on the clinical issues and the type of ethical problem(s). Some committees identify a subgroup or teams of members who are on-call for ECC. Other committees meet as a whole to consider cases. A second model is an ethics consultation service (ECS) with wide variation in membership and patterns of accountability. A third model relies on individual consultants, who may or may not report to an ethics committee or to a source of authority within the HCO. These differences reflect lack of consensus among HCOs and in the field of clinical ethics about the goals of ECC, access to consultation, documentation, and credentialing of consultants.

A conference on ECC, supported by a grant from the Agency for Health Care Policy and Research, convened in 1995 to develop consensus for a long-term project to evaluate ECC.[53] After extensive debate and revisions, the 28 participants reached consensus on a statement of purpose and goals of ECC, as shown in table 17.2.

This consensus statement is a point of departure for regional and statewide bioethics networks and HCOs to discuss standards, education, and training. The interdependence and linkage of different elements of an ethics program is evident in the statement (such as ECC, education, policy development, and being a good bridge to authority when necessary).

2. Indications for an Ethics Case Consultation

When is an ethics consultation indicated? Some typical indications are when the requester finds that she or he is:

* An interested party to a dispute caused by an ethical problem,
* Genuinely conflicted about the moral options,
* Lacking information or informed opinion about an ethical issue, or
* Mistrusted by patients or surrogates, who perhaps have threatened to sue.

The first three reasons could also be reasons for a patient or surrogate to request ECC. Other situations could also call for ECC; for example:

* A rare or novel problem arises.
* The patient is incapacitated, no surrogates or family can be found, and an important decision about treatment must be made.
* A clinician proposes action that colleagues

Table 17.1
Models for Ethics Case Consultation

Model 1: Ethics Committee
    A.   Chair assemble *ad hoc* team of members and others, depending on the features of the case.
    B.   Identified subgroup or teams of members are on call.
    C.   Whole committee meets to consider all cases.

Model 2: Ethics Consultation Service
    A.   ECS is a mixture of committee members and others; it reports to the ethics committee.
    B.   ECS includes members not on the ethics committee; it reports to the ethics committee.
    C.   An independent ECS reports to medical staff or to no one.

Model 3: Individual Consultant
    A.   Under contract to HCO.
    B.   Part of a firm under contract to HCO.
    C.   Under contract to the HCO's ethics committee.

believe is ethically unjustified.

- A patient or surrogate demands a treatment or action that clinicians believe is ethically unjustified.
- An iatrogenic error has harmed a patient, who remains uninformed along with other family members.

Clinicians, although they share important decisions with patients or surrogates, are primarily responsible for moral problem solving in such situations. But to whom can they confidently turn for assistance? Decision makers need assurance that consultants are adequately prepared for such situations and will not dominate decisions of those with standing to make a judgment. Consultants should be familiar with their proper roles through education, training, and experience. However, the reality is that readiness for ECC and quality of performance varies widely.

3. Scope and Quality in Ethics Case Consultation

Issues of scope of ECC and quality of performance can be addressed together. What is the proper scope of ECC? What are examples of role confusion? What counts as a good ethics consultation? What are the legal risks of ECC? ECC's scope is usually limited to requests for help with ethical problems in a "specific clinical case" (that is, involving the care of an identified patient). The scope of ECC is somewhat elastic. It can extend to policy development, especially on very controversial issues. Many of the same skills and knowledge required for ECC in patient care are needed in consultation with groups that must develop policy when their members are divided in their views. Speaking now only of the clinical setting, violations of boundaries occur if an ECC service or consultant formally responds to requests for the following:

- Professional assessment of the benefits/burdens of specific medical tests, treatments, or procedures. Instead, refer to the proper source of expertise),
- Professional assessment of a patient's decision-making capacity. Instead, refer to liaison-consultation psychiatry, clinical psychology, neurology, as appropriate,
- Requests for legal advice. Instead, refer to risk management or the proper attorney,
- Issues of a clinician's competence. Instead, refer to chief of the medical or nursing staff,
- Issues of sexual or emotional harassment. Instead, refer to designated official or supervisor, unless the supervisor is the accused, then go higher,
- Issues of child, spouse, or elder abuse. Instead, refer to the designated protection service,
- An ethical problem in a location outside of the ECC service's designated responsibility. Instead, refer to most suitable ECC service or person.

No boundaries are violated by brief, informal discussion of such requests, while respecting rules

---

Table 17.2

Consensus Statement on Definition and Goals of Ethics Case Consultation

---

Ethics consultation is a service provided by an individual consultant team, or committee to address the ethical issues involved in a specific clinical case. Its central purpose is to improve the process and outcomes of patient care by helping to identify, analyze, and resolve ethics problems.

To guide the evaluation of ethics consultations services, we propose the following goals:

1. To maximize benefit and minimize harm to patients, families, healthcare professionals, and institutions by fostering a fair and inclusive decision-making process that honors patient/proxy preferences and individual and cultural value differences among all parties to the consultation.
2. To facilitate resolution of conflicts in a respectful atmosphere with attention to the interests, rights, and responsibilities of those involved.
3. To inform institutional efforts at quality improvement, appropriate resource utilization, and policy development by identifying the causes of ethical problems and to promote practices consistent with the highest ethical norms and standards.
4. To provide education in healthcare ethics to assist individuals in handling current and future ethical problems.

Source: J.C. Fletcher and M. Siegler, "What Are the Goals of Ethics Consultation? A Consensus Statement," *The Journal of Clinical Ethics* 7, no. 2 (Summer 1996): 125. © 1996. *The Journal of Clinical Ethics.* Used with permission.

of confidentiality ("Please do not mention names"). One must have a sound factual basis for effective referral. There must also be room for "ethics conversations" with persons on an informal basis, while respecting confidentiality.

Issues of quality in ECC can be addressed at two levels: (1) guidelines for HCO ethics programs and (2) standards for consultants in specific cases. These two levels are interactive, but, for purposes of analysis, they may be separated. We recommend for consideration the Virginia Bioethics Network's (VBN) guidelines for HCO ethics consultation programs.[54] Education and training programs for ECC can also consider the usefulness of these guidelines, which respect the diversity in models of ECC. Three premises underlie the VBN guidelines:
1. Diversity among HCOs in the U.S. and Canada requires a variety of approaches to ECC.
2. Multidisciplinary participation is an important value and safeguard.
3. Standards for education and training for ECC must be higher than standards to prepare an ethics committee member for his or her role.

A high standard of education and training for those who are to do ECC is necessary, due to the challenging nature of the activity and its high visibility. A major error by a poorly informed ethics consultant may adversely affect a particular patient, one or more staff members, or the entire institution.

For this and other reasons, the American Society for Bioethics and Humanities (ASBH) published its recommendations concerning the skills and knowledge requirements (tables 17.3 and 17.4) for those who are designated as "ethics consultants." These recommendations are based on a report, *Core Competencies for Health Care Ethics Consultation,* by a task force that spent considerable time in discussion and study prior to issuing final recommendations. This set of guidelines is recognized throughout the U.S. and Canada. The full report of the task force is available from ASBH, and should be required reading for all ethics committee members, and particularly for all who are involved in ethics consultation.[55]

4. Legal Concerns

What are the risks of liability to those who serve in ECC, and how can these risks be minimized? Several recommendations follow.

- It is prudent to assure, in writing, those who provide ECC that the HCO's liability insurance carrier covers them and pays legal fees for defending them, should they be sued for their role in a case.
- There must be a sound process to approve and appoint those who provide ECC. The skills and knowledge of effective professionals from other fields do not directly translate into those needed for ECC. For this reason, an HCO's board needs assurance that those who provide ECC have adequate education and training. The HCO can be a partner in facilitating such opportunities.
- Members of ethics committees should be careful, but not fearful, of adverse legal consequences. There are risks involved for anyone in patient care, but, compared to the risks of physicians and nurses, the risks to ethics consultants are not significant.[56]

Authorities in health law in the U.S.[57] and Canada[58] have described the grounds on which ethics consultants could be sued for negligence or violating the rights of patients. They emphasize the difficulty that exists in establishing a standard of care for ECC, which will persist due to issues of diversity. Lawsuits in clinical ethics are rare, but suits can and do arise.

There are at least four reasons why ethics committees or consultants to date have been named in suits and judicially criticized:
1. A committee or its consultants strongly take sides in cases; the cases may have varying degrees of complexity (for example, *Bouvia, Baby K* — the cases cited here are discussed below).
2. A committee or its consultants give approval to a process in which a physician takes unilateral action to withdraw life-sustaining treatment over the objections of surrogates (for example, *Gilgunn, Rideout*).
3. A committee chairperson intervenes in the plan of care of a terminally ill patient without consultation with surrogates (for example, *Bland*).
4. A committee, backed by hospital policy, is part of a process in which DNR (do-not-resuscitate) orders are written over the objections of the patient's surrogate (for example, *Bryan*).

To date, ethics committees or consultants have been named in at least five lawsuits and criticized by a federal judge in a sixth. Below, each case is described with comments. Except for the *Bouvia* and *Baby K* cases, all were disputes about medical futility. Ethics services and futility disputes are discussed below.

a. *Bouvia v. Superior Court.* Beginning in 1983 at the age of 25, Elizabeth Bouvia, a quadriplegic suffering from cerebral palsy and painfully severe arthritis, was involved in legal proceedings that upheld physicians' forcefully feeding her by artificial means that she refused. The dispute was daily news for months. She became a patient at Los Angeles County High Desert Hospital in 1985. The ethics committee of that hospital, apparently without dissent, supported her physician's decision to force-feed her by a nasogastric tube. Her physicians believed that her failure to eat more was a suicidal attempt to starve herself to death. She claimed that she was eating as much as she could. Bouvia had been examined by a psychiatrist and found to be a capable decision maker. In 1986, a California court of appeals found in her favor and overturned an earlier court decision that sided with her physician and the hospital. The appeals court ordered the feeding tube removed, and stated: "Elizabeth Bouvia's decision to forego medical treatment or life-support through a mechanical means belongs to her. It is not a medical decision for her physicians to make. Neither is it a legal question whose soundness is to be resolved by lawyers or judges. It is not a conditional right subject to approval by ethics committees or courts of law. It is a moral and

Table 17.3
Skills for Ethics Consultation

Ethics consultants must have a variety of "basic" skills, which are used in straightforward cases, and "advanced" skills, which may be required in more complex cases.

Skill Area	Individual/ at least one member of the group needs	Every team member needs	Every committee needs
1. Skills necessary to identify the nature of the value uncertainty or conflict that underlies the need for ethics consultation . . . *	Advanced	Basic	Basic
2. Skills necessary to analyze the value uncertainty or conflict . . . *	Advanced	Basic	Basic
3. The ability to facilitate formal and informal meetings . . . *	Advanced	Basic	Basic
4. The ability to build moral consensus . . . *	Advanced	Basic	Basic
5. The ability to utilize institutional structures and resources to facilitate the implementation of the chosen option . . . *	Basic	Not Required	Not Required
6. The ability to document consults and elicit feedback regarding the process of consultation so that the process can be evaluated . . . *	Basic	Not Required	Not Required
7. The ability to listen well and to communicate interest, respect, support, and empathy to involved parties . . . *	Advanced	Basic	Basic
8. The ability to educate involved parties regarding the ethical dimensions of the case . . . *	Basic	Not Required	Not Required
9. The ability to elicit the moral views of involved parties . . . *	Advanced	Basic	Basic
10. The ability to represent the views of involved parties to others . . . *	Advanced	Basic	Basic
11. The ability to enable the involved parties to communicate effectively and be heard by other parties . . . *	Advanced	Basic	Basic
12. The ability to recognize and attend to various relational barriers to communication . . . *	Basic	Basic	Basic

* Cross references removed.
Society for Health and Human Values — Society for Bioethics Consultation Task Force on Standards for Bioethics Consultation, "Table 1. Skills for Ethics Consultation," *Core Competencies for Health Care Ethics Consultation* (Glenview, Ill.: American Society for Bioethics and Humanities, 1998), p. 15.

philosophical decision that, being a competent adult, is hers alone."[59]

After the tube was removed, Bouvia and her attorney sued the hospital and the physicians for monetary damages. She learned that her physicians had stated that the ethics committee was as responsible as they were, and she filed an amended complaint against each member of the committee as a defendant.[60] Bouvia never served the committee members and voluntarily dropped the suit to avoid publicity.[61]

The main lesson of the *Bouvia* lawsuit for ethics committees is about strongly taking sides in a moral problem. The degree of complexity of the issues in this case is debatable. For many, the case was "easy." A competent patient has a clear, negative right to refuse any form of unwanted treatment, regardless of its lifesaving effect. The case

is harder for those who make distinctions between feeding and hydration and other forms of life-sustaining treatment. Regardless of debate about degrees of complexity, however, ethics committees and consultants should guard against taking sides and being co-opted by physicians. Their role is to provide education and offer consultation about all of the moral options in a case.

b. *In Re Baby K.* In 1992, an ethics committee at Fairfax Hospital in Virginia had a role in the *Baby K* case, and a federal court judge criticized the committee's participation. The critique will alert plaintiff's attorneys and other interested parties to the criticisms that can be made of ethics committees.

At the physicians' request, a team of the ethics committee met with Baby K's mother, who demanded life-sustaining measures for her new-

Table 17.4
Knowledge for Ethics Consultation

Health care ethics consultants require "basic" introductory-level knowledge in some areas and more "advanced" detailed understanding of topics in others. We distinguish between knowledge that individuals or team members must bring to the consultation process ("needs") and knowledge that individuals or team members must have available to the consultation process ("can access"). All consultants should be aware of their limitations so that they know when they need to seek out those who might have specialized knowledge.

Knowledge Area	Individual/ at least one member of the group needs	Every team member needs	Every committee member needs	Individual/ at least one member can access
1. Moral reasoning and ethical theory as it relates to ethics consultation . . .*	Advanced	Basic	Basic	Not Required
2. Bioethical issues and concepts that typically emerge in ethics consultation . . .*	Advanced	Basic	Basic	Not Required
3. Health care systems as they relate to ethics consultation . . .*	Basic	Basic	Basic	Advanced
4. Clinical context as it relates to ethics consultation . . .*	Basic	Basic	Basic	Advanced
5. Health care institution in which the consultants work, as it relates to ethics consultation . . .*	Basic	Basic	Basic	Advanced
6. Local health care institution's policies relevant for ethics consultation . . .*	Advanced	Basic	Basic	Not Required
7. Beliefs and perspectives of patient and staff population where one does ethics consultation . . .*	Basic	Basic	Basic	Advanced
8. Relevant codes of ethics, professional conduct and guidelines of accrediting organizations as they relate to ethics consultation . . .*	Basic	Basic	Basic	Advanced

* Cross references removed.

Society for Health and Human Values — Society for Bioethics Consultation Task Force on Standards for Bioethics Consultation, "Table 2. Knowledge for Ethics Consultation," *Core Competencies for Health Care Ethics Consultation* (Glenview, Ill.: American Society for Bioethics and Humanities, 1998), p. 20.

born who had anencephaly. The staff of the neo-natal intensive care unit viewed these measures as futile and as violations of their professional integrity. A three-person team (family practitio-ner, psychiatrist, and minister) was unsuccessful in resolving the dispute. Their ECC chart note stated that care was "futile" and advised that the hospital "attempt to resolve this through our le-gal system" if, after a waiting period, no change occurred in Baby K's mother's position. Judge Hilton wrote in his opinion, "treating physicians requested the assistance of the Hospital's 'Ethics Committee' in overriding the mother's wishes."[62] He may have put quotation marks around the committee's name to deride their taking sides and their failure to give due attention to the moral ar-guments for the mother's position. Judge Hilton's ruling that the Emergency Medical Treatment and Active Labor Act (EMTALA) required the hospi-tal to provide emergency ventilatory treatment for Baby K's periodic apnea (Baby K was by then re-siding in a nearby nursing home) was upheld by the Fourth Circuit Court of Appeals.[63] The U.S. Supreme Court declined to hear an appeal by the hospital, Baby K's father, and the guardian *ad litem*. Again, the lesson for ECC is to avoid taking sides in a morally complex case.

c. *Bryan v. Stone et al.; Bryan v. Rector and Visitors of the University of Virginia.* Bryan, the executrix of the estate of a 53-year-old patient who died at the University of Virginia (UVA) Hospital on 25 February 1993, brought two lawsuits. The patient had undergone surgery at a regional county hospital on 14 December 1992 for a perforated pyloric ulcer, with peritonitis secondary to inges-tion of mineral oil. Her postoperative course was very poor: acute respiratory distress syndrome, sepsis, bilateral pneumothoraxes, a code followed by stroke, and inability to wean from a ventilator. She was transferred to UVa for evaluation and further treatment on 5 February. Her condition worsened, and computed tomography (CT) scan revealed a massive left cerebrovascular stroke. In addition, her multiple infections were not respon-sive to antibiotics, and she had massive subcuta-neous emphysema and kidney failure. Her fam-ily, speaking through her husband, demanded that "everything be done," including cardiopulmonary resuscitation (CPR). The medical team concluded that CPR for this patient, who by then had seven chest tubes, would be ethically and medically in-appropriate.

The house staff asked for ethics consultation shortly after the patient was transferred to UVa, but the patient's husband and family would not consent to ECC. It is UVa's policy that no formal consultation can be offered without consent of patients or surrogates. However, the Ethics Con-sultation Service (ECS) continued to communi-cate informally with the medical team about the issues in the case.

The dispute about CPR persisted. The house staff strongly resisted the prospect of CPR for this patient. The attending physician attempted to mediate. When the patient's husband refused to meet with the ECS or come to the hospital to dis-cuss the question, the attending physician re-quested formal assistance from the ethics com-mittee. The hospital's policy is that the chair of the committee can, in such a situation, convene an *ad hoc* advisory group to assist clinicians. Fur-ther, acting under a 1992 amendment to the UVa Medical Center's DNR policy, the *ad hoc* group recommended a plan that began with consulta-tion with other noninvolved physicians about the family's request for CPR, and the potential for transferring her care to one of them. If other phy-sicians evaluating the request for CPR deemed it to be futile, the plan included writing a DNR or-der and an order to withhold CPR for reasons of medical futility.

Two other physicians were consulted. Each came to the same conclusion that the attending physician had reached about the futility of CPR. The patient was too critically ill to attempt a trans-fer out of the hospital. Subsequently, the attend-ing physician wrote a DNR order, informed the patient's husband, and documented his objections. The medical team continued to communicate with the patient's husband by telephone. The patient died eight days after the DNR order was written.

Later, a dispute arose between the hospital's billing department and the family. Risk Manage-ment at UVa believed that the aggravation over billing was the primary causation for an ensuing suit. The patient's total bill was approximately $105,000, and her insurance paid for all but about $2,000. The family, already bitter over the out-come of the case, received repeated bills, with a final notice that the unpaid bill would be turned over to a collection agency. They turned the letter over to their attorneys, who sought and received the medical record. Within the report was a re-port from the Ethics Committee chairperson about the consultation and recommendation supporting writing a DNR order.

In a context of this unresolved grievance and the wake of court decisions in the *Baby K* case, the family's attorneys filed two suits. A suit in county court alleged that the attending physician and the members of the *ad hoc* group had violated the patient's religious beliefs, and specifically some conditions of the Virginia Health Care Decisions Act.[64] A second suit, filed in federal court, alleged that the patient had died as a result of withholding emergency treatment in the form of CPR. In the wake of the *Baby K* decisions, the plaintiffs charged that the hospital had violated EMTALA, aided by the Ethics Committee's *ad hoc* advisory group.

The suit in county court was dismissed "with prejudice," meaning that it could not be refiled. The Fourth Circuit Court of Appeals upheld a district court's dismissal of the federal suit. The federal court held that EMTALA was not violated, since the patient died after a 12-day period in the hospital.[65] This important ruling clarified the Fourth Circuit's interpretation of EMTALA following the *Baby K* case. It ruled that the patient had received "stabilizing treatment" during the entire hospital stay, and the court made no comment about the DNR order. The hospital policy that permitted DNR orders in such controversies was adopted when a 1992 amendment to the Virginia Health Care Decisions Act stipulated that physicians are not required to prescribe or render treatment that the physician determines to be "medically or ethically inappropriate."[66] The law requires that a good-faith effort be made to transfer the patient to the care of another physician; because of this patient's hopeless condition, she could not be transferred.

d. *Gilgunn v. Massachusetts General Hospital.* Capron has discussed the ethical and legal significance of this important case.[67] In brief, a 71-year-old woman in very poor health broke her hip in a fall. Before she could undergo orthopedic surgery, she suffered seizures, followed by brain damage and coma. Her daughter, the surrogate of choice, informed physicians that her mother would have "wanted everything done." After several weeks, the medical team desired to stop treatment that they considered futile. The hospital's Optimum Care Committee was one of the earliest types of patient care ethics committees in the nation; it was a small group that confined its scope mainly to intensive care. The committee's chair

was a psychiatrist with a long-standing practice of advocating DNR orders when incapacitated and hopelessly ill patients had lengthy stays in the intensive care unit (ICU) and families demanded that "everything be done."[68] The chair persuaded the attending physician to write a DNR order, which the attending physician later revoked when the daughter protested. The chair then supported a subsequent attending physician's decision to write a DNR order. The chair and committee did not meet with the surrogate. After a DNR was written, the attending physician gradually extubated the patient over the surrogate's objections. The patient died, and her daughter sued for violations of her, rather than the patient's, rights. A trial court jury sided with the hospital.[69] The decision is now on appeal to a higher court.

Capron is correct in his criticism of the intervention of the physician-chairperson of the optimal care committee. The committee did not act as an ethics committee but, in Capron's words, "in the style of a medical consultant." None of the mediational and educational benefits of ECC were evident in the process used in this case.

e. *Estate of James Davis Bland v. Cigna Healthplan of Texas, et al.* This suit was brought by the family of a patient with AIDS for intentional infliction of emotional harm due to decisions made by the chair of the Ethics Committee that were associated with the manner of the patient's death.[70] The case also figured prominently in a 1995 article about managed care and medicine in Texas.[71]

Bland was a registered nurse who understood that he had a terminal illness and would die soon. In July 1993 he was admitted to Houston's Park Plaza Hospital's ICU and placed on a respirator. He was given a paralytic drug to make him comfortable, and the respirator took over his breathing function. Afraid of suffocating if he was taken off the respirator, he asked his physician to allow him to die peacefully while being ventilated. His physician agreed, and the patient soon lapsed into a coma.

The physician explained his plan to the family, who understood and agreed to a DNR order on the condition that the patient remained on the respirator. Bland's physician then withdrew from the case and turned over care to a Cigna primary-care physician. After a few days, the medical director of Cigna contacted the chair of the Ethics Committee, a pulmonologist. The Cigna official raised questions about the patient's stay in the ICU and whether he could be moved. The chair of the Ethics Committee went to the ICU, presumably in the role of a physician — but not the patient's physician — without consulting the patient's original physician or the patient's family. He did discuss the care plan with the Cigna primary-care physician. As a result of the intervention by the pulmonologist/Ethics Committee chair, the patient was removed from the respirator by a respiratory therapist and died shortly thereafter.[72] The circumstances of Bland's death and the involvement of the pulmonologist/Ethics Committee chair were not discussed with the family. They learned the facts from documents prepared for another lawsuit brought by Bland's original physician against Cigna. The suit by Bland's family was settled out of court for an undisclosed amount.

Questions arise about the Cigna official's motives and the actions of the Ethics Committee chair in this case. These questions cannot be answered without more knowledge of the facts. Was the motive for contact cost savings or the appropriate level of care for a moribund patient? If the former, the chair should not have permitted the contact by the official. It is inappropriate for an insurance company official to contact an Ethics Committee except to identify an ethical problem in the care of a patient.

Even if the pulmonologist believed that he was confining his role to that of physician, he appears to have violated the interests of the patient's family. The Cigna primary-care physician may have abdicated his role by permitting the pulmonologist to go to the patient's room and initiate a process leading to removal of the ventilator with no discussion with the family. If this act occurred, it is morally problematic, because it is a well-established social practice that physicians should share such crucial decisions with surrogates. The act was legally questionable in the light of decision-making criteria required by the Texas Natural Death Act.[73] In today's society, physicians do not have the moral authority unilaterally to withdraw life supports, even from a hopelessly ill patient. To be morally valid, this action requires discussion and agreement from surrogates or legally authorized representatives of the patient, because this action contributes to the timing and circumstances of the patient's death.

The legal authority of physicians to withdraw life supports unilaterally is unsettled and controversial, as shown in *Gilgunn*. Physicians' authority to write DNR orders unilaterally is still con-

troversial, as shown by *Bryan*, but is more settled than withdrawing life supports, as shown by the next case, *Rideout*. However, if it is true in *Bland* that an ethics committee chairperson was the main figure in the decision to remove the patient from the ventilator, without consultation with surrogates, this action should be viewed as a serious violation of the role of ethics committees and a failure of the HCO to take precautions to prevent such conflicts. It is a guideline of the Virginia Bioethics Network, for example, that an ethics consultant should make other arrangements and avoid taking a consultation in a unit where he or she regularly practices.[74]

An alternative course of action in *Bland* was that the care plan drawn up by Bland's first physician could have been reviewed in the context of an ethics consultation requested by the Cigna primary-care physician with the consent and participation of the original physician and family (if they were willing to participate in such a meeting). Also, the original physician and the Cigna primary-care physician could have prevented the original problem by supervising a more rapid process of withdrawing life-support measures with control of distress by analgesics.[75]

f. *Rideout v. Hershey Medical Center.* Brianne Rideout, a two-year-old patient with a brain stem glioblastoma (a malignant tumor), had neurosurgery at Johns Hopkins University Hospital. She was admitted to the emergency department of the Hershey Medical Center in Pennsylvania on 6 April 1992. While at Hershey, she lapsed into a stupor and required assistance to breathe. By 13 April, she had a tracheostomy and was placed on a ventilator. Physicians regarded her condition as incurable, but her parents favored aggressive treatment.

Then began a period of negotiation regarding home care or hospital care. Home care was ruled out due to inadequate wiring for a ventilator. By 20 May, the patient's parents learned that her insurance coverage would soon be depleted and Medicaid was needed to cover costs. The next day, the Ethics Committee met at the request of the patient's physician (without the parents present) to discuss the case, and the committee supported a decision to write a DNR order. On 22 May, when they were informed of this decision, the Rideouts stated that they were opposed, because it meant giving up on the child's life. A search began for an appropriate alternate site without success. On 12 July, the child's pupils became fixed and dilated for the first time. On 13 July, her physician decided, based on discussions with the ethics committee and in the light of the patient's deteriorating condition, to remove the ventilator.

On 14 July, her physician informed the Rideouts that he would withdraw the ventilator that day. The chair of the Ethics Committee met with the parents to confirm the decision. Following this meeting, the parents complained to the patient advocate, who persuaded the physician and Ethics Committee chair to delay to allow legal consultation. Nonetheless, the removal was scheduled for 11:00 a.m. on 15 July. The parents sought a judicial order to stop this action and secured the services of an attorney. The hospital had asked local police to be present to prevent disorder. While the parents were in the office of the patient advocate speaking with their attorney by phone, the physician removed the ventilator. The hospital's chaplain communicated the action to the Rideouts. Hearing this, they rushed to her room. They were described in their complaint as being hysterical and crying that their daughter was being murdered. They requested that the ventilator be reconnected, but the physician declined to do so. Mr. Rideout reportedly had an acute asthma attack. The patient died two days later, in the presence of her parents.

The Rideout's 11-count complaint raised common-law, statutory, and constitutional claims, each of which the hospital contested.[76] On 29 December 1995, a three-judge panel overruled the medical center's challenge to claims that by stopping the ventilator over the parents' wishes, the hospital committed an assault and battery on the child, negligently and intentionally inflicted emotional distress on the parents, and impinged parental rights rooted in the free exercise of religion.[77] The panel refused to rule out punitive damages. The hospital won arguments that it did not violate constitutional privacy and liberty interests and that EMTALA was not violated. The panel's decision meant that the parents were free to continue their lawsuit in a jury trial.

The Rideout case has the classic features of a futility dispute. The Hershey Ethics Committee may have erred in the process of the case in two respects. First, was it good practice to meet originally with the physician without notifying and inviting the parents? An opportunity to engage and involve them was missed. Second, later in the case, was it good practice for the chair to meet with the parents for the purpose of notifying them

that the decision to withdraw would be carried out? Closing out morally acceptable options is not the role of an ethics committee. There were two other options available, even at that point: (1) transfer the patient to an alternate site, or, failing that, (2) to seek a court's concurrence with the decision to withdraw.

At the deepest level, the Hershey Ethics Committee appears to have strongly taken sides with a physician and hospital authorities against the patient's parents. The alternative stance is to offer only consultation, education, and mediation about the morally acceptable options. Also, the committee appears to have been a party to a unilateral decision to remove a ventilator over the parents' objections. In such a situation, the ethics committee's role should be confined to searching for other morally acceptable alternatives to such a morally dubious action. If that search fails, then the physician and hospital should seek the help of a court in resolving the dispute. Physicians and ethics committees are not the final arbiters of futility disputes until our society works out fairer approaches to allocation of expensive healthcare resources. The institutions of law must be involved to ensure the highest standards of impartiality.

Bland and *Rideout* pose serious legal challenges to ethics committees or their chairpersons who strongly take sides and who advocate unilateral decision making in situations involving treatment at the end of life. These cases also bear upon the question of the competence and perspective of those who do ECC. A court has not yet asked the question: "For what exactly is an ethics consultant (or a team acting for a committee) responsible and accountable?" Based on the evolution of these cases, such a question can be expected.

5. The Consultant's Competence and Perspective

The consultant's role in each case calls for competence in two areas: moral diagnosis and education. Depending on the circumstances, the role also calls for skills in mediation and being a trustworthy bridge to authority. Every full ethics consultation has a five-part history:

1. The threshold of the case and the consultant's entry,
2. The consultant's assessment,
3. Moral diagnosis and education,
4. Goal setting, decision making, and implementation, and
5. Evaluation.

a. Perspective. The consultant's perspective ought to value a good process in ECC over the "right" solution to the moral problems in the case. The ethics consultant is not the agent of a higher societal power who is authorized to take over disputes and make decisions. Ethics consultants, at most, represent healthcare ethics, an interdisciplinary field with services to offer, one of which is ECC. Ethics consultants serve decision makers who have standing in the case. Their obligation as moral diagnosticians and educators is to probe the complexity of the ethical problems in the case.

Real differences do exist between the views of ECC that emphasize outcomes and views that emphasize process.[78] Pro-active consultants advocate for their point of view and recommend what ought to be done in a case. Process-oriented consultants favor being educators over being moral advocates. They restrain their desires to determine the outcomes of cases and are willing to leave such decisions to those with legitimate moral and legal power to make them. Pro-active ECC is likely to be paternalistic and assumes too much power and responsibility for outcomes. If it is good to avoid the old medical paternalism, why is neopaternalism in ECC desirable except for a rare "ethics emergency"? And, as in *Bland* and *Rideout,* when consultants take sides, a lawsuit may result.

b. Criteria for Entering a Case. If a consultation is indicated, the consultant enters the case using criteria in the HCO's protocol for ECC. Entry criteria for ECC are recommended in the VBN guidelines.[79] The two most important entry criteria are briefly covered below.

1. *Notify the attending physician.* If the attending physician has not requested the consultation, he or she should be promptly notified, preferably by the person who requests consultation. If the person who requests consultation wants anonymity (usually due to fear of the attending physician), this problem should be solved prior to the consultant's entry. An option is to persuade someone else to request the consultation openly, or to persuade the caller of protection by institutional policy on this matter. Some attending physicians may refuse ECC for their own reasons. However, an open-access policy for ECC requires a process for the chairperson of the ethics committee to have authority to respond to refusals of consultation, to review the attending physici-

an's reasons, and to resolve the problem of how the consultation will proceed.

2. *Obtain the consent of patient or surrogate.* In most circumstances, respect for the patient's privacy requires consent for an ethics consultation, prior to the ethics consultant's seeing the patient's chart. The patient's or surrogate's consent is required because ethics consultants are not part of the healthcare team, and they will have access to private and confidential information. Ideally, the attending physician introduces the consultant(s) to the patient or surrogate.

After entry, the ethics consultant should first review the assessment and moral diagnosis made by clinicians, or make a fresh assessment of the issues. The consultant can then guide the process through efforts to resolve the problem(s) and an evaluation. The steps needed for an adequate ECC are outlined in table 17.5. The contents of table 17.5 are comprehensive and cover the relevant issues in the types of cases in which ECC is involved. The consultant needs the knowledge, skills, and experience to use the elements in this outline that are relevant to the case at hand. The consultant must have the competence to use this process in cooperation with decision makers in the case. Again, opportunities for education, training, and supervision must be created regionally by the clinical ethics community.

D. Targeted Research: From Crisis Orientation to Prevention

Strengthened ethics programs create larger opportunities to serve. An advanced service to a HCO and its community is research aimed to prevent chronic ethical problems. So-called targeted research addresses the causes of recurrent problems, rather than on crisis reactions to the symptoms and consequences of these problems. Targeted research is a good example of the influence of quality improvement on healthcare ethics. Wolf has expertly reviewed arguments for quality improvement in ethics.[80] Adapting lessons from the "quality revolution in medicine"[81] will help ethics programs mature and promote more professional relationships with those to be served. Teichholz discussed the relevance of the work of Deming and others in industry to the quality improvement movement in medicine.[82] By focusing on structure, process, and outcome, quality assurance has been transformed from a formerly "policing" function to one in which the "emphasis is now on finding common denominators and asking what the overall process is and whether it can be improved, not on what is wrong in any individual case."[83] This emphasis could help the condition of ethics services evolve from crisis orientation to prevention. Clinical ethics was shaped in the crucible of acute-care medicine of the 1970s and 1980s. It is not surprising that its role has largely been crisis oriented. Clinical ethics must perform well in crises or "ethics emergencies," but it will fail if it remains in this posture.

Ethics services need a two-level strategy that is informed by reliable knowledge about causation. Strategy at the immediate level aims to identify, analyze, and assist in resolving ethical problem(s) that obstruct planning for the care of patients. Strategy at a higher level aims at interim and long-term prevention of remediable causes of ethical problems. Some human conditions underlie and contribute to ethical problems and cannot be "prevented" (for example, contingency, ambiguity, freedom to choose values, finitude, and death itself). However, some causes of ethical problems can be ameliorated:

- Failure to assess promptly the goals of treatment in patients with poor prognosis,
- Toleration of lengthy stays on ventilators without discussion of alternatives,
- Lack of training and practice in advance-care planning,
- Lacking a prior plan to identify and treat surrogate decision makers,
- Structural and power arrangements (for example, leaving decisions about when to initiate discussion about changing the goals of treatment completely to attending physicians), and
- Lack of financial incentives to promote timely discussion and decision making.

Futility disputes are clear examples of the failure of conventional approaches in clinical ethics, and prove the need for a two-level strategy. The lawsuits reviewed above are important in this regard. Even if the lawsuits had been avoided by better communication and mediation, the disputes would not have been prevented. Clinicians and HCOs are attempting to resolve and prevent bedside disputes about futile treatment by means of ethics committees, hospital policies, and the courts. Although well intended, these are interim approaches, and are unstable as true prevention. Ethics consultation or institutional policies that address such disputes have only minor preventive effects, and, when ineptly provided, albeit with good intentions, such efforts can do harm. It is common in futility disputes for the surrogates not to trust ethics consultants or anyone associated with the HCO. For this reason, a better first-level alternative may be to enlist the help of respected leaders in the community as mediators of such disputes and to ask the disputants to abide by their recommendations as a last resort prior to seeking judicial review.

In the long run, futility disputes can only be resolved by reform of allocation of treatments and procedures in healthcare. The root causes of disputes about futile treatment lie in the economic needs of a "supply-state" healthcare policy to support a huge investment in acute-care and critical-care medicine.[84] Failure to reform the policy results in the following:

- The phenomenon of "strangers treating strangers" with desperate life-prolonging measures in acute-care and ICU settings,
- A lack of life-long preventive care and primary-care medicine for Americans, and
- Mistrust of healthcare professionals and medicine as a whole among members of underserved and disadvantaged groups, who are more likely not to believe what physicians say about futile treatment and to demand that "everything be done" in a catastrophic illness or at the end of life.

Remedying these causes requires long-term reform of the healthcare system and higher-quality life-long medical care for all Americans. We will continue to experience futility disputes as long as U.S. health policy remains heavily weighted on the side of supply, and disadvantaged groups are underserved. Reform of allocation and global budgeting, combined with ethically acceptable practices of rationing at the bedside, are sources of prevention of futility disputes.

V. ORGANIZATIONAL ETHICS: WHOSE RESPONSIBILITY?

In addition to a strong ethics program with services, organizational morale is important for moral problem solving. Good organizational morale depends on several factors, which can be rep-

Table 17.5
Elements of an Ethics Consultation

I. **Consultant's assessment**
    A. What is the patient's medical condition?
        1. Identification of medical problems
        2. Diagnosis/diagnostic hypotheses
        3. Predictions and uncertainties regarding prognosis
            a. What are the patient's prospects for full or partial recovery?
            b. Is the patient terminally ill?
        4. Provisional formulation of goals of treatment and care
        5. Recommendations for treatment and reasonable alternative
    B. What are the relevant contextual factors?
        1. Demographic facts: age, gender, education
        2. Life situation and life style of patient
        3. Family relationships
        4. Setting of care: home or institution
        5. Socio-economic factors (such as insurance coverage)
        6. Language spoken
        7. Cultural factors
        8. Religion
    C. Is the patient capable of decision making?
        1. Legally incompetent (for example, child, court determination of incompetence)
        2. Clearly incapacitated (for example, unconscious)
        3. Diminished capacity (for example, depression of other mental disorder interfering with understanding or judgment)
        4. Fluctuating capacity
        5. Prospects for enhancing capacity
    D. What are the patient's preferences?
        1. Understanding of condition
        2. Views on quality of life
        3. Values relevant to decision making about treatment
        4. Current wishes for treatment
        5. Advance directives
        6. Reasons for seeking treatment regarded as medically inappropriate or for refusing treatment regarded as medically indicated
    E. What are the needs of the patient as a person?
        1. Psychic suffering and possible interventions for relief
        2. Interpersonal dynamics
        3. Resources and strategies for helping patient cope
        4. Adequacy of home environment for care of patient
        5. Preparation for dying
    F. What are the preferences of family/surrogate decision makers?
        1. Competence as surrogate decision maker
        2. Judgment and evidence of relevant patient preferences
        3. Opinions on quality of life of patient
        4. Opinions on best interest of patient
        5. Reasons for seeking treatment regarded as medically inappropriate or refusing treatment regarded as medically indicated
    G. Are there interests other than, and potentially competing with, those of the patient?
        1. Interests of family (for example, concerns about burdens of caring for patient, disagreements with preferences of patient)

2. Interests of fetus
3. Scarce resources and competing needs for their use
4. Interests of healthcare providers (for example, professional integrity)
5. Interests of healthcare organization
H. Are there issues of power or conflict in the interactions of the key actors in the case that should be addressed?
1. Between clinicians and patient/family
2. Between patient and family
3. Between family members/surrogates
4. Between members of the healthcare team (for example, attending physicians and house staff, physicians and nurses)
I. Have all the parties involved in the case had an opportunity to be heard?
J. Are there institutional factors contributing to moral problem posed by the case?
1. Work routines
2. Fears of malpractice/defensive medicine
3. Biases favoring disproportionately aggressive treatment or neglect of treatable conditions
4. Cost constraints/economic incentives

II. Consultant's moral diagnosis and educational aims
A. Examine how the moral problems in this case is being framed by the participants. Does this framework need to be reconsidered and replaced by an alternative understanding?
B. Identify and rank the range of relevant moral considerations.
C. Identify any relevant institutional policies pertaining to the case.
D. Consider ethical standards and guidelines, drawing on consensus statements of commissions and interdisciplinary or specialty groups. Educate using these resources.
E. Consider similar cases and discussions in the literature that might shed light on the analysis and resolution of moral problems in the case. Educate using these cases and literature.
F. Identify the morally acceptable options for resolving the moral problem(s) posed by the case. Educate about these options.

III. Goal setting, decision making, and implementation
A. Consider or reconsider and negotiate the goals of treatment and care for the patient.
B. Consider ideas (hypotheses) for possible interventions to meet the needs of the patient and resolve moral problems.
C. Deliberate regarding merits of alternative options for resolving the moral problem.
D. Endeavor to resolve conflicts.
E. Negotiate acceptable plan of action.
F. If negotiations and ethics consultation fail to achieve satisfactory resolution, consider judicial review.
G. Implement plan of action.

IV. Evaluation
A. Current Evaluation
1. Is the plan of action working? If not, why not?
2. Do the observed results of implementing the plan indicate the need for a modification of the plan?
3. Have conditions changed in a way that suggests the need to rethink the plan?
4. Are interactions between clinicians and the patient or surrogate helping to meet the needs of the patient, to respect the patient as a person, and to serve the goals of the plan of care?
5. Are there relevant interests, institutional factors, or normative considerations that have that have not been adequately addressed in planning for the care of the patient?
B. Retrospective Evaluation
1. What opportunities for resolving the moral problem were missed?
2. How did the care received by the patient match up to standards of good practice?
3. What factors contributed to a less than optimal resolution of the problems posed by the case?
4. Was the process of problem solving satisfactory in this case?
5. What might have been done to improve the care of the patient?
6. Are there desirable changes in institutional policy, feasible changes in the clinical environment, or educational interventions that might help to prevent or better resolve the moral problems posed by similar cases?

resented as concentric circles. The largest circle is the way persons are treated in their interactions with those in authority, especially over performance evaluation and job security. The second is the example set by an HCO's leaders in relationship with one another and with those who serve patients. Does trust and openness prevail in relations between the board of directors, the administration, and the medical and nursing staffs? Clinicians find it hard to be open and share decisions with patients where antagonism, secrecy, or a high level of suspicion exists. Another significant factor is the integrity of the business practices of the organization and its interactions with other organizations in the region. A final factor is the organization's responses to larger forces — economic, social, and political — at work in our society. Is the HCO guided by a broad vision of its role and responsibilities? Is there a shared statement of vision and values that is periodically reexamined and renewed?

Healthcare ethics committees to date have mainly addressed issues in patient care. This stance must be balanced by attention to ethical issues raised by organizational and economic forces. As Reiser wrote, "Institutions have ethical lives and characters just as their individual members do."[85] JCAHO has published new rules about "organizational ethics" — issues that concern the integrity of the HCO (see appendix 1).

JCAHO requires members to establish and maintain "structures to support patient rights . . . based on politics, procedures, and their philosophical basis, which makes up the framework that addresses both patient care and organizational ethical issues. . . ."[86] JCAHO rules specifically require a process to examine ethical issues in marketing, admissions, discharge, billing, relationships with third-party payers and managed-care plans, as well as a "code of organizational ethics" to address each of these areas. JCAHO rules can best be met by a HCO's ethics program with two arms: patients' rights and organizational ethics.

Development of effective services in patient care ethics is a useful precedent for services in organizational ethics. Ethical analysis of healthcare systems draws upon some of the ethical concepts used in this text, but requires a different set of skills in describing the context of ethical problems that arise for healthcare and managed-care organizations as such. The tasks of organizational ethics are:

- To provide a forum for discussion and education in issues of organizational ethics for clinical and administrative staff, concerned patients, or their surrogates, and members of the larger community. These issues include:
  - marketing, admissions, transfer, discharge, and billing practices;
  - relationships with healthcare professionals, third-party payers, managed-care companies, and educational institutions;
  - other issues that may arise;
- To do policy studies on request and make recommendations for institutional guidelines to address various ethical issues in the life of the organization and its relationships with others; and
- To provide a process for consultation concerning ethical problems that arise in the life of the organization.

Examples how such ethical issues can arise are:
- An employee, patient, or member of the community questions the veracity of statements the HCO has made in marketing and advertising activities.
- A particular managed-care contract contains restrictions on patient services or treatments that appear to HCO physicians to compromise what in the best medical interests of patients.
- A patient and a primary-care physician complain together that the patient's discharge was premature and based on financial considerations.
- An HCO physician who is removed from the roster by a health insurer's managed-care plan for criticizing the company's policies, and not for poor performance, complains of unfair treatment.
- A patient with significant chronic disease is assigned a new primary-care physician and complains about the lack of continuity of care.

Organizational ethics services could follow some of the practices used by an ECS in patient care:
- Any involved employee, patient, surrogate, or potential patient may ask for consultation regarding an ethical issue in the life of the organization.
- After identifying the ethical issue(s) that need consideration, an organizational ethics subcommittee provides a process for consultation,

education, and mediation (if needed) concerning the morally acceptable options and ways to resolve the problem(s). The consultation is advisory only.

- The organizational ethics subcommittee reports all of its consultations to the ethics committee, respecting rules of confidentiality and privacy when these apply.

HCOs with well-developed ethics programs for patient care already have the experience in moral problem solving that can be used to examine concerns of organizational ethics. Different skills and knowledge of the HCO's business and institutional life are needed, but the process of moral problem solving in these areas is not essentially different from that in patient care settings. In the future, more problems will arise that call for skills and knowledge in both arenas.

VI. EVALUATION

If ethics programs are to be fully effective, recognized aspects of HCOs, they must have a defined reporting procedure and have an understood method or methods for evaluating the work they do. For instance, if an ethics program reports to the institutional board of directors (a structure we favor), this board must approve evaluation methods that guide the program in determining what is or is not appropriate in its activities, as well as open reporting of these evaluations. Most ethics programs submit an outline of their educational activities each year and, as long as this outline is followed, no further reporting on this aspect of the work is needed. Ethics consultations, on the other hand, need to be evaluated more frequently, and should be reported on in a manner that respects confidentiality, yet enables the board to understand what has happened in an ethics consultation. Larger institutions may have a committee of the board to which the ethics program reports, but, whatever the mechanism, timely evaluation and reporting are a necessary part of the work.

In addition, we believe that a yearly or bi-yearly evaluation of the activities of the program itself is indicated, and we suggest that this be accomplished through an outside evaluator. JCAHO inspections can be a stimulus for this type evaluation, but seldom are JCAHO inspections comprehensive enough to fully evaluate an ethics program. Arrangements can be made for a team from one or more closely situated HCOs to spend half of a day in evaluation of a particular program, and a team from that program can reciprocate. Whatever the process, evaluation of the work that is done is a critical aspect of a well-functioning ethics program.

NOTES

1. D. Rothman, *Strangers at the Bedside* (New York: Free Press, 1991).

2. For a discussion of thalidomide, see *Thalidomide* 89th Cong., 2d sess., 1966, S. Rept. 1153, 8-2. For a discussion of the Jewish Hospital for Chronic Diseases Cancer Study, see E. Langer, "Human Experimentations: New York Affirms Patients' Rights," *Science* 151 (1966): 663-5. For a discussion of the baboon-to-human heart transplant, see J.D. Hardy, "Heart Transplantation in Man," *Journal of the American Medical Association* 188 (1964): 1132-5. For discussions of the Willowbrook study, see S. Krugman et al., "Infectious Hepatitis Detection of Virus During the Incubation Period and in Clinically Inapparent Infection," *New England Journal of Medicine* 261 (1959): 729-34; S. Goldby, "Experiments at the Willowbrook State School," *Lancet* 1 (1971): 749. For the Beecher article, see H.K. Beecher, "Ethics and Clinical Research," *New England Journal of Medicine* 74 (1966): 1354-60. For discussion of "Tea Room Trade" (deceptive social research), see L. Humphreys, *Tea Room Trade: Impersonal Sex in Public Places* (Chicago, Ill.: Aldine, 1970); D.P. Warwick, "Tearoom Trade: Means and Ends in Social Research," *Hastings Center Report* 1, no. 1 (1973): 24-38. On fetal research, see "Live Abortus Research Raises Hackles of Some, Hopes of Others," *Medical World News,* 5 October 1973, 32-6; V. Cohn, "NIH Vows Not to Fund Fetus Work," *Washington Post,* 13 April 1973, A1.

3. J.H. Jones, *Bad Blood,* 2nd ed. (New York: Free Press, 1991).

4. Ibid., 204. Jones relates the way Jean Heller, an Associated Press writer, got the story and published it on 25 July 1972 in the *Washington Star.*

5. V. Gamble, "A Legacy of Distrust: African Americans and Medical Research," *American Journal of Preventive Medicine* 9, no. 6 (1993): 35-8 (suppl.).

6. Surgeon-General, U.S. Public Health Service, Department of Health, Education, and Welfare, "Investigations Involving Subjects, Including Clinical Research: Requirements for Review to Insure the Rights and Welfare of Individuals,"

PPO no. 129, Revised Policy, 1 July 1966. In 1974, Congress passed the National Research Act (pub. L. No. 93-348) requiring that all research involving human subjects receive prior group review by an institutional review board.

7. These two norms — professional integrity and informed consent — are the core of the traditional practices embodied in the Nuremberg Code, along with the requirement for previous animal experiments. See P.M. McNeill, *The Ethics and Politics of Human Experimentation* (New York: Cambridge University Press, 1993), 42.

8. National Research Act, (Pub. L. No. 93-348), 88 Stat. 348 (1974).

9. J.C. Fletcher and F.G. Miller, "The Promise and Perils of Public Bioethics," in *The Ethics of Research Involving Human Subjects: Facing the 21st Century,* ed., H.Y Vanderpool (Frederick, Md.: University Publishing Group, 1996), 155-84.

10. Of 125 U.S. medical schools responding to a 1994-1995 survey, 61 had a separate required course in medical ethics, 94 offered medical ethics as part of an existing required course, and all said that there was at least an elective on the topic. Association of American Medical Colleges, *Institutional Profile System Ranking Report* (unpublished report, 1994-1995).

11. P. Singer, *Animal Liberation* (New York: Avon, 1977).

12. R.A. Whitney, "Animal Care and Use Committees: History and Current National Policies in the United States," *Laboratory Animal Science* 37 (January 1987): 18-21.

13. U.S. Department of Health and Human Services, Commission on Research Integrity, *Integrity and Misconduct in Research* (Washington, D.C.: U.S. Government Printing Office, 1995, publication number 1996-746-425).

14. R.E. Bulger, E. Heitman, and S.J. Reiser, ed., *The Ethical Dimensions of the Biological Sciences* (New York: Cambridge University Press, 1993); R.L. Penslar, ed., *Research Ethics: Cases and Materials* (Bloomington, Ind.: University of Indiana Press, 1995).

15. J.D. Moreno, *Deciding Together* (New York: Oxford University Press, 1995), 36.

16. President's Commission for the Study of Ethical Problems in Medicine and Biomedical and Behavioral Research, *Decisions to Forego Life-Sustaining Treatment* (Washington, D.C.: U.S. Government Printing Office, 1983), 153-60.

17. Ibid., 4.

18. *Annotated Code of Maryland,* section 19-

373 (Supp. 1994).

19. *New Jersey Administrative Code,* 8: 43-4.15 (1992); *New Jersey Statutes Annotated,* sec. 2A: 84A-22.10 (West 1994) (establishing privilege).

20. *Hawaii Revised Statutes Annotated,* sec. 663-1.7 (1995) (extending peer review privilege to ethics committee).

21. Joint Commission on the Accreditation of Healthcare Organizations, *Accreditation Manual for Hospitals* (Oakbrook Terrace, Ill.: JCAHO, 1992).

22. Joint Commission on the Accreditation of Healthcare Organizations, *Standards, Rights, Responsibilities, and Ethics* (Oakbrook Terrace, Ill.: JCAHO, 1995).

23. American Hospital Association, *1992 Statistical Guide* (Chicago, Ill.: AHA, 1992). Data were collected in 1989. Of 2,071 hospitals with more than 200 beds, approximately 518 did not have a committee; of 4,649 with fewer than 200 beds, 3,487 did not have a committee. Smaller hospitals were more likely to lack a committee.

24. J.C. Fletcher and D.E. Hoffman, "Hospital Ethics Committees: Time to Experiment with Standards," *Annals of Internal Medicine* 120 (1994): 335-8.

25. G. Glasser, N.R. Zweibel, and C.K. Cassel, "The Ethics Committee in the Nursing Home: Results of a National Survey," *Journal of the American Geriatrics Society* 36, no. 2 (1988): 150-6.

26. D.E. Hoffman, P. Boyle, and S.A. Levenson, *Handbook for Nursing Home Ethics Committees* (Washington, D.C.: American Association of Homes and Services for the Aging, 1995).

27. S. Fry-Revere, J. Sorrell, and M. Silva, ed., *Ethics and Answers in Home Health Care* (Leesburg, Va.: Regis Group, 1995).

28. R.F. Wilson et al., "Hospital Ethics Committees: Are They Evaluating Their Performance?" *HEC Forum* 2 (1993): 449-55.

29. J.W. Ross et al., ed., *Handbook for Hospital Ethics Committees* (Chicago, Ill.: American Hospital Association, 1986).

30. D.E. Hoffman, "Evaluating Ethics Committees: A View from the Outside," *Milbank Quarterly* 71 (1994): 4-40.

31. See note 24 above.

32. B. Lo, "Behind Closed Doors: Promises and Pitfalls of Ethics Committees," *New England Journal of Medicine* 317 (1987): 46-50.

33. S. Fry-Revere, "Some Suggestions for Holding Bioethics Committees and Consultants Accountable," *Cambridge Quarterly of Healthcare*

Ethics 2 (1993): 449-55; S.M. Wolf, "Ethics Committees and Due Process: Nesting Rights in a Community of Caring," *Maryland Law Review* 50 (1991): 798-858.

34. The Health Insurance Portability and Accountability Act was enacted in the late 1990s. It contained provisions concerning the portability of health insurance from one place of employment to another, but also contained several provisions greatly strengthening confidentiality of all patient information. Full application of the confidentiality provisions went into effect in April 2004. Exactly what will be required under this act is still under question (there have been no court challenges to date), but healthcare providers are paying much greater attention to confidentiality issues because of this act.

35. J.A. Tulsky and B. Lo, "Ethics Consultation: Time to Focus on Patients," *American Journal of Medicine* 92 (1992): 343-5.

36. In the *Baby K* case, which did not involve a lawsuit against an ethics committee, federal judge Clarence Hilton ruled that the mother's "treating physicians requested the assistance of the Hospital's 'Ethics Committee' in overriding the mothers' wishes" (see chapter 9). Judge Hilton placed the quotation marks around 'Ethics Committee' in order to deride the committee's actions. *In Re Baby K,* 832 F.Supp. 1022 (E.D. Va. 1993).

37. R. Macklin, *Enemies of Patients* (New York: Oxford University Press, 1993), 212-29.

38. G.J. Annas, "Ethics Committees: From Ethical Comfort to Ethical Cover," *Hastings Center Report* 21, no. 3 (May-June 1991): 18-21.

39. For criticisms of ethics committees, see J.D. Moreno, "Ethics by Committee: The Moral Authority of Consensus," *Journal of Medicine and Philosophy* 14 (1988): 411-32; J.D. Moreno, "What Means This Consensus? Ethics Committees and Philosophic Tradition," *The Journal of Clinical Ethics* 1, no. 1 (Spring 1990): 38-43; M. Siegler, "The Progression of Medicine: From Physician Paternalism to Patient Autonomy to Bureaucratic Parsimony," *Archives of Internal Medicine* 145 (1985): 713-5; J.C. Fletcher, "Ethics Committees and Due Process," *Law, Medicine & Health Care* 20 (1992): 291-3.

40. For criticisms of ethics consultation, see G. Scofield, "The Problem of the Impaired Clinical Ethicist," *Quality Review Bulletin* 18, no. 1 (1992): 26-32; G. Scofield, "Ethics Consultation: The Least Dangerous Profession," *Cambridge Quarterly of Healthcare Ethics* 2 (1993): 417-48;

J.C. Fletcher, "Commentary: Constructiveness Where It Counts," *Cambridge Quarterly of Healthcare Ethics* 2 (1993): 426-34; J. La Puma and D.L. Schiedermayer, "Ethics Consultation: Skills, Roles, and Training," *Annals of Internal Medicine* 114 (1991): 155-60; J. La Puma and E.R. Priest, "Medical Staff Privileges for Ethics Consultants: An Institutional Model," *Quality Review Bulletin* 18 no. 1 (1992): 17-20; J.C. Fletcher, "Needed: A Broader View of Ethics Consultation," *Quality Review Bulletin* 18, no. 1 (1992): 12-4.

41. This statement is based on six years of experience in "Developing Hospital Ethics Programs" (DHEP), an outreach training and education program of the Center for Biomedical Ethics, University of Virginia. An external evaluation of the first group of 10 hospitals (1990) to participate in DHEP, funded by the Greenwall Foundation (New York) in 1992, showed clearly that DHEP had succeeded in eight of the 10 hospitals. M.N. Smith et al., "Evaluation of Effectiveness of Developing Hospital Ethics Programs — A Project to Help Community Hospitals to Strengthen Institutional Ethics Programs," University of Virginia, Center for Biomedical Ethics, 1993. DHEP has served more than 150 hospitals and nursing homes to help them develop stronger ethics programs.

42. J.C. Fletcher et al., "Recommendations for Guidelines on Procedures and Process, and Education and Training to Strengthen Bioethics Services in Virginia," Virginia Bioethics Network, http://www.healthsystem.virginia.edu/internet/bio-ethics/guide.pdf.

43. Ibid.

44. Ibid.

45. Statewide and regional bioethics networks are organized in some parts of the nation. These groups have several functions: (1) to provide public education, (2) to serve as a clearinghouse for regional issues, and (3) to provide mutual support and encouragement for ethics committees. Well-developed networks provide educational and training opportunities for ethics committee members. Some have graduate education in clinical ethics. Networks with efforts of this kind are in Florida, Maryland (Baltimore), Michigan, Minnesota, Ohio, New Mexico, New York City, North Carolina (Charlotte), Pennsylvania (Pittsburgh), Virginia, West Virginia, and Wisconsin.

46. In Virginia, the short-term educational event is "Developing Hospital Ethics Programs," (see note 41 above), a six-day program offered

twice a year. The long-term program is "Programs of Education and Training in Clinical Ethics" (see note 41 above), which will be offered in two regions of Virginia to ethics committee members (six credit hours), to candidates for a certificate in clinical ethics (12 to 15 credit hours plus a one-week summer residency at the University of Virginia), and to individuals enrolled in a master's degree program (24 to 27 credit hours plus two one-week summer residencies at the University of Virginia.)

47. Significant literature on ethics committees includes: E. Doudera and R. Cranford, *Institutional Ethics Committees and Health Care Decision Making* (Ann Arbor, Mich.: Health Administration Press, 1985); R.P. Craig, C.L. Middleton, and L.J. O'Connell, *Ethics Committees: A Practical Approach* (St. Louis, Mo.: Catholic Health Association, 1986); G.A. Kanoti and J.K. Vinicky, "The Role and Structure of Hospital Ethics Committees," in *Health Care Ethics,* ed. G.R. Anderson and V.A. Glesnes-Anderson (Rockville, Md.: Aspen, 1987), 293-307; see note 29 above. See also notes 33 and 34 above for literature on ethics committees in nursing homes and home health agencies.

48. Virginia Bioethics Network, see note 42 above.

49. Information is available from HCOs that have made this transition. These include large, medium-sized, and small hospitals, as well as a few long-term care facilities (Duke University Medical Center, Durham, N.C.; Johnston Memorial Hospital, Abingdon, Va.; Mary Washington Hospital, Fredericksburg, Va.; University of Virginia Medical Center, Charlottesville, Va.; Camelot Health and Rehabilitation Center, Harrisonburg, Va.).

50. The Hippocratic writings direct physicians in doubt about a patient or "in the dark through inexperience" to urge "the calling in of others, in order to learn by consultation the truth about the case, and . . . that there may be fellow workers to afford abundant help." See "Selections from the Hippocratic Corpus," in *Ethics in Medicine,* ed. S.J. Reiser, A.J. Dyck, and W.J. Curran (Cambridge, Mass.: Massachusetts Institute of Technology Press, 1977), 5-9. Thomas Percival's *Medical Ethics,* first published in 1803, urged British physicians to seek help by consultation with others about problems in long and difficult cases; see T. Percival, *Medical Ethics,* 3rd ed. (Oxford, England: John Henry Parker, 1849). Percival prescribes approaches to the resolution of conflict between physicians who disagree, when these conflicts threaten the best interest of the patient. The first (1847) and latest (1990) code of ethics of the American Medical Association also direct physicians to seek consultation. See American Medical Association, "First Code of Medical Ethics," in *Ethics in Medicine,* pp. 26-34; American Medical Association, *Current Opinions of the Judicial Council* (Chicago, Ill.: AMA, 1990). These codes refer to medical problems for which consultation is needed, but they do not exclude seeking help with ethical problems.

51. I.N. Trainin and F. Rosner, "Jewish Codes and Guidelines," in *Encyclopedia of Bioethics,* ed. W.T. Reich (New York: Free Press, 1978), 1428-30; C.E. Curran, "Roman Catholicism," in *Encyclopedia of Bioethics,* 1522-34.

52. A.R. Jonsen, "Can an Ethicist be a Consultant?" in *Frontiers in Medical Ethics,* ed. V. Abernethy (Cambridge, Mass.: Ballinger, 1980); M. Boverman and J.C. Fletcher, "The Evolution of the Role of an Applied Bioethicist in a Research Hospital," in *Research Ethics,* ed. K. Berg and K.E. Traney (New York: Alan R. Liss, 1983), 131-58.

53. Papers from this conference appeared in *The Journal of Clinical Ethics* 7, no. 2 (Summer 1996).

54. Virginia Bioethics Network, see note 42 above.

55. American Society for Bioethics and Humanities was formed in the mid-1990s when three former groups (Society for Bioethics Consultation, American Bioethics Society, and Society for Health and Human Values) merged. One of the first major undertakings of ASBH was the completion and publication of the work of a task force on ethics consultation. This publication, *Core Competencies for Health Care Ethics Consultation,* is available from ASBH, 4700 W. Lake Avenue, Glenview, Ill.

56. L.J. Nelson, "Legal Liability in Bioethics Consultation," in *Healthcare Ethics Services,* ed. M.F. Marshall, J.C. Fletcher, and E.M. Spencer (Dordrecht, the Netherlands: Kluwer, in press).

57. J.A. Robertson, "Clinical Medical Ethics and the Law: The Rights and Duties of Ethics Consultants," in *Ethics Consultation in Health Care,* ed. J.C. Fletcher, N. Quist, and A.R. Jonsen (Ann Arbor, Mich.: Health Administration Press, 1989), 157-72, especially p. 166.

58. L. Lowenstein and J. DesBrisay, "Liability of Health Care Ethics Consultants," in *The Health*

Care Ethics Consultant, ed. F. Baylis (Totowa, N.J.: Humana Press, 1994), 133-61.

59. *Bouvia v. Superior Court,* 179 Cal. App. 3d 1127, 225 Cal. Rptr. 297, (1986). The entire *Bouvia* case is well-reported, except for the involvement and suit against the committee, in G.E. Pence, *Classic Cases in Medical Ethics,* 2nd ed. (New York: McGraw-Hill, 1995), 41-7.

60. "Bouvia Sues Hospital Ethics Committee," *Hospital Ethics* 3, no. 1 (1987): 13-4; L.J. Nelson, "Legal Liability of Institutional Ethics Committees to Patients," *Clinical Ethics Report* 6, no. 4 (1992): 1-8.

61. C. Blades and M. Curreri, "Law, Ethics, and Health Care: An Analysis of the Potential Legal Liability of Institutional Ethics Committees," *BioLaw* 2, no. 33 (1989): S317-26. Nelson, see note 55 above, also cites a personal communication with the late Richard Scott, Bouvia's attorney at the time.

62. *In re Baby K,* 832 F.Supp. 1022 (E.D. Va. 1993). This case and the ethics committee's role is discussed at length in J.C. Fletcher, "Bioethics in a Legal Forum: Confessions of an 'Expert Witness,'" *Journal of Medicine and Philosophy and Medicine* 22, no. 4 (August 1977): 297-324.

63. *In re Baby K,* 16 F.3d 590 (4th Cir. 1994).

64. Virginia Health Care Decisions Act of 1992, *Virginia Code Annotated,* sec. 54.1-2981-2991 (Michie 1994).

65. *Bryan v. Rectors and Visitors of the University of Virginia,* 95 F.3d 349 (4th Cir.1996).

66. See note 59 above.

67. A.M. Capron, "Abandoning a Waning Life," *Hastings Center Report* 25, no. 4 (1995): 24-6.

68. T.A. Brennan, "Incompetent Patients with Limited Care in the Absence of Family Consent," *Annals of Internal Medicine* 109 (1988): 819-25.

69. *Gilgunn v. Massachusetts General Hospital,* No. 92-4820, Suffolk Co., Mass., Super. Ct. (April 1995); G. Kolata, "Court Ruling Limits Rights of Patients," *New York Times,* 22 April 1995, A1.

70. *Estate of James Davis Bland v. Cigna Healthplan of Texas;* Kenneth Lawrence Toppell, M.D.; Milton Thomas, M.D.; and Park Plaza Hospital, District Court of Harris County, Tex., 11th Dist. No. 93-52630 (1995).

71. M. Swartz, "Not What the Doctor Ordered," *Texas Monthly* (March 1995): 86-9, 115-32.

72. In describing his action and the process by which the patient was removed from the respirator, according to the pulmonologist's deposition, he went to the room and changed the settings on the patient's ventilator, observed him breathing on his own, and then returned the ventilator to the previous settings. The pulmonologist testified that a respiratory therapist was called who "put him on a T-tube . . . on twenty-eight percent oxygen." *(Estate of) James Bland v. Cigna Healthplan of Texas,* 2 No. 790732: 118-19.

73. Natural Death Act, *Vernon's Texas Codes Annotated* 672.001 (1992).

74. Virginia Bioethics Network, see note 42 above.

75. T. Gillian and T.A. Raffin, "Withdrawing Life Support: Extubation and Prolonged Terminal Weans Are Inappropriate," *Critical Care Medicine* 24, no. 2 (1996): 352-3.

76. *Marlene and Tyrone Rideout v. Hershey Medical Center,* No. 96-5260, Court of Common Pleas, Dauphin County, Pa. (December 1995).

77. *Rideout v. Hershey Medical Center,* No. 96-5260, Court of Common Pleas, Dauphin County, Pa. (December 1995). The court decision is discussed in W.P. Murphy, "Hospital Faces Liability for Cutting Life Support," *Pennsylvania Law Weekly* 19, no. 3 (1996): 1, 22.

78. For a range of views, see J. LaPuma and D.Schiedermayer, *Ethics Consultation: A Practical Guide* (Boston, Mass.: Jones and Bartlett, 1994); F.E. Baylis, ed., *The Health Care Ethics Consultant* (Totowa, N.J.: Humana Press, 1994); J.C. Fletcher, "The Consultant's Credentials," *Hastings Center Report* 25 (July-August 1995): 39-40; J.C. Fletcher and H. Brody, "Clinical Ethics: Elements and Methodologies," in *Encyclopedia of Bioethics,* 2nd ed., ed. W.T. Reich (New York: Simon & Schuster MacMillan, 1995), 399-404.

79. Virginia Bioethics Network, see note 42 above.

80. S.M. Wolf, "Quality Assessment of Ethics in Health Care: The Accountability Revolution," *American Journal of Law & Medicine* 20 (1994): 107-28.

81. A. Relman, "Assessment and Accountability: The Third Revolution in Medical Care," *New England Journal of Medicine* 319 (1988): 1220-3.

82. L.N. Teichholz, "Quality, Deming's Principles, and Physicians," *Mount Sinai Journal of Medicine* 35 (1993): 350-8.

83. Ibid., 351.

84. L.R. Jacobs, "Politics of America's Supply State," *Health Affairs* 14, no. 2 (1995): 143-57.

85. S.J. Reiser, "The Ethical Life of Health Care Organizations," *Hastings Center Report* 24, no. 6 (1994): 24-45.

86. Joint Commission on the Accreditation of Healthcare Organizations, *Standards on Patient Rights and Organizational Ethics,* reproduced in this volume as appendix 1.

Appendixes

Appendix 1

Joint Commission on Accreditation of Healthcare Organizations: Individual Rights and Organization Ethics

Ethics, Rights, and Responsibilities

Overview

The **goal** of the ethics, rights, and responsibilities function is to improve care, treatment, services, and outcomes by recognizing and respecting the rights of each patient and by conducting business in an ethical manner. Care, treatment, and services are provided in a way that respects and fosters dignity, autonomy, positive self regard, civil rights, and involvement of patients. Care, treatment, and services consider the patient's abilities and resources; the relevant demands of his or her environment; and the requirements and expectations of the providers and those they serve. The family is involved in care, treatment, and service decisions with the patient's approval.

["**M**" in the left margin below indicates the measure of success is one that institutions must meet.]

A hospital's adherence to ethical care and business practices significantly affects the patient's experience of and response to care, treatment, and services. The standards in this chapter address the following processes and activities related to ethical care and business practices:
- Managing the hospital's relationships with patients and the public in an ethical manner
- Considering the values and preferences of patients, including the decision to discontinue care, treatment, and services
- Helping patients understand and exercise their rights
- Informing patients of their responsibilities in care, treatment, and services
- Recognizing the hospital's responsibilities under law

Patients deserve care, treatment, and services that safeguard their personal dignity and respect their cultural, psychosocial, and spiritual values. These values often influence the patient's perceptions and needs. By understanding and respecting these values, providers can meet care, treatment, and service needs and preferences.

[Glossary terms have been omitted from this excerpt.]

Standards

The following is a list of all standards for this function. They are presented here for your convenience without footnotes or other explanatory text. If you have a question about a term used here please check the Glossary.

Note: *A revised standard numbering system is being used with the reformatted standards. This revised numbering system will allow for more flexibility to add standards while maintaining the current label for each standard.*

Organization Ethics

RI.1.10 The hospital follows ethical behavior in its care, treatment, and services and business practices.

RI.1.20 The hospital addresses conflicts of interest.

RI.1.30 The integrity of decisions is based on identified care, treatment, and service needs of the patients.

RI.1.40 When care, treatment, and services are subject to internal or external review that results in the denial of care, treatment, services, or payment, the hospital makes decisions regarding the provision of ongoing care, treatment, services, or discharge based on the assessed needs of the patients.

Individual Rights

RI.2.10 The hospital respects the rights of patients.

RI.2.20 Patients receive information about their rights.

RI.2.30 Patients are involved in decisions about care, treatment, and services provided.

RI.2.40 Informed consent is obtained.

RI.2.50 Consent is obtained for recording or filming made for purposes other than the identification, diagnosis, or treatment of the patients.

RI.2.60 Patients receive adequate information about the person(s) responsible for the delivery of their care, treatment, and services.

RI.2.70 Patients have the right to refuse care, treatment, and services in accordance with law and regulation.

RI.2.80 The hospital addresses the wishes of the patient relating to end-of-life decisions.

RI.2.90 Patients and, when appropriate, their families are informed about the outcomes of care, treatment, and services that have been provided, including unanticipated outcomes.

RI.2.100 The hospital respects the patients right to and need for effective communication.

RI.2.110 Not applicable.

RI.2.120 The hospital addresses the resolution of complaints from patients and their families.

RI.2.130 The hospital respects the needs of patients for confidentiality, privacy, and security.

RI.2.140 Patients have a right to an environment that preserves dignity and contributes to a positive self image.

RI.2. 150 Patients have the right to be free from mental, physical, sexual, and verbal abuse, neglect, and exploitation.

RI.2.160 Patients have the right to pain management.

RI.2.170 Patients have a right to access protective and advocacy services.

RI.2.180 The hospital protects research subjects and respects their rights during research, investigation, and clinical trials involving human subjects.

RI.2.190 In hospitals that provide opportunities for work, a defined policy addresses situations in which patients work.

Individual Responsibilities

RI.3.10 Patients are given information about their responsibilities while receiving care, treatment, and services.

• • •

Standards, Rationales, Elements of Performance, and Scoring

Organization Ethics

Introduction

A hospital has an ethical responsibility to the patients and community it serves. To fulfill this responsibility, ethical care, treatment, and service practices and ethical business practices must go hand in hand. Furthermore, the hospital provides care, treatment, and services within its scope, stated mission and philosophy, and applicable law and regulation.

The hospital's system of ethics supports honest and appropriate interactions with patients. The system of ethics also includes patients whenever possible in decisions about their care, treatment, and services, including ethical issues.

Standard RI.1.10 ▬▬▬▬▬
The hospital follows ethical behavior in its care, treatment, and services and business practices.

Elements of Performance for RI.1.10
1. The hospital identifies ethical issues and issues prone to conflict.
2. The hospital develops and implements a process to handle these issues when they arise.
3. The hospital's policies and procedures reflect ethical practices for marketing, admission, transfer, discharge, and billing.
4. Marketing materials accurately represent the hospital and address the care, treatment, and services that the hospital can provide, directly or by contractual arrangement.

M 5. Patients receive information about charges for which they will be responsible.
6. The effectiveness and safety of care, treatment, and services does not depend on the patient's ability to pay.

M 7. The leaders ensure that care, treatment, and services are not negatively affected when the hospital grants a staff member's request to be excused from participating in an aspect of the care, treatment, and services.

Standard RI.1.20 ▬▬▬▬▬
The hospital addresses conflicts of interest.

Rationale for RI.1.20
Potential conflicts of interest can arise in subtle and obvious circumstances. The hospital needs to be aware of potential conflicts of interest and review relations with other entities carefully to ensure that its mission and responsibility to the patients and community it serves is not harmed

by any professional, ownership, contractual, or other relationships.

Elements of Performance for RI.1.20
1. The hospital defines what constitutes a *conflict of interest.*

M 2. The hospital discloses existing or potential conflicts of interest for those who provide care, treatment, and services as well as governance.
3. The hospital reviews its relationship and its staff's relationships with other care providers, educational institutions, and payers to ensure that those relationships are within law and regulation and determine if conflicts of interest exist.
4, The hospital addresses conflicts of interest when they arise.

Standard RI.1.30 ▬▬▬▬▬▬▬▬▬
The integrity of decisions is based on identified care, treatment and service needs of the patients.

Rationale for RI.1.30
Decisions are based on the patients' care, treatment, and service needs, regardless of how the hospital compensates or shares financial risk with its leaders, managers, staff, and licensed independent practitioners.

Elements of Performance for RI.1.30
1. The hospital has policies and procedures that address the integrity of clinical decision making.

M 2. To avoid compromising the quality of care, decisions are based on the patient's identified care, treatment, and service needs and in accordance with hospital policy.
3. Policies and procedures and information about the relationship between the use of care, treatment, and services and financial incentives are available to all patients, staff, licensed independent practitioners, and contracted providers, when requested.

Standard RI.1.40 ▬▬▬▬▬▬▬▬▬
When care, treatment, and services are subject to internal or external review that results in the denial of care, treatment, services, or payment, the hospital makes decisions regarding the provision of ongoing care, treatment, and services, or discharge based on the assessed needs of the patients.

Rationale for RI.1.40

When an individual requests or presents for care, treatment, and services, the hospital is professionally and ethically responsible for providing care treatment, and services within its capability, mission, and applicable law and regulation. At times, indications for such care, treatment, and services can contradict the recommendations of an external entity performing a utilization review (for example, insurance companies, managed care reviewers, and federal or state payers). If such a conflict arises, care, treatment, service, and discharge decisions are made based on the patients' identified needs, regardless of the recommendations of the external agency.

Elements of Performance for RI.1.40

M 1. The hospital makes decisions regarding the provision of ongoing care, treatment, services, or discharge based on the care, treatment, and services required by the patient.

M 2. The patient and/or the family is involved in these decisions.

Individual Rights

Introduction

A mere list of rights cannot guarantee those rights. Rather, a hospital shows its support of rights by how its staff interacts with patients and involves them in decisions about their care, treatment, and services. These standards focus on how the hospital respects the culture and rights of patients during those interactions. This begins with respecting their right to treatment, care, and service.

Standard RI.2.10 ▬▬▬▬▬

The hospital respects the rights of patients.

Elements of Performance for RI.2.10

1. The hospital's policies and practices address the rights of patients to care, treatment, and services within its capability and mission and in compliance with law and regulation.

M 2. Each patient has a right to have his or her cultural, psychosocial, spiritual, and personal values, beliefs, and preferences respected.

M 3. The hospital supports the right of each patient to personal dignity.

M 4. The hospital accommodates the right to pastoral and other spiritual services for patients.

Standard RI.2.20 ▬▬▬▬▬

Patients receive information about their rights

Elements of Performance for RI.2.20

M 1. Information on rights is provided to each patient.

2. Not applicable

3. Not applicable

4. Not applicable

M 5. Information on the exent to which the hospital is able, unable, or unwilling to honor advance directives is given upon admission if the patient has an advance directive.

M 6. The patient has the right to access, request amendment to, and receive an accounting of disclosures regarding his or her own health information as permitted under applicable law.

Standard RI.2.30 ▬▬▬▬▬

Patients are involved in decisions about care, treatment, and services provided.

Rationale for RI.2.30

Making decisions about care, treatment and services sometimes presents questions, conflicts, or other dilemmas for the hospital and the patients, family or other decision makers. These dilemmas may involve issues about admission; care, treatment, and services; or discharge. The hospital works with patients, and when appropriate, their families, to resolve such dilemmas.

Elements of Performance for RI.2.30

M 1. Patients are involved in decisions about their care, treatment, and services.

M 2. Patients are involved in resolving dilemmas about care, treatment, and services.

M 3. A surrogate decision maker, as allowed by law, is identified when a patient cannot make decisions about his or her care treatment, and service.

M 4. The legally responsible representative approves care, treatment, and service decisions.*

---

* In some states, law dictates that urgent care, family planning, and/or behavioral health services can be provided to a minor without the approval or consent of a parent or guardian.

M 5. The family, as appropriate and as allowed by law, with permission of the patient or surrogate decision maker, is involved in care, treatment, and service decisions.

Standard RI.2.40 ▬▬▬▬▬▬▬▬▬▬

Informed consent is obtained.

Rationale for RI.2.40

The goal of the informed consent process is to establish a mutual understanding between the patient and the physician or other licensed independent practitioner who provides the care, treatment, and services that the patient receives. This process allows each patient to fully participate in decisions about his or her care, treatment, and services.

Elements of Performance for RI.2.40

1. The hospital's policies describe the following:
    *   Which procedures or care, treatment, and services require informed consent
    *   The process used to obtain informed consent
    *   How informed consent is to be documented in the record
    *   When a surrogate decision maker, rather than the patient, may give informed consent
    *   When procedures or care, treatment, and services normally requiring informed consent may be given without informed consent

M 2. Informed consent is obtained and documented in accordance with the hospital's policy.

3. A complete informed consent process includes a discussion of the following elements:*
    *   The nature of the proposed care, treatment, services, medications, interventions, or procedures.
    *   Potential benefits, risks, or side effects, including potential problems related to recuperation.
    *   The likelihood of achieving care, treatment and service goals.
    *   Reasonable alternatives to the proposed care, treatment, and services.

*   The relevant risks, benefits, and side effects related to alternatives, including the possible results of not receiving care, treatment, and services.
*   When indicated, any limitations on the confidentiality of information learned from or about the patient

Standard RI.2.50 ▬▬▬▬▬▬▬▬▬▬

Consent is obtained for recording or filming+ made for purposes other than the identification, diagnosis, or treatment of the patients.

Rationale for RI.2.50

Recording or filming of care, treatment, and services provided to patients can be useful for many purposes, but such recording or filming is likely to compromise the patient's privacy and confidentiality Therefore, the hospital should obtain consent from the patient for recording or filming.

Elements of Performance for RI.2.50

M 1. When recording or filming are to be used only for internal organizational purposes (for example, performance improvement and education), there is documentation of consent, which may be obtained as part of general consent to treatment or another form, if a statement is included in the form regarding the use of recordings or filming for such internal purposes.

M 2. When recording or films are made for external purposes that will be heard or seen by the public (for example, commercial filming, television programs, marketing), there is documentation of a specific, separate consent that includes the circumstances of the use of the recording or film.

M 3. Except for the circumstances set forth in EP 4 (below), there is documentation of consent before recording or filming.

M 4. The following occurs in situations in which the patient is unable to give informed consent before recording or filming:
    *   The recording or filming may occur before consent provided it is within the established policy of the hospital and the policy is established through an appropriate ethical mechanism (for

---

* Documentation of the items listed in EP 3 may be in a form, progress notes, or elsewhere in the record.

+ Recording or filming refers to photographic, video, electronic, or audio media.

example, an ethics committee) that includes community input.

- The recording or film remains in the hospital's possession and is not used for any purpose until and unless consent is obtained.
- If consent for use cannot subsequently be obtained, the recording or film is either destroyed or the nonconsenting patient must be removed from the recording or film.

5. Patients have the right to request cessation of recording or filming.

6. Patients have the right to rescind consent for use up until a reasonable time before the recording or film is used.

M 7. Anyone who engages in recording or filming (who is not already bound by the hospital's confidentiality policy) signs a confidentiality statement to protect the patient's identity and confidential information.

Standard RI.2.60

Patients receive adequate information about the person(s) responsible for the delivery of their care, treatment, and services.

Elements of Performance for RI.2.60

M 1. The information provided includes the following:

- The name of the physician or other practitioner primarily responsible for their care, treatment, and services.
- The name of the physician or other practitioner who will provide the care, treatment, and services.

M 2. The information is given to the patient on a timely basis as defined by the hospital.

Standard RI.2.70

Patients have the right to refuse care, treatment, and services in accordance with law and regulation.

Elements of Performance for RI.2.70

1. Patients have the right to refuse care, treatment, and services in accordance with law and regulation

2. When the patient is not legally responsible, the surrogate decision maker, as allowed by law, has the right to refuse care,

treatment, and services on the patient's behalf.

Standard RI.2.80

The hospital addresses the wishes of the patient relating to end-of-life decisions.

Elements of Performance for RI.2.80

1. Policies, in accordance with law and regulation, address advance directives and the framework for withholding or withdrawing life-sustaining treatment and withholding resuscitative services.

M 2. Adults are given written information about their right to accept or refuse medical or surgical treatment, including forgoing or withdrawing life-sustaining treatment or withholding resuscitative services.

3. The existence or lack of an advance directive does not determine an individual's access to care, treatment, and services.

M 4. Documentation indicates whether or not the patient has signed an advance directive.

5. The patient has the option to review and revise advance directives.

M 6. Appropriate staff are aware of the advance directive if one exists.

M 7. The hospital helps or refers the patients for assistance in formulating advance directives upon request.

8. The hospital has a mechanism for health care professionals and designated representatives to honor advance directives within the limits of the law and the hospital's capabilities.

M 9. The hospital documents and honors the patient's wishes concerning organ donation within the limits of the law or hospital capacity.

10. *For Outpatient Hospital Settings:* The hospital's policies address advance directives and specify whether the hospital will honor the directives.

M 11. *For Outpatient Hospital Settings:* The policies are communicated to patients and families when asked about or as appropriate to the care, treatment and services provided.

M 12. *For Outpatient Hospital Settings:* Upon request, the hospital helps patients formulate medical advance directives or refers them for assistance

13. Through 20. Not applicable.

M 21. The policies are consistently implemented.

Standard RI.2.90 ▬▬▬▬▬▬▬

Patients, and, when appropriate, their families are informed about the outcomes of care, treatment, and services that have been provided, including unanticipated outcomes.

Elements of Performance for RI.2.90

At a minimum, the patient and when appropriate, his or her family is informed about the following (EPs 1.2):

M 1. Outcomes of care, treatment, and services that have been provided that the patient (or family) must be knowledgeable about to participate in current and future decisions affecting the patient's care, treatment, and services.

M 2. Unanticipated outcomes of care, treatment, and services that relate to sentinel events considered reviewable* by the Joint Commission.

M 3. The responsible licensed independent practitioner or his or her designee informs the patient (and when appropriate, his or her family) about those unanticipated outcomes of care, treatment and services (see EP 2 above).+

Standard RI.2.100 ▬▬▬▬▬▬▬

The hospital respects the patients right to and need for effective communication.

Rationale for RI.2.100

The patient has the right to receive information in a manner that he or she understands. This includes communication between the hospital and the patient, as well as communication between the patient and others outside the hospital.

Elements of Performance for RI.2.100

1. The hospital respects the right and need of patients for effective communication.

2. Written information provided is appropri-

ate to the age, understanding, and, as appropriate to the population served, the language of the patient.

M 3. The hospital facilitates provision of interpretation (including translation services) as necessary.

M 4. The hospital addresses the needs of those with vision, speech, hearing, language. and cognitive impairments.

5. The hospital offers telephone and mail service as appropriate to the setting and population.

Additional Elements of Performance for Hospital Settings That Provide Longer Term Care (More Than 30 Days)

M 6. When a hospital restricts a patient's visitors, mail, telephone calls or other forms of communication, the restrictions are determined with the patients participation and, when appropriate, his or her family.

M 7. When a hospital restricts a patient's visitors, mail, telephone calls, or other forms of communication, the restrictions are documented along with justification in the clinical or case record.

M 8. When a hospital restricts a patient's visitors, mail, telephone calls, or other forms of communication, the restrictions are evaluated for therapeutic effectiveness.

Standard RI.2.110 ▬▬▬▬▬▬▬

Not applicable.

Standard RI.2.120 ▬▬▬▬▬▬▬

The hospital addresses the resolution of complaints from patients and their families.

Elements of Performance for RI.2.120

M 1. The hospital informs patients, families, and staff about the complaint resolution process.

M 2. The hospital receives, reviews. and, when possible, resolves complaints from patients and their families.

M 3. The hospital responds to individuals making a significant (as defined by the hospital) or recurring complaint.

M 4. The hospital informs patients about their right to file a complaint with the state authority.

M 5. Patients can freely voice complaints and recommend changes without being sub-

---

* See "Sentinel Events" chapter of this manual for a definition of reviewable sentinel events [not included in this excerpt].

+ In settings where there is no licensed independent practitioner, the staff member responsible for the care of the patient is responsible for sharing information about such outcomes.

ject to coercion, discrimination, reprisal, or unreasonable interruption of care, treatment, and services.

Standard RI.2.130 ▬▬▬▬▬
The hospital respects the needs of patients for confidentiality, privacy, and security.

Rationale for RI.2.130
This standard and its EPs allow flexibility in how a hospital can accomplish this requirement. Privacy, safety, and security can be demonstrated in various ways, for example, via policies and procedures, practices, or the design of the environment.

Elements of Performance for RI.2.130
M 1. The hospital protects confidentiality of information about patients.
M 2. The hospital respects the privacy of patients.
M 3. Patients who desire private telephone conversations have access to space and telephones appropriate to their needs and the care, treatment, and services provided.
M 4. The hospital provides for the safety and security of patients and their property.
   5. Not applicable.
   6. Not applicable.

Additional Element of Performance for Hospital Settings That Provide Longer Term Care (More Than 30 Days)
   7. The number of patients in a room is appropriate to the hospital's goals and the patients' ages, developmental levels, clinical conditions, or diagnosis needs.

Standard RI.2.140 ▬▬▬▬▬
Patients have a right to an environment that preserves dignity and contributes to a positive self image.

Rationale for RI.2.140
The hospital creates a supportive environment for all patients. Because a program or unit at times becomes the patients "home," the hospital provides an atmosphere that supports the patient's dignity. For example, in a long term care unit, patients have space to display greeting cards, calendars, and other personal items important to their well-being.

Elements of Performance for RI.2.140
   1 . The environment of care supports the positive self-image of patients and preserves their human dignity.
   2. The hospital provides sufficient storage space to meet the personal needs of the patients.
   3. The hospital allows patients to keep and use personal clothing and possessions, unless this infringes on others' rights or is medically or therapeutically contraindicated (as appropriate to the setting or service).

Standard RI.2.150 ▬▬▬▬▬
Patients have the right to be free from mental, physical, sexual, and verbal abuse, neglect and exploitation.*

Note: *See standard PC.3.10, which addresses assessing and reporting of abuse, neglect, and exploitation.*

Elements of Performance for RI.2.150
   1. The hospital addresses how it will, to the best of its ability, protect patients from real or perceived abuse, neglect, or exploitation from anyone, including staff, students, volunteers, other patients, visitors, or family members.
M 2. All allegations, observations, or suspected cases of abuse, neglect, or exploitation that occur in the hospital are investigated by the hospital.

Standard RI.2.160 ▬▬▬▬▬
Patients have the right to pain management.

Rationale for RI.2.160
Patients may experience pain. Unrelieved pain has adverse physical and psychological effects. The hospital respects and supports the right of patients to pain management. In accordance with the hospital's mission, this may occur through referral.

Element of Performance for RI.2.160
   1. The hospital plans, supports, and coordinates activities and resources to ensure

---

* Taking advantage of another for one's own advantage or benefit.

that pain is recognized and addressed appropriately and in accordance with the care, treatment, and services provided including the following:

- Assessing for pain
- Educating all relevant providers about assessing and managing pain
- Educating patients and families, when appropriate, about their roles in managing pain and the potential limitations and side effects of pain treatments

Standard RI.2.170
Patients have a right to access protective and advocacy services.

Elements of Performance for RI.2.170
M 1. When the hospital serves a population of patients who often need protective services (that is, guardianship and advocacy services, conservatorship, and child or adult protective services), it provides resources to help the family and the courts determine the patients needs for such services.

2. When appropriate, the hospital maintains a list of names, addresses, and telephone numbers of pertinent state client advocacy groups such as the state authority and the protection and advocacy network.

M 3. The list is given to patients when requested.

4. The hospital develops and implements policies and procedures for the above requirements.

Standard RI.2.180
The hospital protects research subjects and respects their rights during research investigation, and clinical trials involving human subjects.

Rationale for RI.2.180
A hospital that conducts research, investigations, or clinical trials involving human subjects knows that its first responsibility is to the health and well being of the research subjects. To protect and respect the research subjects' rights, the hospital reviews all research protocols. If another institution's Institutional Review Board (IRB) reviews the research protocols, the hospital does not need to perform this activity.

Elements of Performance for RI.2.180
M 1. The hospital reviews all research protocols in relation to its mission, values, and other guidelines and weighs the relative risks and benefits to the research subjects.

M 2. The hospital provides patients who are potential subjects in research, investigation, and clinical trials with adequate information* to participate or refuse to participate in research.

M 3. Patients are informed that refusing to participate or discontinuing at any time will not compromise their access to care, treatment, and services not related to the research.

M 4. Consent forms address the above elements of performance, indicate the name of the person who provided the information and the date the form was signed; and address the participant's right to privacy, confidentiality, and safety.

M 5. Subjects are told the extent to which their personally identifiable private information will be held in confidence.

M 6. All information given to subjects is in the medical record or research file along with the consent forms,

M 7. If a research-related injury (that is, physical, psychological, social, financial, or otherwise) occurs, the principal investigator attempts to address any harmful consequences the subject may have experienced as a result of research procedures.

Applicable Only to Hospital Settings That Provide Longer Term Care (More Than 30 Days)
Standard RI.2.190
In hospitals that provide opportunities for work, a defined policy addresses situations in which patients work.

Rationale for RI.2.190
Patients may be offered the opportunity to perform work for the hospital (for example, work

---

* **Adequate information** includes an explanation of the purpose of the research and expected duration of the subject's participation; a description of the expected benefits, potential discomforts, and risks; alternative services that might prove advantageous to the individual; and a full explanation of the procedures to be followed.

therapy programs in grounds keeping or the library) that does not endanger them, other patients, or staff. If the hospital asks patients to perform such tasks (work), they have the right to refuse.

Elements of Performance for RI.2.190

    1. Policies and procedures address situations in which patients work.

M 2. Policies and procedures are implemented.

M 3. Wages paid to patients are in accordance with applicable law and regulation.

M 4. Work is addressed in the care, treatment, and service plan.

M 5. Work is performed voluntarily.

Appendix 2

A Case Method
for Consideration of Moral Problems

Edward M. Spencer

We have developed a pragmatic formulation for consideration of clinical ethics cases (see table A.2.1).[1] The method is clinical, because it is focused on the circumstances of particular cases of patient care and attentive to the norms and virtues of clinical practice. It is pragmatic because it aims to guide the development, implementation, and evaluation of ethically appropriate and effective plans of action, by means of a collaborative process of problem-solving involving all those concerned with the case. This method can be helpful in the consideration of clinical ethics cases, but there is no guarantee that the use of this, or any other, method of moral problem-solving will generate a satisfactory resolution of a problem. In some cases, moral conflict may remain intractable, and, in spite of the dedicated efforts of skilled and caring clinicians, appeal for judicial review may be required.

The method described in table A.2.1 consists of four steps, with further enumeration of issues under each step. The four steps in the case method involve the following tasks:

1. Assessment of medical facts, contextual factors, the patient's capacity, the patient's preferences and needs, surrogate decision makers, competing interests, institutional factors, and issues of power;
2. Moral diagnosis of the problems posed by the case and options for resolution;

3. Goal setting, decision making, and implementation of a plan of action by means of a shared, deliberative process;
4. Evaluation of results.

To the extent possible, clinicians working with patients and family members should strive to resolve moral problems as they arise. When such efforts fail, owing to interpersonal conflict or perplexity about the right thing to do in a morally complex situation, ethics consultation may be desirable to facilitate resolution.

Table A.2.1 contains a detailed outline of the four steps. Not every item will be relevant in every morally problematic case. Although the method is presented as a linear progression, in practice these steps may occur simultaneously or in a different sequence. The outline should be treated as a flexible guide, rather than a rigid checklist, because the process of problem-solving should be tailored to the particular features of a case as they emerge in clinical practice.

This method is meant for use both prospectively by clinicians who face moral problems in the care of patients and retrospectively for the education of clinicians and ethics committee members. It may also be used to assess the quality of efforts used in moral problem-solving. Ethics committee members and ethicists who use this method in the context of ethics consultation

Table A.2.1
Clinical Pragmatism: A Case Method of Moral Problem-Solving

1. Assessment
- a. What is the patient's medical condition?
  - i. Identification of medical problems and history
  - ii. Diagnosis/diagnostic hypotheses
  - iii. Predictions and uncertainties regarding prognosis (What are the prospects for full or partial recovery? Is the patient terminally ill?)
  - iv. Provisional formulation of goals of treatment and care
  - v. Treatment recommendations and reasonable alternatives
- b. What are the relevant contextual factors?
  - i. Demographic factors (age, gender, education)
  - ii. Life situation and lifestyle of patient
  - iii. Family relationships
  - iv. Setting of care (home or institution)
  - v. Socioeconomic factors (such as insurance coverage)
  - vi. Language spoken
  - vii. Cultural factors
  - viii. Religion
- c. Is the patient capable of decision making?
  - i. Legally incompetent (for example, the patient is a child or a court has determined the patient to be incompetent)
  - ii. Clearly incapacitated (for example, patient is unconscious)
  - iii. Diminished capacity (for example, patient is diagnosed with depression or other mental disorder interfering with understanding or judgment)
  - iv. Fluctuating capacity
  - v. Prospects for enhancing capacity
- d. What are the patient's preferences?
  - i. Understanding of condition
  - ii. Views on quality of life
  - iii. Values relevant to decision making about treatment
  - iv. Current wishes for treatment
  - v. Advance directives
  - vi. Reasons for seeking treatment that is regarded as medically inappropriate or refusing treatment that is regarded as medically indicated
- e. What are the needs of the patient as a person?
  - i. Psychic suffering and possible interventions for relief
  - ii. Interpersonal dynamics
  - iii. Resources and strategies for helping patient cope
  - iv. Adequacy of home environment for care of patient
  - v. Preparation for dying
- f. What are the preferences of family/surrogate decision makers?
  - i. Competence as surrogate decision maker
  - ii. Judgment and evidence of relevant patient preferences
  - iii. Opinions on quality of life of patient
  - iv. Opinions on best interest of patient
  - v. Reasons for seeking treatment that is regarded as medically inappropriate or refusing treatment that is regarded as medically indicated
- g. Are there interests other than, and potentially competing with, those of the patient?
  - i. Interests of family (for example, concerns about burdens of caring for patient or disagreements with preferences of patient)
  - ii. Interest of fetus
  - iii. Scarce resources and competing needs for their use

    iv.   Interests of healthcare providers (for example, professional integrity)

    v.   Interests of healthcare organization

  h. Are there issues of power or conflict in the interactions of the key actors in the case that need to be addressed?

    i.   Between clinicians and patient/family

    ii.   Between patient and family members

    iii.   Among family members/surrogates

    iv.   Between members of the healthcare team (for example, between attending physicians and house staff, between physicians and nurses)

  i. Have all the parties involved in the case had an opportunity to be heard?

  j. Are there institutional factors contributing to moral problems posed by the case?

    i.   Work routines

    ii.   Fears of malpractice/defensive medicine/legal problems

    iii.   Biases favoring disproportionately aggressive treatment or neglect of treatable conditions

    iv.   Cost constraints/economic incentives

2. Moral diagnosis

  a. Examine how the moral problems in this case are being framed by the participants. Determine whether this framing should be reconsidered and replaced by an alternative understanding.

  b. Identify and rank the range of relevant moral considerations.

  c. Identify any relevant institutional policies pertaining to the case.

  d. Consider ethical standards and guidelines, drawing on consensus statements of commissions or interdisciplinary or specialty groups.

  e. Consider similar cases and discussions in the literature that might shed light on the analysis and resolution of moral problems in the case.

  f. Identify the morally acceptable options for resolving the moral problems posed by the case.

3. Goal setting, decision making, and implementation

  a. Consider or reconsider and negotiate the goals of treatment and care for the patient.

  b. Consider ideas (hypotheses) for possible interventions to meet the needs of the patient and resolve moral problems.

  c. Deliberate regarding merits of alternative options for resolving the moral problems.

  d. Endeavor to resolve conflicts.

  e. Assess whether ethics consultation is necessary or desirable.

    i.   Is there persistent conflict between clinicians and patients/surrogates or among clinicians regarding how to resolve the moral problems posed by the case?

    ii.   Would ethics advice be helpful in understanding or providing guidance on moral issues presented by the case?

  f. Negotiate acceptable plan of action.

  g. If negotiations, including ethics consultation, fail to achieve satisfactory resolution, consider judicial review.

  h. implement plan of action.

4. Evaluation

  a. Current evaluation

    i.   Is the plan of action working? If not, why not?

    ii.   Do the observed results of implementing the plan indicate the need for a modification of the plan?

    iii.   Have conditions changed in a way that suggests the need to rethink the plan?

    iv.   Are interactions between clinicians and the patient or surrogate helping to meet the needs of the patient, to respect the patient as a person, and to serve the goals of the plan of care?

    v.   Are there relevant interests, institutional factors, or normative considerations that have not been adequately addressed in planning for the care of the patient?

  b. Retrospective evaluation

    i.   What opportunities for resolving the moral problem were missed?

    ii.   How did the care received by the patient match up to standards of good practice?

    iii.   What factors contributed to a less than optimal resolution of the problems posed by the case?

    iv.   Was the process of problem solving satisfactory in this case?

    v.   What might have been done to improve the care of the patient?

    vi.   Are there desirable changes in institutional policy, feasible changes in the clinical environment, or educational interventions that might help to prevent or resolve the moral problems posed by similar cases?

should function as facilitators of moral problem-solving by the clinicians, patients, and family members involved in the case. Ethics consultants should not act as moral arbiters called on to render authoritative judgment on what to do. Rather, they should promote careful consideration of the range of reasonable options that are available, ensure that all concerned parties have an opportunity to be heard, and endeavor to mediate conflicts.

The case presented below is a composite of a number of real cases.[2] This case has been used as a mock consult (see appendix 3) for the training of ethics consultants, and a number of important, but often unexpected, issues have arisen during these training sessions. Because of the "richness" of this case, it is used here to illustrate the case analysis method described in table A.2.1. The case and analysis are set in sans-serif type (Helvetica), to make it easier for readers to review the tasks of the case method separate from the specifics of this case.

I. THE CASE REPORT

John J. was brought to the emergency room of a 350-bed community hospital following an auto accident. John was found lying outside of the vehicles involved in the two-car accident. The rescue squad that initially arrived at the scene of the accident noted that John had some contusions of his chest wall, a number of superficial lacerations on his extremities, and a large laceration and hematoma on the left side of his skull. His breathing was shallow, he had a heart rate of 40, and blood pressure of 140/110 when first seen by the rescue squad personnel. John was intubated, an IV begun, and he was immediately transported to the emergency room.

John was initially evaluated by an emergency room nurse who was concerned that he may have sustained a severe intracranial injury. She relayed her concerns to the emergency room physician who was busy with others injured in the same accident, and he advised that John be watched closely and a stat CT scan of the head be obtained. John was sent to radiology with an orderly and, while there, stopped breathing and his heart rate became unobtainable. He was immediately resuscitated and taken to the operating room, where the neurosurgeon on call drilled a burr hole in his skull and evacuated a large amount of blood from the space surrounding his brain. The neurosurgeon noted significant brain swelling and began treatment for this edema. John was transferred from the operating room to the ICU. One hour later John's wife and father arrived at the hospital and asked to talk to the neurosurgeon.

The neurosurgeon told John's wife and father that John had had a severe injury to his brain and that it was possible

that he would not survive. He explained that John was being treated for his brain swelling, and although he hoped this would be effective, he could not be sure of the prognosis. John's wife was particularly distraught and his father was noncommittal. The neurosurgeon told the family members that he would keep them informed of any change and left to check on other patients. Later that morning the neurosurgeon informed the risk managers at the hospital of John's case, as a potential liability case since John had not been initially evaluated by a physician on admission to the ER.

John's condition remained stable for the next few hours. He was intubated and ventilated, and his circulatory system was closely monitored. John's wife and father visited frequently, and the wife remarked how good his color was and how this was a good sign, and that God would surely take care of John, since he was a good Christian. Both the wife and father mentioned that John's mother, who had remarried after divorcing John's father when John was a child, was on a cruise to Antarctica and that they were trying to inform her of John's condition. John and his mother had always been very close.

After 10 hours in the ICU, John's cerebral edema became much worse and he became totally unresponsive. An EEG done three hours later showed essentially a flat line. A repeat EEG and necessary tests for a diagnosis of brain death the next day revealed that John met all of the criteria for brain death. John's wife and father were informed that John was "dead," even though he continued to maintain cardiac output with the physiologic support his body was receiving. A nurse inadvertently mentioned the possibility of donating his organs, and John's wife became almost hysterical and screamed, "He can't be dead. Look at him. He is still breathing and his heart is still beating. You have to keep treating him and God will heal him." John's father seemed to accept that John was dead, but asked that "treatment" be continued until John's mother could be found and she could come to the hospital. The neurosurgeon gave no specific assurances, but told John's father that he would continue physiologic support for John's body until "things could be worked out."

The chief nurse in the ICU questioned the neurosurgeon's decision in a private conversation shortly after his meeting with John's wife and father. Her objections were based on her knowledge of an acute need for beds in the ICU, as well as the open-ended commitment to continued treatment for a dead patient and the psychological problems this could entail for the staff. The neurosurgeon told her he understood her objections, but that he knew of other instances in which brain-dead patients were maintained on physiologic support until a distant relative arrived. He also told her of his fear that the hospital could be liable for the delay in treating John in the ER. He asked for her cooperation and asked that the staff do nothing further that could upset John's family. By the next morning a few of the staff in the ICU were beginning to ask questions as to how and when this matter would be resolved.

II. FOUR-PART CASE METHOD

A. Assessment

1. Patient's Medical Condition

The first step in the case method is to assess the patient's medical condition and set some provisional goals for treatment and care. The initial tasks for which all clinicians are trained are to identify the patient's basic medical problems, to make a diagnosis, and to predict a prognosis.

This case presents a number of difficult but important questions:

1. *Does this case represent a clinical ethics problem?* The issues of the differing definitions of death, the question of obligation to John's remaining family members, and the tension between the hospital's and clinicians' obligations to John and his family and the needs of other patients and society in general all point to this being a case with a number of ethical issues imbedded in it.
2. *Who is the patient, John, John's family, or some combination?* If the patient is John alone, he is, by definition, "dead," and medical obligations to him have ceased. But what are the obligations to John's family, particularly his wife and absent mother? Are there medical issues here related to the wife? How can the hospital staff show appropriate respect for John's present condition (a dead body) and fulfill the obligations to the other members of the family?

2. Contextual Factors

The next step, admittedly difficult in emergencies, is to assemble the best set of facts about the patient and his or her life situation. In a hospital, a special effort is needed to discover the patient as a person. Who was he or she before the illness? What is known about his or her life plans? This information is related to the diagnosis and treatment plan. The illness disrupts a life story to which clinicians aim to restore the patient. With a thorough history and good information about the patient's family and values, clinicians will have done much to accomplish this step.

Again, this case is made more difficult because of the questions mentioned in the previous section.

At the time of the accident, John was a 23-year-old laborer living with his wife of seven months in a rented mobile home. He had been raised by his mother in a nearby town after his parents had divorced when he was five years old. He seldom saw his father during his childhood and he had resented this perceived lack of attention. Two days prior to the accident, his father had arrived for a visit (the first in three years) and some progress in resolving old problems between the two had begun. John attended church (a fundamentalist congregation) with his wife, but had never seemed to be particularly religious.

He had never considered the possibility of his early demise, so had not discussed his beliefs and wishes concerning death and dying with anybody. John and his wife had been married seven months and had been sweethearts since high school. Since the marriage there had been a number of adjustment problems for both John and his wife, and just prior to his leaving home on the day of the accident, they had had a prolonged argument concerning how John had been spending their limited income.

John's father is devastated by John's death, even though he and John had not been particularly close. He had been invited for a visit by John and his wife so they could all "get to know each other better." He had welcomed this invitation and had arrived two days prior to the accident. He and John had just begun to talk about their estrangement and the reasons for it when the accident occurred. He accepts that John is really dead, but understands his daughter-in-law's reluctance to accept this. He believes that more time is needed for his daughter-in-law to come to terms with John's present condition and for John's mother to return.

John's wife is 20 years old and has been married to John for seven months. They had been high school sweethearts, and she had never had another serious boyfriend. Their marriage had had its ups and downs with frequent arguments about John's spending too much of their meager income on decorative additions for their six-year-old car. They had also had arguments about religion, since she was a member of a fundamentalist church and John had not been particularly religious. Recently John had seemed more interested and involved in the church and its activities, and she had been very pleased with this turn of events. Just prior to John's leaving for the last time, she and John had had a major argument concerning how money was being spent. Both were very angry and she had yelled that she wished she had never married him just before John stormed out of the house. She believes that this argument was the cause of the accident and feels very guilty about it. She knows that John has been seriously injured, but cannot accept that John is "dead" since his color is good, his heart continues to beat, and he continues to breathe with the help of machines. She firmly believes that miracles can occur, and that if she prays hard enough John will be saved. She was very upset when the possibility of organ transplantation had been mentioned, since she believes this is contrary to God's will.

The attending neurosurgeon finds himself in a difficult situation. He understands the feelings of the family members, but also understands the need to stop maintaining the brain dead body for the sake of the family, the staff, and the hospital. Even so, he has concerns about the ER physician's and the hospital's potential liability in this case and would like to avoid a possible lawsuit.

The ICU nurse sees her role as using her resources wisely so that the most good for the most people will result. She does feel sorry for John's wife, but doesn't believe this sympathy should have any bearing on the appropriate use of the ICU resources.

The hospital is a community hospital, and its management and staff are proud of its reputation as being devoted to excellent medical care and concern for the individual patient. It has strong support throughout the community and has never been held liable for an adverse outcome in a malpractice trial.

The community has a small town atmosphere and is considered to be a good place to live and raise children. It has a strong religious community that is mainly Protestant.

3. Capacity of the Patient

If the patient is John, he has no decision-making capacity, nor does he have any rights to make decisions, since he gave no prior instructions concerning what should happen after his death. If the "patient role" is extended to the family, the wife's capacity may be questionable and should be explored further. There is no evidence to indicate that John's father is not a capable decision maker. But this begs the question of who should have the authority to make decisions concerning the future treatment or nontreatment of John's brain-dead body.

Our society has determined that death can be diagnosed by using neurological criteria (as happened with John), and no further discussion or interventions are needed or indicated. But what of the family unit and its desires? Is there a place for considering these issues?

4. The Patient's Preferences

John can have no preferences as to maintaining his brain dead body. John's wife desires continued full treatment. John's father has asked for continued support until his daughter-in-law accepts the situation and until John's mother returns.

5. The Needs of the Patient as a Person

John has no needs as a person except that his body be treated with respect, since John is no longer a living person. John's wife needs support from her family and friends and likely from her church. She may need outside counseling.

6. Preferences of the Family

See item 4, immediately above.

7. Competing Interests

A case can be made that John's interest in having his dead body respected and his family's interest in having physiologic support for his body continue are at odds, and this raises the question of which should take precedence. Obviously, the wife's interest in maintaining John's body competes with the hospital's and the community's interest in efficient use of medical resources. The hospital's interest in avoiding a lawsuit may induce it to support the family's desires, even though this would not usually be the case.

8. Issues of Power or Conflict

There are clearly issues of power and status in this case. The surgeon caring for John has greater status and power than the ICU head nurse but she may have champions within the administration who balance the surgeon's expected power. The potential lawsuit may be an issue here too since avoidance of the suit enhances the power of those who support continuation of physiologic support. The church and its minister may have significant power and may be a strong influence on John's wife.

9. Opportunity for All Parties to Be Heard

Communication among all involved in the case seems to be adequate, and continuation of effective communication should be a primary goal, even though there are significant areas of disagreement.

10. Institutional and Legal Factors

See items 7 and 8, above.

B. Moral Diagnosis

1. Framing the Moral Problems

How can moral problems be framed clearly and accurately? It is not helpful to define a problem initially as a conflict between ethical principles (for example, "there is a conflict in this case between justice and beneficence"). Such framing is too abstract and mechanical to be of much help at this early stage of deliberation.

2. Identify and Rank Moral Considerations

In this case, there are several ethical problems of essentially equal importance. Included in these ethical problems are:

1. Are John's family's demands that full treatment be continued valid ethically? What supports this position and what does not?
2. What are the obligations of the physicians and hospital staff to John's family? To the memory of John and his body? To the community, which expects efficient use of medical resources?
3. How much weight should be given to religious beliefs that contradict science?
4. Who are the major decision makers in this case? How can this be decided?

5. Should risk to the institution be a part of the decision making concerning individual patients?

3. Identify Institutional Policies

There is no institutional policy in the hospital where John was treated regarding requests for delay in removing physiologic support from a brain dead body.

Many healthcare organizations (HCOs) are developing such policies. Whether they will be of help in similar situations is an open question.

4. Identify Guidelines for Clinicians on Models of Good Practice

Often guidelines from one or more authoritative sources are available, but there are no known guidelines concerning the major issues in this case.

5. Consider Similar Cases

After framing the ethical problems in a case, one ought to ask: "What cases are most similar, factually and morally, to my case?" Cases can be found in the legal realm, in the ethics literature,[3] or in clinicians' own experience. Comparing similar and different cases helps with decisions about whether the case fits with other well-settled cases or whether a unique facet or circumstance of the case makes it truly different from others. Also, when reviewing past cases, the question should arise: "What principles or other sources of appeal were used to resolve the case?"

This case, although similar in certain respects to other cases, is difficult to compare with other cases since it has a number of unique features, and no published similar cases are known. We have been told of cases in which there were requests for continued physiologic support for a brain-dead patient until distant relatives could gather. In two of these cases, the request was granted, but with a specific time limit.[4]

C. Goal Setting, Decision Making, and Implementation

1. Reconsider the Goals of Treatment

The third step begins with the recognition that moral and ethical problems often disrupt the plan of care for the patient. Reconsideration about and negotiation of the goals of treatment and the plan of care cannot be divorced from the task of considering various options to resolve the moral problems in the case. Moral problem-solving and planning for the care of patients go hand in hand. For this reason, moral problem-solving should not take place "behind closed doors" in an ethics committee, but at or near the bedside.

It is worth recalling that ethics is not an alien force, outside clinical practice, but an integral part of the competent practice of medicine and nursing. Clinical medicine involves planning throughout. Medicine is a consulting profession in which patients bring bodily or mental problems (or potential problems) to the attention of clinicians. The diagnosis and therapy for such problems call for systematic and continuous planning in the light of medical knowledge and clinical experience. The plan of care encompasses the entire encounter between clinicians and patients, even if such an encounter spans years or decades, as it often does in private practice.

In this particular case, a decision as to whether the family unit as a whole is to be considered the "patient" should be a part of this consideration. We believe that most clinicians would favor this approach.

2. Consider Ideas for Intervention

At this stage, the discussion of the problems in the case should refocus on the needs of the patient and on ideas (hypotheses) for possible interventions to resolve moral problems. If disputants in the case have taken sides and are still defending their positions strongly, it is crucial to attempt to reframe the debate by focusing on potential solutions.

3. Weigh the Merits of the Options

Deliberating the merits of alternative options to resolve the moral problem involves:
1. Stating and ranking morally acceptable options to resolve the problems;
2. Weighing the merits of alternative options, giving justification (the best ethical reasons) for the preferred resolution of the problems (drawing on ethical principles and other resources from ethical theory for this step is clearly appropriate);
3. Making a decision (a judgment) about which option is best, under the circumstances.

Each of these points merits further discussion.
a. State and rank the ethically acceptable options. Participants may offer options that are clearly unacceptable or intolerable in this society. These options ought not be included for decision-making, although they are useful for teaching purposes, in order to frame the parameters within which society permits choices about the problem at hand. For example, agreement to unlimited

continued support of John's brain-dead body would be unacceptable, even though John's wife would likely favor that option at the moment. However, our society has determined that dead persons should be treated in a certain manner, and unlimited continued physiologic support of the dead body is not allowed. A controversial option is not the same as a morally indefensible option. No matter what option is chosen in this case, it is likely to be considered controversial by one or more of those involved in the case.

Stating options is not the same as ranking them. By ranking options, decision makers open themselves to challenge from different ethical claims that need to be further heard for their persuasiveness and relevance. To decide to rank the options evokes specific ethical commitments of decision makers and also considerations of the needs and relationships of the persons in the case. One can always re-rank options, if arguments to do so prevail.

What are the options in this case? How should they be ranked? There are only two options:

1. To explain again to the family members that John is dead and his body must be treated as such, so all physiologic support will be withdrawn immediately;
2. To allow a specific limited time during which physiologic support will be continued, after which support will be withdrawn. During this time it is expected that counseling for John's wife will occur and that his missing mother will likely be able to return to see John before physiologic support is withdrawn.

b. Weigh and justify the options. *Option 1* is to withdraw support immediately. What ethical reasons can be given to support this option? This option would assure that the traditional manner of respecting dead bodies was upheld. More importantly, it would insure that scarce medical resources in the ICU were not being squandered and would seem more just to the community. It is interesting to note that until the definition of death was expanded to include the diagnosis of death by neurological criteria, this option would not have been considered as long as John's wife urged continued treatment.

Option 2 is to allow a time-limited continuation of physiologic support. This option is based on a beneficent consideration of the serious concerns of John's wife. It would allow time for some counseling and for consultation with trusted friends and religious leaders. This option has the disadvantage of unnecessary use of scarce resources, but at least there is a specified time-limit to this unnecessary cost. This option also would please those who are concerned about possible liability for the hospital and the ER physician. A case can be made that main-

taining the hospital's stellar reputation is of benefit to all its patients and the community at large. It might be possible to move John's body to a less costly part of the hospital during the continued support.

4. Endeavor to Resolve Conflicts

Once a decision has been made about the ethically preferable option, clinicians need to discuss how the resolution is to be effected and who will be involved in attempting it. They should discuss what dialogue and meetings between themselves, the patient, and surrogates (family or others) are needed to resolve the ethical and/or legal problems and to implement a satisfactory plan of care for the patient.

Readers should note that the clinicians who are involved in the care of the patient, working with the patient or a surrogate decision maker, can accomplish all of the steps of moral problem-solving themselves. Clinical ethics is part of clinical practice. At times the level of conflict around an ethical problem may require ethics case consultation and/or judicial review. If there is persistent conflict regarding how to resolve the ethical problems posed in a case, the responsible clinicians should ask whether ethics consultation would be helpful. The HCO (see chapter 3) should have the resources available to help with such problems. In addition to the question of appropriate ethics consultation, the case may pose questions that require judicial review, which should be sought by the legal officers of the institution, rather than by the clinicians themselves.

5. Assess Whether Ethics Consultation Is Necessary or Desirable

If consultation is sought from a hospital ethics committee or its consultants, their work can build upon the earlier efforts of clinicians to analyze and resolve the ethical problems in the case. If clinicians have thoroughly covered the first three parts of the four-step method, the consultants can build upon their work. The role of the consultant is to facilitate meetings, to ensure (if needed) participation of all parties with vital interests in the outcome and moral standing in the case, and to encourage dialogue open to different ethical views. The goal of consultation is to continue to educate the key decision makers in the case, and to assist their process in resolving ethical and legal problems. It is not to impose a decision on them.

6. Assess Whether Judicial Review Is Necessary or Desirable

Clearly, judicial review is necessary in cases involving incapacitated patients who have no surrogate decision makers, when the welfare of children and their parents' interests conflict, or when there are novel legal questions posed by the case. Courts should also be consulted if the disputes are serious and cannot be resolved by ethics consultation or other good-faith efforts.

D. Evaluation

Evaluation, the fourth part of the case method, is most directly linked to the plan-of-care approach. Evaluation in such cases begins from two different points in time:

1. Evaluation of the plan for intervention in the ethical and/or legal problems(s) that arise within the plan of care, and
2. Retrospective evaluation of opportunities that were missed early in the case or in the institution itself to prevent such problems.

1. Current Evaluation

When evaluating the current plan of action to resolve the ethical and/or legal problems, these questions should be asked:

- Is the plan working? If not, why not?
- Do the observed results indicate a need to modify the plan?
- Have conditions changed in a way that suggests a need to rethink the plan?
- Are interactions between clinicians and the patient meeting the needs of the patient, respecting the patient as a person, and serving the therapeutic goals of the plan of care?

2. Retrospective Evaluation

In this evaluative step, decision makers should look back to the origins of the case and to the setting of the institution and its policies. The following questions then can be asked:

- What opportunities were missed? How did the care received by the patient match up to standards of good practice?
- What factors contributed to a less than optimal resolution of the case?
- What might have been done to improve the care of the patient?
- Are there desirable changes in institutional policy, feasible changes in the clinical environment, or educational interventions that might help to prevent or better resolve the ethical problems posed by similar cases?

We do suggest that HCOs would do well to consider the issues raised by this case to ascertain whether a hospital policy should be developed to address these issues prospectively.

NOTES

1. Much of the explanatory text for this appendix was taken from chapter 2 of the previous edition of this book, J.C. Fletcher et. al., ed., *Introduction to Clinical Ethics,* 2nd ed. (Hagerstown, Md.: University Publishing Group, 1997). Chapter 2 was written by Franklin G. Miller, John C. Fletcher, and Joseph J. Finns.

2. This case and several others in appendix 3 were written by the author as "mock consults" for the training of ethics consultants.

3. A good collection of cases in clinical ethics is in G.E. Pence, *Classic Cases in Medical Ethics: Accounts of the Cases that Have Shaped Medical Ethics, with Philosophical, Legal, and Historical Backgrounds* (New York: McGraw-Hill, 1990). Other case anthologies include C. Levine, *Cases in Bioethics* (New York: St. Martin's Press, 1989); R.M. Veatch and S.T. Fry, *Case Studies in Nursing Ethics* (Philadelphia: J.B. Lippincott, 1987). The following textbooks have rich case reports and analyses: B. Brody, *Life and Death Decision Making* (New York, Oxford University Press, 1989); R.M. Zaner, *Ethics and the Clinical Encounter* (Englewood Cliffs, N.J.: Prentice-Hall, 1988); R.M. Zaner, *Troubled Voices: Stories of Ethics and Illness* (Cleveland, Ohio: Pilgrim Press, 1993); C.M. Culver, *Ethics at the Bedside* (Hanover, N.H.: University Press of New England, 1991); B.J. Crigger, ed., *Cases in Bioethics,* 2nd ed. (New York: St. Martin's Press, 1992); J.C. Ahronheim, J. Mareno, and C. Zuckerman, *Ethics in Clinical Practice* (Boston: Little, Brown, 1994).

4. Ellison Conrad, MD, chair of the ethics committee at Johnston Memorial Hospital, Abingdon, Va., and Earl White, MD, chair of the ethics committee at Sentara Hampton Hospital, Hampton, Va., each shared similar cases with the author on separate occasions.

Appendix 3

Training for Ethics Consultation: Mock Consultation Scenarios

Edward M. Spencer

Ethics consultants' comfort and effectiveness are increased by ongoing training using scenarios written expressly for this purpose. Four of these scenarios are included here, and we invite our readers who are involved in ethics consultation to use the mock consults as written, or to modify them as needed for their purposes.

CASE 1:
"STEP BY STEP"

Joe B, a 55-year-old male, was transferred to a university hospital from a community hospital 200 miles away. Joe had been admitted to the community hospital three days prior to his transfer because of symptoms of severe gastroenteritis (severe vomiting, moderate diarrhea, dehydration, and electrolyte imbalance). The diagnostic work-up at the community hospital revealed that Joe had a fulminant hepatitis, so he was transferred to the university hospital for further care. Joe's attending physician at the university hospital, a gastroenterologist, told Joe and his wife, Becky, that Joe's disease was rare and its outcome was uncertain. The prognosis in the few cases reported had varied from complete recovery after a prolonged medical course to death in a few days to a few weeks. The only known treatment was supportive care and corticosteroids.

Joe and Becky, when told of the uncertain prognosis and lack of definitive treatment, seemed overwhelmed, but both immediately told the physician that they wanted "everything done" no matter the cost. The attending physician assured them that Joe would receive optimum care and that he would talk with them daily or more often if conditions changed.

The following morning, while discussing Joe's case at the bedside, one of the senior gastroenterology residents asked the attending physician whether the "transplant people" had been consulted, and the attending physician answered that transplantation had never been tried for this type of hepatitis since infection of the transplanted organ by the hepatitis virus was virtually certain. Nothing more was said by the resident at that time. Joe mentioned this conversation to Becky when she visited, and they questioned the resident about the possibility of a transplant when he visited that afternoon. He explained that liver transplantation for a patient like Joe would be highly experimental, but, depending on past experience with similar viruses, might offer some hope. Joe and Becky asked the attending about this possibility later that day and he explained that this was an experimental intervention that had little chance of working but, when pressed, agreed to ask for a consult from the transplant surgeons.

The senior transplant surgeon, when he saw Joe the next morning, was more optimistic than the attending gastroenterologist, and, although he made no specific guarantee, assured Joe that liver transplantation "could be the answer" and at that time was Joe's "only hope." Both Joe and Becky were heartened to hear what the transplant surgeon said, and agreed to being listed for an "emergency liver transplant." Later that day Joe's attending physician reiterated his position that transplantation could only be considered a "last-ditch" intervention, and that he was still uncertain of the prognosis for Joe with medical treatment. Because Joe and Becky had been impressed with the transplant surgeon and because a cousin had had a successful kidney transplant, they decided to accept the surgeon's recommendation. Joe was immediately transferred to the transplant service although his former attending gastroenterologist continued to act as consultant.

Three days later a liver became available and Joe had a liver transplant. His post-op course was difficult. He developed significant coagulation difficulties and required 48 units of blood during the first post-op week. He also had difficulty with the anti-rejection drugs and developed kidney failure, requiring dialysis. He became depressed and repeatedly told the surgeons, "Just let me die. I can't stand to live like this." Because of his depression, he was considered mentally incapacitated and Becky was asked to give permission for all medical interventions. She was assured that all of Joe's difficulties were treatable and that he still had a chance for complete recovery. Based on these assurances, Becky continued to agree to the treatments recommended by the transplant surgeon. She did overhear an argument between the transplant surgeon and the gastroenterologist, with the gastroenterologist arguing that Becky be asked to think about how far she wanted to go with Joe's treatment. Becky interrupted this argument by saying that Joe had said he wanted everything possible done.

Joe and Becky had two adult children who came to see Joe every weekend (They each lived 200 miles away). Six weeks following Joe's transplant with Joe still in the ICU requiring blood transfusions and dialysis, both children began to question the treatment and mentioned to Becky that they did not believe their father would want to live this way. Becky replied that Joe had said he wanted everything done and that she "couldn't let him die when there is still hope."

On the seventh post-op week, Joe developed acute rejection of his liver and a second emergency transplant was completed in the middle of the night. His post-op course following the second transplant was somewhat better than that following his first transplant. His anti-rejection drugs were changed and his renal failure subsided. He continued to have some bleeding problems, but this subsided after two weeks. He was doing well enough to move to the floor on the third week after the second transplant. He continued to be clinically depressed and pleaded with Becky to "stop all this and take me home to die." On the day following his transfer from the ICU, he developed a high fever and signs of infection and so was re-admitted to the ICU. He was found to have pneumonia. In spite of adequate treatment for the pneumonia, his fever continued, and further testing revealed that the transplanted liver had become infected with the hepatitis virus. A third transplant was recommended to Becky and she was told this was the only chance Joe had. Becky asked that she be able to talk with her children prior to making this decision. The transplant surgeon urged her to act quickly.

The following day Becky and her two children talked at length about the situation. Becky told them she was exhausted and did not know what to do. She asked that they make any future decisions concerning Joe's treatment. Before agreeing, the daughter, who was a social worker, asked that an ethics consultation be requested.

Case 1: Assigned Roles

Becky:

You are 52 years old. You and Joe have been married since you were 20, and you have had a good marriage. You completed one year of business school and worked as an executive secretary for the president of a local furniture company until Joe's illness. You have been on a leave of absence since Joe became ill. You and Joe have two grown children and you are quite proud of them. Joe completed college with a degree in agriculture, and has been a successful farmer until his illness. You and Joe belong to the local Methodist Church and believe in God, but have not defined your beliefs more specifically. Joe's illness has been devastating to you and you are no longer sure what to do. You want Joe to have every chance to live, but you question whether what is being done is really giving him a chance or just making his last days miserable. You have faith in your local physician and in physicians in general, but wonder about the motivation of the transplant surgeon. You and Joe had a retirement plan containing $240,000, but, in spite of your insurance, your savings and the retirement money have been depleted. You hope you do not have to sell the farm to pay for Joe's medical care, but you are willing to do that if Joe can recover. You asked your children to make future decisions, but if they should decide to stop all treatment, you are not certain that you could allow this to happen now.

Daughter:

You are the 28-year-old daughter of Joe and Becky. You are a social worker and work for the state. You are married to a medical laboratory technician who works in the local hospital. You have never considered what a serious illness or death of one of your parents would mean to you until Joe's illness. When Joe first became ill you believed that he would recover, but as he has not responded to the most advanced high-tech care, you have become convinced that further treatment is futile and that any further treatment is just punishing your father as well as depleting his savings. Joe had always told you and your brother that he wished to be able to leave something for you after his death. You are familiar with hospitals and ethics committees because of your work, and are not particularly intimidated by physicians or others who work in hospitals. You believe prolonged high-tech care can be harmful as well as beneficial. You accept that it is your responsibility (along with your brother) to help your mother make difficult decisions about your father's future care.

Son:

You are the 25-year-old son of Joe and Becky. You are a graduate student at the state university studying history. You plan to teach at the university level after the completion of your studies. You have been overwhelmed by your father's sudden illness and his rapid decline. You hate to see him in his present condition and know that he hates it too. You are not convinced that he is not coherent and believe he should be able to make his own decisions. You are not comfortable with making decisions for him and hope your mother and sister do not force you to participate. You are strongly religious and believe only God should decide the moment of one's death.

Transplant Surgeon:

You are the chief of a highly regarded transplant service. You believe that organ transplantation offers hope for many who would have no other hope and you believe Joe fits this category. You understand that Joe's prognosis is not good, but you know that you and your service offers him his only chance, and you believe that is an appropriate reason to continue with full treatment for Joe. You will not give up when there is still some hope, no matter how slight. You think your gastroenterologist colleague has negatively influenced Joe's family into prematurely considering stopping treatment. You believe that Joe's prognosis is no worse now than when he received his first transplant, and therefore believe that the only possible realistic decision is to continue treatment. You are apprehensive about the ethics consultation, but will participate fully and try to explain to the family that to stop treatment now would be a crime.

Gastroenterologist:

You are the chief of the gastroenterology service. You support organ transplantation in circumstances where benefit has been proven. You question the value for individuals and particularly for society of highly experimental transplantation. You and the transplant service chief have had a number of arguments concerning this issue. You believe that the best chance for a full recovery for Joe would have been to continue medical treatment. You understand why Joe and Becky made the decision they did, but wonder whether you should have been more forceful in making your case for medical treatment. Presently you believe that Joe's prognosis is hopeless and that further treatment is likely to be harmful rather than beneficial. You are willing to articulate this view in the ethics consultation, even though it may lead to further animosity between you and the transplant surgeon.

Nurse:

You are the head nurse in the ICU where Joe has spent the last two months. You have gotten to know Becky quite well and Joe's children less well. You have also spent a lot of time trying to talk with Joe. In spite of the diagnosis of depression, you believe Joe retains some capacity for decision making and believe he should be listened to by everybody. You are uncertain as to what you would recommend be done in reference to further treatment for Joe. You understand both points of view, but tend to favor the transplant surgeon's view, since it is the only chance Joe has.

Consultant A:

You are a nurse in the medical center and a member of the ethics consultation service for the past three years. You enjoy your work for the ethics committee and hope to be of help in this situation. You have had some previous disputes with the transplant surgeon concerning withdrawing what you considered overly aggressive care. The decision makers in the previous situation decided to continue with the care, and the patient died after a prolonged course.

Consultant B:

You are a chaplain resident in the medical center and have been a member of the ethics consultation team for 18 months. You believe ethics consultation is similar to the counselling and mediation work you do as a chaplain. You have talked with all of the participants in this consultation except for the transplant surgeon who was "too busy."

CASE 2:
"IS THIS HOW WE SHOW OUR LOVE?"

Baby R was delivered at a tertiary care hospital after a 23 to 24 week gestation complicated by early labor and premature delivery. At delivery her apgar score was 1 (heart rate of 60, but no other vital functions noted). She was immediately intubated, and taken to the NICU, where she was begun on full monitoring and maximum intensive care. Her condition stabilized on life support and she seemed to do as well as could be expected for an infant this premature. A CT Scan on the second hospital day revealed a Grade II Intraventricular hemorrhage (bleeding into brain tissue)

Baby R's parents are unmarried, although the father and paternal grandmother were present at the time of birth and have been very interested in Baby R's condition and prognosis. Baby R's mother is 19, employed as a waitress in a fast food restaurant, and is estranged from her family. There is no insurance coverage for Baby R's treatment.

The attending neonatologist responsible for Baby R's care talked with Baby R's parents and paternal grandmother at length following Baby R's birth. She explained that it is difficult to predict whether Baby R will survive, and, if so, whether she will have any mental or other developmental deficiencies. She explained that statistically Baby R had between a 60 and 80 percent chance of survival and, of those infants who survived, there is the expectation that up to 50 percent could have serious developmental problems and another 30 percent have some less serious developmental problems. She explained that if Baby R survived, there would be a prolonged and costly course. When asked by the grandmother what she would recommend, the neonatologist replied that she was devoted to saving these very small babies, if possible, and that she saw no other reasonable course than to continue treating Baby R. The grandmother queried whether there were not other considerations such as cost and strain on the family that could be considered, and the neonatologist replied that these matters were important but not as important as saving Baby R's life. Baby R's parents asked no questions at the initial meeting with the neonatologist.

During the next few hours, both parents visited the NICU both together and separately and began asking the neonatal nurse a number of questions. The neonatal nurse reiterated the statistical outlook for Baby R, and told the parents that the attending neonatologist was a very good neonatologist and that she was strongly committed to saving the life of each of her patients. The father asked the nurse if that was always the "right thing to do," and the nurse replied that this was not her decision to make.

On the second hospital day, Baby R's physician told the parents and grandmother about the intraventricular hemorrhage. When asked if this changed the outlook for Baby R, she replied that it made the outcome more doubtful, but did not change it so drastically that they could "give up" on the baby. Both parents questioned whether Baby R was suffering, since she was attached to so many machines, and the neonatologist replied that she hoped not. The three family members present continued to question the neonatal nurse about the outlook for Baby R and her possible pain. On the third hospital day, the grandmother asked if the doctors could continue treating Baby R even if the parents wanted to "let her go to God" and the nurse replied that the parents had the authority to decide on appropriate treatment for their child, but that they usually listened to their doctor. The mother began crying at the end of this conversation and stated, "We have to give the baby every possible chance," and walked away from the grandmother and father.

Shortly thereafter Baby R began having problems because of the lack of development of her skin and began bleeding when she was handled. The grandmother saw this and asked, "Is this how we show our love?" and, shortly thereafter, the grandmother and the father asked to talk with the attending physician for the purpose of demanding that she stop all treatment for Baby R and let her go. The nurse asked the mother if this is what she wanted, and she replied that she didn't know. After talking briefly with the neonatologist, the nurse asked for an ethics consultation.

Case 2: Assigned Roles

Paternal Grandmother:

You are the 45-year-old grandmother of Baby R. You are divorced and have been a highly successful real estate broker for the past 20 years. You were shocked and upset three months ago when your only son told you that his girlfriend was pregnant with his baby. Since your son's girlfriend is estranged from her family, it became your responsibility to help with the necessary decisions concerning this pregnancy. There was an initial consideration of an abortion, but, mainly because of your strong religious beliefs, this option was soon discarded. Neither your son nor his girlfriend wanted to get married at that time, so it was decided that you would help pay for the expenses of the pregnancy and that your family would accept financial responsibility for the baby after it was born. The premature delivery of the infant and the subsequent course in the NICU have added to your concerns both for Baby R and for her parents. You have never believed that the parents were ready to accept full responsibility for the infant, even before you knew Baby R would likely be handicapped. You believe that abortion is wrong, but also believe that there is too much high-tech treatment that often leads to a prolongation of suffering rather than to any real benefit. You believe that continued treatment of Baby R fits this definition, and that the only reasonable decision is to stop treatment and let her die naturally. Since you are financially responsible for Baby R and her mother's medical care, you believe you should be the primary decision maker in this situation.

Mother:

You are the 19-year-old mother of Baby R. You graduated from high school last year and since that time have supported yourself by working as a waitress. You are estranged from your parents and have lived at the home of a friend since the beginning of your final year in high school. You met Baby R's father while working and began dating him one week later. You dated him exclusively until you discovered you were pregnant, three months after you began dating him. When you discovered you were pregnant, you talked with him about the pregnancy and your future. He is a college sophomore and plans to go to law school and refused to consider marriage, so both of you favored an abortion. However, when the two of you talked with his mother, she was strongly opposed to abortion and promised to pay all of your medical bills and to take care of the baby financially. Since then she has been making most of the decisions concerning the pregnancy and the baby's future. You had not seen Baby R's father for three weeks prior to the premature delivery of Baby R, and you had begun a relationship with another young man who seemed genuinely interested in you and your future. Baby R's birth and subsequent course in the NICU has been very difficult for you. If Baby R had been stillborn, everybody's problems would have been solved. However Baby R is alive and you want her to have a chance to have a future. You resent Baby R's father and grandmother making all the decisions and are not sure you agree that treatment should be stopped at this stage. On the other hand, you are not prepared to care for a handicapped infant. You don't know what the best course is now.

Father:

You are the 20-year-old father of Baby R. You are a sophomore at the state university (located in the town where you live) and plan to go to law school. You started dating Baby R's mother because she is very pretty and you wanted to have a good time. When she became pregnant, you wanted to pay for an abortion, but your mother refused and worked out an agreement which allowed you to continue in school. You subsequently lost interest in Baby R's mother. When Baby R was born prematurely and you were apprised of the future considerations, you were very concerned. You felt sorry for Baby R and her mother, but hoped that the baby would not survive. As her condition has gotten worse and as your mother has advocated withdrawal of treatment, you have become convinced this is the best solution. You do not believe Baby R's mother should be able to override this decision.

Neonatologist:

You are the chief of the neonatology service at the university hospital. You believe that your duty is to save all of the infants whom you can, unless it is obvious that the infant has no chance for a meaningful life (as with anencephaly). You believe treatment of very small premature infants should be continued until it is obvious that further treatment can not possibly lead to a prolongation of meaningful life. You believe that physicians, because of their superior medical knowledge, should decide when withdrawal of treatment is indicated. You understand that such decisions belong to the parents, but are uncomfortable when the parents' decision leads to "premature" withdrawal of treatment. You have gone to court on a number of occasions to attempt to have an outside guardian appointed to override parents' decisions to withdraw. You are convinced that Baby R has a chance for complete recovery and a healthy life and believe everything should be done to enhance this chance.

NICU Nurse:

You are the NICU nurse responsible for Baby R's care. You understand the positions of all of the people involved in the problem. You are concerned that Baby R's mother has not been allowed any decision-making authority concerning Baby R's care, and hope to support her during the ethics consultation. You believe that Baby R's grandmother and the neonatologist are both advocating what they believe is best for Baby R, but do not believe the father is very involved.

Consultant A:

You are a 30-year-old attorney-ethicist. You are a part-time employee of the hospital who was hired three years ago to help with ethics consultations. Prior to your employment, there was no formal process for ethics consultation and you have been instrumental in developing this process. You have a good relationship with most of the staff and believe you are respected by them.

Consultant B:

You are an internist and joined the consulta-

tion service six months ago. You believe each consultation should have a physician as one of the consultants. You respect the other consultant, but believe she should be more respectful of physicians.

CASE 3:
"NOBODY HAS THE AUTHORITY TO STOP TREATING THIS PATIENT"

Betty K, a 73-year-old woman, was transferred to a 250-bed community hospital from a nursing home affiliated with the hospital. Betty had been a "resident/patient" in the skilled nursing area of the affiliated nursing home for the previous two years and had been admitted to the hospital once before, three months ago.

Arrangements for admission to the nursing home two years earlier had been made by Betty's two nieces who were her closest living relatives and, according to the nieces, the only people with whom Betty had a close relationship. The physician who had admitted Betty to the nursing home had seen her only twice before the admission to the nursing home. The admitting diagnoses at the time of admission to the nursing home had been "malnutrition secondary to early Alzheimer's disease." Both the admitting physician and Betty's nieces had warned the nursing home personnel that Betty would be a difficult patient, since she was not only somewhat demented and combative for that reason, but also had always been fearful and mistrustful of medical personnel and medical institutions. Both nieces stated that Betty would "hate" being in the nursing home. They were, however, unable to care for her at her home or at either of their homes. When she had been told that she had to live in the nursing home, Betty had cried and then become uncommunicative.

After her admission to the nursing home, she actually did better than expected. She seemed to like several members of the nursing home staff and allowed them to feed her, and her malnutrition was slowly corrected over the next two months. Just before Betty seemed ready to move from the skilled nursing area to the assisted care area, she sustained a fall while walking in the hallway and refused to walk after the fall. The nursing home staff believed that Betty was not seriously injured by the fall and was using this as an excuse to remain in the skilled nursing area where she was comfortable with the staff. Her dementia was also gradually becoming more severe and she often refused to get out of bed for several days at a time and again began to refuse to eat. During the remainder of her nursing home stay her condition gradually got worse. Three months before this admission to the hospital, Betty had attempted to get out of bed and had fallen and broken her left hip. She was hospitalized at that time for surgical repair of her hip. The surgery went well, but, because she refused to eat, she had a nasogastric tube inserted for the purpose of feeding her. She was transferred back to the nursing home with the nasogastric tube in place after her attending physician had promised that the tube would be removed in "a short time."

After Betty's return to the nursing home, she seemed totally confused and responded only occasionally to her favorite staff members. She did seem to enjoy having her hair brushed and often this was the only way to keep her from being disruptive. She made several attempts to pull the nasogastric tube out and was successful on two occasions. However, her attending physician re-inserted the tube on these occasions when it became obvious that Betty was not going to eat. Six days prior to this admission, Betty developed a large decubitus ulcer over her left hip. This ulcer became worse rapidly, so that at the time of the hospital admission it was 16 centimeters in diameter and extended deeply into her tissue, almost reaching the bone. Her physician re-admitted her to the hospital for treatment of the ulcer with debridement and antibiotics and for insertion of a gastrostomy tube for future feeding. Betty's physician ordered the re-admission, and it took place prior to the physician's talking with Betty's nieces.

Both of Betty's nieces came to the hospital on the afternoon of her admission and talked with the attending physician. Both were concerned that the contemplated treatment was not what Betty would have wanted and that it was time to stop all treatment and allow Betty to die. The older niece was more adamant that no further treatment be instituted, but both seemed to agree that this was the proper course. The older niece explained to the attending physician that Betty had been a semi-recluse even before developing Alzheimer's, and that she had always hated hospitals and doctors. Even though she had been relatively content initially in the nursing home, this was no longer the case, and her dementia precluded her having any meaning for her life. The niece concluded by saying, "I know this is what I would want, and I think she would want it too."

Betty's physician explained to the nieces that she believed that Betty's medical problems could be effectively treated and that, although her dementia was getting worse, she still showed signs of pleasure, especially when her hair was brushed. The physician stated that she couldn't "give up" so soon. The older niece told the physician they would refuse to give permission to do the surgery. The physician replied that she hoped they would reconsider, and she would talk with them again the next morning. In a discussion with the nurse caring for Betty, the physician stated, "Nobody has the authority to stop treating this patient, and, if necessary, I will go to court to get permission to continue needed treatment." The nurse suggested an ethics consultation prior to going to court and suggested that one or more nursing home staff members be invited to the consultation.

Case 3: Assigned Roles

Physician:

You are a 47-year-old general/orthopedic surgeon. You have been primarily responsible for Betty's care since her first fall in the nursing home. You did the surgery following her hip fracture. Betty's previous physician retired six months ago, so you agreed to be her primary physician at that time. You talked with both of Betty's nieces on a number of occasions and both impressed you that they were very interested in Betty's well-being and were trying to do everything possible for her. You were therefore surprised when Betty's nieces refused to give permission for the necessary surgery. Betty is not terminally ill, so you do not believe stopping treatment should even be considered. You also know that Betty's care is covered by Medicaid, so you believe that the nieces do not have the authority to withhold needed treatment from a non-terminal patient. You talked with your friend, the hospital attorney, about this matter, and he advised that the only way you can proceed is to get a court to appoint another guardian. You asked him to be present for the ethics consultation.

Older Niece:

You are a 54-year-old school teacher. Betty is your mother's older sister. After your mother died 10 years ago, Betty asked you to "keep in touch," and since she had never married and had no other close relatives except you and your younger sister, you gradually became more responsible for her care. You frequently urged her to find a doctor she trusted and have regular medical check-ups. She always refused and told you she didn't need doctors, since God would take care of her. You never talked specifically about her wishes should she not be able to make decisions for herself, but you do remember her saying on a number of occasions that God would decide when it was time for her to go, and no doctor or hospital should have anything to say about it. You have recently completed a living will for yourself. You believe that you and your sister have the authority to make medical decisions for Betty, and think that Betty's physician is wrong to question your authority.

Younger Niece:

You are a 43-year-old housewife. You have never worked outside your home. You and your sister have never been particularly close because of the age difference, but you have always admired and respected her, particularly her assertiveness. Your older sister has consistently made decisions concerning Betty's care and you have gone along with these decisions without much thought. Your sister has talked with you about her recently completed living will and advised you to complete a living will for yourself. You agree that Betty has little reason to continue living. You are still uncomfortable with withdrawing all treatment and, if the decision were left to you, you would probably follow the physician's advice.

Nursing Home CNA:

You have worked in the nursing home since just before Betty was admitted there two years ago. Betty is actually the first patient for whom you had responsibility after your beginning work at the nursing home. Betty reminded you of your recently deceased grandmother and she seemed to respond well to you. You have cared for Betty since that time and believe you have a good relationship with her, and that you understand her better than her nieces do. You brush her hair anytime you have time to do so and she always enjoys it. You believe she does have some self awareness and derives pleasure from your company and from the hair brushing. You do not dispute that Betty's nieces are trying to do what is best for her, but you are convinced that they are not with Betty often enough to realize that she is occasionally more aware than they think. You believe it would be a crime not to treat Betty for her present difficulties and believe the gastrostomy tube placement will allow her to be more comfortable.

Hospital Attorney:

You are the attorney for the hospital and nursing home and a good friend of the attending physician. When the attending physician first told you of the difference of opinion concerning Betty's future treatment, you were concerned that there could be some degree of liability for the hospital if everything was not done for Betty. You also realize that in your state the nieces are the legally accepted decision makers for Betty. You told the attending physician that, if the nieces continued to insist that no treatment be instituted, the only possible legal way to institute treatment would be to ask the court to appoint a legal guardian for Betty. You hope that the ethics consultation will resolve the issue before one or both parties in the dispute goes to court.

Consultant A:

You are a nurse in the ICU of your hospital and you presently are the chairperson of your ethics committee. You know the attending physician quite well and respect her medical judgment. You have noted that she is rather dogmatic, and, like most surgeons, does not like to withdraw treatment. You have interviewed all of the participants in the consultation meeting and believe you understand the problem. You have noted that the younger niece does not seem as adamantly opposed to treatment as her sister, and you hope to draw her out during the consultation meeting.

Consultant B:

You are the chaplain at your hospital and have been a member of the ethics consultation group for five years. You have spoken to all of the participants in the consultation prior to the consultation meeting.

CASE 4: "JENNY JONES"

Jenny Jones, a 13-year-old White female, was referred to your hospital for "diagnostic work-up and treatment of aplastic anemia" two days ago. She had been referred from an adjacent state by the family pediatrician. The history revealed that she had had a prolonged nosebleed, requiring hospitalization, two days prior to her referral to your facility. Laboratory studies at the local hospital revealed a severe anemia, low white blood cell count, and low platelet count. A bone marrow done there revealed "aplastic anemia with essentially no blood-forming cells seen."

Family and social history revealed that Jenny lives at home with both parents and a younger brother. She has an older brother (age 20) away at the state university in a pre-med course of study. The Jones family belongs to the Jehovah's Witness religion. Jenny's father is in a position of authority in their local church and spends much of his spare time in church activities. Jenny is nominally in the seventh grade, but for the past two years she and her younger sister have been being instructed at home by their mother. When asked to explain this situation further, the father stated, "We had a lot of problems with what the local schools were teaching our older son, so decided to enable our other children to postpone exposure to some of the less desirable things happening in our world now." Jenny seemed pleased with her school situation and, when asked about friends, stated she had plenty of friends in the church.

On physical examination, Jenny was found to be basically healthy except for some bruising on her legs and arms and generalized pallor. Laboratory studies, including a review of the bone marrow slides from the referring hospital, confirmed the diagnosis of aplastic anemia. Jenny was admitted to the hematology service at your institution and her attending hematologist, after consultation with her colleagues, recommended immediate transfusion of blood and a bone marrow transplant to be completed as soon as a suitable donor is found. Jenny's attending physician met with Jenny's parents on the morning following her admission and gave these recommendations. The hematologist told the parents that with the treatment which she was recommending, Jenny had over 90 percent chance of survival and a normal lifespan, but without the treatment her chances for recovery were less than 5 percent, and that she would likely die within two weeks.

Both parents seemed shocked and dismayed and asked to talk together for awhile and get back to the physician; 90 minutes later they asked that the physician explain the situation to Jenny and the minister from their church who had accompanied them to your facility. The physician readily agreed and the meeting with the parents, Jenny, and their minister occurred later that afternoon. During that meeting the minister asked a number of questions concerning possible alternative means of treatment. Jenny cried briefly at the beginning of the meeting and was subdued, and clung to her mother during the rest of the meeting. She made no comments during the meeting.

Jenny's father thanked the attending physician and told her that they would let her know their decision the next morning. The attending physician mentioned that in cases involving minor Jehovah's Witness patients, local judges frequently allowed treatment over the objections of the parents in life-threatening situations. The minister and Jenny's father seemed concerned with this statement, and the minister stated that he had heard of this happening in other areas, but that it had never happened in an area where he had a congregation, and that a 13-year-old should, along with her parents, have "control of her destiny."

Two hours later the attending physician was called at home by Jenny's parents and was told that they had all decided that the only possible course of action for them was to pursue any and all alternative treatments. The attending physician expressed her dismay and told Jenny's parents that she would talk to hospital authorities and talk with them again the next morning.

The attending physician returned to the hospital later that evening in the hopes that she could speak to Jenny alone. When she arrived at Jenny's room a young man was in Jenny's room arguing quietly with her and Jenny was crying. The young man introduced himself as Jenny's brother. He told the attending physician that he had been raised as a Jehovah's Witness and still was "religious," but that discussions with teachers and students while in high school had led him to question the tenets of his family's religion and that he had left the church prior to entering college. He also stated that he respected his parents, but that they had no right to refuse lifesaving treatment for Jenny. Jenny interrupted him and said, "But I don't want it." He was adamant that Jenny could not know the real consequences of this decision and asked if something could be done. The attending physician told the brother that the first people usually consulted in a case of this sort is the Ethics Consultation Group and gave Jenny's brother the number.

He called the consultant on call and requested a consultation "as soon as possible."

Case 4: Assigned Roles

Jenny:

You are the patient in this scenario. You are a 13-year-old girl who was entirely well until about one week ago, at which time you developed a nosebleed that just wouldn't stop. You saw your pediatrician, whom you have known for as long as you can remember, and he admitted you to your local hospital. While in the hospital your nose was "packed" and you had a lot of blood tests. The worst thing that happened in the hospital was the "bone marrow" test. It really hurt when that test was done. You heard your doctor and your parents talking about what the tests showed, but when you asked about this, they told you that you had to come to this big hospital for more tests and treatment. On the morning you left to come here, your pediatrician did tell you that your bone marrow was not making enough blood cells and that he was sending you to the bigger hospital to get treatment for this condition. You asked him if the treatment would hurt, and he answered that he did not know.

You have always been healthy and have never been in a hospital before. You live at home with both parents and your eight-year-old sister. You have an older brother whom you look up to and who is presently at the state university in your state studying to be a doctor. Your family is very religious and belongs to the Jehovah's Witness Church. You have been told about religion for as long as you remember. You consider yourself a Christian and understand and subscribe to the unique aspects of the Jehovah's Witness Church. You know that your older brother had a number of arguments with your parents (particularly your father) before leaving for college two years ago. He has not attended church with the rest of your family since that time, even when he is home for vacations. When you asked him about what had happened, he told you that he would talk with you later about what happened when "you can understand the whole thing better." When you asked your father the same question, he replied that your brother had "gotten a bunch of weird ideas at high school" and that he (your father) hoped your brother would "come to his senses" soon. Your mother told you that your brother no longer had all of the same religious beliefs as the rest of the family. In spite of this, your relationship with your brother has continued the same. Because of your brother's change in religious

ideas, your parents decided that you and your sister would no longer go to public school, and made all arrangements necessary for your mother to teach you at home.

You have felt frightened since coming to the bigger hospital. Your new doctor (the hematologist) is nice enough and seems to know what she is doing, but you just don't know her the same way you know your pediatrician back home. You know your parents are very worried too. The last 24 hours have been particularly frightening. Yesterday afternoon your doctor, your parents, and your minister from back home met with you and talked with you about your illness. Your doctor told you that you had a disease in which all of the cells in your bone marrow (which make the cells in your blood) are not functioning and are therefore not making blood cells, which you need to live and function. She told you that unless proper treatment is begun soon that you will likely die. When you heard this you became really scared and the only thing you remember her saying after that was that the only good treatment for this is blood transfusions and a bone marrow transplant (taking bone marrow cells from somebody else and putting them in your bones or blood). You knew that this would be against the teachings of your religion. Later you asked your mother whether there is another treatment and she told you she didn't know. You told her then that you did not want to have the transfusions and the bone marrow transplants and that you were willing to "leave it in God's hands." A short time later your brother came to visit you and told you that you should ask to have the treatment and that "God wouldn't mind." You told him you couldn't do that because you believed that allowing blood to be put in your body would be a sin.

During the night you had frightening dreams about leaving your family. This morning when you awoke, you felt more resigned to placing your future in God's hands and believe that you and your parents have made the only choice you could in refusing to allow blood to be transfused into your body. Two strangers came to see you this morning and told you they were from the Ethics Consultation Service and that they had been asked to help with the decisions to be made in your case. You told them the decisions had already been made, and that you did not need them. They said that some of the people on the staff, including your doctor, were not comfortable with the decisions that were made and want to discuss it further. They asked if you would help with this process and you reluctantly agreed.

Brother:

You are the 20-year-old brother of Jenny Jones. You are presently a sophomore at your state university in a pre-med course of study. Your family consists of your parents, yourself, Jenny, aged 13, and Julie, aged eight. Your family have been devout Christians for all of your life and have belonged to the Jehovah's Witness Church. During your senior year in high school you had a number of conversations with your close friends about the "no blood" tenet of the Jehovah's Witness Church, and came to the conclusion that, for you, this tenet really made no sense. You therefore left the Jehovah's Witness congregation to which the rest of your family still belongs. You had a number of discussions with your parents at that time and they were both dismayed with your choice and believed that you had been "brainwashed in that liberal public school." In spite of this, your relationship with your parents has remained cordial. Jenny has always been particularly close to you and you have had a great influence on her. At the time you left the Jehovah's Witness congregation you promised your parents that you would not attempt to influence Jenny or Julie to doubt the tenets of the church.

Your mother called you when Jenny was admitted to the hospital in your hometown and called again when she was referred to the larger hospital. You called your parents yesterday and they explained Jenny's condition and the recommended treatment. You told them at that time that they "couldn't let Jenny die." Your father told you that Jenny did not want the treatment and that it would be left "in God's hands." Rather than argue with your parents over the phone, you decided to come to the hospital and drove all yesterday afternoon and arrived at the hospital last night. You went to see Jenny immediately after arrival. She appeared frightened and tired. You talked with her briefly about whether she should agree to the treatment, but upon seeing how much this upset her, decided to wait until the next day. Jenny's doctor arrived while you were in her room and, after your visit with Jenny, she explained the medical situation.

You believe that your parents, although sincere, have no right to impose their religious values on Jenny. You believe that she has not had a chance to be exposed to, and thereby to under-

stand, other ways of looking at the "no blood" tenet of your family's church. You base this belief on the fact that she and Julie have been taught at home and have not had friends from outside the church community. You therefore believe that Jenny should be given the needed treatment over your parents' objections. You believe that you can convince Jenny that she should get the recommended treatment. Jenny's physician agrees that, if Jenny decides to accept the treatment, your parents' wishes for no treatment should be overridden. When Jenny's doctor mentioned the Ethics Consultation Service and its function, you decided to call on this group for help in the hopes that some consensus concerning the proper treatment course could be reached. You called the ethics consultant on call and asked for a consultation.

Nurse:

You are the head nurse on the pediatric hematology ward. You were filling in for one of the floor nurses when Jenny was admitted, so you admitted her to the hematology service. Since her admission you have followed her course closely because you have a 14-year-old daughter, and Jenny reminds you of her in a number of ways.

You have been involved with a few patients from Jehovah's Witness families. Usually court orders to authorize treatment over the objections of the parents have been sought and obtained. These cases all involved children much younger than Jenny who had little or no idea as to the likely benefits of the recommended treatments. It has been your observation that, after the decision has been taken from the family, the family members often seem somewhat relieved and seldom protest further. You know of no Jehovah's Witness child who was treated over the objections of the family who has been ostracized or overtly punished by any family member. You have maintained contact with two of these children and know that they are still members of their church in spite of having received blood or blood products.

You are personally troubled after talking to Jenny because she seems to be a capable decision maker in spite of her age, and you believe that capable people have the right to make their own medical care decisions. You have also talked briefly with Jenny's parents and her brother. The parents seem to be concerned and caring. The brother has presented a different point of view, that Jenny is really not capable of making an informed decision because of her lack of exposure to alternatives, which you believe must be considered.

You have been a part of three previous ethics consultations and have a generally favorable opinion of this activity. You do believe that the ethics consultants could sometimes be of more help if they just told the participants what is the right thing to do. You also realize that the ethics consultants may not always have the "answers" and understand why they do not wish to impose their values on others. You are pleased that an ethics consultation has been requested, but have little hope that it will be of any help in resolving the problem. You expect the attending physician to ask for a court order no matter the result of the ethics consultation.

Attending Physician:

You are a 38-year-old pediatric hematologist at the major teaching hospital in your state. You have had your present position since completing your hematology fellowship seven years ago. You have a special interest in aplastic anemia and consider yourself one of the major experts on this condition in this country.

Jenny Jones was referred to you by a pediatrician in a neighboring state. You have received several previous referrals from this physician and respect his work as a general pediatrician. Jenny's bone marrow exam has convinced you that she has a particularly virulent and severe form of aplastic anemia that is very unlikely to respond to any treatment other than bone marrow transplant. You also know that she will require one or more transfusions while preparing for the bone marrow transplant. The referring pediatrician mentioned to you that Jenny and her family were members of the Jehovah's Witness church.

You have explained fully to Jenny's parents her present condition and her prognosis. At the end of your explanation you acknowledged that you understood that they belonged to the Jehovah's Witness church and that their beliefs may present a problem in Jenny's treatment. You urged the parents to consider that transfusion and bone marrow transplant are likely the only possible treatments which can save Jenny's life. You also told the parents that you have occasionally attempted to get a court order to give treatment over parents' objections in life threatening situations. At that juncture Jenny's mother, who had been quietly crying, looked up and said to her husband, "That might be the answer." Her husband had then said to his wife, "Jenny will never agree to that."

You do not believe that a 13-year-old patient has the capacity, nor should she have the responsibility, to make serious healthcare decisions for herself. However, at the urging of the parents, you did explain the situation to Jenny, and she did seem to understand her medical condition and what refusing your recommendations would mean.

You met Jenny's brother last evening and he told you that Jenny cannot be a capable decision maker because of her lack of exposure to others with different religious perspectives. You mentioned the possibility of an ethics consultation and he immediately called the consultant on call.

You have been involved in two previous ethics consultations and found both to be helpful, particularly in clarifying issues and options. In neither consultation was a recommendation made as to the "best" outcome. You welcome this consultation, but believe that you will likely go to court for permission to override the wishes of the parents (and possibly Jenny) and to go forward with your recommended treatment. You understand that the parents can remove Jenny from your care unless they agree to abide by the court's permission, if granted.

Mother:

You are the 46-year-old mother of Jenny Jones. You graduated from the state university of your state with a bachelor's degree in education and taught school for five years after graduation. You married your husband two years after receiving your college degree. You had met your husband at the Jehovah's Witness church in the town where the state university is located. You both had been raised in Jehovah's Witness families and had always found comfort in your faith, in spite of its being the cause for your lack of acceptance in certain activities in your town. Shortly after your first child was born, you resigned your school teaching position and have not worked outside the home since that time.

You believe that you and your husband have a good marriage and consider your faith as a major factor in maintaining your marriage and family. Your husband has always been a good and thoughtful man. He has maintained a job throughout your marriage. You have been particularly proud of his achievements in your church, such that presently he is looked to by the congregation for help and advice often as soon as your minister.

You are particularly proud of your children, all of whom are intelligent and thoughtful. Many of your friends have mentioned how mature Jenny seems, and she does seem to you to be able to understand situations and make appropriate decisions far beyond what is usually expected of a child of her age. Your oldest child did disappoint you when he questioned some of the basic tenets of your church and ultimately left the congregation two years ago. In spite of this, you have maintained a good relationship with him and have continued to hope that he will see the error of his thinking and return to your congregation. Because of your son's leaving the congregation, you and your husband decided that it would be better for Jenny and Julie if they were taught at home by you and if their major friends were confined to families you know from your church.

When Jenny became ill you had no idea that this could be a severe test of your faith. As you have discovered, Jenny's illness presents your family with a stark choice: Maintain your church's admonitions against the use of blood and likely see your beloved child die, or renounce your religion's tenets and leave the church, which has been the most important aspect of your family's life. You have elected to allow your husband to make the decisions to this time and he has maintained the importance of staying with the church. Jenny has agreed with this position.

When Jenny's doctor told you that she may try to get a court order to treat Jenny over your objections, you at first believed that this was God's way of allowing Jenny to be treated without approval from you. Your husband quickly told you that this was a cop-out, and that the family had to place Jenny's care in God's hands and continue to abide by the teachings of the church.

The arrival of your son, his vehement disagreement with your position, and his subsequent request for an ethics consultation was considered one more cross to bear at this difficult time. However, after thinking about it, you have come to the conclusion that the ethics consultation may represent a way out of your dilemma and you therefore welcome it. You really don't know what to expect during the consultation but will cooperate fully. You are not sure what you would do if a court order is obtained, but believe that you would likely accept it and see Jenny treated without your permission.

Father:

You are the 47-year-old father of Jenny Jones. You graduated from the state university of your state with a bachelor's degree in finance, and, since graduation, have worked for the bank in your hometown. You are presently one of three vice-presidents of this bank and believe that you have an excellent chance of becoming president at the time the present president retires. You have been a devout member of the Jehovah's Witness church since you were a child.

You met your wife at a church function while you were in college. You have always had a good marriage and believe that a major determinate of the quality of your marriage has been your church affiliation and activities. You have become one of the more important members of your church and are often consulted by other church members for advice. One of the issues about which you have been asked for advice is the question of accepting blood in a life-threatening situation. You have consistently advised those asking for your advice to maintain the tenets of your church and leave the outcome in "God's hands."

You have three children, all of whom have been a cause for celebration until two years ago. At that time your oldest son began to question the basic tenets of the church and ultimately left the congregation. You were very upset and disappointed when this happened, but you have continued to maintain a cordial relationship with your son in hope that he will return to the congregation after college. Because of your son's betrayal of your basic beliefs, you and your wife decided that your other children, Jenny and Julie, should be taught at home to remove them from possible corruption at the public school. This has seemed to work well, in that both of the younger children seem happy and well-adjusted and have a number of friends. Their friends are all from families who are members of your church.

Jenny's illness has been a great shock and worry for you. You have, however, not wavered in your faith and believe that you are acting in Jenny's best interest when you refuse the recommended treatment. You do believe that a mature 13 year old, such as Jenny, should have decision-making authority. You would be gravely disappointed if Jenny decided she wished to be treated. You are certain this will not happen. When Jenny's doctor told you that she may try to get a court order to treat Jenny over your objections, you became angry that she was attempting to take this very important decision from you. Your wife seemed to be pleased with this turn of events, so you did not express your anger at that time. You did mildly berate your wife for her "lack of faith."

The arrival of your son and the request for the ethics consultation added to your dismay that the decision-making authority properly belonging to you was being wrested from you. You see no need for an ethics consultation, since you do not see that there is anything to discuss. You initially thought you would refuse to participate in the consultation, but reconsidered when the consultants told you that they were not there to make decisions.

You hope that the consultation will convince the physician not to ask for a court order. To support your belief that no court order is needed, you want Jenny to be a part of the consultation so that everybody can see she really will refuse treatment if given the authority to do so.

CPSIA information can be obtained
at www.ICGtesting.com
Printed in the USA
BVHW01s1231070818
523444BV00012B/1/P